NURSING
PRACTICE and
the Law

Avoiding Malpractice and
Other Legal Risks

DEDICATION

To my three daughters,
Liz, Katie, and Heather,
whom I love and adore.

FOREWORD

My law firm's relationship to health care began several decades ago. Established by William Pitt Ballinger in 1848, when he received the first law license issued by the State of Texas, our firm for many years did no more than share firsts with its Galveston Island neighbor, the John Sealy Hospital (now University of Texas Medical Branch), the oldest medical school in Texas. Early in this century, the firm's relationship with the Medical School began with a partner, R. Waverly Smith, one of the initial directors of the Sealy & Smith Foundation for the John Sealy Hospital, and a member of the family that created the foundation. Over the years, seven members of the firm have served as directors of that foundation and have seen that small medical school grow into a major institution for treatment, teaching, and research.

During my 38 years of the practice of law, the relationship between law and health care continued to expand—in some senses for better and in some possibly not. In personal injury litigation, medical treatment must be presented to the trier of fact through depositions and medical records. As health care and law have both become more specialized and as medical treatment has become many times more complex, the lawyer must consult with several health care providers in a single case. Our firm is fortunate in being able to consult on a wide range of medical questions with Mary O'Keefe, who combines a nursing degree with a law degree. Many firms on both "sides of the docket" retain the services of nurses either as consultants or as in-house members of a litigation team. Few lawyers can give the in-depth analysis of medical records and medical claims that a nurse can.

My perspective is that of the defense bar, which includes insurance company clients and the representation of professionals, including doctors, dentists, and nurses. The public purpose served by malpractice litigation is to clarify the duties owed by health care providers to patients. The patient has benefited from the greater responsibility accepted by health care professionals. At times, the system seems also to impose burdens on those professionals, both in terms of the added expense of malpractice insurance and a sense that some procedures and practices must be followed, not for cogent medical reasons but simply for protection against possible claims.

Nursing Practice and the Law: Avoiding Malpractice and Other Legal Risks will give nurses and nursing students a valuable tool in gaining insight on the relationship between law and health care. It is essential that nurses today be aware of this relationship. It will help the reader gain a better understanding of the legal duties of a nurse, as well as an understanding of the legal system and how to live with it while engaged in the practice of nursing. This book will give the reader a better knowledge of the law and the standards of practice. It will identify ethical considerations for the practitioner and will suggest areas of nursing that are still in need of greater definitions of standards.

John Eckel
Senior Partner
Mills, Shirley, Eckel, and Bassett, LLP
Galveston, Texas

NURSING

PRACTICE and THE LAW

Avoiding Malpractice and Other Legal Risks

MARY E. O'KEEFE RN, PHD, JD

Nurse Attorney
Mills, Shirley, Eckel, and Bassett, LLP
Galveston, Texas

Assistant Professor
Texas Tech University Health Science Center
School of Nursing
Lubbock, Texas

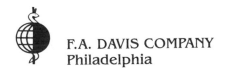

F.A. DAVIS COMPANY
Philadelphia

F. A. Davis Company
1915 Arch Street
Philadelphia, PA 19103

Printed in the United States of America

Last digit indicates print number: 10 9 8 7 6 5 4

Acquisitions Editor: Joanne Patzek DaCunha, RN, MSN
Developmental Editor: Diane Blodgett
Production Editor: Elena Coler
Designer: Maria Karkucinski
Cover Designer: Louis Forgione

As new scientific information becomes available through basic and clinical research, recommended treatments and drug therapies undergo changes. The author(s) and publisher have done everything possible to make this book accurate, up to date, and in accord with accepted standards at the time of publication. The authors, editors, and publisher are not responsible for errors or omissions or for consequences from application of the book, and make no warranty, expressed or implied, in regard to the contents of the book. Any practice described in this book should be applied by the reader in accordance with professional standards of care used in regard to the unique circumstances that may apply in each situation. The reader is advised always to check product information (package inserts) for changes and new information regarding dose and contraindications before administering any drug. Caution is especially urged when using new or infrequently ordered drugs.

Laws change rapidly. Although each chapter was carefully researched in good faith, laws referenced in this book may have changed by the date of publication. Also, not all laws relevant to an issue may have been included within the chapter. Further, individual attorneys may reach different conclusions regarding the application of a law to a unique set of facts. For these and many other reasons, this book is not a substitute for the advice of an attorney regarding the scope of any issue discussed within this book.

Library of Congress Cataloging in Publication Data

O'Keefe, Mary E.
 Nursing practice and the law: avoiding malpractice and other legal risks / Mary E. O'Keefe.
  p. cm.
 Includes bibliographical references and index.
 ISBN 0-8036-0602-8 (alk. paper)
 1. Nursing—Law and legislation—United States.   2. Nurses—Malpractice—United States.
I. Title.
KF2915.N8 038 2000
344.73'0414—dc21

00-022791

PREFACE

The conceptual framework of this book is based on the principles of law that The American Association of Nurse Attorneys (TAANA) has recommended for inclusion in nursing educational programs (TAANA requirements). The rationale for this book is to provide an updated, in-depth presentation of the principles of law as outlined by TAANA requirements. The purpose of this book is to make the student or nurse aware of the principles of law that guide nursing practice. The goal of this book is to provide the student nurse with a source for, and education about, the principles of law as outlined by TAANA requirements.

This book may be described as either a legal text for student-nurses or a legal reference for nurses or other health care workers in all levels of practice. The approach of this book is to provide six distinct sections, each building on the other. The sections progress from legal principles that guide the nurse in general practice to legal principles that guide the nurse in specialized areas of practice. For example, Part I is an introduction to nursing law and ethics; Part II relates nursing practice and the legal system; Part III relates nursing law and the patient; Part IV relates nursing law and management; Part V relates nursing law and specialization; and Part VI relates nursing law and forensics.

This book is designed as a basic legal text for student-nurses. It also serves as a reference for nurses and health care workers in various levels and areas of practice. The following subcategories are included in each chapter: chapter objectives, an introduction placing the chapter topic in its historical perspective, issues and trends in nursing practice and law, ethical considerations and conflicts, recommendations for research and malpractice prevention, a summary, a bibliography, additional suggested references, and/or appendices (for example, references landmark cases).

The subject matter of this book consists of TAANA requirements. These are principles of law that guide nursing practice and that according to TAANA, should be a component of professional nursing education. This book also examines law that is relevant to certain specialized areas of nursing practice, including advanced practice nurses in general, home health care, long-term care, psychiatric care, and emergency care. Other legal principles discussed refer to forensic aspects of nursing, including basic forensics, life care planning, violence, telecommunications, and correctional facilities. The scope of these principles of law encompasses relevant constitutional, federal, and state law, including both statutory and common or case law affecting nursing practice.

This book will be appropriate for: (1) junior- and senior-level nursing students; (2) graduate nursing, medical, and law students; (3) health care professionals, such as general or advanced practice nursing, physicians, lawyers, and health care providers in general; and (4) correctional facility personnel or anyone working with correctional facility staff. No prerequisite is necessary for using this book, which may also be used in continuing education courses for any of the four areas listed above.

The following graphic enhancements are used throughout the text: tables used, for example, to highlight landmark legal cases; boldface type to denote special terms, definitions, and key words; and box inserts to identify, for example, the authors of standards relevant to practice area and/or legal issue addressed.

Learner aids in the workbook include: (1) chapter study guides and/or test questions, (2) critical thinking exercises, and (3) case studies.

ACKNOWLEDGMENT

I wish to acknowledge the extensive help provided to me by Diane Blodgett, who rewrote, revised, and edited each chapter way above and beyond the call of a developmental editor. She has been an invaluable support to me and a joy to work with.

CONTRIBUTORS

Victoria Berry, MSN, RN, CNS
Legal Nurse Consultant/Clinical Nurse Specialist
Medical/Legal Resources
Austin, Texas

Barbara Scott Cammuso, RNCS, PhD, EdD
Professor
Fitchburg State College
Fitchburg, Massachusetts

Doreen Casuto, RN, MRA, CRRN, CCM
Rehabilitation Nurse, Case Manager
Rehabilitation Care Coordination, LLC
San Diego, California

Anne Marie K. Catalano, RN, PhD, CS
Assistant Professor
Graduate Department of Nursing
Fitchburg State College
Fitchburg, Massachusetts

Shirley Chater, RN, PhD, FAAN
Regent's Professor
School of Nursing
University of California
Institute for Health and Aging

Anthony K. Cutrona, JD
Attorney at Law
Houston, Texas

Patricia Fedorka, RNC, PhD
Assistant Professor
Duquesne University
School of Nursing
Pittsburgh, Pennsylvania

Daniel Hall, RN, BSN, JD
Attorney at Law
Corpus Christi, Texas

Jacquelyn K. Hall, RN, MEd, JD
Nurse Attorney
Private Practice of Law and Morality in Illness Care
Amarillo, Texas
Clinical Faculty
Texas Tech University Schools of Medicine and Pharmacy
Lubbock, Texas

Elizabeth L. Higginbotham, RN, JD
Nurse Attorney
Browder and Higginbotham, LLP
Austin, Texas

Roselyn Holloway, RN, MSN
Lead Instructor, Leadership and Management
Covenant School of Nursing
Lubbock, Texas

Taralynn R. Mackay, RN, JD
Nurse Attorney and Partner
McDonald, Mackay and Weitz, LLP
Austin, Texas

Barbara Power Madden, RN, EdD, SANE
Forensic Nurse Educator, Adjunct Faculty
Fitchburg State College
Fitchburg, Massachusetts
Staff nurse, per diem
Newton-Wellesley Hospital
Massachusetts Department of Public Health
Newton Lower Falls, Massachusetts
SANE
Self-employed, Legal Nurse Consultant
Boston, Massachusetts

David V. Marchand, MS, JD
Assistant Managing Partner
Morgan and Weisbrod, LLP
Dallas, Texas

Leanna Marchand, RN, JD
Nurse Attorney and Junior Partner
Morgan and Weisbrod, LLP
Dallas, Texas

M. Dena Matthews, RN, BSW, LNC
Legal Nurse Consultant
Medical-Legal Consultants, Inc.
Lubbock, Texas

Rosemary Conlon McCarthy, BSN, MS, JD
Nurse Attorney
Gallagher, Young, Lewis, Hampton & Downey
Houston, Texas

Patricia McCollom, RN, MS, CRRN, CDMS, CCM, CLCP
Nurse Consultant/President
Management Consulting and Rehabilitation Services, Inc.
Life Care Economics Ltd.
Ankeny, Iowa

Mary E. O'Keefe, RN, PhD, JD
Nurse Attorney
Mills, Shirley, Eckel, and Bassett, LLP
Galveston, Texas
Assistant Professor
Texas Tech University Health Science Center
School of Nursing
Lubbock, Texas

Cheryl Pozzi, RN, BSN, MS, Postgraduate Certificate in Forensic Nursing, DABFN
Forensic, Safety and Legal Nurse Consultant
Vice President
Sandia Safety Sciences
Cedar Crest, New Mexico

Nancy E. Purtell, RN, BSN
Area Director, Behavioral Health Services
University of New Mexico Health Sciences Mental Health Center
Albuquerque, New Mexico

Lenore Kolljeski Resick, MSN, RN, CS, CRNP
Assistant Professor
Director, Nurse-Managed Wellness Clinics
Duquesne University
School of Nursing
Pittsburgh, Pennsylvania

Susan Sportsman, RN, PhD, CNA
Dean, College of Health Sciences
Midwestern State University
Wichita Falls, Texas

Ana M. Valadez, RN, EdD, CNAA, FAAN
Director of Undergraduate Program and Professor in the Roberts Practiceship
Texas Tech University Health Sciences Center
School of Nursing
Lubbock, Texas

Andrea J. Wallen, EdD, RN
Professor and Chairperson
Graduate Program in Forensic Nursing
Department of Nursing
Fitchburg State College
Fitchburg, Massachusetts

Cynthia J. Weiss-Kaffie, RN, C, CNS, PhD
Associate Professor/Legal Consultant
Texas Tech University Health Sciences Center
School of Nursing
Lubbock, Texas

CONSULTANTS

Barbara Acello, RN, MS
Executive Director
Innovations in Health Care
Denton, Texas

Diane H. Blanchard, RN, PhD
Associate Professor
Southeastern Louisiana University
Baton Rouge, Louisiana

Janis Campbell, RN, PhD
Associate Professor of Nursing
The University of Akron
College of Nursing
Akron, Ohio

Eileen K. Dvorak, RN, MSN
Staff Nurse, Cardiac Catheterization Laboratory
St. Joseph's Medical Center
South Bend, Indiana
Adjunct Professor
Bethel College
Mishawaka, Indiana

Dolores Eitel, RN, MA
Instructor
Bloomfield College
Bloomfield, New Jersey

Diane Kjervik, RN, JD, FAAN
Professor and Associate Dean for Community Outreach and Practice
University of North Carolina
Chapel Hill, North Carolina

Linda Linc, RN, PhD
Professor
The University of Akron
College of Nursing
Akron, Ohio

Dee McGonigle
Associate Professor
Pennsylvania State University

CONTENTS

INTRODUCTION

This textbook, which provides a framework for preventing malpractice and other legal risks, is based on Goren's three-prong approach, or preventive law paradigm, for health care. The three prongs of the preventive law paradigm serve to (1) prevent health care problems from occurring, (2) prevent health care problems from becoming larger, and (3) prevent health care losses.

Goren noted that to prevent problems in health care, nursing law must anticipate future problems; plan for them; have specific objectives to achieve and/or successfully deal with the problems; be able to address the problems in clear, understandable language; and ultimately, reflect the client's rights and wishes. Goren also believed that to minimize problems in health care, nursing law must know the forseeable risks of liability, know which risks carry greater liability than others know what other health care problems may surface, and prepare health care workers for their roles.

Finally, Goren wrote that to prevent or cut losses in health care, nursing law must look to a win/win format (that is, a winning outcome for both patient and nurse); identify, examine, understand, and support health care issues critical to the client; utilize alternative means of dispute resolution; and clearly reflect the complexities of health care issues.

This textbook is organized in sections designed to address Goren's three-prong preventive law paradigm for health care. Preventing problems in health care is addressed in Parts I and II; minimizing problems in health care is addressed in Parts III and IV; preventing or cutting losses in health care is addressed in Parts V and VI.

In Part I, Introduction to Nursing Law and Ethics, the principles of preventing health care problems are addressed in Chapter 1, American Jurisprudence, by demonstrating the legal principles from which both the client's rights and parameters of nursing practice are derived. Chapter 2, Legal Terminology, provides the nurse with the basis with which to address health care issues in clear, understandable language. Chapter 3, The Nurse and the Legal System, provides the nurse with the understanding of the legal process necessary for planning to deal with health care issues within the legal system and identifying specific objectives and mechanisms to achieve successful resolution of the health care problem. Finally, Chapter 4, Ethics in Nursing, identifies ethical issues in health care that the nurse may face within the practice setting.

In Part II, Nursing Practice and the Legal System, principles of preventing problems in health care are also addressed, but with the focus on nursing practice. Chapter 5, Defining Nursing Practice, helps the nurse plan for practicing nursing within its legal parameters, by identifying the roles and responsibilities within the practice of nursing. Chapter 6, Elements of Nursing Negligence, helps the nurse plan for and effectively deal with the client's rights and wishes, to prevent the occurrence of any of the elements of nursing negligence. Then Chapter 7, Negligence Specific to Nursing, prepares the nurse to anticipate and plan for future problems or issues that commonly arise in nursing practice. Chapter 8, Vicarious Liability, examines legal concepts related to preventing liability that may result from actions of another health care provider. Finally, Chapter 9, Documentation, addresses the legal issues surrounding the duty to record nursing practice in clear and understandable language.

In Part III, Nursing Law and the Patient, the principles of minimizing problems in health care are addressed from the viewpoint of the patient. Chapter 10, The Nurse-Patient

Relationship, focuses on and prepares the nurse for the role of provider within the health care relationship. Chapter 11, Patient Rights, outlines the patient's rights, the loss of which may result in a risk of liability for the health care provider. Finally Chapter 12, Informed Consent, identifies elements of the nurse's role when informed consent is provided, which if not properly executed, results in one of the greatest risks for malpractice.

Part IV, Nursing Law and Management, addresses principles of minimizing problems in health care from the viewpoint of management. Chapter 13, Nursing Law and Employment Issues in Nursing, identifies employment issues that cause the greatest risk of liability within management. Chapter 14, Managed Care and the Law, identifies economic issues that cause the greatest risk of liability for health care providers. Chapter 15, Alternate Dispute Resolution in Nursing, identifies a cost-effective non-adversarial mechanism that patient and provider may utilize to address and/or minimize risks and issues of health care outside the court system. Within the preventive law paradigm, Goren also identifies alternate dispute resolution as a mechanism that facilitates cutting losses. Chapter 16, the Legislative Process, identifies another mechanism that patient and provider may use to address and/or minimize risks and issues of health care: the political and legislative processes.

In Part V, Nursing Law and Specialization, the principle of preventing or cutting losses in health care is addressed within specialized areas of nursing practice. Chapter 17, Advanced Nursing Practice, identifies and examines the roles and issues related to advanced practice nursing so that the nurse can clearly understand the complexity of problems that arise in this practice arena. Chapter 18, Home Health Nursing: (1) identifies and examines the roles and issues related to home health care nursing, so that the nurse can clearly understand, anticipate, and plan for the complexity of problems that may arise; (2) provides an understanding of rights and needs of home health care patients, promoting a win/win philosophy; and (3) provides a basis to support issues critical to home health care patients when utilizing alternative dispute mechanisms to negotiate their rights and needs. Chapter 19, Long-Term Care Nursing, encompasses the same three areas of discussion as Chapter 18, but with respect to long-term care. Likewise, Chapter 20, Psychiatric Nursing, and Chapter 21, Emergency Nursing, deal with those two areas of practice.

In Part VI, Nursing Law and Forensics, the principle of preventing or cutting losses is addressed within nursing practice areas that have more traditionally been associated with the legal system or have frequently raised evolving legal issues. Chapter 22, Forensic Nursing, and Chapter 23, Life Care Planning, identify and examine the roles and issues related to these types of forensic nursing, so that the nurse can clearly understand the complexity of problems that arise in these practice arenas. Chapter 24, Violence, as well as the following two chapters, is structured like those in the previous part. It identifies issues related to the occurrence of violence, outlines the rights of both nurses and patients, and discusses issues that arise when utilizing alternative dispute mechanisms. Chapter 25, Telecommunications, has been included in this section because it is an area where legal issues are evolving and frequently arise and it is commonly used by the correctional system. Finally, Chapter 26, Correctional Nursing, gives a comprehensive overview of the legal issues involved in this specialized nursing practice.

Many of the legal concepts are repeated throughout various chapters, to reinforce their utilization in a variety of settings. For example, although the Patient Self-Determination Act is introduced in Part I, it is also discussed throughout the remainder of the book, as it relates to a variety of nursing and health care situations.

Goren, W. D. (1996/1997, Winter). Preventive techniques and health care: Health care and preventive law: Utilization of the three prong paradigm. *Preventive Law Reporter*, 39-40.

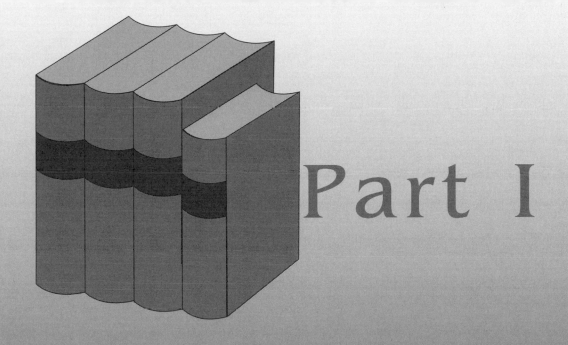

Part I

INTRODUCTION TO NURSING LAW AND ETHICS

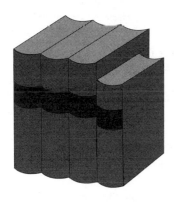

Chapter 1

AMERICAN JURISPRUDENCE

David V. Marchand

OBJECTIVES

Upon completion of this chapter, the reader will be able to:

- Describe the basic structure of our government and explain where its various branches get their power.
- Identify the four sources of law enforced in our court system.
- Describe the basic structure of our state and federal court systems.
- Identify the participants in our court system and explain their roles in the judicial process.

INTRODUCTION

Nurses have chosen a calling that bears directly on people's health and, ultimately, on people's lives. The governmental entities that licensed nurses have, therefore, established criteria, rules, and procedures for granting licensure, regulating nursing practice, reviewing complaints, and disciplining licensees. Patients who believe they have been injured at the hands of their health care providers can bring suit in the courts. And nurses must regularly make decisions regarding patient care in situations where employer protocols, sound nursing judgment, licensure considerations, and the potential for malpractice claims may be in tension. These dilemmas in patient care are common, and familiarity with nursing rules of ethics is essential if the practitioner is to carry out his or her duty to the patient without violating those rules. Thus, although a nurse's primary duty is to the patient, every act of providing health care is done in a much broader context of licensure, ethics, and the law. Disputes between nurse and patient over duties, rights, and remedies are ultimately subject to resolution in the courts. In many states, disputes over licensure issues are also resolved in the courts.

From high school civics lessons and college courses in government or political science, most readers are aware that their local county courthouse is part of their state's judicial system, that there is also a system of federal courts, and that there are different kinds of cases, such as criminal, civil, and administrative. But the law, as it is practiced and enforced in the courts, is quite complex. The nurse who is introduced to the legal system by being handed papers stating that she has been sued will have an unpleasant, confusing, and perhaps even frightening experience, in large part as the result of having no idea where in the bigger medicolegal picture she fits.

This chapter introduces the reader to the way the American legal system makes and administers law—our system of **jurisprudence**—as well as how our court system came about, how it is structured, and how it works. All of these elements are designed to help resolve some of the problems that may arise due to a nurse's unfamiliarity with our legal system.

HISTORICAL PERSPECTIVE

The roots of the American legal system can be traced back to the Battle of Hastings in 1066. Edward the Confessor had died childless; and an earl, the king of Norway, and William of Normandy, Edward's cousin, all claimed England's throne for themselves. The earl, Harold Godwinson, was crowned king and then defeated the king of Norway, Harold Hardraade. The next month, William of Normandy defeated Harold Godwinson in the Battle of Hastings. The legal system that developed during and subsequent to William's rule was, therefore, influenced heavily by Norman, French, and Roman principles and practices. In fact, some courts are called to order each day by the bailiff crying "oyez," a Norman-French expression usually taken to mean *hear ye*, just as the courts were called to order in England centuries before the American Revolution.

Much of American **common law**, that is, law created by judges, can trace its roots to the laws created by English judges during the 600 years after William captured the throne. Likewise, our state and federal legislatures have many of their roots in the British parliamentary system. To be sure, English monarchy and American democracy are diametrically different concepts of sovereignty, but the laws enforced in their respective courts are similar in many respects.

The right of a person to bring suit when she is served unfit food that makes her sick, or the farmer whose crops are eaten by a neighboring rancher's trespassing cattle, or of a patient who is injured by a doctor or nurse who rendered patient care that fell below applicable standards, as well as the rights of those harmed in their person or property in countless other scenarios, have been recognized by English and then American courts for hundreds of years. The courts of our original 13 states, and now of the 50 states, continue to a great extent to embrace and develop causes of action conceived in English courts. But the laws invoked and enforced in the courts come from several sources.

SOURCES OF LAW

Each case brought before a court in this country is decided by applying the law to the facts of the case. There are *four basic sources of law*: (1) the constitutions of the federal and state governments; (2) the laws passed by the federal and the state legislatures; (3) the common law; and (4) administrative rules and regulations. Each of these sources provides specific statements of law. For example, the Constitution declares that we are to be secure in our homes and in our person from unreasonable searches and seizures (U.S. Constitution, 4th Amendment). Likewise, the U.S. Congress has declared that individual citizens may sue the federal government, but only under certain circumstances (Federal Tort Claims Act of 1946). But what is an unreasonable search or seizure? And who is to say whether the proper circumstances exist such that a private citizen can sue the government? The answer is the courts. So not only do the courts, both federal and state, continue to develop the common law as they have for hundreds of years, but they also interpret the laws passed by legislatures and administrative bodies. And they determine whether the legislatures and administrative bodies had, in the first place, the authority to pass the laws or rules in question, that is, courts decide whether a challenged law or regulation is constitutional. The process by which a court reviews a decision of a lower court, a decision of an administrative body, or the constitutionality of a law passed by a legislature is called **judicial review**. Before examining these more detailed functions of the courts, it is helpful to understand the basic constitutional underpinnings of our judicial system.

CONSTITUTIONAL LAW

The most fundamental principle of American government is that the power to govern is held by the people. The President, the Congress, and the courts govern the American people only because the American people have *consented* to be governed by them. The Constitution is the fundamental document by which the American people have granted this consent.

Originally ratified in 1787, the Constitution has seven Articles. Article I creates the Congress, consisting of a Senate and a House of Representatives, and vests all federal legislative powers in that body. In ten separate sections, Article I sets forth the powers and duties of the House and the Senate. Article II establishes the presidency and vests all federal executive power in that office. Article III establishes the Supreme Court and vests in it all federal judicial power of the United States. And these powers of the three branches of government are separate. The President cannot enact a law, like the Congress, or declare one unconstitutional like the courts; the Congress cannot sign a treaty, like the President, or interpret the Constitution, like the courts; and the courts cannot veto a bill, like the President, or propose an amendment to the Constitution, like the Congress.

Article IV contains the full faith and credit clause and the privileges and immunities clause. The former specifies that each state shall give the laws, records, and proceedings of every other state **full faith and credit**. Under this provision, the courts of one state must recognize, for example, a divorce decree issued by a court of another state. Similarly, the **privileges and immunities** clause entitles the citizens of each state to all privileges and immunities of citizens of the other states. Under this provision, for example, states recognize the validity of drivers' licenses issued by other states. Article V sets forth the procedure for amending the Constitution. Article VI contains the **supremacy clause**, which declares that the Constitution and laws of the United States are the supreme law of the land. Thus, if there is a conflict between a state's law and federal law, the courts will follow federal law. Finally, Article VII required ratification by nine states for establishment of the Constitution.

As most readers are probably aware, the Founding Fathers built a system of **checks**

and balances into this governmental framework. Under this scheme, the President can veto a bill passed by Congress, therefore preventing it from becoming law; and Congress can in turn override the President's veto with a two-thirds majority vote in both the House and the Senate. If challenged in the courts, laws passed by Congress can be struck down as unconstitutional, that is, the courts—and in the ultimate instance, the Supreme Court—can declare that the Congress did not have the authority to pass a given law in the first instance. However, the most important check provided by the Constitution is the people's power to amend it.

Amendments may be proposed by two-thirds of both the House and the Senate or by the legislatures of two-thirds of the states. Proposed amendments become effective if ratified by the legislatures of three-fourths of the states or by constitutional conventions in three-fourths of the states (U.S. Constitution, Article V). There are currently 26 amendments to the Constitution, the first ten are known as the Bill of Rights, which were ratified in 1791.

In 1865, after the Civil War, the Thirteenth Amendment was ratified, followed shortly by the Fourteenth Amendment in 1868. The Civil War and these two amendments marked our country's fundamental shift away from a state-dominated union and toward one with a strong federal government. The Thirteenth Amendment abolished slavery. The Fourteenth Amendment provided the people with virtually the same protection from their state governments as the Bill of Rights had given them from the federal government for almost 100 years, although the Supreme Court had to hash out the extent of that protection over the next 100 years. Because the Constitution is the supreme law of the land, the Fourteenth Amendment, as interpreted by the Supreme Court, sets a minimum level of protection; and the states may grant their citizens greater protection under their own laws than does the Constitution.

A great deal of constitutional litigation arises from the rights conferred by the first ten amendments. These include freedom of religion, speech, and the press, and the right to peacefully assemble, to keep and bear arms, and to be free from unreasonable searches and seizures. The right to equal protection under the law has also been the basis of much civil rights litigation.

In deciding cases involving so-called fundamental constitutional rights, the courts look at the right at issue, the nature of the class of persons affected, as well as the state's interest in regulating certain conduct. Where **fundamental rights**, such as privacy, speech, religion, or liberty, are involved, or where issues specific to a certain class of persons, such as racial minorities or persons of a given national origin, come into play, the courts apply a **strict scrutiny test** (*Yick Wo v. Hopkins*, 1886). Under this analysis, a court will decide whether the law alleged to impinge on fundamental rights is the least restrictive mechanism by which the state can accomplish a compelling state interest. If there are less restrictive means by which a state could accomplish its goals in advancing its compelling interest, then the challenged law will be found unconstitutional (*Cruzan v. Director, Missouri Department of Health*, 1990). Where a law is challenged because it supposedly discriminates based on classifications such as gender, the courts examine the law to see whether it is substantially related to a legitimate state interest (*Craig v. Boren*, 1976). This test of **"intermediate scrutiny"** has also been applied to non-marital children (*United States v. Clark*, 1980). But where a challenged law regulates and affects only economic or property interests, the courts will strike down such a law only if it bears no rational relationship to a conceivable legitimate state purpose. This is known as the **rational relationship test** (*Minnesota v. Clover Leaf Creamery Co.*, 1981).

Although there is no right to privacy provided expressly in the Constitution, the U.S. Supreme Court has nevertheless held that the Constitution does offer protection to such a fundamental right. For example, the high court has held that the right to privacy prohibits a state from passing a law that prohibits a doctor from giving a married couple information regarding contraception (*Griswold v. Connecticut*, 1965). As put by Justice William O. Douglas, the Court had, prior to *Griswold*, recognized in the Fourth Amendment a "right to privacy, no less important than any other right carefully and particularly reserved to the people"

(*Griswold v. Connecticut*, 1965, p. 485 [quoting *Mapp v. Ohio*, 1961, p. 656]). *Griswold*

"concern[ed] a relationship lying within the zone of privacy created by several fundamental constitutional guarantees. And it concern[ed] a law which, in forbidding the *use* of contraceptives rather than regulating their manufacture or sale, [sought] to achieve its goals by means of having a maximum destructive impact upon that relationship" (*Griswold v. Connecticut*, 1965, p. 485).

The Court called the marital right of privacy at issue in *Griswold* "older than the Bill of Rights" (*Griswold v. Connecticut*, 1965, p. 486).

Eight years after *Griswold*, the Court decided *Roe v. Wade* (1973), which involved a state's right to criminalize abortion. The *Roe* court held, in effect, that a state may not interfere with a woman's right to abortion prior to viability of the fetus, which the court recognized as commencing at approximately the beginning of the third trimester of pregnancy. According to the *Roe* Court,

"[t]his right of privacy, whether it be founded in the Fourteenth Amendment's concept of personal liberty [as] we feel it is, or [in] the Ninth [Amendment], is broad enough to encompass a woman's decision whether or not to terminate her pregnancy" (*Roe v. Wade*, 1973, p. 153).

Another important area in which the courts have found constitutional rights to privacy is where a patient refuses medical treatment, either for himself or herself or for a child. Courts generally afford great deference to a patient's refusal to undergo medical treatment on religious grounds, regardless of the consequences of that decision, because it is the patient that bears those consequences (*In re Brooks' Estate* [reversed order of the trial court appointing a conservator of the person to consent to unwanted blood transfusions], 1965; *In re Osborne*, 1972; *Mercy Hospital, Inc. v. Jackson*, 1985 [affirming denial of petition to appoint a guardian to consent to Jehovah's Witness blood transfusion during cesarean section where fetus not at risk]).

One such case involved a woman with dysfunctional uterine bleeding who would, in all medical probability, die if she did not receive a blood transfusion (*Public Health Trust of Dade County v. Wons*, 1989). The

patient, a Jehovah's Witness with two small children, refused the transfusion. The hospital petitioned the court for an order permitting it to give the transfusion against the patient's wishes. The court granted the petition, the hospital gave the transfusion, and the patient subsequently gained consciousness and refused further such transfusions, although she needed them because of the recurrent nature of her condition. But the hospital asserted that "[her] children's right to be reared by two loving parents is sufficient to trigger the compelling state interest [in protection of innocent third parties]" (*Public Health Trust of Dade County v. Wons*, 1989, p. 97). The *Wons* court, in reaching its decision, turned to one of its prior opinions in which it adopted four criteria wherein the right to refuse medical treatment may be overridden by a compelling state interest. These factors are:

1. Preservation of life
2. Protection of innocent third parties
3. Prevention of suicide
4. Maintenance of the ethical integrity of the medical profession (*Public Health Trust of Dade County v. Wons*, 1989, p. 97)

But the court took the position that while "the nurturing and support by two parents is important in the development of any child, it is not sufficient to override fundamental constitutional rights" (*Public Health Trust of Dade County v. Wons*, 1989, p. 97). The court also quoted with approval the opinion of the district court:

Surely nothing in the last analysis, is more private or more sacred than one's religion or view of life, and here the courts, quite properly, have given great deference to the individual's right to make decisions vitally affecting his private life according to his own conscience. It is difficult to overstate this right because it is, without exaggeration, the very bedrock upon which this country was founded (*Public Health Trust of Dade County v. Wons*, 1989, p. 98).

As can be seen, *Wons* illustrates how important an individual's constitutional rights are, even when their own lives, or indirectly, the lives of children, are put in jeopardy by the exercise of those rights. *Wons* also illustrates how a compelling state interest in the protection of innocent third parties, here an interest in maintaining a home with two parents for the minor children, did not override the patient's constitutional rights of privacy and freedom of religion.

In *Superintendent of Belchertown State School v. Saikewicz* (1977), the court considered the four factors discussed in *Wons* in determining whether an incompetent, mentally retarded patient could refuse medical treatment necessary to prolong his life. In considering a state's interest in the preservation of human life, the *Saikewicz* court noted that "[t]here is a substantial distinction in the State's insistence that human life be saved where the affliction is curable, as opposed to the State interest, where, as here, the issue is not whether but when, for how long, and at what cost to the individual that life may be briefly extended" (*Superintendent of Belchertown State School v. Saikewicz*, 1977, pp. 425–426). In tension with the state's interest, the court found the constitutional right to privacy to be "an expression of the sanctity of individual free choice and self determination as fundamental constituents of life" (*Superintendent of Belchertown State School v. Saikewicz*, 1977, p. 426). The court concluded "the value of life as so perceived is lessened not by a decision to refuse treatment, but by the failure to allow a competent human being the right of a choice" (*Superintendent of Belchertown State School v. Saikewicz*, 1977, p. 426). But these constitutional rights are not absolute.

In *Application of the President & Directors of Georgetown College, Inc.* (1964), the Supreme Court granted the hospital permission to transfuse a patient who was unwilling to consent owing to religious reasons. The state's interest in protecting the patient's minor children from "abandonment" by their parent was an overriding factor in the decision. In *Commissioner of Corrections v. Myers* (1979), the court considered whether a prisoner could refuse life-saving kidney dialysis unless the state moved him to a less secure prison. In holding that he could not, the court found that the state's interest in "orderly prison administration" outweighed the prisoner's constitutional right to privacy (*Commissioner of Corrections v. Myers*, 1979, p. 457).

These cases illustrate that the Constitution touches directly on health care providers when they are confronted with a patient exercising choice regarding the care he or she will receive. Although these so-called right-to-die cases are an extreme example of the more general legal theory of informed consent, the practitioner must be aware that she or he works in an environment occupied by some of the most fundamental rights recognized in the courts.

STATUTORY LAW

The federal and state legislatures enact laws that touch on virtually every aspect of our lives. Such a law passed by a legislature is called a **statute**. When legislatures organize laws into a logical group and systematically arrange them, such as into chapters, sections, and subsections, this group of laws is called a **code**. For example, a state may have a penal code, a code of criminal procedure, a property code, a highway code, as well as many other codes relating to the functions of its government or regulating the conduct of its citizens. Laws passed by Congress are contained in the U.S. Code. Volumes of codes and statutes passed by state legislatures, as well as the U.S. Code, can be found in local law libraries. Most such libraries also have volumes of codes and statutes that contain short summaries of court cases in which the listed statutes were at issue. These lists of summaries, called **annotations**, which can go on for dozens of pages, can provide a good start toward understanding how the courts interpret a particular law under various factual scenarios.

In addition to federal and state statutes and codes, local governmental entities, such as cities, counties, and parishes, pass their own rules and regulations affecting government and citizens within their borders. This type of law, commonly called an **ordinance**, may affect traffic, parking, construction, curfews, trash burning, control of animals, and many other aspects of activity taking place within a city's or county's limits. As discussed in the preceding sections, all laws passed by legislative bodies are subject to review in the courts. And depending on the nature of the challenge to a given law, the courts use various standards in deciding whether the law is proper and enforceable.

Because the American people granted only a certain amount of their power to govern to the federal government, the states retain broad powers to legislate in many areas. This power, known as the states' **police power,** includes the power to legislate in the area of public health. It is by this authority that the states have enacted their respective medical and nursing practice acts, under which the states license and regulate health care providers. Under this power, a state may also authorize formation of a board of health. Typically, state legislatures then delegate to such boards the authority to adopt rules necessary for the effective administration of their legislative mandates, which may, for example, include prevention of communicable diseases (Communicable Disease Prevention and Control Act of 1983). In response, a board of health may require a nurse to report certain communicable diseases to the state's health department, or in the case of a school nurse, to ensure that children have certain immunizations before they are permitted to attend school (*Staffel v. San Antonio School Board of Education*, 1918).

COMMON LAW

As discussed previously, another source of law is the courts themselves. For hundreds of years, judges have been creating and modifying legal duties, rights, and remedies. Although federal and state codes and statutes are voluminous, the vast majority of law was created and shaped by the courts. Certain causes of action, such as the right to bring suit against a restaurant for serving unfit food, have remained essentially unchanged for hundreds of years. Courts developed the **common law** very gradually, making minor changes as societal needs, public policy, and, on occasion, compelling factual situations demand. The most fundamental concept to this development of the common law is that prior decisions should be followed when courts are presented with the same legal questions. This idea of **precedent**, in Latin **stare decisis,** which means "let the decision stand," helps provide predictability to the outcome of legal disputes. Although this process of accretionary law-

making is the rule, courts have occasionally engaged in rapid revision of whole areas of the common law. For example, during the mid-1990s, the high courts of many states engaged in wholesale revision, and even abolition, of many duties, rights, and remedies available to personal injury plaintiffs. This revolution in the common law of many states, together with similar efforts in the various legislatures, is collectively referred to as **tort reform.**

In general, tort reform in both the courts and legislatures has been aimed at restricting liability and imposing limits on money damages. For example, many states have traditionally permitted a plaintiff, under certain circumstances, to collect an entire judgment from a single defendant that a jury found negligent, even if the jury also found several other defendants negligent, and even if the jury found them to have contributed more to the plaintiff's injuries. The only recourse the paying defendant had was to look to the other defendants the jury had found negligent for reimbursement for their share of the judgment. This is called **joint and several liability**. Some states have enacted legislation to abolish joint and several liability, whereas other states have chosen to narrow it. In states that have abolished this provision, each defendant is liable only for his or her proportionate share of the damages awarded by the jury.

The tort reform movement has also been aimed at limiting the amount a plaintiff can recover, regardless of a jury's verdict. These types of provisions are called **damage caps**. Florida, for example, limits the amount a medical malpractice plaintiff can recover for noneconomic damages such as pain and suffering to $350,000 (Florida Damage Statute, 1986), and Texas limits punitive damages, which can be awarded when the jury finds a defendant was grossly negligent (Texas Exemplary Damages Statute of 1987).

In addition to permitting someone to sue for money damages, the common law provides a system of laws based on fairness, or, in legal parlance, **equity**. For example, people can bring suit to have a court declare that a city's busing program is illegal, that an insurance policy does or does not provide certain coverage, or that a patent is invalid.

Equitable remedies include restraining orders, injunctions, and orders directing parties to do or refrain from doing certain things. Nevada's Board of Nursing, for example, may seek an injunction to preclude violation of certain provisions of that state's nurse practice act (Injunctions Against Violations of Chapter, 1995).

ADMINISTRATIVE LAW

Administrative bodies, such as the Food and Drug Administration, the Social Security Administration, and the Equal Employment Opportunity Commission, provide yet another source of law for the courts. Examples of administrative bodies at the state level include Workers' Compensation Commissions, Employment Commissions, and Boards of Medical and Nurse Examiners. These bodies get their power from the federal or state legislatures. The legislatures delegated this rule-making authority because these various bodies have the experience and expertise to regulate in a given area. The body of law created by these agencies, which includes rules, regulations, and orders, to carry out their regulatory function is called **administrative law**. The rules promulgated by federal administrative bodies, such as the Federal Aviation Administration or the Food and Drug Administration, can be found in the Code of Federal Regulations.

At the state level, such rules are commonly organized into an administrative code, which may include medical, nurse, and physician's assistants practice acts. The boards of nurse examiners of the various states have a number of purposes, such as to interpret the state's nurse practice act, establish standards of nursing practice, and regulate the practice of professional nursing (Texas Examining Boards, 1998). State boards of nurse examiners are also empowered to grant licensure to qualified applicants, to investigate and discipline violators, and to enforce the nurse practice act and rules and regulations (Florida Administrative Code, 1993; Kansas Administrative Regulations, 1988).

Typically, licensees who have been disciplined, or whose licenses have been encumbered or revoked, must exhaust all administrative appeals before filing suit in the courts (Florida Board of Nursing, 1998). This may involve hearings before administrative law judges or some other form of appellate administrative review. Often the courts cannot hear these types of disputes until the affected party has exhausted all administrative remedies. Once administrative decisions are placed in litigation in the courts, claimants often do not have a right to trial by jury. Instead, the applicable law may require the judge to review the evidence that was put before the administrative body and determine whether the administrative decision is supported by substantial evidence. In *Lunsford v. Board of Nurse Examiners* (1983), the Texas Board of Nurse Examiners found that the nurse's failure to assess a patient's condition, and her failure to inform the attending physicians of the life and death nature of the patient's instability, which resulted in the patient's death, constituted unprofessional conduct likely to injure the public. The Court upheld the Board's finding that there was sufficient evidence to revoke the nurse's license for 1 year. As can be seen, the law gives great deference to the proceedings of administrative bodies.

CIVIL VERSUS CRIMINAL LAW

Most readers are aware of the dichotomy in our judicial system between civil cases and criminal cases. In **criminal law**, the federal or state government is attempting to deprive an individual of life or liberty for something the law considers an offense against society in general. By contrast, **civil law** seeks to resolve disputes between private parties, which often results in the payment of money damages. Perhaps the most striking difference between the two types of cases can be seen in the difference in burden of proof. In criminal law, where all of the might and resources of the government are directed at depriving someone of life or liberty, the prosecution is required to prove its case beyond a **reasonable doubt**. By way of example, Texas defines reasonable doubt as that degree of doubt that would cause a reasonable person to hesitate to act if the decision involved the most important of his or her own affairs (*Geesa v. State*, 1991). Note that this does not require the fact-finder not to act, it only requires hesitation to act. Similarly, California defines reasonable doubt as "that state of the case, which, after the entire comparison and consideration of all the evidence, leaves the minds of jurors in that condition that they cannot say they feel an abiding conviction of the truth of the charge" (Presumption of Innocence; Effect; Reasonable Doubt, 1998).

In stark contrast to the burdens of proof in a criminal case, a litigant in a civil case must simply satisfy the jury that, more likely than not, the allegations he or she has made are true. To do this, a plaintiff must persuade the jury that a **preponderance of the evidence** is in his or her favor (Keeton, Dobbs, Keeton, & Owen, 1984, p. 239). In a case of medical malpractice, for example, a plaintiff must show that, more likely than not, had the health care rendered not fallen below the standard of care the patient would not have suffered the injuries alleged.

Criminal and civil cases differ in several other fundamental ways. In criminal cases, the accused is not required to give testimony and can invoke the right against self-incrimination contained in the Fifth Amendment to the Constitution. Furthermore, the accused's silence may not be held against him or her or commented on by the prosecution (LaFave & Israel, 1985, p. 884; *Griffin v. California*, 1965). However, if called to the stand, a defendant in a civil case must give testimony. If she or he refuses to testify and invokes the Fifth Amendment right, the jury can consider that in their deliberations. Moreover, all criminal defendants enjoy the right to trial by jury (U.S. Constitution, Article VI), whereas parties to a civil action are not always entitled to a jury. Although the Constitution guarantees a criminal defendant the right to counsel (U.S. Constitution, Article VI), parties to civil actions do not have such a right.

The various avenues for appeal are also different between criminal and civil law. Although this is described in more detail later, the basic levels of appeal are the same for criminal and civil cases, but those convicted of crimes have an additional set of procedures available for review of their convictions, that is, a convicted person may, in addition to appealing conviction, file a petition asking a court to issue an order to the warden, or other person responsible for the petitioner's incarceration, to release the petitioner (Lafave & Israel, 1985). The order, which actually takes the form of a letter, is called a **writ of** *habeas corpus*, a Latin expression meaning, "you have the body." A writ of *habeas corpus,* sometimes referred to as the great writ of liberty or the great writ (Lafave & Israel, 1985), will issue only when a petitioner can show that she or he is being held in violation of the Constitution, treaties, or statutes of the United States (Habeas Act of 1867, 1997).

SUBSTANTIVE VERSUS PROCEDURAL LAW

There are extensive rules of procedure and evidence governing the conduct of litigation in the courts. This myriad of rules establishes the step-by-step process that litigants must follow in filing and defending civil or criminal cases. For example, the rules of civil procedure govern how lawsuits are filed and answered, how parties obtain documents and pretrial testimony from one another, how parties may attempt to have their opponent's claims thrown out of court before trial, and what evidence may be presented at trial. These rules are embodied in the Federal Rules of Civil Procedure, the Federal Rules of Evidence, and the analogous rules promulgated by the courts of each state. The goal of these rules is to bring order to a dispute so that it will be resolved fairly and expediently.

For example, when a plaintiff files a complaint in federal court, he or she must serve each defendant with a summons, which orders them to appear in court, and also with a copy of the complaint (General Provisions Governing Discovery; Duty of Disclosure, 4(b), 1998). The plaintiff must do so because the Fourteenth Amendment to the Constitution provides, among other things, that it would be fundamentally unfair for a defendant to have claims made and tried against him or her without giving him or her notice of the lawsuit and an opportunity to be heard. The act of formally delivering lawsuit papers to a defendant, called **service of process**, is legally sufficient to charge the defendant with notice of the lawsuit (*Volkswagenwerk Aktiengesellschaft v. Schlunk*, 1988). This and other rules of civil procedure, called **procedural law**, in both state and federal courts seek to maintain an orderly and fair progression of the lawsuit from filing to dismissal.

In contrast to these rules of procedure are the actual laws under which claims are brought and defended. For example, a person may bring a lawsuit under a wrongful death statute claiming that the defendant doctor or nurse was negligent in providing care to a patient, which resulted in the patient's death. The applicable laws regarding who may file a wrongful death claim and the time period within which someone can file such a lawsuit, called a **statute of limitations**, are examples of **substantive law**. Similarly, a plaintiff who alleges that a nurse's negligence caused him injury may sue a hospital under the theory that because the nurse was an employee of the hospital, the hospital is responsible for the nurse's negligence. This is the theory of *respondeat superior*. Also, a plaintiff may sue an independent contractor nurse or physician and claim that he or she was an agent of the hospital, and that the hospital is, therefore, liable for the defendant physician's or nurse's actions under the theory of **agency**. These are further examples of substantive law.

Although procedural rules may seem at first glance to be rather ministerial in comparison to the applicable substantive law, rules of procedure can actually provide tools for prosecuting, defending, and even disposing of cases that are sometimes more powerful than the applicable substantive law. In fact, in some situations, the rules of civil procedure are arguably substantive in their effect. This can be seen readily in the wake of the tort reform movement of the mid-to-late 1990s. For example, if a medical malpractice plaintiff in Texas does not, within 180 days of filing suit, provide the defendant with an expert report setting forth how the defendant failed to meet the applicable standards of care and how such failure caused the plaintiff's injuries, the plaintiff's case can be dismissed (Medical Liability and Insurance Improvement Act of Texas, 1998). Even though this provision is listed in the statute under the heading "Procedural Provisions," it can clearly result in the dismissal of the plaintiff's case, which is a rather substantive result.

JUDICIAL SYSTEM

Each year, there are approximately 17 million civil cases filed in the courts across this country, only about 2% of which are filed in the federal courts (National Center for State Courts, 1991; "Annual Report of the Director," 1984–1990). This includes divorce and custody, will probate, contract disputes, disputes over deed restrictions, sexual harassment, personal injury, and countless others. To understand where in this vast landscape the practitioner may find herself or himself during the course of a malpractice suit, the practitioner must understand the basic types of courts that constitute our judicial system.

TYPES OF COURTS

Although each state is different, there are basically three types of courts: trial, appellate, and supreme. This basic court system exists at the local, state, and federal levels. When a civil action is filed, the court in which the case is litigated is referred to as the **trial court**. This is because, should the case not settle or be dismissed, it will proceed to trial, either before the judge alone or before a judge and jury.

If a party is dissatisfied with the judgment of the trial court, it can appeal to the next highest court. In many states this type of court is simply called a **court of appeals**, or court of civil appeal. Unlike the trial courts, appellate courts have no juries. Instead, they consist of a panel of judges who review the transcript of the trial, as well as all exhibits, pleadings, motions, and orders, to determine whether there were errors made in the trial. If these errors materially affected the outcome, the appellate court can take several different types of action: (1) it can reverse the judgment of the trial court, either in whole or in part, and can send the case back for another trial; (2) it can reverse the judgment of the trial court and render judgment in favor of the appealing party; or (3) it can affirm the trial court's finding.

In addition to hearing appeals from final judgments in the trial courts, courts of appeal can also hear appeals from trial court orders entered during the course of litigation. An **interlocutory appeal**, as this type of appeal is called, is heard usually only where there would be irreparable harm to the appealing party, or his or her case, if the trial court's order were complied with. These appeals typically arise when a trial court has granted an opposing party access to information that the appealing party feels should not be disclosed. For example, a court may order a hospital to turn over certain peer review committee documents that the hospital feels would do it irreparable harm. In such a case, the hospital may appeal to the appellate court for an order directing the trial court to vacate its order.

For example, in *Terrell State Hospital of the Texas Department of Mental Health and Mental Retardation v. Ashworth* (1990), a mother sued a hospital alleging that the hospital's negligence led to her 16-year-old son's suicide. During the case, the trial judge ordered the hospital to turn over a psychological autopsy its peer review committee had performed after the boy's suicide. Despite the fact that the Hospital Committee Privilege (1989) protects information generated by a hospital in its investigation process, the court ordered the document produced, because it held that the hospital had waived the privilege by disclosing significant parts of the document. The hospital, unsuccessfully, filed an interlocutory appeal seeking to have the court of appeals order the trial court to vacate its order.

Another such example would be when a trial court orders an individual party to turn over federal income tax returns, psychiatric records, diaries, notes or communications from his or her attorney, or other such information that, under the law, should not be disclosed because it is considered to be protected by privilege or a **qualified immunity** (General Provisions Governing Discovery: Duty of Disclosure, 1998). In such a situation, a party has a right to ask an appellate court to intervene.

If a party is dissatisfied with the ruling of a court of appeals, it may appeal to the next level, which is typically the highest court in a given state. In the case of appeals to a state's highest court, as well as to an intermediate court of appeals, the reviewing court may decline to hear the appeal, that is, just because a litigant is unhappy with the result in a lower court does not mean there were errors made that, in the opinion of the higher court, merit review. Once a higher court reviews an appealing party's allegations of errors made in the lower court, the legal briefs filed by the appellant and appellee, as well as pertinent portions of the transcript of the proceedings in the lower court, it may set the appeal for oral argument or simply rule based on the papers on file. If the case is of significance to the law, the court may decide to publish a written opinion explaining why it ruled as it did.

If a party is dissatisfied with the ruling of the highest court in the state, it has the option of petitioning the U.S. Supreme Court for review of the actions of the state's highest court. However, the U.S. Supreme Court will review the actions of a state's Supreme Court only where those actions involve rights or duties under the Constitution of the United States.

The system of federal courts is similar to that of the states. In the federal system, the trial courts are the U.S. District Courts. Congress configured the districts for these trial courts based on population, distance, and caseload (Ferguson & McHenry, 1973). In small states such as Rhode Island, there may be only one district court for the entire state. In large states such as Texas, not only are there district courts for different parts of the state, but there are also different divisions of district courts in a given district. For example, in Texas there are United States district courts for the Western District, Southern District, Eastern District, and Northern District of Texas.

Appeals from the U.S. District Courts are made to the U.S. Circuit Courts of Appeals. Currently there are 13 Courts of Appeals, one in each of 12 geographic regions, known as circuits, and one court for patent cases, called the U.S. Court of Appeals for the Federal Circuit (Wright, 1983, p. 10). Each circuit hears appeals from the district courts of various states. For example, the U.S. Court of Appeals for the Fifth Circuit hears appeals from U.S. District Courts for the districts of Texas, Louisiana, and Mississippi. The Ninth Circuit is the largest circuit, encompassing nine states and Guam. A panel of not more than three judges (Assignment of Budgets; Panels; Hearings; Quorum, 1948) hears most cases appealed to the Circuit Courts of Appeals.

The Courts of Appeals also hear most appeals from orders of federal administrative agencies (Wright, 1983, p. 716).

If a party is dissatisfied with the ruling of a circuit court of appeals, they can appeal to the U.S. Supreme Court. Such an appeal is usually made by a petition to the Supreme Court for a **writ of** *certiorari* (Wright, 1983, p. 14). Like writs of error in the state systems, a writ of *certiorari* is an order from the U.S. Supreme Court to the circuit court of appeals below to send the record of the case up for review. And as with appeals from state supreme courts, the U.S. Supreme Court will review the actions of the lower courts only for errors that implicate constitutional rights and duties.

LOCAL, STATE, AND FEDERAL SYSTEMS

Most readers have had some contact with a local court system. Traffic citations, typically classified as the lowest grade of criminal offense, are often issued and prosecuted by counties, parishes, or municipalities. Although conviction on a speeding ticket normally involves only monetary penalties, it nevertheless entails a governmental entity engaging in a criminal prosecution of an individual. All of the rights and privileges available under the federal Constitution are, therefore, available to the accused, including trial by jury. Municipal courts and justice of the peace courts hear such other cases as landlord-tenant disputes, including eviction, and they often perform ceremonial functions.

Judges at the local and state levels are usually elected officials, although the role of partisan politics in their campaigns for office varies widely from state to state. Federal judges, by contrast, are nominated by the President of the United States and are confirmed by the Senate (Appointment and Number of District Judges, 1948). Unlike their state and local counterparts, whose terms of office are typically limited to a number of years, federal judges are appointed for life.

JURISDICTION

In order for parties to a lawsuit to bring their case in a given court, that court must have authority to hear that particular case. This is called **jurisdiction**. Typically, a family court cannot hear a medical malpractice case, nor can a tax court hear a dispute over an insurance policy. Similarly, a trial court in one state typically cannot hear a dispute between citizens of a different state. Nor can a trial court hear a dispute between one of its citizens and a citizen or business of another state where the events giving rise to the dispute all occurred in the other state, and where the out-of-state party has never set foot in, or had any dealings with, the state in which the lawsuit is intended to be brought. To hear a particular case, a court must have **subject matter jurisdiction** over the dispute, such as where a family court hears a divorce or child custody case, or a probate court hears a dispute over a will (Wright, 1983, p. 25).

Courts must also have jurisdiction over the parties, called *in personam* **jurisdiction**, or personal jurisdiction. To exercise jurisdiction over a given party, that party must have had what the law refers to as **minimum contacts** with the state in which the court sits. For example, if someone is involved as a driver in an automobile accident in another state, he or she may be sued in the courts of that state even if that is the only time he or she has ever been or will ever be in that state. Similarly, courts typically have jurisdiction over persons or businesses in other states that solicit or conduct business in that court's state. The limits of a state court's jurisdiction over non-resident parties is defined by the constitutional law of due process (U.S. Constitution, 14th Amendment), and by the state's statutes governing jurisdiction over out-of-state defendants.

Although a detailed discussion of the concepts of substantive and procedural due process are beyond the scope of this introduction to jurisprudence, the reader should be aware that the Constitution itself affords parties to a lawsuit certain fundamental procedural rights. As discussed previously, these include the right to be given notice of the lawsuit and an opportunity to be heard (U.S. Constitution, 14th Amendment). Courts cannot hear cases involving subject matter or parties over which they have no jurisdiction. States have, therefore, enacted what are known as **long arm statutes**, which set out the limits of a court's jurisdiction over parties from other states or other countries (Presumption of Innocence; Effect; Reasonable Doubt, 1998; Texas Long Arm Statute, 1985). A state court may assert personal jurisdiction over a non-resident defendant only if the requirements of both the Due Process Clause of the Fourteenth Amendment to the U.S. Constitution and the state's long arm statute are satisfied. Although *in personam* jurisdiction issues can arise where, for example, a patient from another state files suit in his or her home state against a practitioner from another state, these jurisdictional challenges are relatively rare in malpractice actions.

VENUE

Not only does a court have to have jurisdiction over both subject matter and the parties before it, but that court must also be a proper place, or **venue**, to hear a given lawsuit. Obviously, a medical negligence case that arises solely out of care rendered at a hospital in Miami to a patient from Miami, and where all of the family members and health care providers are in Miami, would generally not properly be brought in Tallahassee.

As an example, Texas's venue statute provides that a suit may be brought "(1) in the county in which all or a substantial part of the events or omissions giving rise to the claim occurred; (2) in the city of defendant's residence at the time the cause of action accrued if defendant is a natural person; (3) in the county of the defendant's principal office in this state if the defendant is not a natural person" (Texas General Venue Statute, 1997).

ADVERSARIAL SYSTEM

Courts use a relatively short cast of characters to host litigation and conduct trials. The parties, their attorneys, the judge, and the jury together determine the outcome of a given case. The system places parties in adversarial roles and equips them with the same rules of procedure and evidence, with the goal of the proceedings being to discover the truth about the claims and defenses involved. The **judge** acts as a neutral overseer of the proceedings and controls the parties' access to evidence under their opponents' control, as well as their presentation of evidence to a jury. Judges also decide certain issues not meant for juries. These would include such questions as whether a county hospital can or cannot be sued in a malpractice action under a given state's statutes; whether a nurse-patient relationship existed at the time of an alleged act of malpractice, thus giving rise to a legal duty for the nurse to provide certain care to the patient; whether a defendant hospital's nurses were acting as its vice-principals at the time they allegedly committed malpractice, thus exposing the hospital to punitive damages; and whether a plaintiff has obtained sufficient evidence that can be admitted at trial to support a jury's finding that a given nurse was an employee of a defendant hospital or clinic, as opposed to merely being an independent contractor.

By contrast, the **jury** decides issues of fact, that is, the jury is the sole judge of the credibility of witnesses, and the jury answers such ultimate questions as whose negligence caused the plaintiff's injuries and how much money will fairly and reasonably compensate the plaintiff. Courts are reluctant to disturb jury findings of fact, even where there is evidence that jurors did not follow instructions given them by the judge. Typically, the only circumstances that warrant disregard of a jury's findings are when the jury has been subject to an improper outside influence (*Texas Employers' Insurance Association v. McCaslin*, 1958). In this regard, jury deliberations take place in a metaphorical black box.

Attorneys are hired to represent the parties in the lawsuit. Although attorneys, being members of their state's bar, are officers of the court, their duty is to their clients. The **attorney-client relationship,** which dates back hundreds of years, is one of the most sacred relationships in our society. Communications between a client and his or her attorney are privileged and cannot be disclosed without the client's consent, or unless there is a showing that the communications were made in furtherance of a crime or fraud (*In re Burlington Northern, Inc.* [the work product privilege does not protect information from discovery related to the commission of a crime or fraud], 1987; *Cox v. Administrator U.S. Steel & Carnegie*, 1994). Limited only by rules of professional responsibility, the lawyer's duty is to zealously advocate his or her client's case, subordinating even personal wants and desires should they come into conflict with the legal needs of the client (American Bar Association, 1995). Although opposing counsel in a given case may work with one another on a regular basis, a lawyer can make no concessions to opposing counsel or their client if that would in any way compromise his or her own client's case (American Bar Association, 1995, Rule 1.6). And it is also an attorney's duty to fully disclose to the client any conflict of interests that may arise during the course of representation of that client (American Bar Association, 1995).

ADMINISTRATIVE LAW SYSTEM

As already mentioned, Congress and the state legislatures have delegated considerable rule-making and enforcement authority to such governmental bodies as the Social Security Administration, Workers' Compensation Commissions, and boards of nurse examiners.

Individuals making claims for benefits from these entities typically initiate the process by making some type of written application for benefits. In the case of workers' compensation proceedings, an injured worker will be examined by a physician and given an impairment rating. If the applicant is dissatisfied with the agency's initial response, she or he usually may then employ an attorney for representation throughout the remainder of the administrative and postadministrative process.

Individuals seeking disability benefits from the Social Security Administration initially fill out an application for benefits. If that application is denied, or denied in part, the applicant may hire an attorney to file a Request for Reconsideration and Hearing before an administrative law judge. The applicant's local Office of Hearings and Appeals will then set the matter for hearing before an administrative law judge. Before the hearing, the applicant or attorney may file additional medical records and reports to support the claim of disability. At the hearing before the administrative law judge, which is nonadversarial, the applicant puts on evidence that he or she is unable "not only to perform his or her previous work but cannot, considering his or her age, education, and work experience, engage in any other kind of substantial gainful work that exists in the national economy" (*Oldham v. Schweiker*, 1981, p. 1083). The applicant and the federal government, which is represented by the judge in these proceedings, not separate counsel, may both produce expert witnesses to give testimony regarding the claim of disability. Subsequent to the hearing, the administrative law judge issues a written opinion setting forth in detail why the claim should or should not be allowed.

If the applicant is dissatisfied with the judge's decision, he or she may file an appeal with the Appeals Counsel in Falls Church, Virginia. At this level, the applicant may file briefs of fact and law to support the claim that the administrative law judge erred in the decision. Only after the applicant has exhausted this final appeal may he or she then invoke the jurisdiction of the federal courts to review the administration's decision (*Hines v. Weinberger*, 1975). Such a lawsuit is brought against the Commissioner of Social Security, and the claimant is not entitled to trial by jury. Rather, the federal district court judge who reviews the administration's actions will decide simply whether the administration's decision was based on substantial evidence (*Casey v. Cohen*, 1968). As with all cases filed in federal court, the claimant may appeal the district court's decision to the applicable federal circuit court of appeals, and even to the United States Supreme Court.

At the state level, boards of nurse examiners may discipline applicants and licensees for a number of reasons. Idaho, for example, sets forth nine grounds for disciplining applicants for nursing licensure or renewal, including practicing under an assumed name, conviction of a felony or crime of moral turpitude, gross negligence, habitual drug use, and violating the state's nurse practice act (Disciplinary Action, 1977). Nevada has similar provisions (Nevada Revised Statutes § 632.320, 1995). Every nurse who is subjected to disciplinary proceedings in Idaho is afforded an opportunity for hearing after reasonable notice (Idaho Board of Nursing, 1977). After the hearing, it is the hearing officer, not the Idaho Board of Nursing, who makes the initial decision as to guilt or innocence; and the Board can only approve or disapprove a guilty decision.

In *Tuma v. Board of Nursing* (1979), a clinical instructor of nursing (Tuma) at the College of Southern Idaho provided care to a patient who was dying of cancer. The patient was scheduled to undergo chemotherapy. Tuma agreed to meet with the family and discuss alternative treatments using natural products. A student nurse testified that Tuma told the patient that the discussion "wasn't exactly ethical . . . [or] legal." (*Tuma v. Board of Nursing*, 1979, p. 713). Tuma and a student nurse then commenced the patient's chemotherapy. But the chemotherapy was temporarily discontinued that evening at the patient's request so that Tuma could meet with the patient and family. The patient died 2 weeks later.

After a hearing was held, the hearing officer determined that Tuma's actions interfered with the physician-patient relationship, among other things. The decision was appealed to the district court, where Tuma requested a new trial, which was denied.

Although the district court affirmed the Board's suspension, the Idaho Supreme Court reversed the district court and the order suspending Tuma's license. The Idaho Supreme Court held that the Board of Nurse Examiners must promulgate rules and regulations to adequately warn licensees of prohibited conduct, which it had not done.

Florida's license revocation procedures are similar and have, for example, been invoked to revoke the license of a nurse who failed to use proper technique in inserting a catheter, failed to respond in a timely manner to a patient in distress, and failed to properly assess and report a patient's condition (*Holmes v. Department of Professional Regulation, Board of Nursing*, 1987).

ISSUES AND TRENDS

Although the basic structure of our system of jurisprudence is essentially constant, its substantive and procedural laws undergo constant change to keep pace with the evolving and shifting values and public policies of our democratic society. The tort reform movement and the response by both courts and legislatures to the growth of managed care in the marketplace are of particular significance to the health care practitioner.

TRENDS IN NURSING PRACTICE AND HEALTH CARE MANAGEMENT

As the reader is all too well aware, the cost of health care has increased at an alarming rate over the past several decades and has outstripped the general rate of inflation. **Managed care,** in the form of health maintenance organizations (HMOs), preferred provider organizations (PPOs), and a myriad of other organizations, has been the marketplace's response to these spiraling costs. These health care provider systems seek to control costs and preserve profits in several nontraditional ways.

First, managed care systems attempt to monitor in detail their members' utilization of the resources available. Second, these systems integrate management decision-making and medical decision-making much more closely than has been done in the past. Third, these systems educate health care providers about utilization management and involve them in more closely monitoring and regulating utilization of resources. Some managed care entities have even tied the income of their health care providers to utilization goals. In 1996, Texas Supreme Court Justice Gonzalez wrote:

Recent developments in the health care industry have diffused the medical chain of authority for the sake of containing costs and increasing profits. For example, there are reports that in managed care systems like health maintenance organizations (HMOs), physicians are subjected to gag orders and are given financial incentives not to perform certain procedures or make referrals to outside specialists. Some HMOs hire bargain-rate labs and allow non-physicians to decide what is or is not appropriate treatment based solely on economic considerations, not on the best interests of the patient . . .Unless the Legislature acts in a comprehensive way to address this issue, courts will be forced to rethink traditional notions of duty and standards of care, leading to fundamental doctrinal shifts gauged both to protect victims of medical malpractice and to shield physicians from frivolous malpractice claims (*Jennings v. Burgess*, 1996, p. 796).

Finally, as part of their overall efforts to contain costs and deliver health care in as economic a fashion as possible, managed care organizations have expanded the use of advanced nurse practitioners and physician's assistants in the delivery of patient care. Practitioners in these settings work with an entirely new set of constraints unknown to their predecessors. Advanced nurse practitioners, sometimes referred to by managed care entities as physician extenders, must regularly balance their employer's charter of cost-efficient health care with the patient's needs as determined by their best nursing judgment.

LEGAL ISSUES AND GENERAL TRENDS

In the past, medical malpractice claims against managed care organizations that involved allegations that the malpractice was motivated in part by financial incentives often ended up in federal court. This is because despite the fact that medical negligence claims typically arise under the common law of the states, and thus are litigated in state court, allegations that are tantamount to claims of denial of benefits fall under the auspices of the Employee Retirement Income Security Act **(ERISA),** a federal law that preempts state law claims. Thus, in the past, a medical malpractice plaintiff who alleged "bad medicine due to financial incentives" would find the lawsuit removed from state court to federal court, and the state tort claims of medical negligence preempted. One Federal District Court judge wrote that the court had no choice but to "pluck [the] case out of state court . . . and then at the behest of Travelers, to slam the courthouse doors in [the wife's] face and leave her without any remedy" (*Andrews-Clark v. Travelers Insurance Co.*, 1997, p. 65). Judge Young further wrote, "ERISA has evolved into a shield of immunity that protects health insurers . . . from potential liability for the consequences of their wrongful denial of health benefits" (*Andrews-Clark v. Travelers Insurance Co.*, 1997, p. 65). Federal courts have begun to read ERISA much more narrowly and have consequently remanded many such actions to state court after declaring the state common law medical negligence claims not to be preempted by ERISA (*Martco Partnership v. Lincoln National Life Insurance Co.*, 1996).

In addition to this trend in judicial opinion, legislatures have begun to pass statutes aimed directly at managed care entities. In 1997, Texas was one of the first states to pass this type of legislation, which consisted of six managed care bills, the most significant being the HMO liability portion of Senate Bill 386 (Texas HMO Liability Bill, 1997). These statutes contain several novel provisions, including abolition of a defense traditionally used by corporate entities faced with allegations of medical negligence. In this situation, managed care organizations would make a motion to the court to throw out claims of medical negligence levied against it on the grounds that the managed care organizations were prevented by statute from practicing medicine, that is, the essence of their motion for summary judgment would be that because they were prevented by law from practicing medicine, they could not have committed medical negligence (*Williams v. Good Health Plan Plus, Inc.*, 1987). Under the new HMO statutes, this is no longer a defense. However, Aetna Insurance Company and its affiliated entities filed suit against the Texas Department of Insurance in June 1997 to obtain a declaratory judgment that the liability provisions of Senate Bill 386 are preempted by ERISA. But the judge presiding over the case ruled that the law is not preempted by ERISA (*Corporate Health Insurance, Inc. v. Texas Department of Insurance*, 1998).

On the national level, the president of the American Nurses Association, Beverly Malone, testified in April 1998 at a joint federal-state hearing on managed care reform and liability legislation (Hemlinger & Reed, 1998). In that testimony, she advocated that (1) nurses must be able to advocate for their patients without fear of retribution; (2) health care consumers have a right to full and comparable information about staffing and outcomes in health care institutions; and (3) consumers must have access to a full range of health care providers (Hemlinger & Reed 1998).

ETHICAL CONSIDERATIONS AND CONFLICTS

Ethics has been defined as the "rules or principles that govern right conduct" (*Dorland's Illustrated Medical Dictionary*, 1974). Not only are ethical decisions inherent in daily nursing practice, but they are also increasing almost as rapidly as medical technology progresses. When coupled with requirements imposed by law, a nurse often finds herself struggling with the question: What is the right thing to do?

As discussed previously, nurses face dilemmas involving such issues as right-to-die, abortion, genetic testing, HIV-infected health care workers, genetic research, euthanasia, organ transplantation, and intrauterine surgical intervention (see Chapter 4, Ethics in Nursing). Not uncommonly, these issues are

ultimately resolved in the courts. The advent of managed care organizations has opened the floodgates to even more complex ethical decisions. In the new environment of managed care, nurses find themselves delivering patient care while their employers look over their shoulder to see how cost efficiently they do so. This creates an ongoing ethical tension for the nurse, and sometimes gives rise to outright dilemmas.

The role of advance practice nursing is growing rapidly as a partial response to the need for more economical health care. At the same time, nurses must balance the increased use of **unlicensed assistive personnel (UAP)**. The American Nurses Association has defined UAP as an "unlicensed individual who is trained to function in an assistive role to the licensed registered nurse in the provision of patient/client care activities as delegated by the nurse" (American Nurses Association, 1992). Increasingly, licensed nurses are being replaced by lesser-trained UAPs who perform increasingly complex tasks while under the supervision of the nurse. This creates more opportunities for ethical issues to arise, as nurses delegate UAPs tasks that the nurse feels is appropriate given the UAP's training. However, should her or his judgment be in error, the nurse still retains accountability for the UAP's actions.

The professional nurse must balance the roles as an employee, nurse, and member of society who is required to comply with the law. A basic understanding of the judicial system and its legal terminology and workings will serve the nurse when working her or his way through the medicolegal scenarios that present themselves throughout each day.

POINTS TO REMEMBER

- American common law traces its roots to laws created by English judges during the 600 years after William of Normandy captured the throne.
- The four sources of law are (1) constitutions of the state and federal governments, (2) laws passed by state and federal legislatures, (3) common law, and (4) administrative rules legislation.

- The American people consent to be governed by the President, Congress, and the courts through the Constitution.
- The first 10 Amendments to the Constitution, known as the Bill of Rights, protect individual rights to freedom of religion, speech, and the press; to peaceful assembly; to keep and bear arms; and to be free from unreasonable search and seizure.
- Although no right to privacy is specifically expressed in the Constitution, it is a right recognized by the Supreme Court under the Fourth, Ninth, and Fourteenth Amendments.
- Under the rights to privacy and religious freedom, patients have a right to refuse medical treatment.
- There are three types of courts: trial, appellate, and supreme.
- The U.S. Supreme Court reviews only those actions of a state supreme court that involve rights and/or duties under the Constitution.
- In federal courts, the trial courts are the U.S. District Courts.
- Appeals from the U.S. District Courts are made to one of 13 U.S. Circuit Courts of Appeals.
- The judge determines issues of law.
- The jury decides issues of fact.
- Communications between attorney and client are privileged and cannot be disclosed unless (1) the client consents or (2) there is a showing that the communications were made to further a crime or fraud.

REFERENCES

American Bar Association. (1995). *ABA model rules of professional conduct*, New Providence, New Jersey: Martindale–Hubbell.

American Nurses Association. (1992). *ANA position statement: Registered nurse utilization of unlicensed assistive personnel* [On-line]. Available: www.nursing.org.com.

Andrews-Clark v. Travelers Insurance Co., 984 F. Supp. 49, 65 (D. Mass. 1997).

Annual report of the Director, Administrative Office of the United States Courts. (1984–1990). Washington, DC: U.S. Government Printing Office.

Application of the President & Directors of Georgetown College, Inc., 331 F.2d 1000, certiorari denied, 377 U.S. 978 (1964).

Appointment and Number of District Judges, 28 U.S.C. § 133 (1948).

Arkansas Long Arm Statute, Arkansas Code of 1987 Annotated 16-4-101 (Michie 1987).

Assignment of Budgets; Panels, Hearings; Quorum, 28 U.S.C. § 46 (1948).

Board of Nursing; Membership; Appointment; Terms, Florida Administrative Code Annotated, 59A-18.00 (1993).

Casey v. Cohen, 295 F. Supp. 561 (D.C. Va. 1968).

Commissioner of Corrections v. Myers, 399 N.E.2d 452 (Mass. 1979).

Communicable Disease Prevention and Control Act of 1983, Texas Health & Safety Code Annotated § 81.002 (Vernon's 1998).

Corporate Health Insurance, Inc. v. Texas Department of Insurance, 12 F.Supp.2d 597 (S.D. Tex. 1998).

Cox v. Administrator U.S. Steel & Carnegie, 17 F.3d 1386, 1422 (11th Cir. 1994).

Craig v. Boren, 429 U.S. 190 (1976).

Cruzan v. Director, Missouri Department of Health, 497 U.S. 261 (1990).

Dorland's illustrated medical dictionary (25th ed., p. 548). (1974). Philadelphia: WB Saunders.

Disciplinary Action, Idaho Code § 54-1412(a) (1977).

Federal Tort Claims Act of 1946, 28 U.S.C. §§ 1346, 1402 *et seq.*

Florida Board of Nursing, Florida Statutes Annotated § 464. 004 (West. Supp. 1998).

Florida Damage Statute, Florida Statutes Annotated § 766.209(4)(a) (1986).

General Provisions Governing Discovery: Duty of Disclosure, Federal Rule of Civil Procedure 26(b)(3) (West 1998).

Geesa v. State, 820 S.W.2d 154, 162 (Tex. Crim. App. 1991) (en banc).

Griffin v. California, 380 U.S. 609, 85 S.Ct.1229 (1965).

Griswold v. Connecticut, 381 U.S. 479, 486 (1965).

Grounds for Denial or Suspension of License or Certificate of Other Disciplinary Action, Nevada Revised Statutes Annotated, § 632.480 (Michie 1996).

Habeas Act of 1867, 28 U.S.C.§§ 2241–2255 (1997).

Hemlinger, C., & Reed, S. (1998). Managed care legislation: ANA testifies in federal-state hearing. *American Journal of Nursing*, 98(6), 16.

Hines v. Weinberger, 395 F.Supp. 1215 (D.C. Wyo. 1975).

Holmes v. Department of Professional Regulation, Board of Nursing, 504 So.2d 1338 (Fla. Dist. Ct. App. 1987).

Hospital Committee Privilege, Texas Health & Safety Code § 161.032(a) (1989).

Idaho Board of Nursing, Idaho Code § 54-1403 (1974).

Injunctions Against Violations of Chapter, Nevada Revised Statutes Annotated, § 632.320 (Michie 1995).

In re Brooks' Estate, 32 Ill.2d 361, 205 N.E.2d 435 (1965).

In re Burlington Northern, Inc., 822 F.2d 518, 524-25 (5th Cir. 1987).

In re Osborne, 294 A.2d 372 (U.S.App.D.C. 1972).

Kansas Administrative Regulations, 60-3-101 (1988).

Keeton, W.P., Dobbs, D.B., Keeton, R.E., & Owen, D.G. (1984). *Prosser and Keeton on the law of torts.* St. Paul, Minnesota: West.

LaFave, W.R., & Israel, J.H. (1985). *Criminal procedure.* St. Paul, Minnesota: West.

Lunsford v. Board of Nurse Examiners, 648 S.W.2d 391 (1983).

Mapp v. Ohio, 367 U.S. 643, 656 (1961).

Martco Partnership v. Lincoln National Life Insurance Co., 86 F.3d 459 (5th Cir. 1996).

Medical Liability and Insurance Improvement Act of Texas, Tex. Rev. Civ. Stat. Ann. Art. 4590i § 1301 (Vernon 1998).

Mercy Hospital, Inc. v. Jackson, 489 A.2d 1130 (Md. App. 1985), vacated on other grounds, 510 A.2d 562 (1986).

Minnesota v. Clover Leaf Creamery Co., 449 U.S. 456 (1981).

National Center for State Courts. (1991). *State court caseload statistics: Annual report.* Washington, DC: U.S. Government Printing Office.

Nursing Registries Standards and Licensing, Ferguson, J., & McHenry, D. (1973). *The American system of government* (12th ed., p. 431).

Oldham v. Schweiker, 660 F.2d 1078 (5th Cir. 1981).

Presumption of Innocence; Effect; Reasonable Doubt, California Penal Code § 1096 (West 1998).

Public Health Trust of Dade County v. Wons, 541 So.2d 96 (Fla. 1989).

Requirements for Licensure & Standards of Practice, Jennings v. Burgess, 917 S.W.2d 790, 796 (Tex. 1996).

Roe v. Wade, 410 U.S. 113, 153 (1973).

Staffel v. San Antonio School Board of Education, 201 S.W. 413 (Tex. Civ. App.-San Antonio 1918).

Superintendent of Belchertown State School v. Saikewicz, 370 N.E.2d 417 (Mass. 1977).

Summons. General Provisions Governing Discovery: Duty of Disclosure, Federal Rule of Civil Procedure 4(b) (West 1998).

Terrell State Hospital of the Texas Department of Mental Health and Mental Retardation v. Ashworth, 794 S.W.2d 937 (Tex.App.–Dallas 1990).

Texas Employers' Insurance Association v. McCaslin, 317 S.W.2d 916 (Tex. 1958).

Texas Examining Boards, 22 Tex. Admin. Code 211.2 (West Jan. 1, 1998).

Texas Exemplary Damages Statute of 1987, Tex. Civ. Prac. & Rem. Code § 41.008 (Vernon 1987 & Supp. 1998).

Texas General Venue Statute, Tex. Civ. Prac. & Rem. Code 15.002(a)(1)-(3) (Vernon 1997).

Texas HMO Liability Bill, Senate Bill 386 (1997).

Texas Long Arm Statute, Tex. Civ. Prac. & Rem. Code § 17.041-17.045 (Vernon 1985).

Tuma v. Board of Nursing, 593 P.2d 711 (Idaho 1979).

United States v. Clark, 445 U.S. 23 (1980).

Volkswagenwerk Aktiengesellschaft v. Schlunk, 486 U.S. 694, 700 (1988).

Williams v. Good Health Plan Plus, Inc.-Health America Corp. Of Texas, 743 S.W.2d 373 (Tex. App.–San Antonio 1987, no writ).

Wright, C.A. (1983). *The law of federal courts* (4th ed.). St. Paul, Minnesota: West.

Yick Wo v. Hopkins, 118 U.S. 351 (1886).

SUGGESTED READINGS

Texas Nurses Association (TNA). (1988). *The Texas APN: The resource guide for advanced practice.* Austin, TX: Author.

Werth, B. (1997). *Damages.* New York: McGraw-Hill.

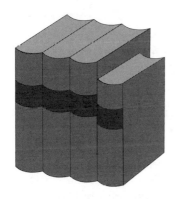

Chapter 2

LEGAL TERMINOLOGY

Leanna Marchand

OBJECTIVES

Upon completion of this chapter, the reader will be able to:
- Define legal terms that are commonly used in litigation involving health care providers.
- Identify the various claims that may be brought by the patient against a nurse.
- List the forms of discovery available to the patient and the nurse in civil litigation.

INTRODUCTION—
HISTORICAL PERSPECTIVE

Although the subject of legal terminology is as broad as an entire legal education, a nurse needs to be familiar primarily with terminology pertaining to the field of torts, of which medical malpractice is a small subset. The law of **torts** is "a body of law which is directed toward the compensation of individuals, rather than the public, for losses which they have suffered within the scope of their legally recognized interests generally, rather than one interest only, where the law considers that compensation is required" (Keeton, Dobbs, Keeton & Owen, 1984, p. 6). For example, someone involved in a car wreck can file a lawsuit against those he believes at fault in causing the accident, and through that lawsuit may seek compensation for, among other things, the damage to his car, his medical bills, and his lost wages. The person bringing such a lawsuit is called a **plaintiff**, and the person being sued is called a **defendant**. Early English common law recognized only two types of lawsuits between private individuals: trespass and trespass on the case (Keeton, Dobbs, Keeton & Owen, 1984).

Trespass, which dealt with criminal type behavior, was the remedy for "forcible, direct and immediate injuries, whether to persons or to property" and was available regardless of whether there were actual injuries (Keeton, Dobbs, Keeton & Owen, 1984, p. 29). Damage awards to plaintiffs were incidental to this type of action. The action of trespass on the case came along a bit later and grew out of the action of trespass. **Trespass on the case** provided redress for injuries that were not necessarily forcible, as was the case in trespass (Keeton, Dobbs, Keeton & Owen, 1984). Although it might seem that the two actions were distinguished by intentional and negligent conduct, the real difference lay in the connection between the act and the injury. The requirement in today's law of negligence—that injuries be foreseeable to be compensable—appears to have its roots in this core concept of the old action of trespass on the case.

Today, the field of torts encompasses a myriad of harms or wrongs. These include such intentional acts as **assault and battery,** negligent acts, which involve the breach of a duty such as to provide undue nursing care, and torts involving speech, such as **libel** and **slander**. Although lawsuits brought by someone to recover damages for injuries are generally brought in civil court, the same conduct can also be the basis of criminal charges if it constitutes what the law refers to as **wanton and willful conduct,** or if the conduct shows a reckless disregard for the rights, welfare, or safety of others. Most importantly, the law of torts is fluid, with courts and legislatures recognizing new causes of action and elements of damages, and abolishing long-standing ones, each year.

A patient's right to bring a tort action against a nurse, a doctor, or other health care provider has its roots in the common law, but the bounds of such actions, as well as the details of how they are litigated in the courts, are relatively well defined by laws passed by legislatures. It is essential that nurses have a basic understanding of these laws, under which they may someday be held accountable, as well as how they are applied and enforced in the courts. Although practitioners should leave the intricacies, nuances, and strategies of a malpractice claim to an attorney, they should nevertheless familiarize themselves with the basic terminology involved in a tort action. A nurse must understand that patient care is far removed from a written assignment in nursing school that has long since been graded and forgotten, that is, caring for the sick means assuming legal and ethical responsibilities by which a nurse may someday be judged. Thus, a nurse must be aware of the legal aspects of the profession, which are far broader than the medical malpractice claims that most nurses have read about in the newspapers. Legal issues confronting nurses include disciplinary actions, employment disputes, informed consent issues, intrastate licensure regulation, and telenursing, just to name a few. To understand these concepts, the nurse must first have a basic understanding of certain legal terminology.

BASIC LEGAL TERMINOLOGY

It would be a gross understatement to say that legal terminology can be confusing, incomprehensible, and even daunting to the nonlawyer, just as medical terminology is to the general public. However, legal jargon is the currency of lawyers and judges, and all nurses should be familiar with the words and phrases a lawyer may someday use to counsel them through a disciplinary proceeding, a medical malpractice case, or a criminal proceeding. Similarly, to help prevent malpractice, a hospital's risk manager will often use legal terminology to educate nurses about their legal duties and responsibilities.

The law touches on a wide range of possible nursing conduct, including obtaining a patient's informed consent to treatment, failing to render care that meets applicable standards, and acting in a manner that is intentionally harmful to the patient. Although there are numerous legal claims that may be brought against a nurse, the most prevalent claim is negligence. Once the reader has a basic understanding of the concept of negligence and how such claims are made in a medical malpractice case, she or he must then become familiar with some of the legal procedures lawyers use to litigate such a claim.

NEGLIGENCE AND NURSING MALPRACTICE

The **standard of conduct** in a negligence case is based on "what society demands generally of its members" (Keeton, Dobbs, Keeton & Owen, 1984, p. 169). Although the legal definition of **negligence** varies from state to state, it can generally be described as the failure to use ordinary care. **Ordinary care** is that degree of care that a reasonable and prudent person would exercise under the same or similar circumstances (*Palsgraf v. Long Island Railroad Co.*, 1928). Therefore, a person is negligent if he or she fails to do something that a reasonable and prudent person would do under the same or similar circumstances, or if he or she does something that a reasonable and prudent person would not do under the same or similar circumstances. Obviously, this definition can be used to judge almost any type of conduct, including that of motorists, landlords, manufacturers of consumer products, as well as doctors and nurses. Someone making a claim of negligence must prove (1) the existence of a legal duty, (2) breach of the duty, (3) causation, and (4) damages (Keeton, Dobbs, Keeton & Owen, 1984, p. 164).

Malpractice is professional negligence, and as such it is a subset of negligence. Specifically, malpractice is negligence committed by a person in his or her professional capacity, such as nurses, attorneys, accountants, and physicians. Medical malpractice differs from simple negligence in that it involves specialized medical skill and training not possessed by the average person (*Gilinsky v. Joseph Rosario Indelicato*, 1995, p. 90 [patient's absence of knowledge concerning consulting physician's identity is not a fatal flaw to the existence of a physician-patient relationship]; *Gould v. New York City*

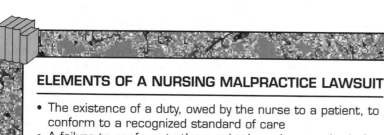

ELEMENTS OF A NURSING MALPRACTICE LAWSUIT

- The existence of a duty, owed by the nurse to a patient, to conform to a recognized standard of care
- A failure to conform to the required nursing standard of care
- Actual injury
- A reasonable close causal connection between the nurse's conduct and the patient's injury

Health and Hosp., 1985). **Medical malpractice** occurs when a doctor or nurse fails to do that which a reasonable, prudent doctor or nurse would do under the same or similar circumstances, or does that which a reasonable, prudent doctor or nurse would not do under the same or similar circumstances (*Byrd v. Hospital*, 1932; *Jernigan v. King*, 1993; *Laskowitz v. CIBA Vision Corp.*, 1995). To recover damages in a nursing malpractice action, the person making such a claim is required to prove:

1. The existence of a duty, owed by the nurse to a patient, to conform to a recognized standard of care
2. A failure to conform to the required standard of care
3. Actual injury
4. A reasonably close causal connection between the nurse's conduct and the patient's injury (*Complete Family Care v. Sprinkle*, 1994; *Poluski v. Richardson Transp.*, 1994, p. 713; *Tilotta v. Goodall*, 1988)

A plaintiff must prove these four elements by a **preponderance of the evidence**, that is, the plaintiff must prove that the defendant nurse's negligence, more likely than not, caused the plaintiff's injury. By contrast, in a criminal action the law requires the jury to find the defendant guilty beyond a reasonable doubt.

EXISTENCE OF A LEGAL DUTY

The duty a nurse owes to a patient arises from the **nurse-patient relationship.** A nurse owes no duty to a patient with whom she has not formed a nurse-patient relationship. Generally, a nurse must have performed some affirmative act to establish the relationship with a patient. Where the patient has not sought care and treatment from the nurse, the nurse does not owe a duty of care that would subject the nurse to liability. In *Clough v. Lively* (1989), the Georgia Court of Appeals held that an emergency room nurse's mere taking of a blood sample to obtain a blood alcohol level in compliance with an arresting police officer's written request did not constitute a nurse–patient

relationship. In *Weaver v. University of Michigan Board of Regents* (1993), the plaintiffs' child suffered from hydrocephalus. The child's pediatrician had told the parents to get a second opinion about a shunt that had been placed. The parents, following the pediatrician's advice, called a new doctor for an appointment and related to the clerical staff that the pediatrician did not think the condition was an emergency. When the new doctor saw the child about 2 weeks later, he scheduled the child for emergency surgery, but the child suffered permanent and nearly total loss of vision. The parents sued the new doctor for the delay in seeing the child, but the Michigan appellate court held that "a telephone call merely to schedule an appointment with a provider of medical services does not by itself establish a physician–patient relationship where the caller has no ongoing physician–patient relationship with the provider and does not seek or obtain medical advice during the conversation" (*Weaver v. University of Michigan Board of Regents*, 1993, p. 266).

Similarly, in *St. John v. Pope* (1995), a patient who had recently undergone back surgery and epidural injections presented to an emergency room with back pain, fever, and an elevated white blood cell count. The emergency room physician who examined the patient called the on-call physician, Dr. St. John, a board–certified internist, and recounted the presentation to him. Because he was not a neurologist or neurosurgeon, and the hospital was not equipped to handle those types of cases, Dr. St. John recommended that the patient be referred to a hospital that had those capabilities. However, for reasons that are unclear in the record, the receiving hospital refused to accept the patient. The patient's wife then took her husband home. The next day, the patient was transported by ambulance to another hospital where a lumbar puncture revealed the patient had meningitis.

The patient filed suit against the emergency room physician and the on-call physician, among others. Dr. St. John, the on-call physician, filed a motion asking that the claims against him be dismissed on the grounds that he owed no duty to the patient because he had not formed a physician–

patient relationship with the patient. The Texas Supreme Court agreed. Although the court said that a physician-patient relationship can be formed even where the physician does not deal directly with the patient, Dr. St. John did not form such a relationship because he had not agreed to examine or treat the patient. Rather, he listened to the presentation by the emergency room physician for the purpose of evaluating whether he should take the case, not to diagnose or prescribe treatment. The court, therefore, dismissed the claims against the on-call physician.

Although it is not necessary for nurse and patient to enter into a contract, or even for there to be direct contact between them, in order for a nurse-patient relationship to exist, it is the plaintiff's legal burden to show the existence of such a relationship. Generally, this may be done, thus establishing the existence of a legal duty owed by the nurse, by proving that the nurse was an employee of the hospital and that the plaintiff was a patient of the hospital. Whether or not a defendant nurse owed a legal duty to a plaintiff is an issue to be determined by the judge, not a jury.

BREACH OF THE LEGAL DUTY—FAILING TO MEET THE STANDARD OF CARE

Once the existence of a legal duty is established in a malpractice claim, the plaintiff must then prove that the nurse breached that duty. The plaintiff proves a **breach** by showing that the nurse's conduct fell below the applicable standard of nursing care, that is, the plaintiff must show that the nurse did not act as would a reasonable, prudent nurse under the same or similar circumstances (*Harris v. Groth*, 1983; Reasonable Prudent Health Care Provider, § 7.70.040). In particular, the plaintiff must show that the nurse did not exercise that degree of care, diligence, and skill that nurses of reasonable and ordinary prudence would have exercised under the same or similar circumstances. Obviously, then, the plaintiff must first establish the applicable standard of care required of a nurse under the circumstances

at issue (*Malooley v. McIntyre*, 1992; *Rodriguez v. Reeves*, 1987). In *Harrington v. Rush-Presbyterian-St. Luke's Hospital* (1990), the patient was voluntarily admitted to an inpatient detoxification program for her dependency on Darvocet. After several days in the program, the patient was found dead in her room from combined drug toxicity. The plaintiff, the deceased patient's husband, presented evidence of the standard of care required of a psychiatric nurse. The evidence showed that the nursing staff failed to document that the patient had collapsed in the bathroom, failed to notify the physician of a change in the patient's status, failed to check on the patient for more than 6 hours, and failed to give the patient her prescribed medication on two occasions.

Although a plaintiff may establish the standard of care in a number of ways, the law generally requires that he or she do so by expert testimony, because medical and nursing knowledge is not within the knowledge and experience of jurors. Without expert testimony, a plaintiff's claims may be dismissed. In *Vassey v. Burch* (1980), a claim against a hospital based on the conduct of one of its nurses was dismissed because the plaintiff failed to provide expert testimony at trial that stated either the accepted standard of nursing care for an emergency room nurse or whether the nurse violated that standard. Thus, parties to medical malpractice cases generally hire **experts** to serve as witnesses on their behalf. These witnesses must be qualified by reason of education, training, or experience to render expert opinions about a given subject (Testimony by Experts, 1998). They may, by virtue of their qualifications, provide testimony establishing what the standard of care is for a given set of clinical circumstances (*Poluski v. Richardson Transp.*, 1994). In *Belmon v. St. Francis Cabrini Hosp.* (1983), the Louisiana Court of Appeals held that an assistant professor of nursing at Northwestern University with a specialty in cardiovascular nursing in the intensive care area was qualified to render opinions about the nursing standard of care for a patient receiving heparin in an intensive care unit (ICU) setting. The nurse expert testified that the ICU nurse "failed to recognize and respond properly to the signs of hemorrhage in a heparinized patient . . . a nurse should be especially vigilant in monitoring a patient receiving a heavy dose of heparin. . ." (*Belmon v. St. Francis Cabrini Hosp.*, 1983, p. 545). She further testified that "the duty of care increases as the Prothrombin Time (PTT) value increases" (*Belmon v. St. Francis Cabrini Hosp.*, 1983, p. 545).

The **testifying expert** may also establish applicable standards by relying on the state's nurse practice act, the nurse's job description, the clinic or hospital's policies, procedures and protocols, standards and guidelines adopted by professional organizations, or textbooks taken by the witness as authoritative. Nursing organizations such as the American Nurses Association, Emergency Nurses Association, American Association of Nurse Anesthetists, and American Association of Critical Care Nurses, which formulate position statements and policies that they expect nurses to follow, are another source for establishing standards of care. For example, the Association of Women's Health, Obstetric and Neonatal Nurses (AWHONN) publishes *Standards & Guidelines for the Professional Nursing Practice in the Care of Women and Newborns* (AWHONN, 1998), which discusses a variety of guidelines such as breastfeeding support and resuscitation of the pregnant woman and newborn. Evidence of standards of appropriate care pertaining to such activities as charting, staffing, and patient observation can also be obtained from the Joint Commission on Accreditation of Healthcare Organizations (JCAHO), as well as in the **Code of Federal Regulations** (Sweeney, 1991), which establishes requirements for facilities receiving Medicare and Medicaid funding. In *Koeniguer v. Eckrich* (1988), for example, a nurse expert "[r]eferring to standards published by the American Nurses Association and various general nursing practice treatises" testified that in her opinion the defendant nurse's actions did not meet the standard of care for postoperative urologic patients (*Koeniguer v. Eckrich*, 1988, p. 602).

Although expert testimony is almost always required to establish the standard of care, there are situations where the situation itself provides the conclusion that the standard of care was not met. For example, where (1) the event is of a kind that ordinarily does not occur in the absence of negligence; (2) other responsible causes, including the conduct of the plaintiff and third persons, are sufficiently eliminated by the evidence; and (3) the indicated negligence is within the scope of the defendant's duty to plaintiff, then it may be inferred that the plaintiff's injuries were caused by the negligence of the defendant (Restatement (Second) of Torts § 328D, 1965). This type of claim is referred to as *res ipsa loquitur*, or "the thing speaks for itself" (*Ramage v. Central Ohio Emergency Serv., Inc.*, 1992). An example of such a situation would be when a surgeon removes a healthy lung instead of a diseased one.

Another situation where no expert testimony is required to establish the applicable standard of care is when the defendant's conduct violates some law that is designed to protect the class of persons of which the plaintiff is a member. This occurs, for example, where a student nurse administers anesthesia, in violation of a state statute, and injures the patient (*Central Anesthesia Assoc., P.C. v. Worthy*, 1985). This is called **negligence per se**. Yet another situation in which the plaintiff would not have to establish a standard of care by expert testimony is where the conduct at issue falls within the common knowledge and experience of jurors. For example, where a patient falls from a bed because the side rails are not raised, no expert testimony need be offered regarding a standard of care (Greenlaw, 1982).

Nevertheless, expert testimony is almost always required in medical malpractice cases, and practitioners are generally held to standards applicable to their area of specialty and level of qualifications. Thus, a nurse specialist or advanced nurse practitioner (ANP) will be held to the standard of care appropriate to persons of superior knowledge and skill (*Ewing v. Aubert*, 1988; *Fein v. Permanente Medical Group*, 1981). A nurse who performs a task generally performed by a physician will be required to exercise that degree of care, diligence, and skill that a physician of reasonable and ordinary prudence would exercise under the same or similar circumstances (*Thompson v. Brent*, 1971). In *Planned Parenthood of Northwest Indiana, Inc. v. Vines* (1989), the plaintiffs alleged that a nurse practitioner improperly inserted an intrauterine device (IUD). The Dean of the School of Nursing at Purdue University testified that the insertion of an IUD by a nurse practitioner required the same minimum standard of care applicable to IUD insertion by a physician.

Finally, the law requires expert testimony to establish in what way the conduct of the defendant doctors or nurses failed to meet that applicable standard of care (*Hiatt v. Groce*, 1974; *Northern Trust Co. v. Upjohn Co.*, 1991).

THE CAUSAL CONNECTION BETWEEN THE INJURY AND THE FAILURE TO MEET THE STANDARD OF CARE

Proving that a nurse has failed to meet the applicable standard of care is just one step in the process of proving a claim of nursing negligence. There must also be proof that such failure caused the patient to be injured, that is, someone claiming to be injured because of nursing negligence must show that the nurse's acts or omissions complained of actually resulted in their injuries. In *Jarvis v. St. Charles Medical Center* (1986), the physician ordered neurovascular checks every hour on a patient with a fractured leg because of potential compartment syndrome. Expert testimony showed that the failure of the nurses to perform neurovascu-

lar checks on the patient for more than 4 hours caused injury to the muscle tissue in the patient's leg.

The law in some states, in addition to this showing of **cause in fact**, requires a showing that the injuries complained of, or some similar injury, were a **foreseeable** consequence of the conduct complained of. This two-part showing of causation—namely, cause in fact and foreseeability—is referred to as **proximate cause** (*Dixon v. Taylor*, 1993). The nurse does not need to foresee events that are merely possible, but only those that are reasonably foreseeable (*Adams v. Mills*, 1984). Causation is often regarded as the most difficult element for the plaintiff to prove in a malpractice claim.

The plaintiff must also prove **damages** to recover in a malpractice claim. For example, if a nurse administers the wrong drug to a patient in violation of the standard of care but there are no adverse consequences or injury, then the plaintiff does not have a cause of action.

INTENTIONAL TORTS

Although most personal injury lawsuits are based primarily on claims of negligence, a person may also sue someone for intentionally injuring them. For example, a person who strikes someone may not only be charged with criminal assault, but he or she may also be sued by the injured person for money damages. Similarly, someone who kidnaps a person, or holds that person captive without legal justification, is not only

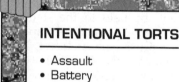

INTENTIONAL TORTS

- Assault
- Battery
- False imprisonment
- Intentional infliction of emotional distress

subject to criminal prosecution but can be sued for money damages as well. The obvious difference between this type of intentional conduct and negligence is the defendant's state of mind. Unlike the concept of failure to use ordinary care, as in a claim of negligence, intentional conduct is designed to bring about a particular result. The law, therefore, calls these acts **intentional torts**. Although the law varies considerably from state to state, there are four generally recognized intentional torts: assault, battery, false imprisonment, and intentional infliction of emotional distress.

ASSAULT AND BATTERY

When a person intentionally places another in apprehension or fear that they will suffer harmful or offensive contact, that person has committed an **assault** (Keeton, Dobbs, Keeton, & Owen, 1984). For example, it is an assault to shake a fist under someone's nose (*Stockwell v. Gee*, 1926). To constitute assault, it is essential that the plaintiff be aware of the threat of contact (*State v. Barry*, 1912). The law also recognizes the tort of **battery**, which is "harmful or offensive contact with a person, resulting from an act intended to cause the plaintiff or a third person to suffer such a contact, or apprehension that such a contact is imminent" (Keeton, Dobbs, Keeton, & Owen, 1984, p. 39). Put another way, a battery is intentional contact that is harmful or offensive, or creating the apprehension that such contact is imminent. It is no defense that the defendant did not intend a particular type of injury; rather, to be held liable, it is sufficient that the defendant intended only the act that resulted in the harmful or offensive contact (*Vosburg v. Putney*, 1981).

Health care providers are occasionally sued for assault and battery. For example, a patient may make such a claim against a nurse or doctor for performing a medical or surgical procedure without informed consent. This occasionally occurs where surgery is performed on the wrong patient, or where a surgeon removes a healthy kidney or lung, although intending to remove a diseased one. Nurses are occasionally sued for battery, although such claims usually arise in the context of an allegation of lack of informed consent. In *Schloendorff v. Society of New York Hospital* (1914), Justice Cardoza stated:

Every human being of adult years and sound mind has a right to determine what shall be done with his own body; and a surgeon who performs an operation without his patient's consent commits an assault, for which he is liable in damages. This is true except in cases of emergency where the patient is unconscious and where it is necessary to operate before consent can be obtained (p. 93).

A patient has also sued a male nurse for seeing and touching her naked body when she had communicated to the hospital her religious opposition to such conduct (*Coehen v. Smith*, 1995). Nursing home and mental health patients have also brought suits for assault and battery against their health care providers.

FALSE IMPRISONMENT

False imprisonment consists of willful detention, without consent and without authority of law (Keeton, Dobbs, Keeton, & Owen, 1984, p. 49). If someone is arrested or detained with the permission of a court that has proper authority, such as pursuant to an **arrest warrant**, there is no action for false imprisonment (*James v. Brown*, 1982). Although claims of false imprisonment arise infrequently in the area of health care claims, doctors and nurses do occasionally find themselves defending such allegations, especially where mental health or nursing home patients are involved (*Cook v. Highland Hospital*, 1915; *Lord v. Clayton*, 1940). The practitioner should be aware that there may be liability for false imprisonment even though he or she believes in good faith that he or she was acting for the patient's own good (*Maxwell v. Maxwell*, 1920). In *Marcus v. Liebman* (1978), the plaintiff contended that her psychiatrist falsely imprisoned her on a psychiatric ward. Although she had voluntarily committed herself to the ward, she alleged she was falsely imprisoned because her psychiatrist threatened to transfer her involuntarily to a state hospital if she were to check herself out of the hospital.

INTENTIONAL INFLICTION OF EMOTIONAL DISTRESS

The law also recognizes a cause of action for what is called **intentional infliction of emotional distress** (*Labrier v. Anheuser Ford, Inc.*, 1981; Restatement (Second) of Torts, 1965). As its name implies, this cause of action permits a plaintiff to sue someone who has intentionally caused that person to suffer emotional distress. But what constitutes legally cognizable emotional distress? And what type of conduct is society willing to deem sufficiently objectionable so as to give rise to the right to bring such an action? Is an insult sufficient, or must the offensive behavior be truly outrageous? And must a plaintiff's emotional suffering be so severe that he or she develops physical symptoms before the law will permit him or her to bring such a claim? The law has grappled with these and other questions in connection with this particular cause of action, and the answers are as diverse as the states (Keeton, Dobbs, Keeton, & Owen, 1984). Generally, the defendant must have engaged in outrageous conduct that inflicts emotional distress on the plaintiff (Restatement (Second) of Torts § 46, 1965). Unfortunately, there are a number of cases involving the handling of dead bodies. For example, in *Johnson v. Woman's Hospital* (1975), a woman returned to the hospital 6 weeks after the loss of her stillborn child to inquire about the disposition of the child's body. A hospital employee presented the mother with a jar of formaldehyde containing the body of the child. The Tennessee appellate court held that sufficient evidence existed such that a jury could find that the employee's actions constituted outrageous conduct.

Conversely, in *C.M. v. Tomball Regional Hospital* (1997), the nurse allegedly treated a 15-year-old rape victim and her mother "like dirt, and told them 'we do not like to deal with rape victims' " (*C.M. v. Tomball Regional Hospital*, 1997, p. 244). The nurse also allegedly implied the victim may have lost her virginity and sustained her physical injuries from something other than rape or sex. The plaintiffs sued the nurse claiming intentional infliction of emotional distress; but the court held that, although rude, insensitive, and uncaring, the remarks did not rise to the level of intentional infliction.

In *Boney v. Mother Frances Hospital* (1994), a plaintiff alleged that overhearing a nurse's conversation with another patient regarding the complications that arise from anesthesia, namely that some patients die, constituted the intentional infliction of emotional distress. The plaintiff alleged the conversation should have been held in a private room out of earshot. But the court upheld dismissal of the plaintiff's claim because there was no evidence that the remark was intentionally made such that the plaintiff would hear it. Without evidence of intent, there is no cause of action for intentional infliction of emotional distress.

QUASI-INTENTIONAL TORTS

In addition to negligence and intentional torts, the law recognizes a family of torts involving speech. These torts are called **quasi-intentional torts**, where the word *quasi* means "resembling," because they are based on speech that, although harmful, may not be intentional in the same sense that assault and battery are. Because nurses write texts, journal articles, and editorials; speak in public; and take on roles in the political arena, they should be familiar with this area of the law.

DEFAMATION

Defamation is a communication that "tends to hold the plaintiff up to hatred, contempt or ridicule, or to cause him to be shunned or avoided" (Keeton, Dobbs, Keeton, & Owen, 1984, § 111; citing *Kimmerle v. New York Evening Journal*, 1933). Defamation has also been defined as "a communication [that] tends so to harm the reputation of another as to lower him in the estimation of the community or to deter third persons from associating or dealing with him" (Keeton,

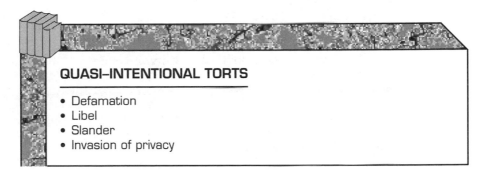

QUASI–INTENTIONAL TORTS

- Defamation
- Libel
- Slander
- Invasion of privacy

Dobbs, Keeton, & Owen, 1984). A person may sue someone who makes false statements about him or her, either orally or in writing, if those statements are made to a third person and are harmful. If the statements are made orally, the legal claim is one for slander; and if the statements are in writing, the claim is called libel.

To be held accountable for the tort of libel, a plaintiff must show that the defendant published a defamatory statement about the plaintiff. Obviously, a defendant may not have intended to communicate a given statement to anyone; she or he may not have intended the statement to be defamatory; the statement may be inoffensive on its face, but may still be defamatory when taken together with facts unknown to the person who made it; the defendant may not have intended the statement to be about the plaintiff at all; or she or he may reasonably have believed the statement to be true. In the first instance, where the defendant did not intend to publish the statement, the law will not impose liability (*Olson v. Molland*, 1930; *Weidman v. Ketcham*, 1938). However, where the defendant's fault with respect to the truth or falsity of the statement is at issue, the law has developed a myriad of rules and balancing tests that vary from situation to situation and from state to state.

The U.S. Supreme Court began to give some definite structure to this area of the law beginning in 1964 with its opinion in *New York Times v. Sullivan*. This was the first in a series of opinions by the high court that defined special protection for people using mass media to disseminate information to the general public. In particular, the Supreme Court developed different rules to be fol-

lowed in defamation actions involving "private" plaintiffs as opposed to those involving "public" plaintiffs. If a plaintiff in a defamation action is a public figure, there is a higher standard of proof than for a plaintiff who is not a public figure. Similarly, a defendant in a defamation case who is a member of the press will enjoy more legal protections for her or his speech than will such a defendant who is not a member of the press.

In particular, the U.S. Supreme Court has held that a plaintiff's status as a **public figure** applies only to someone who has assumed a role of importance in the resolution of specific public affairs or affairs of general importance to the public (*Gertz v. Robert Welch, Inc.*, 1974), that is, there are people who the law recognizes as public figures for all purposes, because they have achieved such pervasive fame or notoriety; and there are people who the law recognizes are public figures for a limited range of issues, because they have voluntarily injected themselves, or have been drawn, into a particular public controversy (*Gertz v. Robert Welch, Inc.*, 1974). Where a defendant can show that the plaintiff is a public figure with respect to the allegedly defamatory statement the defendant made about the plaintiff, the plaintiff must prove by clear and convincing evidence that the defendant made the statement knowing that it was false or with reckless disregard to the statement's truth or falsity (*New York Times v. Sullivan*, 1964).

Also, the defendant in a defamation action can always claim that the statements made were true. Such a defendant may also be able to claim absolute immunity for statements made during the course of judicial proceedings (*Ginger v. Bowles*, 1963), legislative proceedings (*Cochran v. Cousins*, 1930), executive communications (*Hackworth v. Larson*, 1969), and certain political broadcasts (*Farmers Educational and Co-Op Union of America, North Dakota Division v. WDAY, Inc.*, 1959).

In *Cohen v. Advanced Medical Group of Georgia, Inc.* (1998), Dr. Cohen was accused of communicating false information to patients of Advanced Medical Group (AMG), with which Dr. Cohen had previously been affiliated. A Georgia trial court ordered Dr. Cohen not to communicate false information about AMG to its patients, but Dr. Cohen, arguing that he had a right of free speech, appealed the order. The Georgia Supreme Court reversed the trial court and found that AMG failed to show it would be irreparably harmed by Dr. Cohen's statements so as to justify an injunction that violated Dr. Cohen's right of free speech.

INVASION OF PRIVACY

The law also recognizes a cause of action for **invasion of privacy**, which can take one or more of three basic forms. The first of these occurs when the defendant, for his or her own benefit, appropriates the plaintiff's name or likeness (*Carlisle v. Fawcett Publication, Inc.*, 1962). In the second form of invasion of privacy, the defendant makes an unreasonable and extremely offensive intrusion upon the plaintiff or his or her personal affairs (Restatement (Second) of Torts, 1965). In the third type of invasion of privacy, the defendant places the plaintiff in a false light in the public eye (*Martin v. Johnson Publishing Company*, 1956). Patient information is generally considered to be personal and confidential, and its disclosure could subject the person doing so to a claim of invasion of privacy (*Hammonds v. Aetna Casualty & Surety Company*, 1965; *McCormick v. England*, 1997). For example, Alabama law permits a patient to sue his or her doctor for invasion of privacy if the doctor, against the patient's express instructions, discloses confidential information about the patient to the patient's employer (*Horne v. Patton*, 1973).

In addition to a claim of invasion of privacy, many states have recognized a cause of action against a physician for breach of a duty of confidence that he or she owes to a patient. If a health care provider discloses confidential patient information to some third person without the patient's consent, the courts will permit the patient to bring suit (*Hague v. Williams*, 1962; *McCormick v. England*, 1997). For example, where a woman's psychiatrist, in the course of a child custody dispute with her former husband, delivered a detailed affidavit regarding her mental health status to her former husband's attorney, the court held that the woman could maintain an action against the psychiatrist for breach of a statutory duty of confidentiality (*Schaffer v. Spicer*, 1974). Maryland has held it to be a violation of confidentiality pursuant to its Medical Records Act for a physician to obtain another physician's patient's records for use in an unrelated medical malpractice action (*Warner v. Lerner*, 1998). In *Warner v. Lerner* (1998), Dr. Lerner and Dr. Schirmer were both urologists who were treating the same patient. That patient sued Dr. Lerner for malpractice and retained Dr. Schirmer as an expert witness against Dr. Lerner. Dr. Lerner then obtained, without consent, confidential information about one of Dr. Schirmer's other patients who was not involved in the litigation. Dr. Lerner used this confidential information about Dr. Schirmer's other patient to discredit Dr. Schirmer as an expert witness. That other patient then sued Dr. Lerner for breach of the state's confidentiality statute. The Maryland Court of Appeals held that Dr. Lerner had no authority under state statute to obtain and disclose the other patient's confidential medical records.

This area of confidentiality of patient information has received much legislative attention in recent years in the area of patients' human immunodeficiency virus (HIV) status. For example, an Alabama statute requires physicians, dentists, and certain other persons to report cases or suspected cases of notifiable diseases and health conditions, such as HIV infections and acquired immunodeficiency syndrome (AIDS) cases, to the Alabama State Board of

Health (Health, Mental Health, and Environmental Control Reporting Notifiable Diseases, 1975). Although this statute was challenged on constitutional grounds by an infectious disease physician who refused to disclose the names and addresses of his patients with HIV and AIDS to the Board of Health, the Alabama Supreme Court nevertheless found the provisions not to constitute an impermissible invasion of privacy and not to be violative of equal protection (*Middlebrooks v. State Board of Health*, 1998).

Similarly, the Texas legislature has passed a law that permits release of test results to a spouse "if the person tests positive for AIDS or HIV infection, antibodies to HIV, or infection with any other probable causative agent of AIDS" (Communicable Disease Prevention and Control Act, 1989). In *Santa Rosa Health Care Corp. v. Garcia*, 1998, the wife of a hemophiliac who was HIV positive sued a health care provider for negligently failing to notify her that her husband might be HIV positive. Although the case turned on the wording of the statute and the question of when the patient actually tested positive for the virus, the court held that the health care provider had no statutory or common-law duty to notify the patient's wife that her husband might be infected because the husband was not tested. As these cases so clearly demonstrate, the practitioner must be familiar with the law in her or his state regarding confidentiality and disclosure of patient information, particularly where that information concerns mental health or HIV status.

LITIGATION AND THE DISCOVERY PROCESS

After a lawsuit has been filed, and the defendants have been served with a copy of the lawsuit, which is referred to in various jurisdictions as a **petition** or a **complaint,** the plaintiff and the defendants may request information from each other, or from people or businesses who, although not involved in the lawsuit, may have knowledge of facts pertaining to the allegations made. This process is called **discovery.** Discovery serves many purposes in the litigation process, such as to avoid surprise and to clarify the issues so that each party may prepare for trial.

INTERROGATORIES

These requests for information take several forms, one of which is a list of questions, called **interrogatories**, which usually seek general information about the opposing party and their claims or defenses. For example, a plaintiff may ask a defendant questions about his or her insurance coverage, employment status, and relationships, as well as questions about the defendant's experts who will testify in the case. A defendant, on the other hand, may ask a plaintiff about his or her marriage, children, residence and work history, prior medical conditions, and the plaintiff's experts who will testify at trial. Interrogatories must be answered in writing and under oath. In

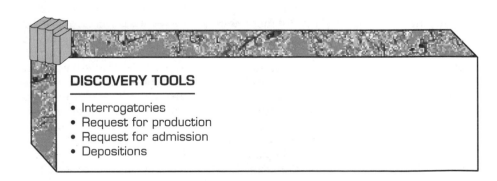

DISCOVERY TOOLS

- Interrogatories
- Request for production
- Request for admission
- Depositions

federal court, certain information, such as information about expert witnesses, must be voluntarily disclosed without the need for a discovery request (Required Disclosures; Methods to Discover Additional Matter, 1998).

REQUESTS FOR PRODUCTION

Parties to a lawsuit can also send opposing parties requests for documents and other tangible items, called **requests for production**. If served with a proper request, parties must disclose all documents and tangible items within their possession, custody, or control that are relevant to the facts of the case. Plaintiffs may want copies of a hospital's protocols, bylaws, work schedules, and employment records for the doctors or nurses who rendered care to the plaintiff. Defendants might ask plaintiffs for their personnel file from work, records from prior workers' compensation claims, prior medical records, and diaries or notes made about the events giving rise to the lawsuit.

REQUESTS FOR ADMISSION

In addition to interrogatories and requests for production, parties to a lawsuit may also send one another a list of requests that the opposing party admit or deny the truth of certain statements of fact. This discovery tool, called **requests for admission**, is typically used later in the discovery process to narrow the issues over which there remains a dispute. For example, a plaintiff might request a defendant hospital to admit or deny that a particular nurse was acting within the course and scope of her employment with the hospital at the time she rendered health care to the plaintiff.

Additionally, a party may be required to submit to a physical or mental examination if the physical or mental condition of the party is in controversy. This form of discovery requires a court order. In an obstetrical malpractice case, for example, the defendant may request an examination of the baby by a defense expert to determine the severity of the baby's brain damage. In federal court there is not an absolute right to have the person examined by a physician of the requesting party's choice. However, unless the person to be examined has a valid objection to the selected physician, the examination should be conducted by a physician identified by the requesting party.

DEPOSITIONS

Parties to a lawsuit can also take sworn testimony from other parties, or from nonparties who have knowledge of facts pertaining to the case. This type of sworn testimony, which is taken somewhere other than the courtroom, is referred to as a **deposition**. Typically, an attorney for one of the parties will issue a notice of deposition in which he or she informs all the attorneys involved in the case that he or she intends to take the deposition of a given party or witness. The notice specifies where and when the deposition will take place, and it identifies anyone who will attend the deposition other than the parties, the attorneys, and the witness. The depositions of the parties are usually taken in their attorneys' offices, but depositions of fact witnesses and experts may be taken anywhere and at any time that is reasonable (Required Disclosures; Methods to Discover Additional Matter, 1998). Medical experts may give their depositions in their office, a conference room in the clinic where they work, in an attorney's office, or any other convenient location. Depositions may be taken in a hospital room, someone's home, or in any other place that the attorney noticing the deposition desires, as long as it is reasonable. When an attorney issues a notice of deposition for a party to the lawsuit, that notice carries the force and effect of a subpoena (*Monks v. Marlinga*, 1991). However, if an attorney wishes to depose someone who is not a party to the lawsuit, the only way he or she can truly compel the appearance of that person for deposition is to have that person served with a **subpoena** (*Westmoreland v. CBS, Inc.*, 1985). Deposition notices and subpoenas may also contain a list of items that the deponent is to bring with him to the deposition. Such a list is called a *duces tecum*.

At a deposition, the witness is sworn in by a **court reporter,** who is there to transcribe all that is said during the course of the deposition. The attorney who issued the notice of deposition begins the examination of the witness, and when she or he is through with initial questioning, permits the other attorneys in the case to also examine the witness. When the other attorneys have finished their questioning, the initial attorney may ask more questions, as may the other attorneys; and the process continues in this fashion until all attorneys have taken all the testimony they desire at that time. During the course of the deposition, attorneys may make objections to either a question posed, or an answer given. Under the Federal Rules of Civil Procedure, an attorney may object only to the form of the question or the responsiveness of the answer. For example, an attorney may object that a question assumes facts not in evidence, mischaracterizes prior testimony, or is vague and ambiguous. Likewise, an answer may not be responsive to the question posed and, therefore, may also draw an objection. When the transcript of the deposition is prepared, the witness has an opportunity to review it and make changes.

During a deposition, an attorney may ask the witness about any subject as long as the question appears reasonably calculated to lead to the discovery of admissible evidence (Required Disclosures; Methods to Discover Additional Matter, 1998). In the case of a nurse or physician, an attorney will typically spend some time reviewing the person's background, education, training, and experience. The attorney will also want to learn the witness's version of the chronology of events surrounding the incident at issue in the lawsuit. In this regard, deposition examination can become extremely detailed and at times repetitive, because the attorney will not only be attempting to learn as much about the facts and circumstances of the health care at issue, but will also be attempting to pin the witness down to a specific version of events. This will necessarily include going over all conversations the nurse had with doctors, other nurses, and family members during the period at issue.

The attorney will also want to discuss at length the witness's assessment of the patient, her or his nursing diagnosis and care plan, and the basis for those decisions (i.e., use of the nursing process). The witness will also have to discuss when and how she or he instituted certain interventions and will have to explain the basis for doing so. She or he will also likely have to explain why she or he did not intervene in certain respects. One of the most important areas touched on in depositions is the nurse-witness's knowledge of the policies, procedures, and protocols of the institution where she or he practices. Although most nurses are well versed in the practices used at their hospital or clinic, they all too often are unfamiliar with the specific contents of the official practices and procedures promulgated and printed by the hospital or clinic. The witness may also be examined regarding knowledge of the state's nurse practice act.

Although an attorney may examine the witness regarding any matter that appears reasonably calculated to lead to the discovery of admissible evidence, this broad latitude is not absolute, as there are certain subjects that are off limits. For example, communications between an attorney and client are confidential and not subject to disclosure. Likewise, communications made between a husband and wife that are intended to be confidential, or to a member of the clergy, may not be disclosed. An attorney's thought processes, mental opinions, and impressions, commonly referred to as **attorney work product**, are also exempt from disclosure. The work product of, or an attorney's communication with, **consulting expert** retained purely for consultation and who will not testify at trial, is not subject to disclosure. And under federal law, a medical staff or hospital review committee's inquiries regarding an armed forces patient are protected from discovery (*In re United States of America*, 1989; *Maynard v. United States*, 1990). The foregoing types of information, although not an exclusive list, all are examples of what the law calls **privileged**

information. If an attorney asks a witness a question that calls for disclosure of privileged information, the witness's attorney may object to the question on that grounds and may instruct the witness not to answer. If the witness does not have an attorney, the witness may do so herself or himself. However, because the purpose of discovery is to seek the truth, a party or witness resisting discovery, by way of objection and refusal to answer, may later be required to prove to the court the existence and applicability of a particular privilege. This is usually done only when the party asking the question files a motion seeking to have the court compel the witness to answer further. In that situation, the witness must prove the existence of the privilege either by affidavit or by further testimony at a hearing.

Depositions are used by attorneys in several ways. As already discussed, they help the parties develop the evidence needed to prosecute or defend their case. At time of trial, should the witness testify in a manner that is inconsistent with his or her prior deposition testimony, an attorney may **impeach** his or her credibility by confronting the witness with that inconsistency. If a witness is unavailable to testify live at trial, either part or all of his or her deposition may be read to the jury. If the deposition was recorded on videotape, that tape may be played to the jury. As part of their efforts to get a case settled short of trial, attorneys often prepare videotapes that in essence tell the plaintiff's story in summary fashion. These tapes may include segments depicting a day in the life of the plaintiff both before and after he or she was injured, may show enlarged and highlighted versions of important medical records or documents in the case, and commonly include excerpts from videotaped depositions in which defendant doctors, nurses, or other health care providers give testimony favorable to the plaintiff's case.

STATUTES OF LIMITATIONS

As one might expect, the law does not allow someone to take forever to bring a lawsuit, and each state has its own **statutes of limitations**, which specify how long a plaintiff has to bring a particular cause of action. Personal injury plaintiffs typically have 1, 2, or 3 years from the date of injury to file a legal claim, whereas disputes over contracts or real estate may be brought as late as 4 or 15 years after the dispute arises, respectively. The obvious purpose of such laws is to avoid unfair and unduly costly situations that may arise when a lawsuit is brought so long after the injury that evidence has been lost or altered and memories have faded. Such laws also allow individuals and businesses to make plans for the future, including evaluating their needs to carry liability insurance. Because the law provides that these statutes of limitations begin to run when the injury occurs, there is a vast amount of litigation regarding just what constitutes the injury and when the injury actually occurred. This is especially true in medical malpractice cases.

As with such general personal injury cases as car wrecks, the date of negligence in some medical malpractice cases can be clearly determined. However, quite often a patient does not discover the possible malpractice until well after the applicable statute of limitations has run out. For example, if a surgeon leaves a sponge in a patient or fails to diagnose the patient's cancer, it may be years before the patient discovers his or her potential claim against the provider. Although the law has at times been harsh to such plaintiffs in dismissing their cases for not being timely brought (*Shearin v. Lloyd*, 1957), many courts have adopted what is referred to as the **discovery rule**. Under this rule, a statute of limitations will begin to run only when the plaintiff actually discovers, or in the exercise of ordinary care should reasonably have discovered, his or her injuries (*Schiele v. Hobart Corp.*, 1978). The discovery rule typically will apply not just to medical malpractice cases but to personal injury claims in general. But medical negligence claims often involve what is described as a **continuing tort**, as where a patient continues under a physician's care for an extended period of time, but the physician nevertheless negligently fails to detect the patient's illness.

Texas, for example, provides that a medical malpractice plaintiff must file his or her lawsuit within 2 years of the date of the occurrence of the negligence, or the date of completion of the medical or health care treatment or hospitalization made the basis of the claim (Texas Medical Liability & Insurance Improvement Act, 1997). However, the statute is **tolled,** or suspended, for 75 days when the plaintiff notifies the potential defendants of intent to file a health care claim under the statute. Although some states have adopted the discovery rule legislatively, medical malpractice plaintiffs in Texas wishing to invoke such a rule must turn to what is known as the **open courts provision** of their state's constitution (Texas Constitution, Art.1 § 13). This provision precludes the Texas legislature from passing legislation that would cut off claims and causes of action that had been available to Texas citizens as common law. Because medical negligence plaintiffs in Texas had been able under the common law to file suit even though they had discovered their injuries and the defendant's potential negligence after the applicable statute of limitations had run out, such plaintiffs still have that right, notwithstanding statutes that would otherwise bar their claims (*Hellman v. Mateo*, 1989; *Neagle v. Nelson*, 1985).

Minors and incompetent individuals who would be plaintiffs in personal injury actions present special problems in applying statutes of limitation. Because most states consider minors and incompetent individuals not to have legal capacity to bring suit, the law in most states provides that statutes of limitation are tolled during a would-be plaintiff's period of **legal incapacity,** that is, statutes of limitation generally do not run against a child until he or she turns 18, nor do they run against an incompetent person (Limitations of Personal Actions, 1987). The specific rules on when and how these tolling provisions operate vary widely from state to state, and their interpretation is best left to legal counsel. Although these tolling provisions can permit minors and incompetent individuals to bring suit many years after an alleged negligent act, the provisions have been almost universally held constitutional.

On the other hand, the common law of many states also recognizes a legal argument that proposes it would be unfair to permit certain claims to go forward if it has been so long since the act that evidence has been lost, memories have faded, and the defendant would be unduly prejudiced by such a claim. This legal doctrine, which can operate to bar a lawsuit even though the applicable statute of limitations has not run out because the plaintiff was a minor or was incompetent, is referred to as *laches* (*National Association of Government Employees v. City Public Service Board*, 1994). However, application of this doctrine is rare.

ISSUES AND TRENDS

As the scope of nursing practice expands, so will the scope of liability. For example, advanced practice nurses in most states now have limited prescriptive authority. This limited authority to prescribe medications carries with it liability once held only by physicians. Similarly, nurse practitioners in various practice areas are expanding their scope of practice, and physician oversight is decreasing. The trend toward autonomy leaves many questions unanswered. How will advanced nurse practitioners be compensated? How much oversight will be required, if any, by physicians?

POINTS TO REMEMBER

- Torts are the body of law directed toward compensation of individuals for losses suffered to legally recognized interests.
- The field of torts encompasses the following actions (1) intentional acts such as assault and battery or false imprisonment, (2) negligent acts, and (3) quasi-intentional acts such as defamation, invasion of privacy, and breach of confidentiality.
- Conduct that is the basis of a civil claim may also be the basis of a criminal charge.
- Elements of negligence include (1) a legal duty, (2) breach of that duty, (3) causation, and (4) damages.

- The duty to the patient arises within the nurse-patient relationship.
- A breach of a legal duty occurs when the nurse fails to meet the standard of care as identified in (1) the state's nurse practice act, (2) job description, (3) policies and procedures, (4) professional standards, and/or (5) treatises.
- Expert testimony is almost always required to establish the standard of nursing care.
- Expert testimony is not required in the following instances: (1) *res ipsa loquitur*, (2) negligence per se, and (3) conduct that falls within the common knowledge of the jurors.
- Nurse specialists are held to a standard of care appropriate to nurses with advanced knowledge and experience.
- To prove proximate cause, evidence must be provided of (1) cause in fact and (2) foreseeability.
- Intentional torts include (1) assault, (2) battery, (3) false imprisonment, and (4) intentional infliction of emotional distress.
- Quasi-intentional torts involve (1) defamation and (2) invasion of privacy.
- An action for invasion of privacy may also include an action for breach of a duty of confidentiality.
- Forms of discovery include (1) interrogatories, (2) requests for production, (3) requests for admission, and (4) depositions.
- During the deposition of a health care provider, questions usually relate to (1) background, education, training and experience; (2) chronology of events relevant to the case; (3) use of the nursing process; (4) any failure to act; (5) policies, procedures, and protocols of the employing institution; and (6) knowledge of the state's nurse practice act.
- Communications that are privileged include (1) attorney-client, (2) husband-wife, (3) clergy-parishioner, and (4) attorney-consulting expert.
- The statute of limitations begins to run in a medical malpractice case in three instances (1) the date the injury occurred, (2) the date injury was discovered or reasonably should have been discovered, or (3) in the case of a minor, after the child turns 18.

REFERENCES

Actions for Injuries Resulting from Health Care, Reasonable Prudent Health Care Provider, West's Revised Code Wash. Ann. § 7.70.040.

Adams v. Mills, 312 N.E. 181, 322 S.E.2d 164, 172 (1984).

Association of Women's Health, Obstetric and Neonatal Nurses (AWHONN). (1998). *Standards & guidelines for the professional nursing practice in the care of women and newborns* (5th ed.). Washington, DC: Author.

Belmon v. St. Francis Cabrini Hosp., 427 So.2d 544 (La. Ct. App. 1983).

Boney v. Mother Frances Hospital, 880 S.W.2d 140 (Tex. App.—Tyler 1994, writ refused).

Byrd v. Hospital, 202 N.C. 337, 162 S.E. 738 (1932).

Carlisle v. Fawcett Publication, Inc., 201 Cal.App.2d 233 (1962).

Central Anesthesia Assoc. P.C. v. Worthy, 333 S.E.2d 829 (Ga. 1985).

Cochran v. Cousins, 42 F.2d 783 (D.D.C.), certiorari denied, 282 U.S. 874 (1930).

Clough v. Lively, 387 S.E.2d 573, 574 (Ga. Ct. App. 1989).

Coehen v. Smith, 648 N.E.2d (Ill.App.Ct. 1995).

Cohen v. Advanced Medical Group of Georgia, Inc., 496 S.E.2d 710 (Ga. Mar 9, 1998).

Communicable Disease Prevention and Control Act, 1983, Texas Health & Safety Code, § 81.103 (1989).

Complete Family Care v. Sprinkle, 638 So.2d 774, 777 (Ala. 1994).

Cook v. Highland Hospital, 84 S.E. 352 (N.C. 1915).

C.M. v. Tomball Regional Hospital, 961 S.W.2d 236 (Tex. App.–Houston [1st Dist.] 1997).

Dixon v. Taylor, 111 N.C. App. 97, 431 S.E.2d 778 (1993).

Ewing v. Aubert, 532 So. 2d 876 (La.Ct.App. 1988).

Farmers Educational and Co-Op Union of America, North Dakota Division v. WDAY, Inc., 360 U.S. 525 (1959).

Fein v. Permanente Medical Group, 121 Cal.App.3d 135, 175 Cal.Rpt. 177 (1981).

Gertz v. Robert Welch, Inc., 418 U.S. 323 (1974).

Gilinsky v. Joseph Rosario Indelicato, D.C 894 F.Supp. 86, 90, 93 (E.D. N.Y. 1995).

Ginger v. Bowles, 120 N.W.2d 842 (Mich.), certiorari denied, 375 U.S. 856 (1963).

Gould v. New York City Health and Hosp., 490 N.Y.S.2d 87, 89 (N.Y. Sup. Ct. 1985).

Greenlaw, J. (1982, June). Failure to use siderails: When is it negligence? *Law, Medicine & Health Care, 10,* 125-128.

Hackworth v. Larson, 165 N.W.2d 705 (S.D. 1969).

Hague v. Williams, 181 A.2d 345 (N.J. 1962).

Hammonds v. Aetna Casualty & Surety Company, 243 F.Supp. 793 (N.D. Ohio 1965).

Harrington v. Rush-Presbyterian- St. Luke's Hosp., 569 N.E.2d 15 (Ill. Ct. App. 1990).

Harris v. Groth, 99 Wash.2d 438, 663 P.2d 113 (Ct. 1983).

Health, Mental Health, and Environmental Control

Reporting Notifiable Diseases, Alabama Code § 22-11A-2 (1975).

Hellman v. Mateo, 772 S.W.2d 64 (Tex. 1989).

Hiatt v. Groce, 215 Kan. 14, 523 P.2d 320 (Ct. 1974).

Horne v. Patton, 287 So.2d 824 (Ala. 1973).

In re United States of America, 864 F.2d 1153 (5th Cir. 1989).

James v. Brown, 637 S.W.2d 914 (Tex. 1982).

Jarvis v. St. Charles Medical Center, 713 P.2d 620 (Or. Ct. App. 1986).

Jernigan v. King, 440 S.E.2d 379, 381 (S.C. App. 1993).

Johnson v. Woman's Hosp., 527 S.W.2d 133 (Tenn. App. 1975).

Keeton, W.P., Dobbs, D.B., Keeton, R.E., & Owen, D.G. (1984). *Prosser & Keeton on the law of torts.* St. Paul, Minnesota: West.

Kimmerle v. New York Evening Journal, 186 N.E. 217 (N.Y. 1933).

Koeniguer v. Eckrich, 422 N.W.2d 600 (S.D. 1988).

Labrier v. Anheuser Ford, Inc., 612 S.W.2d 790 (Mo. App. 1981).

Laskowitz v. CIBA Vision Corp., 632 N.Y.S.2d 845, 847 (N.Y. App. Div. 1995).

Limitations of Personal Actions, Tex. Civ. Prac. & Rem. Code § 16.001 (1987).

Lord v. Clayton, 8 S.E.2d 657 (Ga. App. 1940).

Malooley v. McIntyre, 597 N.E.2d 314 (Ind. App. 1992).

Marcus v. Liebman, 59 Ill. App.3d 337, 16 Ill. Dec. 613, 375 N.E.2d 486 (Ct. 1978).

Martin v. Johnson Publishing Company, 157 N.Y.S.2d 409 (Ct. 1956).

Maxwell v. Maxwell, 177 N.W. 541 (Iowa 1920).

Maynard v. United States, 133 F.R.D. 107 (D. N.J. 1990).

McCormick v. England, 494 S.E.2d 431 (S.C. Ct. App. 1997).

Middlebrooks v. State Board of Health, 1998 WL 4751 (Ala. Jan 9, 1998).

Monks v. Marlinga, 923 F.2d 423 (6th Cir. 1991).

National Association of Government Employees v. City Public Service Board., 40 F.3d 698, 708 (5th Cir. 1994).

Neagle v. Nelson, 685 S.W.2d 11 (Tex. 1985).

New York Times v. Sullivan, 376 U.S. 254 (1964).

Northern Trust Co. v. Upjohn Co., 572 N.E.2d 1030 (Ill. App. Ct. 1991).

Olson v. Molland, 232 N.W. 625 (Minn. 1930).

Palsgraf v. Long Island Railroad Co., 248 N.Y. 339, 162 N.E. 99 (1928).

Planned Parenthood of Northwest Indiana, Inc., v. Vines, 543 N.E.2d 654 (Ind. Ct. App. 1989).

Poluski v. Richardson Transp., 877 S.W.2d 709, 713 (Mo. Ct. App. 1994).

Prohibitions Against Excessive Bail or Fines and Against Cruel or Unusual Punishment; Open Courts; Remedy by Due Course of Law, Sweeney, P. (1991). Proving nursing negligence. *Trial, 27,* 34-40.

Ramage v. Central Ohio Emergency Serv., Inc., 592 N.E.2d 828 (Ohio, 1992).

Restatement (Second) of Torts, §§ 46, 328D, 652B, comment a (1965).

Required Disclosures; Methods to Discover Additional Matter, Federal Rule of Civil Procedure 26(a), 30(b)(1) (1998).

Rodriguez v. Reeves, 730 S.W.2d 10 (Tex. 1987).

Santa Rosa Health Care Corp. v. Garcia, 964 S.W.2d 940 (Tex. 1998).

Schaffer v. Spicer, 215 N.W.2d 134 (S.D. 1974).

Schiele v. Hobart Corp., 587 P.2d 1010 (Or. 1978).

Schloendorff v. Society of New York Hospital, 105 N.E. 92, 93 (N.Y. 1914).

Shearin v. Lloyd, 98 S.E.2d 508 (N.C. 1957).

St. John v. Pope, 901 S.W.2d 420 (Tex. 1995).

State v. Barry, 124 P. 775 (Mont. 1912).

Stockwell v. Gee, 249 P. 389 (Okla. 1926).

Testimony by Experts, Federal Rule of Evidence 702 (1998).

Texas Constitution, Art. 1 § 13.

Texas Medical Liability & Insurance Improvement Act of 1977, Tex. Rev. Civ. Stat. Ann. Art. 4590i § 10.01.

Thompson v. Brent, 245 So. 2d 751 (La. Ct. App. 1971).

Tilotta v. Goodall, 752 S.W.2d 160, 161 (Tex. App.–Houston [1st Dist.] 1988, writ denied).

Vassey v. Burch, 262 S.E.2d 865, 867 (N.C. 1980).

Vosburg v. Putney, 50 N.W.2d 403 (Wis. 1981).

Warner v. Lerner, 705 A.2d 1169 (Md. 1998).

Weaver v. University of Michigan Board of Regents, 506 N.W.2d 264, 267 (Mich. App. 1993).

Weidman v. Ketcham, 15 N.E.2d 426 (NY 1938).

Westmoreland v. CBS, Inc., 770 F.2d 1168 (D.C. Cir. 1985).

SUGGESTED READINGS

Fifoot, C. H. S. (1949). *History and sources of the common law: Tort and contract.* London: Stevens & Sons Limited.

Gorlin, R. A. (1990). *Codes of professional responsibility* (2nd ed.). Washington, DC: Georgetown University Press.

Hicks, L. L., Stallmeyer, I. M., & Coleman, J. R. (1992). *Role of the nurse in managed care.* Kansas City, Missouri: National Center for Health Care Administration.

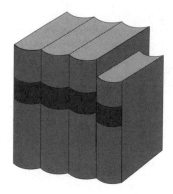

Chapter 3

THE NURSE AND THE LEGAL SYSTEM

M. Dena Matthews
Patricia Fedorka

Accountability	Interrogatories
Actual Damage	Jurisdiction
Aggregate	Jury Instructions
Appeal	Life-Care Plan
Assumption of Risk	Litigation
Bad Baby Case	Loss of Consortium
Benefits	Malpractice Insurance
Case Number	Mediation
Causation	Medical Malpractice
Challenge for Cause	Motion in Limine
Claims Made Insurance	Negligence
Comparative Negligence	Notice of Intent
Compensatory Damages	Occurrence Insurance
Complaint	Opening Statement
Contributory Negligence	Peremptory Challenge
Cross-Examination	Plaintiff
Damages	Plaintiff's Petition
Deposition	Prelitigation or Medical
Direct Examination	Review Panel
Discovery Phase	Rebuttal Evidence
Docket Number	Request for Admission
Duty	Request for Production
Exceptions	Risk Management
Exemplary or Punitive	Sovereign Immunity
Damages	Standard of Care
Expert Witness	Statute of Limitations
Exposure	Tail
Fact Witness	Trial
Feasibility	Unavoidable Accident
Good Samaritan Statutes	Voir dire
Indemnified	Willful Conduct
Independent Medical	
Examination (IME)	

OBJECTIVES

Upon completion of this chapter, the reader will be able to:
- Identify factors to consider when buying malpractice insurance.
- Explain the four elements of malpractice.
- Identify the steps of a medical malpractice lawsuit.
- Describe the defenses to a medical malpractice claim.
- Describe the role of various witnesses testifying in a malpractice lawsuit.

INTRODUCTION

In a perfect world, every nurse would provide perfect care and treatment for each patient in his or her care, and the medical outcome would be perfect. In a perfect world, each patient would accept and appreciate the care and treatment rendered by every nurse with whom he or she is in contact. But in our imperfect world, bad things happen to patients under the care and treatment of nurses. These bad outcomes may be the result of inevitable disease process or injury or noncompliance on the part of the patient or family caregivers, but sometimes they are the direct or indirect result of decisions and/or actions of a nurse. It is generally accepted that the members of society today are more reluctant to accept a negative outcome and, more importantly, more likely to try to affix blame for that outcome and seek redress in a manner that involves the legal system. The party who brings the matter in a civil action or suit is called a **plaintiff**. Negligence claims are not new in the medical world; however, what is new is the reporting by both plaintiff and defense attorneys of a distinct increase in the inclusion of nurses as malpractice defendants.

Although a part of the reason for this increase is no doubt the desire on the part of plaintiffs and attorneys to broaden and increase the potential for monetary recompense, there are other issues that should be considered. One of these is the notable shift of registered nurses into the highly technical and increasingly responsible and independent positions that have developed with changes in the health care delivery system. With expanding responsibility and independence comes the corresponding increase in accountability for the nursing treatment provided. Not only doctors are accountable for those who work at their direction; with the advent of increased use of nonlicensed personnel to perform direct treatment tasks, the registered nurse who provides immediate supervision is held accountable for the work product of those under his or her direction. The issue of **accountability** for nursing standards of care, particularly na-

tional standards of care, is becoming a factor in court rulings as a result of the speed and proliferation of all types of information, including information that relates to nursing diagnosis, care, and treatment. The nurse in clinical practice today should include professional **risk management** activities as a necessary part of preparation to minimize the risk of encountering the legal system sometime during his or her professional career. This chapter, therefore, will familiarize the nurse with the process of a malpractice lawsuit, liability insurance, and other issues involved when nursing meets the law.

PROFESSIONAL LIABILITY INSURANCE

To begin, let us examine the idea of medical malpractice insurance. First, it is important to know that **medical malpractice** is another term for professional liability in the medical field. This is based on the concept of **negligence**, a legal term defined as *a breach of duty, a departure from the recognized* **standard of care**—*what is reasonable and prudent for someone with the same or similar knowledge and skills to do in the same or similar circumstances* (Black, 1979), or what a reasonable person, guided by ordinary considerations would do or not do under the same or similar circumstances. The type of insurance that protects professional people against claims of negligence is called **malpractice insurance**. It is often carried by physicians, attorneys, accountants, engineers, and nurses. As defined by state nurse practice acts, nurses now function under their own license, and, therefore, can now be considered as professionals at risk for claims that arise from the daily practice related to the duties of the profession. Today, nurses are bombarded from the moment of entry into the nursing classroom, and throughout their career in professional nursing, with information that suggests a need to consider whether to carry individual professional liability (malpractice) insurance. This text provides a strong base of information that will allow a professional nurse to make a reasoned decision about his or her need to contract for an individual professional liability policy.

REASONS TO CONSIDER PURCHASE OF MALPRACTICE INSURANCE

The most important elements in that decision-making process are _cost_ for the policy, potential _exposure_ to malpractice litigation, and _benefits_ offered by the insurance company if one is named as a defendant and the policy comes into force. Individual professional liability coverage has an annual cost based on the practice base and setting of the nurse. In other words, an obstetrical nurse practitioner has a higher risk or chance of being the target of a malpractice suit than the nurse who works as a consultant in a case management firm; therefore, the premium cost for the insurance would be greater. Current annual rates may range from less than $100 for the general duty registered nurse (RN) or educator to just less than $1000 for a self-employed RN who is an advanced practice nurse. The most popular policies today carry liability limits that are specific for each individual incident and another limit for an aggregate. (The term **aggregate** is defined as the total amount that can be paid out in a single year.)

Exposure indicates the likelihood for a malpractice action to be filed against the nurse. As is evident from the earlier example, the nurse who is in solo practice or self-employed has greater exposure than the one who is employed within a hospital or clinic structure. The nurse in the latter situation should approach the employer and determine whether that employer has liability coverage that will include the individual nurse. If so, the individual nurse may choose not to purchase separate insurance, but he or she should at least ask for a copy of the declaration page for the policy. Even though a nurse has been assured of coverage under the umbrella of the employer, he or she may consider purchasing individual coverage. This ensures that the nurse's best interests, rather than that of the employer, is the primary focus of the defense process. If the attorney retained to represent the hospital also is named to represent the nurse, a conflict of interest may occur. The nurse might find herself or himself outside the umbrella of coverage by the employer because of failure to follow hospital policies and procedures. Another exposure risk for nurses is acts performed outside the scope of employment. This can include work in a moonlighting job and even care or advice provided to friends or neighbors. This risk will almost always fall outside the limits of the corporate policy of the employer.

The third issue in consideration of purchase of individual liability insurance is the **benefits.** There are a number of benefits in the individual liability policy that are routine and some that will cover expenses not found in the corporate policy. These include legal fees and court costs in addition to liability limits (even if the suit is groundless, false, or fraudulent), reimbursement of defense costs (up to a specified limit) for licensing or governmental regulatory board hearings, and reimbursement to the nurse for lost earnings for time away from work owing to depositions, court time, and the like.

TYPES OF POLICIES

Once a nurse has decided to purchase professional liability insurance, the decision-making process has just begun. One of the first considerations to be made is what _type of policy_ to purchase. There are two basic types of malpractice insurance policies available: _occurrence_ and _claims made_ (Shinn, 1997). **Occurrence insurance** is most often recommended for physicians and nurses. This type of policy covers any injury or damage that occurs during the time the policy is in force, regardless of when the claim is made. This is very important in the medical field because the statute of limitations for medical malpractice is complicated by such issues as date of discovery of the injury and the rights of a minor to sue up to and after they reach their majority. (The statute of limitations for medical malpractice is discussed more fully later in the chapter.) The other type of insurance, **claims made insurance**, provides coverage only for claims made during the time the policy is in force, and perhaps for an extension of the policy coverage. Thus, a labor and delivery nurse who has purchased occurrence malpractice insurance, then allowed it to lapse after leaving the workforce, is still covered years later for an injury involving an infant for whom suit is brought at age of majority. It is more likely that the claims made policy would not provide coverage when the policy has not been maintained. It would be important for a nurse who decides to purchase a claims made policy to consider a **"tail,"** or extension of the policy period that would be in effect until there is no longer any possibility of a claim being made against his or her professional practice.

FACTORS TO CONSIDER WHEN BUYING A POLICY

There are a number of factors to consider when buying a professional liability policy. Prior to purchase, the nurse should carefully examine the following elements of the policy in question.

- *Types of injuries covered* usually include bodily injury, mental anguish, property damage, and economic injury. Later in the chapter the explanation of types of damages awarded provides the rationale for types of injuries covered by the policy.
- *Exclusion* is another consideration. Most policies exclude coverage for what is called **willful conduct.** This means the policy will not cover injury or damage sustained as a result of sexual abuse of a patient, caused when the nurse is under the influence of drugs or alcohol, or occurring during the commission of criminal activity. These are sometimes lumped under the term *failure to render professional services.*
- *Policy limits and deductibles* are another important part of the coverage, with a rule of thumb that the coverage limit exceeds the highest amount awarded to an injured party in a recent malpractice case against a nurse in the geographic area. (This information can be obtained from the state nursing association.)
- *Deductibles* may or may not be a part of a

policy; they should be considered when choosing a policy if one wishes to limit out-of-pocket expenses.
- *Right to select an attorney* is an important consideration for some individuals. Most reputable liability insurance firms have relationships with attorneys and law firms that have extensive experience in handling medical malpractice claims for nurses. However, if selection of his or her own attorney is important to the nurse, he or she should make sure it is provided for in the policy that is purchased.
- *Right to consent to settlement or trial of the suit* can be another important element of malpractice insurance. Some policies allow the nurse to refuse to settle the claim, others do not. This becomes a factor when the company deems the cost of settlement of the suit to be less than the cost to defend. With national data banks now available to the public and to potential employers, the settlement of a lawsuit might play an important role in future professional employment opportunities.

INSURER'S ROLE IN A LAWSUIT

Whether a nurse has made a decision to purchase individual professional liability insurance or has decided to rely on coverage provided by an employer, it is important to understand the role of the insurer in the event of a lawsuit. The nurse should anticipate activities that focus on a number of considerations.

- *Multiple insurers* may occur when an individual policyholder has had coverage by more than one company over the years. The insurers will determine exactly which policy was in force at the time of the alleged occurrence, and all others will deny claims responsibility. Multiple insurers often do occur when the plaintiff includes more than one defendant in the lawsuit. If the insurance company is the same, two law firms and two adjusters may be used to represent two different defendants. When the insurance companies are different, there is a strong incentive for cooperation to provide a mutual defense. However, a nurse's insurance company should provide legal representation that maintains his or her interests as the number one priority.

- *Indemnification suits* occur if an individual is under contract to an organization (e.g., hospital, clinic) and as part of the contract is **indemnified** or covered for any liability that is related to the provision of services stated in the contract. This might occur in the case of a nurse practitioner that is hired to staff a clinic. It does not necessarily mean that the individual does not need individual separate coverage, but it should be a consideration.
- *Provisions for defense* are the activities that the insurer is bound to provide in the event of a malpractice claim against the insured individual, including handling of all presuit activities, providing adequate defense by a competent and experienced law firm, meeting all demand letters from the plaintiff, settling in good faith if indicated, agreeing to any mediation that is ordered, and establishing adequate reserve funds to pay for all legal expenses and outcomes.
- *Stipulations denying coverage* are conditions of practice and behavior that, if breached, allow the insurance company to deny coverage of the policy. Stipulations are often related to the following: maintaining standards of practice and maintaining current state licensure, practicing in an approved setting, functioning within the legal scope of practice, and refraining from acts that would be deemed illegal.

THE NURSE AND THE LAWSUIT

ELEMENTS OF A MALPRACTICE CLAIM

One of a nurse's worst nightmares is to find that he or she has been named as the subject of a medical malpractice lawsuit. It is important to remember that any patient can sue any health care provider for any reason. This does not mean that the case has merit. It will be the responsibility of the plaintiff to prove the merit of the suit with the presence of the four essential elements of the personal liability/medical malpractice claim (Black, 1979).

- **Duty** presumes a relationship between the provider (defendant) and the patient (plaintiff). It says the provider has accepted a duty to care for that patient.
- **Negligence** is a breach of duty, a departure from the recognized standard of care. The term *standard of care* is defined as what is reasonable and prudent (ordinary) for someone with the same or similar knowledge and skills to do in the same or similar circumstances.
- **Damages/injuries** to the patient of a physical, emotional, psychological, and/or economic nature have occurred.
- **Causation** shows that the damage suffered by the patient/plaintiff was caused by the negligence of the provider. It includes **feasibility**—but for the negligence, the injury would not have happened.

The jury in a medical malpractice lawsuit will consider both the plaintiff's allegations and the defendant's answers to the allegations based on the four elements.

INITIATION OF THE LAWSUIT

STATUTE OF LIMITATIONS

One of the first considerations in the filing of the lawsuit is the time frame within which the alleged events occurred. This is viewed in the context of the statute of limitations. The **statute of limitations**, a part of the state or federal rules of court, establishes a specific time period within which a lawsuit must be filed (Richardson & Regan, 1992). For instance, a statute may state that a lawsuit for a personal injury must be filed within 2 years of the date the injury occurred. If the lawsuit is not filed within that time frame, the plaintiff may *never* bring suit. Even a case with merit may face summary judgment, or dismissal as a point of law, if it is filed even 1 day beyond the applicable statute of limitations. Many, if not most, states have a

2-year statute of limitations for medical malpractice. This means that the suit must be filed prior to the second anniversary date of the occurrence in question. However, as is often the case with law, there are **exceptions.** Common exceptions include delay in the 2-year time clock until the deviation from accepted practice is found or revealed. An example of this exception may be the discovery on x-ray examination or exploratory surgery of an instrument left in the body cavity at the time of a previous surgery more than 2 years prior to the discovery. Another common exception is one that delays the start of the statute of limitations clock for a minor child until that child is 18 to 21 years old. That is why the so-called **bad baby case** may not be filed until the child has reached a legal majority, or perhaps 2 years from the death after the alleged birth trauma.

PRELITIGATION PANELS

The **plaintiff** (the person who is claiming to have been damaged and who is seeking redress from the court) and his or her attorney will begin a prescribed sequence of events called litigation. Some states have statutory requirements that force the plaintiff to go through a **prelitigation or medical review panel** (Bogart, 1998). The length of time required and the makeup of the panel vary from state to state. The panel will likely consist of health care providers, attorneys, and/or judges. Based on the documentation supplied to them, they will decide whether negligence has indeed occurred. This process has been developed with a declared purpose of eliminating lawsuits with little or no merit. Opponents of prelitigation panels contend that the process delays the plaintiff's day in court and adds to the cost for both plaintiff and defendant. However, in cases in which the panel deems that the case does have merit, the process often provides incentive for a settlement. Some states without prelitigation requirements have addressed the need to limit and/or eliminate questionable cases by requiring the affidavit of an appropriate expert within a set number of days after filing the suit or by requiring

that the filing attorney post a substantial bond in lieu of an expert report.

FILING OF THE CLAIM

When all prelitigation requirements have been met, the suit is initiated by a filing process. This is done by taking a document to the office of the clerk of court, where it is assigned a **case number** that then appears on every subsequent filed document related to the suit. The initial document filed is called a **complaint** or **plaintiff's petition** (Richardson & Regan, 1992). This document has a number of elements and will always include:

- A statement of **jurisdiction**—including the identity and capacity of the parties and their addresses, the jurisdiction of the court over the controversy, and the personal jurisdiction of the court over the defendant
- A statement of the plaintiff's cause of action, which in a medical malpractice suit is most likely a claim of negligence
- The demand for judgment for the relief sought

The purpose for the filing of the petition is to provide fair notice to the defendant(s) of the claims made against them and the relief being sought. In a medical malpractice suit, which is one type of professional liability case, the relief sought is monetary compensation for the damages suffered. Later in this chapter, the types of damages are discussed in more detail.

Once the complaint or petition is prepared, it is then filed with the clerk of the designated court, who assigns the case a number called a **docket number**. At this point, the petition is served on the named defendants, either by a sheriff or by a private process server. In some states a notice of intent to file suit is required. The preliminary notice of filing must be sent to the defendant within a predetermined number of days before the petition is filed with the court.

The formal process of the lawsuit begins with the filing of the claim as just described.

This service of the complaint (or **notice of intent)** may be the first indication to the nurse that he or she is being named as a defendant. It is the point at which panic threatens. At this time the nurse will want to move quickly to notify the liability insurance company, engage the services of an appropriate attorney if without insurance, and also notify his or her employer. This allows the beginning of defense action to limit or even eliminate the actions of the lawsuit. It is also likely that the defense attorney will advise the nurse to refrain from discussing the case with anyone not approved by his or her attorney.

PHASES OF THE LAWSUIT

DISCOVERY PHASE

The first phase of the lawsuit is the **discovery phase**. It begins immediately with the filing of the lawsuit, and in most states continues until 30 days before trial. The purpose of discovery is the same for both sides. It is to discover or gather information that will better define the issues of the case (Bogart, 1998). Discovery also functions to define legal and factual issues, determine the opposing side's allegations, obtain the information at least cost possible, preserve testimony of witnesses who may not be available for trial, and prevent any surprise element at the time of the trial itself. As both parties learn more details about the opposing case strengths and weaknesses, discovery may lead to mediation or settlement. Each side is allowed to *discover* information that is not considered privileged, and determination of whether or not requested information is privileged may require a ruling by the court/judge. Good attorneys often push the limits of accepted procedures in attempting to get information that might be legally considered privileged if they think they can obtain it from an unsuspecting or naive source. For this reason, it is important for the nurse defendant to reply to requests for production of information only after consulting his or her attorney. In fact, that defendant attorney will likely advise his or her client

never to speak with the opposing attorney or staff without defense counsel present. The five methods of discovery are covered below (Richardson, 1992).

1. **Interrogatories**—written questions submitted by one party to another. They require written responses under oath and may relate to any matter not privileged that is relevant to the subject matter of the litigation. There is a strict time frame for the answering of interrogatories. According to federal rules, answers must be served to opposing counsel within 30 days of service of the interrogatories, or within 45 days if served along with the original complaint. A notarized signature sheet attached to the interrogatory answers provides that the client swears that his or her answers are true and correct.

2. **Request for production**—a formal written request for copies of relevant, nonprivileged documents, such as medical records, personnel records, correspondence, or any written information to be introduced into evidence. It may also include a request for access to a place or production of tangible items such as equipment that are relevant to the case. In a medical malpractice case the medical records, personnel records, policies, and procedures are commonly requested.

3. **Request for admission**—a tool used to develop in writing the agreement by both parties to certain uncontroverted facts. Again, the request for admission is a written document from one party asking the other party to agree to the truth of certain facts or the authenticity of certain materials. It requires a written response or objection within 30 days, and the answer must admit parts that are true, deny any other parts, or give a detailed reason why there can be no admission or denial. A request for admission might ask that the defendant admit as true that he or she was employed by Hospital X on a certain date and was on duty on Ward Y for the hours of 1 to 5 P.M. The defendant would then admit in writing to those facts as true. This is a good tool to narrow the issues either of fact or law in the case to

simplify the matter before it goes to trial. It is also a way to authenticate documents that have been obtained in the discovery phase of production.

4. **Physical or mental examination**—done by an impartial doctor. This is called an **independent medical examination (IME)** and is used by the defense when the physical or mental condition is an issue in the lawsuit. This is not often seen in medical malpractice, but it might occur if there is a question of the validity of claims of an injury resulting from the alleged negligence.

5. **Deposition**—an oral questioning of relevant witnesses by an attorney for the opposing side. The deposition is taken under oath, without a judge present, outside the courtroom. A court reporter is used to record the proceedings. A deposition allows the opposing attorney to assess the strength of the case (plaintiff or defense) and to judge the impact this witness may have in the courtroom. In many instances, the deposition will be videotaped so that it may be played for the jury during the trial. This might be done in lieu of an appearance by the witness, or when a dispute occurs at the time of the trial. A defendant will be deposed by the plaintiff's attorney; the defendant's attorney will depose the plaintiffs. A nurse's attorney should prepare him or her for this process and will be with the nurse for the deposition. The nurse will be allowed to attend all depositions related to the case and should plan to be an active listener and advising participant to his or her attorney.

MEDIATION AND SETTLEMENT AGREEMENTS

There is an increasing attempt on the part of judges, attorneys, and insurance companies to find agreement without going to trial. Because the cost of defending a malpractice case through the trial process can range from $15,000 to more than $100,000 (depending on the complexity of the case), some malpractice attorneys estimate that more than 90 percent of those cases settle prior to going to

court. Akin to the prelitigation panels, there are other formalized procedures whose goal is to move the dispute between plaintiff and defendant to an agreed conclusion. These programs fall under the category of **mediation**, or moderated settlement conferences. They may come at any time in the process of the lawsuit prior to the opening of the trial. Many judges order a mediation or settlement conference to ensure that every effort has been made to bring the parties to closure without resorting to the time and expense of the trial process. Mediation or moderated settlement conferences utilize a person who is trained as a go-between and who provides a strictly impartial viewpoint to the disputed claims. This moderator or mediator may be an attorney, but in some settings may have no formal legal training, instead being trained in the moderator or mediator role. Although judges may mandate a mediation or settlement conference, the parties may not be compelled to settle or mediate the final outcome. They have the right to a day in court.

TRIAL

Motions in Limine

After the discovery process, and if no settlement is reached, the case proceeds to **trial**. The first hurdle for the nonlegal layperson to cross is the incredible time required to reach the trial date. In today's legal arena court dockets are crowded, and delays are inevitable before judge, jury, attorneys, plaintiff, and defendants are ready and available to enter the courtroom. One of the first things that may happen in the court is the filing of a **motion in limine**. This is the request by one or the other of the attorneys to limit inclusion of specified evidence and is done to prevent the jury from seeing information that may be damaging to the case prepared by that attorney.

Jury Selection

The next phase of the trial is jury selection. Each attorney has been given basic information on the potential jurors, filled out in advance of jury service. One of the most important parts of any trial begins with what is called **voir dire** (Black, 1979), which literally means speak the truth. The purpose of voir dire is for the attorney to question and then select a jury that he or she believes will be most receptive to his or her client's version of the case. Each attorney is allowed to ask questions of the individual jurors and will likely include some very general demographic type questions along with others more specific to the elements and nature of the case. This allows the attorney to identify any bias that might be either a positive or negative factor in presenting the case. In some instances, a question may elicit an answer that requires immediate ruling by the judge as to the suitability of the prospective juror. After the questioning is completed, each attorney issues challenges (or requests) that a juror candidate be exempted from service on that jury. There are two types of challenges. The first type is a **peremptory challenge**, in which the attorney is allowed to excuse a juror without stating a reason. Each attorney has a limited number of peremptory challenges. The second type of challenge is the **challenge for cause**. To excuse a jury candidate for cause, the attorney must state the reason for excluding that person from the jury. Common challenges for cause include relationship to one of the parties, friend of one of the attorneys, or a prejudice regarding one of the parties or the allegations in the case. After all questioning and challenges are completed, the jury is seated from the first of the remaining candidates. To fully appreciate the judicial system, one should embrace the opportunity to serve as a juror. If an individual finds himself or herself as a defendant (or a plaintiff) in a trial, knowledge of the legal system and jury process will be a great asset.

Opening Statements

Once a jury has been selected and sworn in, the attorneys begin the work of presentation of the case from the viewpoint of their client. Each attorney begins with an **opening statement**. The purpose of this statement is to give a comprehensive summary of the nature of the case, including a succinct account of the evidence that he or she will present, and includes an explanation of the points that he or she will prove with that evidence. Beginning with the plaintiff's attorney, each counsel seeks to plant within the minds of the jurors the version of the case that best represents his or her client. Most often, the defense attorney follows the plaintiff's attorney immediately, but he or she may choose to reserve the opening statement until just before he or she begins to present evidence. Attorneys know that opening statements can be crucial to the outcome of the case, as it often provides an initial bias about the case that will color all further evidence and/or testimony. Opening statements are not arguments for the case, instead they are an attempt to explain who the parties are, develop the theory of the case, and present his or her client in a sympathetic light to the jury.

Presentation of Plaintiff's Case

The courtroom trial continues with presentation of the plaintiff's case. This is done with the use of witnesses and exhibits that will tell the story to the jury. There can be three types of witnesses utilized in a civil trial: (1) the principals (plaintiffs and defendants), (2) fact witnesses, and (3) expert witnesses. Each witness has a specific role in the telling of the story and establishing the required burden of proof. In a civil trial, such as a malpractice case, the plaintiff's burden of proof is to provide evidence to the jury to prove that by the preponderance of the evidence the facts support the essential elements of the plaintiff's claims for relief. Unlike in a criminal trial, it is not necessary that the evidence prove beyond a reasonable doubt that the facts support the claims. This is a significant difference, as it does not require that there be no doubt whatsoever, but that it is more probable than not that the facts are true. Also, unlike in a criminal trial, no party in the case is exempt from required testimony. Therefore, the plaintiff will be called for testimony and examination by the defense if he or she has not been presented by the plaintiff's attorney. In most instances, the plaintiff will be one of the first witnesses called by his or her attorney to personalize the case for the jury as the plaintiff tells the story of the alleged negligence and damages. This is called **direct examination**. Questions asked by the plaintiff's attorney are carefully crafted to elicit the information desired to be placed before the jury, but must not be "leading" questions. Both the judge and the defense attorney will listen as carefully to the form of the question as to the answer, and that form may provoke an objection by opposing counsel, or a ruling by the judge, who will either sustain or overrule the objection. During the questioning of the plaintiff, some documentary evidence may be introduced, as it undoubtedly will be during questioning of fact or expert witnesses.

Another type of witness being increasingly utilized in professional liability actions is the **fact witness**. Historically, a fact witness was one who had actually been present to see or perceive a thing, and has been called an eyewitness. In today's medical malpractice trials, a fact witness may be called to present information found in documentation. The use of a fact witness is becoming increasingly popular in medical malpractice cases. This is an individual (usually a nurse) who is considered by the court to be capable and qualified to summarize and explain complex and voluminous medical records and medical terminology to the jury.

The last type of witness to be discussed is the **expert witness**. Nurses have been serving as experts since the 1900s but have been only formally accepted by the courts since 1980 (Josberger & Reis, 1985). Now it is the norm to have nurse experts testify in malpractice litigation.

The expert witness plays an important and unique role in the legal process. The expert's role consists of presenting the nursing standards that were in force at the time the incident took place and giving an opinion as to whether the defendant nurse adhered to said standards by acting as a reasonable and prudent nurse would have done in the same or similar circumstances. If a nurse failed to

meet the standards of care and breached her or his duty, by definition, she or he was negligent (Aiken & Catalano, 1994).

A nurse is considered an expert based on his or her education, clinical expertise, research activity, publications, professional activities, and participation in continuing education (Strickland & Fishman, 1994). An expert witness is one whose specialized knowledge of a subject allows him or her to draw conclusions and form opinions about the facts that are presented in the discovery documents, including medical records, depositions, and the like. In addition to giving an opinion as to whether the defendant nurse was negligent in the nursing care given, experts play another important role in medical malpractice litigation. Because of the highly complex nature of health care, an expert attempts to present the pertinent case information in a manner in which the judge and jury can understand. At the deliberation portion of the trial, the jury will consider the facts of the case, which include expert testimony. Then it is up to the jury to decide whether the nurse did or did not adhere to said standards. In addition, the causation factor must also be proved, for a nurse is not considered negligent if the breached duty did not cause the particular injury in question. As stated previously, a bad outcome is not always an indication of negligence nor does not adhering to standards always result in damages.

In determining whether a nurse has breached his or her duty, the expert nurse may review a number of standards to form an opinion. These sources may include a variety of national, state, and institutional standards, guidelines, and publications. They can originate from national professional nursing organizations, state nurse practice acts, and the Joint Commission for Accreditation of Healthcare Organizations (JCAHO) manuals. In addition, the expert will usually request the pertinent hospital policies and procedures relevant to the case. Texts and other authoritative material from the period of time in which the incident took place may also be reviewed and used as an additional basis for whether the nurse met or breached standards.

Occasionally there are published guidelines that are very specific in such areas as the intervals for assessing and evaluating patients, which makes determination of adherence to standards relatively simple. However, in many instances there are no specific standards or guidelines that address the exact nursing issues in the case. In these instances when guidelines are broad, the expert witness for the defense may have an opinion that differs drastically from that of the plaintiff expert. In *Fraijo v. Hartland Hospital* (1979), the court upheld the opinion that a nurse is not bound do to exactly what another nurse would do, only to conduct herself or himself as a reasonable and prudent nurse. If there is more than one recognized method of diagnosis or treatment, and not one of them is used exclusively by all practitioners, a physician or nurse is not negligent if when exercising his or her best judgment, he or she selects one of the approved methods that later turns out to be a wrong selection, or one not favored by other practitioners. There might be a variety of options that would fulfill the nurse's duty to the patient. The nurse's best defense to a charge of negligence is a thorough knowledge of applicable nursing standards and strict adherence to them.

As has been previously mentioned, another part of the plaintiff case presentation is the use of *evidentiary documents and materials*. It is well known by both plaintiff and defense attorneys that because of the complexity of professional liability cases (particularly medical malpractice), illustrative evidence can significantly impact a jury's understanding of elements of a case. The effective attorney uses as much graphic material as possible to enhance and explain the facts of the case he or she feels are most important for jurors to understand and remember. Each piece of evidence, whether documents such as medical records, illustrations, graphs, or videotapes, is introduced and identified with a number that also indicates whether it is presented by plaintiff or defense. Both sides of the case have full access to the documentary evidence, and the opposing side has probably seen and agreed to introduction prior to the beginning of the trial.

Presentation of Defendant's Case

The next part of the trial is the presentation of the defendant's case. Indeed, the defendant's case has already begun during the presentation of witnesses by plaintiff's attorney. At the conclusion of direct examination, the defense attorney is permitted to do **cross-examination** of the witness. At this time, an attorney not only can but also doubtless will ask leading questions that will seek to call forth a desired answer, particularly a "yes" or "no" answer without opportunity to explain or qualify the answer. It is a rule of thumb that an attorney never asks a question on direct or cross-examination to which he or she does not already know the answer. The formal presentation of the defendant's case follows the same procedure as that of the plaintiff. The defense attorney presents witnesses and documentary evidence and does direct examination. The plaintiff's attorney then cross-examines the defense witnesses. For both sides, there may follow re-direct and re-cross-examination.

As a defendant in a medical malpractice case, the nurse must be prepared for the intense spotlight that will be focused on him or her. The good defense attorney has spent sufficient time with the defendant to ensure that the nurse knows what to expect from the attorneys, both plaintiff and defense. This may take the form of role-play with expected direct and cross-examination questions being asked. The deposition that has preceded the trial is a good example of the questions and the behavior that may be expected from the opposing counsel in the trial setting. No matter how uncomfortable the trial may be, the nurse defendant will be required to be present throughout the entire proceedings. As one of the principals of the case, he or she can expect to be under scrutiny of jurors, spectators, and perhaps even the press at all times. For this reason, courtroom demeanor is very important. The kind of appearance presented and the impression to be made by dress and behavior is considered carefully.

This should be discussed in advance with the defense attorney, so that the nurse is prepared to be seen as professional, competent, and human. The nurse will also want to be comfortable in the courtroom and in transit to and from the courthouse.

Closing Statements and Rebuttal

At the completion of presentation of the defense case, all defense witnesses and evidence have been brought before the jury. It is the goal of the defense attorney to show that the defendant's version of the facts is true. All documentary evidence is entered into evidence, and the defense rests. It is at this time that the plaintiff's attorney has one more chance to bolster his or her case. This may be done by presenting **rebuttal evidence**. This is not an opportunity to present additional general evidence, but to rebut or contradict specific points raised by the defendant attorney. Additional witnesses may be called to contradict or dispute testimony by a defense expert witness. Any rebuttal witness is subject to cross-examination by opposing counsel.

After all evidence and rebuttal, the attorneys complete the presentation of the evidence with closing arguments or statements. The purpose of closing statements is to summarize the evidence to the jury in a way that will persuade them that their client's version of the facts is true. The attorneys are not allowed to go beyond the evidence already presented, but will try to provide an amalgam of the evidence with their theory of the case. The plaintiff's attorney generally gives the first closing argument, followed by the defense attorney, with an opportunity for the plaintiff's attorney to briefly rebut the defense. These are the final words by the attorneys and are followed by the judge's charge to the jury.

Jury Instructions

Jury instructions by the judge explain which laws are relevant and apply in this particular case. Prior to closing arguments, the judge and the attorneys may discuss any specific instructions that the attorneys wish included. This generally takes place in judge's chambers outside the hearing of the jury. Procedural matters are explained, including the burden of proof, and the essential elements that the plaintiff must establish. The judge will also instruct the jury on the effect of affirmative defense, such as contributory negligence and the effect of comparative negligence. Once jury instructions are completed, the jury retires for deliberation. This allows the jury to collectively consider all of the evidence presented and to even ask for clarification or hear portions of the transcript. In a civil case it is rare for the jury to be sequestered. Once the conclusion has been reached by the jury, the judge is notified in writing and reads the verdict in the open court. In the medical malpractice case, the jury must determine whether the plaintiff has proved negligence by one or more of the defendants and then must determine the percentage of negligence attributed to each defendant. In some jurisdictions the jury must also consider comparative or contributory negligence on the part of the plaintiff. This is of particular importance when the jury determines the damages or monetary award to the plaintiff.

APPEAL PROCESS

Once the jury verdict has been given, both parties have the opportunity to present post-trial motions, to move for a new trial, or to appeal either verdict or damages. The party who is challenging the court's decision **(appeal)** must show that the trial court committed an error during the trial and that such error was harmful to or biased the outcome of the case. The appellate court must accept the appeal or uphold the judgment. If the appellate court decides to review the case, it does not hear witnesses nor hear new evidence. Presentations to the appellate court will primarily be written briefs, but may include oral arguments. This means that the litigation process may go on for some time before a final outcome is derived.

THE NURSE AND THE LEGAL SYSTEM **55**

DEFENSES TO A MALPRACTICE CLAIM

In any medical malpractice case, the defense attorney will consider a number of possible defense strategies (Black, 1979).

- **Contributory negligence** indicates that the plaintiff or injured party failed to take reasonable care to prevent the injury that happened. A finding of contributory negligence may prevent the injured party from any recovery in a tort action.
- **Comparative negligence** is a similar and more often seen defense that assigns a percentage of fault for the injury to more than one individual, and may likely include the injured party or plaintiff. This also means that damages are assigned in the same proportion as fault, and, therefore, reduces the monetary compensation to the plaintiff accordingly.
- **Statute of limitations,** as stated earlier in the chapter, establishes a specific time period within which a lawsuit must be filed.
- **Assumption of risk** is another defense strategy that may be seen, particularly utilizing such documentation as signed informed consent for procedures or treatment. Assumption of risk requires that the plaintiff has knowledge of the facts that constitute a dangerous condition, knows the condition is dangerous, appreciates the nature or extent of the danger, and voluntarily exposes himself or herself to the danger.
- **Good Samaritan statutes** provide protection for a person who gives aid to an individual in imminent and serious peril and who acts with good faith and reasonable care to minimize or prevent injury, no matter the outcome.
- An **unavoidable accident** is one in which casualty occurs without negligence, and all reasonable and common means have been used to prevent it. An unavoidable accident suggests that nothing could have been done by the defendant to keep this event from happening. If an otherwise competent patient falls out of a wheelchair in an earthquake and fractures an arm, it could be considered an unavoidable accident.
- The issue of **sovereign immunity** is considered when the defendant is an agent of a government entity. Government immunity requires an expressed waiver, which is usually accompanied by a cap limit on tort actions. Thus a public hospital in a state with sovereign immunity may be sued for negligence, but there is a cap on the monetary damages that may be awarded.

TYPES OF DAMAGES

When a personal liability or medical malpractice case has been tried with findings for the plaintiff, the second phase of jury process is the assignment of damages. **Damages** in the civil court system are monetary and may include past damages for actual expenses, past wage loss, and future damages for expenses and wage loss. There may also be damages awarded for pain and suffering, but these may be limited by law in some jurisdictions. The types of damages assigned are:

- Actual or **compensatory damages** are the amount of money that compensates the injured party for the injury sustained and nothing more. In a medical malpractice case this will most likely include all past medical care, loss of wages, future medical care, necessary equipment to restore the individual to as close to a preinjury life as possible, and even the inability to continue normal marital relations, called **loss of consortium** (Black, 1979). **Actual damages** are based on bills for care, calculation of lost wages, and in some cases a **life-care plan** prepared by a medical expert with the assistance of an economist to forecast future costs.
- **Exemplary or punitive damages** is an amount of money assigned to the plaintiff that will stand as punishment of the defendant's actions (Black, 1979). It is under exemplary damages that awards for pain and suffering and mental anguish are

given. There is a significant difference in the process that assigns exemplary damages, and this is a much more subjective consideration of the jury.

RECOMMENDATIONS FOR RESEARCH

- Determine which factors play a role in determining whether a patient files a lawsuit.
- Determine whether and how much legal content is taught in basic nursing curricula.
- Determine whether there is a need for more continuing education in legal topics for professional nurses.
- Determine what practicing nurses know about the legal process and how to minimize their chances of being found negligent.

SUMMARY

Nurses are constantly being challenged by the rapid changes in medical technology and the impact of an evolving health care delivery system. As nurses function in more independent roles and assume more responsibilities in their present positions, they are at increased risk for encountering the legal system. Although it is unlikely that a nurse will be named as an individual defendant in a medical malpractice litigation, he or she will come under scrutiny if the hospital in which he or she works is named as a defendant. Although many lawsuits are frivolous and never proceed to a court trial, they are nevertheless stressful for the defendants. In today's suit-conscious society, it is impossible to protect health care professionals from all litigation, but a sound understanding of the legal process can decrease the stress from interacting with an unknown entity. In addition, nurses must be aware from their first clinical experience that they will be held to applicable national standards regardless of the setting or geographic area. As professionals, nurses have a legal respon-

sibility to be competent in their area of practice. Lack of knowledge will never be an acceptable defense for substandard or negligent nursing care.

POINTS TO REMEMBER

- Nursing practice today carries a higher risk of professional liability lawsuits, and many nurses may need to consider individual professional liability insurance.
- A nurse considering purchase of professional liability insurance should consider the types of policies available and factors related to individual needs and policy elements.
- A plaintiff in a malpractice lawsuit must prove four elements—duty, negligence, damages, and causation.
- The statute of limitations on initiation of a malpractice case is set by the federal or applicable state government.
- Discovery phase of the lawsuit provides the opportunity for both plaintiff and defense to determine the strengths and weaknesses of the opposing side's case.
- Today there is an increasing push to conclude malpractice claims prior to court appearance through mediation or settlement agreements, and such mediation may be court mandated.
- Nurses play a growing role in medical malpractice claims as either expert or fact witnesses.
- Preparation for court appearance as a defendant is crucial to positively influencing the jury.
- There are a number of valid defenses to a malpractice claim.
- Damages awarded in a malpractice case are either actual/compensatory or exemplary/punitive.

REFERENCES

Aiken, T., & Catalano, J. (1994). *Legal, ethical, and political issues in nursing*. Philadelphia: F.A. Davis.

Black, H. C. (1979). *Black's law dictionary*. St. Paul, MN: West Publishing.

Bogart, J. B. (Ed.). (1998). *Legal nurse consulting principles and practice*. New York: CRC Press.

Fraijo v. Hartland Hospital, 99 Cal. Rept. 3d 331, 160 Cal. Rept. 246 (1979).

Josberger, M. C., & Ries, D. T. (1985, June). Nurse experts. *Trial*, 68–71.

Richardson, E. C., & Regan, M. C. (1992). *Civil litigation for paralegals*. Dallas: South-Western Publishing.

Schulmeister, L. (1998, April). Individual professional liability insurance: Who needs it? *Clinical Journal of Oncology Nursing*, 67–69.

Shinn, L. J. (Ed.). (1997). *Take control: A guide to risk management*. Chicago: Kirke-Van Orsdel.

Strickland, O. L., & Fishman, D. J. (1994). *Nursing issues in the 1990s*. Albany, NY: Delmar.

SUGGESTED READINGS

American Nurses Association. (1973). *Standards of nursing practice*. Washington, DC: Author.

American Nurses Association. (1980). *Nursing: A social policy statement*. Washington, DC: Author.

American Nurses Association. (1985). *Code for nurses with interpretive statements*. Washington, DC: Author.

American Nurses Association. (1990). *Liability prevention & you: What nurses & employers need to know*. Kansas City, MO: Author.

American Nurses Association. (1991). *Standards of clinical nursing practice*. Washington, DC: American Nurses Publishing.

Bernzweig, E. P. (1996). *The nurse's liability for malpractice* (6th ed.). St. Louis: Mosby.

Brent, N. (1997). *Nurses and the law: A guide to principles and applications*. Philadelphia: W.B. Saunders.

Cangelosi v. Our Lady of the Lake Regional Medical Center, et al., 564 2d 654 (La. 1989).

Catalano, J. T. (1996). *Contemporary professional nursing*. Philadelphia: F.A. Davis.

Commonwealth of Pennsylvania, State Board of Nurse Examiners v. Rafferty, 508 Pa. 566, 499 A.2d. 289 (Sup. Ct. Pa. 1984).

Dorsaneo, W. V., & Griggs, S. K. (1993). *Civil litigation*. New York: Matthew Bender.

Gardner, S., & Hagedorn, M. (1997). *Legal aspects of maternal-child nursing practice: Concepts and strategies in risk management*. Menlo Park, CA: Addison Wesley Longman.

Guido, G. W. (1997). *Legal issues in nursing*. Prentice Hall, NJ: Appleton and Lange.

Huycke, L. I. (1992). *A primer for the medical expert witness*. CODES. Oklahoma: Med-Law Case Review of America.

Joint Commission for Accreditation of Healthcare Organizations. (1997). *Comprehension accreditation for hospitals: The official handbook*. Oakbrook Terrace, IL: Author.

Moniz, D. (1992). The legal danger of written protocols and standard of practice. *Nurse Practice, 17*, 58–60.

Poynter, D. (1987). *Expert witness handbook: Tips and techniques for the litigation consultant*. Santa Barbara, CA: Para Publishing.

Prosser, W. (1971). *Handbook of the law of torts* (4th ed.). St. Paul, MN: West Publishing.

Santa Rosa Medical Center v. Robinson, 560 S.W.2d 751 (Tex. 1977).

Trandel-Korenchuk, D. M., & Trandel-Korenchuk, K. M. (1997). *Nursing & the law* (5th ed.). Gaithersburg, MD: Aspen Publications.

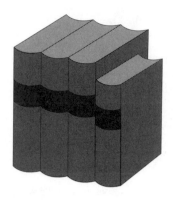

Chapter 4

ETHICS IN NURSING

Mary E. O'Keefe

Abortion
Act Deontology
Active Euthanasia
Act Utilitarianism
Advance Directive
Anencephalic Infant
Artificial Insemination
Assisted Suicide
Autonomy
Beneficence
Bioethical Change
  Process
Bioethics
Biomedical Ethics
Brain Death
Caring
Casuistry
Categorical Imperative
Clinical Ethics
Compassion
Deontology
Discernment
Distributive Justice
Do Not Resuscitate
  (DNR) Order
Durable Power of
  Attorney
Embryonic Stem Cells
Ethical Dilemma
Ethics
Euthanasia
Exposure-Prone
  Procedure
Extraordinary Medical
  Treatment
Feminist Ethics
Fidelity
Focal Virtues
In vitro Fertilization
Integrity
Involuntary Euthanasia

Justice
Law
Life-Sustaining Medical
  Treatment
Living Will
Medically Futile
  Treatments
Morals
National Organ
  Transplant Act of
  1984
Nonmaleficence
Nonvoluntary Euthanasia
Normative Decisions
Nursing Code of Ethics
Obligations
Ordinary Medical
  Treatment
Paradigm Cases
Passive Euthanasia
Paternalism
Patient Self-
  Determination Act
Principled Ethics
Procedural Justice
Rights
Rule Deontology
Rule Utilitarianism
Safe Harbor Law
Slow Code
Surrogate Mother
Trustworthiness
Uniform Anatomical Gift
  Act
Uniform Determination of
  Death Act
Utilitarianism
Veracity
Voluntary Euthanasia
Whistle-Blowing

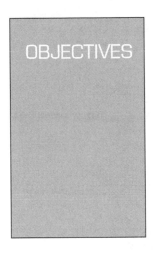

Upon completion of this chapter, the reader will be able to:
- Discuss the historical significance of ethics in nursing.
- Discuss the relationship between law and ethics.
- Define ethical terminology.
- Describe ethical decision-making models used in nursing practice.
- Discuss major ethical issues in nursing.
- Identify current issues and trends in nursing.
- Identify recommendation for future research and malpractice prevention surrounding ethical issues in nursing.

INTRODUCTION

The very essence of nursing practice requires a continuous evaluation of ethical duties while providing patient care. **Ethics** is a process of making decisions based on one's moral beliefs. **Morals** are one's sense of good and bad, right and wrong. Ethical duties may or may not be based on or correlate with the **law**, or set of enforceable principles and/or rules established to protect society (Aiken, 1994, p. 22; Burkhardt & Nathaniel, 1998, p. 390). The purpose of this chapter is to provide a basic knowledge and framework within which nurses may make ethical decisions.

HISTORICAL PERSPECTIVE

The evolution of the **nursing code of ethics,** or professional values and standards of nursing practice (Aiken, 1994, p. 22), has been of historical significance to the development of health care, and thus nursing practice. Burkhardt and Nathaniel (1998) hypothesized that spiritual beliefs and religious practices and the evolution of the role of women have specifically influenced the moral foundation of nursing practice. According to Burkhardt & Nathaniel (1998,

p. 110) "... laws represent an attempt to codify ethics."

RELATIONSHIP BETWEEN LAW AND ETHICS

Ethics is a set of formal or informal rules that guide behavior. The law consists of rules, which are enforced to govern society (Burkhardt & Nathaniel, 1998, p. 109). The four basic functions of law within society are (1) to define relationships between its members, thus defining permissible and impermissible actions; (2) to define how rules may be enforced and by whom; (3) to provide problem resolution; and (4) to redefine relationships during change (Kozier & Erb, 1988, p. 244).

Laws are based on what society defines as right or wrong, structured on an ethical or moral foundation (Burkhardt & Nathaniel, 1998, p. 110). Burkhardt and Nathaniel (1998, p. 110) have identified four major reasons why there are discrepancies between what is legal and what is ethical. First, differences exist between ethical points of view. For example, the deontologist would make decisions based on certain fixed principles, whereas utilitarians would look only to actions that produce good consequences.

Second, Burkhardt and Nathaniel (1998, p. 110) proposed that human behavior and motivation are more complicated than laws reflect. For example, although a woman has a right to choose abortion, the provider has a right to choose not to participate in the abortion procedure.

The third discrepancy between law and ethics is that laws judge rather than motivate. For example, the nurse may be motivated under a professional code of ethics to maintain the confidentiality of the patient but is legally bound to disclose the patient confidence in a criminal proceeding (Burkhardt & Nathaniel, 1998, p. 110).

Finally, ethics change slowly, whereas laws change more rapidly. For example, nurses have had a long-standing duty to provide nursing care to protect the mother and developing fetus; yet laws are changing regarding the right of the mother to choose abortion or use the fetus as an organ donor (Burkhardt & Nathaniel, 1998, p. 110).

ETHICAL TERMINOLOGY

The nurse's ability to make an ethical decision requires a working knowledge of ethical terminology and the ethical frameworks or systems within which these terms are used. The purpose of this section is to provide a definition of basic ethical terminology and discuss ethical systems within which these ethical terms may be organized and applied.

DEFINITIONS OF BASIC ETHICAL TERMINOLOGY

According to Aiken (1994, p. 21), the ethical principles handed down by the ancient Greeks, such as Hippocrates, are used today by nurses in making ethical decisions involving patient care. Nurses make these ethical decisions often within an **ethical dilemma**, which occurs when the nurse has a choice between two or more alternatives with two equally unfavorable outcomes.

Within an ethical dilemma the nurse identifies the key ethical terms, principles, and/or concepts whose understanding and application are fundamental to the nurse's

ethical decision-making process. These key ethical terms or principles include (1) autonomy, (2) beneficence, (3) fidelity, (4) justice, (5) nonmaleficence, and (6) veracity.

Autonomy is the freedom to be self-regulating. According to E.K. Dvorak (personal communication, November 22, 1998), the principle of autonomy has two distinct features, which allow (1) the patient the right to be left alone or untreated and/or (2) the patient to be considered the best judge of the best treatment for his or her needs. This ethical concept is perhaps the first and the most important consideration in patient care. Although the right is not absolute, it may be ignored or refused only in special circumstances. For example, although the terminally ill patient may have a right to commit suicide, the nurse has no duty, and may refuse, to assist the patient to commit suicide (Aiken, 1994, p. 23; Burkhardt & Nathaniel, 1998, pp. 40–42).

Fidelity is an ethical principle that embodies the nurse's duty to be loyal, faithful, and keep promises. The nurse is faithful to the practice of nursing through promises made to the state via nursing licensure. The monitoring of the nurse's ability to keep those promises is conducted through various administrative laws and codes of ethics, established by the state nursing boards and professional nursing organizations, respectively (Burkhardt & Nathaniel, 1998, p. 58). Fidelity is the basis for accountability, and ethical dilemmas arise when the nurse must be loyal, and thus accountable, to two opposing interests (Aiken, 1994, p. 24). For example, the nurse may be forced to discharge a patient from outpatient care because the patient can no longer pay for services. Thus a conflict exists between duties and loyalties to the patient and the economic needs of the employer.

Justice encompasses the nurse's duty to be fair and equitable and provide access and appropriate care to all patients (Aiken, 1994, pp. 21–22; Burkhardt & Nathaniel, 1998, p. 57). **Distributive justice** contemplates the fair and equitable distribution of health care goods and nursing services (Burkhardt & Nathaniel, 1998, p. 57). Decisions about distributive justice are made on the governmental, organizational, and individual levels. The nurse participates with other providers in determining who will get limited or scarce health care resources and services. Aiken (1994, p. 23) suggests that the key question the nurse should ask to provide distributive justice is "Who is entitled to these goods and services?"

E.K. Dvorak (personal communication. November 22, 1998) defined **procedural justice** as a known, fair process within which distributive justice occurs. For example, the organ procurement system, although seemingly unfair to waiting patients, is an accepted process because the participants become familiar with it and know what to expect.

Beneficence means to do good for the patient. Within this concept is the duty of the nurse to act as the patient's advocate. According to Burkhardt and Nathaniel (1998, p. 47), beneficence lays the groundwork for the trust placed in nursing practice. Society expects the nurse to act in ways that help the patient. Underlying this ethical concept is the belief that the nurse not only must do good, but also must prevent evil or harm to the patient (Burkhardt & Nathaniel, 1998, p. 48).

The principle of **nonmaleficence** contemplates that the nurse will do no intentional or unintentional harm to the patient (Aiken, 1994, p. 24). The principle of nonmaleficence is related to the principle of beneficence, in that the nurse must avoid any risk of harm that may occur when doing beneficial nursing acts (Burkhardt & Nathaniel, 1998, p. 48).

Under the umbrella of the principle of nonmaleficence, the nurse must protect those who cannot protect themselves, such as the mentally challenged, unconscious, weak, and/or debilitated (Aiken, 1994, p. 24). This principle also prohibits (1) experimental health care research that may have a negative outcome and/or (2) the performance of unnecessary procedures as learning experiences (Burkhardt & Nathaniel, 1998, p. 48).

Veracity is an ethical and legal principle, simply defined as truthfulness. Again this principle is not absolute. For example, under therapeutic privilege, patients may not be given information about health care if the information would cause further harm to the patient (Aiken, 1994, p. 25). Most of the literature identifies truth as an important component of nursing practice. Not telling the truth may show lack of respect for others and nontrustworthiness of the person telling the lies (Burkhardt & Nathaniel, 1998, pp. 50–53).

ETHICAL SYSTEMS

Nurses make decisions every day that involve conflicts between **rights**, something that can be claimed by another, and/or **obligations**, something that is owed to another. These types of decisions are called **normative decisions** and take place within the context of **bioethics**, which is an ethical framework involving not only everyday health care issues but also moral questions regarding the quality of life and death (Aiken, 1994, p. 26–27). According to E.K. Dvorak (personal communication, November 22, 1998), bioethics includes medical, nursing, and other health care issues that involve "should we"-type questions.

There are three fundamental theories or systems within which the nurse makes bioethical decisions: utilitarianism, deontology, and virtue ethics (Burkhardt & Nathaniel, 1998, pp. 27–28).

UTILITARIANISM

Under the moral theory or system of **utilitarianism**, a nursing action is judged on the outcomes or consequences (Aiken, 1994, p. 27; Burkhardt & Nathaniel, 1998, p. 394). Specifically, the nurse chooses the action which has the greatest utility or usefulness for the greatest number of people (Burkhardt & Nathaniel, 1998, p. 28). The nurse's actions are weighed in the context of risks versus benefits to the patient. The two types of utilitarianism are act utilitarianism and rule utilitarianism.

According to the definition of **act utilitarianism**, which is synonymous with situational ethics, the action taken by the nurse depends on the situation. Under this ethical theory, acts selected depend on their consequences, assessing the risks versus benefits. Actions taken at one time may be the opposite of actions taken at another time (Aiken, 1994, p. 27; Burkhardt & Nathaniel, 1998, p. 29). For example, one patient may be given full informed consent regarding a procedure, whereas another patient may not because of the detrimental effects the information would have on the patient.

Rule utilitarianism presents the idea that nurses select actions according to rules that result in the greatest happiness and the least unhappiness. These rules are selected from past experience (Aiken, 1994, p. 27; Burkhardt & Nathaniel, 1998, p. 30). The rule is strictly adhered to, with what may appear to be less respect for the rights and/or autonomy of the patient. For example, strict adherence to rule utilitarianism would require the nurse to tell the truth in all situations; thus, providing informed consent to all patients would be viewed as having the greatest benefit.

DEONTOLOGY

Under the ethical system of **deontology**, the action of the nurse is right or wrong based on ethical principles, not the consequences. *Deontology* is a Greek term, which stands for duty. Deontology is a system of ethics within which ethical decisions are made based on the duty of the nurse, as specified within ethical principles (Aiken, 1994, p. 29; Burkhardt & Nathaniel, 1998, p. 31).

Within the system of deontology there are also subsystems, identified as act deontology and rule deontology. The nurse functioning within **act deontology** bases nursing actions on personal moral values or rules. The ethical decisions the nurse would make would also depend on the situation; thus, the nurse would determine the duty to the patient based on the situation (Aiken, 1994, p. 30). For example, state law may not require the nurse to obtain informed consent from an adolescent's parents prior to performing an abortion. But the health care provider may decide to obtain the parental consent, based on personal belief that a 13-year-old adolescent is not as mature and capable of making this decision as a 16-year-old adolescent would be in similar circumstances.

Rule deontology is premised on the belief that the ethical decision-making of the nurse is based on rules or standards that are fixed and inflexible (Aiken, 1994, p. 30). The nurse identifies duties strictly based on nursing standards and/or rules of law. For example, the nurse working with the previously mentioned pregnant adolescent would obtain informed consent regarding the abortion only in compliance with state law, regardless of personal belief that the adolescent was not mature or capable enough to make the decision alone.

According to Kant (1959, p. 39; see also, Burkhardt & Nathaniel, 1998, p. 31), knowledge of the rightness or wrongness of an action can be determined by following the **categorical imperative**. The term *categorical* denotes a moral rule with no exceptions, such as a nursing standard. The term *imperative* denotes this rule must be followed, such as the nursing standards established by the state board of nursing (Burkhardt & Nathaniel, 1998, p. 31).

VIRTUE ETHICS

Virtue ethics is synonymous with character ethics and is based on the assumption that nursing actions are determined by innate moral virtues (Burkhardt & Nathaniel, 1998, p. 33). According to Aristotle, there are three criteria for a virtuous character: (1) choosing virtuous acts for their nature; (2) choosing virtues stemming from a firm, unchangeable character; and (3) choosing the "golden mean," that is, a virtuous act that is not an excess or a deficiency (Burkhardt & Nathaniel, 1998, p. 34).

Burkhardt & Nathaniel (1998, p. 35) identify four **focal virtues,** or character traits, that are central to a virtuous person. The first focal virtue is **compassion**, or "the ability to place oneself in the situation of another." For example, the nurse will demonstrate insight when internalizing and practicing the golden rule. The second focal virtue is **discernment**, which involves "sensitive insight involving acute judgment and understanding, and eventuates in decisive action" (Burkhardt & Nathaniel, 1998, p. 35). For example, a nurse demonstrates discernment when distinguishing between the patient's need for sleep hygiene measures versus sleep medication. The third focal virtue, **trustworthiness**, involves (1) belief in, and reliance on or by, another; (2) acting within moral norms; (3) consistency and reliability; and (4) reputation (Burkhardt & Nathaniel, 1998, p. 35). The final focal virtue is **integrity**, often called the cardinal virtue. The nurse demonstrates integrity through soundness, reliability, wholeness, fidelity, and consistency of convictions (Burkhardt & Nathaniel, 1998, p. 35). For example, the nurse demonstrates integrity by refusing to violate the patient's confidentiality.

Burkhardt and Nathaniel (1998) proposed that principled ethical decision-making is more likely to occur in the presence of an ethical nurse (p. 35). Nursing ethics is a subcategory of biomedical ethics. Veatch and Fry (1987) define **biomedical ethics** as "the ethics of judgments made within the biomedical sciences" (p. 1). Nursing ethics then becomes the ethics of nursing judgments or decisions made within ethical decision-making models.

ETHICAL DECISION-MAKING MODELS

The most common forms of ethical analysis and ethical decision-making in nursing practice are conducted through the following models: (1) principled ethics, (2) clinical ethics, (3) feminist ethics, and (4) casuistry.

PRINCIPLED ETHICS

Kantian or **principled ethics** is based on "the equal and uncompromising application of fixed principles" (Bandman & Bandman, 1995, p. 70). Principled morality and deontological ethics are synonymous. Kant believed that an act is good if everyone ought to act the same way in similar circumstances (Bandman & Bandman, 1995, p. 70).

In the application of principled ethics, the nurse assists in the determination of which of the following major ethical principles are in conflict, including patient autonomy, beneficence, nonmaleficence, or justice. Then an argument is made regarding which one of the principles controls (Beauchamp & Childress, 1994; Ross, Glaser, Rasinski-Gregory, Gibson, & Bayley, 1993, p. 21).

Within the model of principled ethics, whether analyzed within a deontological or utilitarian ethical system, the principle of autonomy is often viewed as the priority ethical principle. Therefore, when analyzing a bioethical dilemma, the nurse (1) determines whether the patient understands the risks and benefits of the procedure or treatment; and if so, (2) allows the patient to choose whether or not the offered health care will be accepted or refused (Ross et al., 1993, pp. 21–22).

The patient may choose to give up a right to make final decisions regarding health care. The decision will then be made by the health care provider, an ethical principle that is called **paternalism.**

The patient may be unable to make health care decisions; then health care providers consider the principles of (1) beneficence, the duty to do good for the patient, and (2) nonmaleficence, the duty to do no harm to the patient. Health care providers also consider the principle of justice, basing ethical decisions on (1) policy and procedure, such as do not resuscitate (DNR) orders, and/or (2) federal and state laws, such as enforcing the patient's advance medical directives.

CLINICAL ETHICS

The model of ethical analysis utilizing clinical ethics was developed in 1982 by Jonsen, Seigler, and Winslade (1986). The four-step **clinical ethics** model utilizes principled ethics, as does the Beauchamp and Childress model (1994), but organizes the ethical principles in a different manner, considering the impact of socioeconomic factors on the final decision (Ross et al., 1993, p. 22).

Jonsen et al. (1986) also believe that patient autonomy is the priority principle within the clinical ethics model, if the patient can make preferences known. If the patient's prefer-

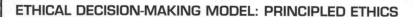

ETHICAL DECISION-MAKING MODEL: PRINCIPLED ETHICS

Step 1: Does/did the patient understand the risks and benefits of the treatment/procedure?
Step 2: Does/did the patient want to make the decision?
Step 3: Which ethical principles are at issue?
a. Patient autonomy
b. Beneficence
c. Nonmaleficence
d. Justice
Step 4: Which ethical principles are at conflict?
Step 5: Propose alternative resolutions.
Step 6: What decision will accomplish the health care goals?

Source: Ross et al., 1993.

ences are known, then the outcome of both the principled and clinical ethics models of decision-making will typically be the same. For example, under both models, if the patient has executed an advance directive requesting to remain on life support, then that request is the foremost consideration of the ethics committee in providing patient autonomy.

But when the patient cannot make preferences known, other ethical principles are considered, such as (1) beneficence, analyzing the patient's quality of life, and/or (2) distributive justice, analyzing relevant socioeconomic factors (Ross et al., 1993, pp. 22–23). For example, when the patient has no advance directive, the costs of maintaining the patient on life support will be weighed against the long-term benefits that may be obtained by the patient.

FEMINIST ETHICS

The feminist or caring model of nursing ethics was developed by medieval Christian philosophers, such as St. Thomas Aquinas (Bandman & Bandman, 1995, p. 13). **Caring** means that the person, place, thing, or event actually matters. Caring within the context of a feminist framework was first presented by Gilligan (1982) and Noddings (1984).

Gilligan (1982) proposed that ethical writ-

ers "who focus on rights, justice, and fairness. . . appeal to a masculine orientation in ethics." In contrast, the ethic of care developed by women has an underlying logic based on the psychology of relationships (Bandman & Bandman, 1995, p. 14).

Noddings (1984, p. 14) proposed that a mother's ethical decision-making is guided by an ethic of caring, rather than an ethic of equality, universality, or impartiality. The ethic of caring is derived from virtue ethics, appealing to qualities of courage, generosity, commitment, and responsibility (Bandman & Bandman, 1995, p. 14).

Within the **feminist ethics** framework of ethical decision-making, the nurse considers the ethical alternatives or principles that will best preserve the patient's existing relationships. Patient preferences may not have the same force in the feminist model. The feminist ethics model does not view patient autonomy as the priority, instead relationships are the priority (Ross et al., 1993, p. 23).

Ross et al. (1993, pp. 23–24), describes relationships and connections within the feminist ethics model of decision-making in terms of "webs" or "networks." These networks or relationships are most frequently analyzed in ethics committees, where health care providers routinely consider the patient as a family member rather than an isolated individual. For example, a patient may have an advance directive that contradicts the

ETHICAL DECISION-MAKING MODEL: CLINICAL ETHICS

Step 1: Gather health care facts to determine the patient's condition and prognosis.
Step 2: Considering those facts, determine the patient preferences.
Step 3: If the patient's preferences are known, from the patient's perspective, determine what the patient's quality of life will be with or without treatment.
Step 4: Consider the impact of socioeconomic factors, or burdens and benefits for all parties, with each decision.

Source: Ross et al., 1993.

QUESTIONS REGARDING ALLOCATION OF RESOURCES OR DISTRIBUTIVE JUSTICE

1. Is the patient entitled to these services?
2. What services should the patient receive?
3. How much service should be provided?
4. Should the patient receive minimum services or everything there is to offer?
5. Who should pay for the services?
6. Is the patient able to pay for the services?
7. Are services being denied to other patients because this patient is receiving these particular services?
8. What are the risks versus the benefits of the services?
9. What is the cost in relation to the predicted benefits?
10. Are the services ordinary, extraordinary, or futile?

Source: Burkhardt & Nathaniel, 1998, pp. 273–276.

wishes of his or her immediate family. The health care providers may attempt to obtain approval of the family before implementing the patient's advance directive, placing family relationships above patient autonomy.

CASUISTRY

Jonsen and Toulmin (1989) proposed an ethical decision-making model based on **casuistry**, or the use of paradigm cases to consider not only principles and rules of ethics but also consequences (see also, Ross et al., 1993, pp. 24–25). According to the ethical decision making model of casuistry, there are **paradigm cases**, or classic cases, about which everyone can agree on a right or wrong solution. A paradigm is a standard example (Bandman & Bandman, 1995, p. 88). Paradigms or standard case examples may be used to show how rights and/or obligations function within health care. Paradigm cases may be used to either support or refute a specific ethical position (Bandman & Bandman, 1995, p. 88).

ETHICAL DECISION-MAKING MODEL: FEMINIST ETHICS OR CARING MODEL

Step 1: Collect, analyze, and interpret the data and facts, according to the parties who have a relationship with the patient.

	Parties:	**Data/Facts:**
1.		
2.		
3.		
4.		
5.		

(Were there other data/facts to be considered for the parties?)

Step 2: State the ethical dilemma for each party who has a relationship with the patient (e.g., X vs. Y/may be a question).

	Parties:	**Dilemma:**
1.		
2.		
3.		
4.		
5.		

(Were there other ethical dilemmas for the parties?)

Step 3: Consider the choices of action for each of the parties who has a relationship with the patient.

	Parties:	**Choices of Action:**
1.		
2.		
3.		
4.		
5.		

(Were there other choices of action for the parties?)

Step 4: Analyze the advantages/positives and disadvantages/negatives of each course of action for each of the parties who has a relationship with the patient.

	Parties:	**Course of Action:**
1.		Positive:
		Negative:
2.		Positive:
		Negative:
3.		Positive:
		Negative:

(Continued)

The casuistry model is also called case-based ethics, a process that requires the health care provider to find a similar paradigm case and then determine how this case is similar or different. On points where the ethical case is similar to the paradigm case, the health care provider may take a similar course of action. On points on which the ethical case is different from the paradigm case, new solutions and/or decisions must be developed. For example, a paradigm case has been developed regarding criteria for the

**ETHICAL DECISION-MAKING MODEL:
FEMINIST ETHICS OR CARING MODEL** *(Continued)*

4.   Positive:
                                               Negative:
5.   Positive:
                                               Negative:
(Were there other advantages or disadvantages for each course of action?)
Step 5: Identify potential decisions for each of the parties who has a relationship with
the patient.

Parties:	Decision:	Your Decision:
1.		
2.		
3.		
4.		
5.		

(Were there other decisions that were made by the parties or that you would have
made?)

Source: Ross et al., 1993.

ETHICAL DECISION-MAKING MODEL: CASUISTRY

Step 1: Gather health care facts to determine the patient's
condition and prognosis.
Step 2: Identify a paradigm class within which this case occurs.
Step 3: Identify a paradigm case within this class to which this case
is similar.
Step 4: Identify how this case is similar.
Step 5: Identify how this case is different.
Step 6: Propose alternative resolutions.

Source: Ross et al., 1993.

removal of life support, when the comatose, brain-dead patient is on a respirator. Clinical cases involving comatose, brain-dead patients who are being considered for removal of life support would be compared with this paradigm case.

Points of dissimilarity between the paradigm case and the clinical case will proba-bly raise a variety of ethical issues. The use of paradigm cases in nursing ethics is discussed in *Case Studies in Nursing Ethics* by Veatch and Fry (1987). Points of dissim-ilarity in the clinical cases are presented to raise for discussion a variety of major ethical issues that the practitioner may face within nursing practice.

MAJOR ETHICAL ISSUES

Ethical issues are a major source of conflict and dilemmas within nursing practice. The purpose of this section is to identify the major ethical issues that the nurse may find in the clinical area, including (1) organ donation, (2) human immunodeficiency virus (HIV) and acquired immunodeficiency syndrome (AIDS), (3) surrogate motherhood, (4) abortion, (5) artificial insemination and in vitro fertilization, (6) right to live or die, and (7) advance directives, including living wills and durable power of attorney.

ORGAN DONATION

The process of organ donation is controlled by the **National Organ Transplant Act of 1984** (NOTA), which (1) provides for the creation of a system for organ sharing on a national basis, (2) prevents the sale of organs, and (3) funds grants for agencies that obtain and provide organ transplantation services. Some states have a mandatory policy for requesting organ donations from families (Andrews, Goldberg, & Kaplan, 1996, p. 300).

Although in most hospitals there is an assigned person to request the donation of the organ, nurses continue to be surrounded by ethical dilemmas related to the issue of organ donation, including (1) child donors, (2) cadaver donors, (3) the donation of organs of anencephalic babies, and (4) the selection of the transplant recipient (Andrews et al., 1996, pp. 297–304).

CHILD DONORS

Under law, the consent for organ donation by a child must be provided by the child's parents, because the child is a minor, and only a legal guardian can give a valid consent for such a procedure. The ethical dilemma of justice versus nonmaleficence arises when the nurse believes the decision of the parent to allow an organ donation by

the child is not in the best interest of the child. For example, the nurse may believe a bone marrow transplant from a newborn infant to an older sibling may severely compromise the infant's immune system. Or, the nurse may question the ability of an adolescent child to comprehend the risks and benefits of donating a kidney to an older brother or sister.

CADAVER DONORS

Ethical dilemmas surrounding cadaver donors may include issues related to (1) determination of death, (2) informed consent, and (3) utilization of fetal tissue. Ethical dilemmas arise because some organs can be transplanted after cardiac arrest, such as bone, skin, and cornea, whereas other organs can be transplanted only after brain death, but not before cardiac arrest, such as the heart, lung, liver, pancreas, and kidneys (Andrews et al., 1996, pp. 298–299).

The definition of brain death has been stated in the **Uniform Determination of Death Act** (UDDA) but is not universally accepted by all members of the health care professions. Under the UDDA, the criteria for defining death is **brain death:** ". . . the irreversible cessation of brain functioning accompanied by ongoing biologic functioning in all other parts of the body, maintained on life-support measures" (Andrews et al., 1996, p. 290).

When approaching the family regarding the donation of organs, the following procedure must be followed: (1) a neurologist, not the doctor involved in the organ removal and donation, should have determined brain death according to the criteria established under the UDDA; (2) the family must be provided informed consent, including a clear understanding of the definition of brain death; and (3) the family must clearly understand that brain death is a final state, and irreversible (Andrews et al., 1996, p. 299).

Under the **Uniform Anatomical Gift Act** (UAGA), a patient is allowed to give informed consent to donate body organs. According to Andrews et al. (1996, p. 299), a patient may orally give informed consent to an organ donation prior to death. But the patient must be given an opportunity to withdraw informed consent. The final consent is left up to the family, however, before the procedure is performed. Even with an organ donation as allowed under the UAGA, the gift may be excluded if the donation causes severe emotional distress to the family (Andrews et al., 1996, p. 299).

Fetal tissue donors are also cadaver donors. Working with a fetal tissue donor is an area of great ethical conflict and dilemma, including autonomy versus nonmaleficence. Not only must the nurse respect the mother's right to autonomy and decision to have the abortion, but he or she must also protect the fetus, which may be born alive. The nurse then has a duty to maintain the potential donor, but must look to the physician for instructions on when to discontinue any medications that may damage the organs, raising issues of beneficence versus paternalism (Andrews et al., 1996, p. 299).

ANENCEPHALIC INFANT DONORS

The **anencephalic infant** is one born without cerebral hemispheres, with a brain stem only. A great source of ethical dilemmas within nursing is the use of these infants as organ donors. Anencephalic infants have beating hearts and functioning brain stems, so are not brain dead. These infants remain in vegetative states. Laws have been proposed to expand the definition of brain death to include these infants. But currently, nurses are faced with a duty to care for these infants while being faced with consideration of their potential as an organ donor (Andrews et al., 1996, p. 301).

SELECTION OF TRANSPLANT RECIPIENTS

Nurses are often involved in the critical decisions regarding the placement of a patient on a transplant recipient list. According to Andrews et al. (1996, p. 302), many donation matches may be ruled out by medical and/or physical factors. But most medical transplant centers have a set of guidelines for determining who will receive an organ donation, which includes (1) coordination of transplants, (2) determining the need for the transplant, and (3) determining the potential for survival of a transplant (Andrews et al., 1996, p. 302).

Organ donations are coordinated through regional transplant centers. Although the center may look to the recipient who is first on the list, there are other criteria. A committee, composed of a doctor, nurse, lawyer, religious leader, and expert layperson, may make the decision about who will be placed on the transplant recipient list. This committee may be supervised by a neutral organization, such as the Red Cross. The committee may consider (1) the priority of need, usually those who are dying; (2) the best potential for survival or those who do not have other debilitating diseases, such as emphysema (Andrews et al., 1996, p. 303); (3) the value of the recipient to the community (for example, James Earl Ray, who was convicted of assassinating Dr. Martin Luther King, did not receive a liver transplant because he was a convict); and (4) whether or not the intended recipient has received other transplants (Andrews et al., 1996, p. 304).

HIV/AIDS

A variety of ethical issues surround the patient with human immunodeficiency virus (HIV) or acquired immunodeficiency syndrome (AIDS). These issues relate to (1) the nurse as carrier of HIV, (2) the patient as carrier of HIV, (3) and the prevention of the transmission of HIV.

THE NURSE WITH HIV

Currently, no law mandates the testing of the nurse who is HIV positive, but ethical issues of autonomy versus beneficence and nonmaleficence may arise as to the nurse's duty to protect the patient from unreasonable risk of exposure to disease. The nurse must be especially aware of the duty to protect the patient when conducting an **exposure-prone procedure**, defined as an invasive procedure that may directly expose or risk transmission of a disease to the patient (Murphy, 1995, p. 145).

The nurse may be asked to voluntarily be tested for exposure to contagious diseases in the case of accidental exposure to contaminated body fluids, such as with a pin prick. Or the testing may be a requirement of employment, such as for those working with populations for which there is a higher duty to protect from unreasonable risk of exposure to contagious diseases (Murphy, 1995, p. 146).

Nurses with HIV may continue to work in patient care areas, but have a duty to follow specific practice restrictions. These restrictions include (1) following universal precautions, (2) performing only noninvasive procedures, (3) doing invasive procedures that do not cause exposure of the patient, (4) working in emergency situations, and (5) providing services to HIV patients, including those that cause exposure (Murphy, 1995, p. 147).

The nurse with HIV is protected from employment discrimination under the Americans With Disabilities Act of 1990, unless the nurse is unable to do the job. The nurse with HIV is further protected from employment discrimination under the Rehabilitation Act of 1973 when employed at any facility receiving Medicare funds (Murphy, 1995, p. 149).

Any decisions regarding the nurse's right to work is made by an expert review panel, whose proceedings are strictly confidential. All records are kept in the nurse's medical file, not the employee file (Murphy, 1995, p. 150).

THE PATIENT WITH HIV

A number of patient care issues also arise when caring for the patient who is HIV positive. These issues relate to (1) mandatory testing, (2) the use of universal precautions, and (3) refusal to provide nursing care.

Other than diagnostic testing for HIV, a patient may be asked to test for AIDS only in two situations: (1) the patient will undergo diagnostic testing that may expose the health care provider to HIV, and/or (2) the health care provider believes he or she may have been exposed to HIV by contamination with the patient's body fluids. In the event either nurse or patient test positive for HIV, neither can be told until face-to-face counseling is available (Murphy, 1995, pp. 150–151).

Universal precautions must be used when working with the patient with HIV. This involves using gloves, gowns, and goggles to prevent contact with body fluids. According to Andrews et al. (1996, p. 310), few nurses follow the use of universal precautions, unreasonably exposing themselves and their patients to the risk of HIV.

Nurses may refuse to care for the HIV patient, based on religious values and/or fear of contacting the disease. Although the American Nurses Association Code for Nurses, (1985) (see Appendix 4–C) instructs the nurse to care for the patient, regardless of health problems, the duty to care for the HIV patient is not absolute. According to Andrews et al. (1996, p. 310), when deciding whether or not to provide care for the HIV patient, the nurse may ask "If the risk . . . is greater than the potential benefit to the patient, [then] . . . ethically refuse to take that risk."

SURROGATE MOTHERHOOD

A **surrogate mother** is one who carries for another an artificially implanted embryo or an embryo that has been created by artificial insemination by the sperm of a donor. Ethical issues related to surrogate motherhood are becoming more common, although they are generally specific to nursing settings that provide obstetrical and gynecological care. These ethical issues are generally related to (1) a conflict of parental rights, (2) parental rejection of the child, (3) exploitation of surrogate mothers, and (4) lack of clarity in the governing laws.

Courts may refuse to enforce a surrogacy agreement, if the surrogate mother decides she wants to keep the child. In the case of *R.R. v. M.H.* (1998), from the state of Massachusetts, R.R. negotiated a surrogacy contract with M.H. (1) to be inseminated with his sperm and carry the baby to term; (2) to give R.R. full parental rights; (3) to allow R.R. to take the child home from the hospital to live with him and his wife, and consequently M.H.'s parental rights would not be terminated; (4) for periodic monetary payments, from conception to birth; (5) to enforce her parental rights via court order; and (6) to reimburse R.R. for all expenses, if M.H. sought custody or visitation rights (*R.R. v. M.H.*, 1998; "Surrogate Parenting," 1998).

M.H. decided she wanted to keep her baby at the sixth month of pregnancy. She returned a portion of the money given to her by R.R. After the birth of the child, R.R. sued M.H. (1) to establish his paternity, (2) for breach of contract, and (3) as declaration of his rights under the surrogacy agreement (*R.R. v. M.H.*, 1998).

In Massachusetts, ". . . consent [for adoption] . . . is not to be executed 'sooner than the fourth calendar day after the date of birth of the child to be adopted'" ("Surrogate Parenting," 1998, p. 252). Further, the state of Massachusetts prohibits the sale of a child for adoption.

The Massachusetts Supreme Judicial Court refused to enforce the surrogacy agreement, because (1) the surrogate mother was not allowed a sufficient amount of time after the child's birth to consent to loss of custody, that is, 4 days; and (2) the payment of money to the surrogate mother, for relinquishing her custody for adoption, was illegal. The Massachusetts court held the surrogacy agreement could have been enforced if it had been executed 4 days after the birth of the child. Regardless, the court noted, any payment of money for the child would have made the contract void (*R.R. v. M.H.*, 1998; "Surrogate Parenting," 1998).

Several other classic well-publicized lawsuits have arisen over conflicts between the rights to the child of the surrogate parents and the contracting parents. For example, surrogate mother Mary Beth Whitehead negotiated a financial contract with the biological father and his wife for carrying Baby M to term. Although Whitehead refused to give up the child, the child was awarded to the contracting parents by the courts, with Whitehead being given visita-

tion rights (Bandman & Bandman, 1995, pp. 133–134).

In some cases, both contracting and surrogate parents have rejected the surrogate child. For example, a contracting father rejected a deformed infant born to a surrogate mother with whom he had contracted. Biological testing revealed that the surrogate mother's husband was the father. Subsequently, both the real father and the surrogate mother rejected the child (Bandman & Bandman, 1995, p. 134).

All parties involved in issues related to surrogate motherhood are affected by the ethical dilemmas presented. All parties have rights and obligations. For example, the nurse may be caught in an ethical dilemma involving the implementation of justice, through which the courts determine the rights to access the child, and/or autonomy, or the right of the surrogate or contracting parents to either demand or refuse the surrogate child.

Surrogate motherhood is often viewed as an exploitation of the surrogate parents and/or the contracting parents. For example, the surrogate parent may be poor and desperately need the money the financial contract for the surrogate child will bring. Exploiting childless couples is an age-old problem, as these contracting parents are desperate to have a child at any cost (Andrews et al., 1996, p. 318). But some surrogate mothers are blood relatives and ask for no payment. For example, a mother may agree to carry the embryo of her daughter and her son-in-law, so that the daughter can be a mother, and the surrogate mother can become a grandmother.

Other ethical issues that arise regarding surrogate motherhood involve questions about the basic definition of parenthood, the duties and rights of parents, and providing justice, beneficence, and nonmaleficence for the child. The laws affecting the surrogate parent's and contracting parent's rights to the child vary from state to state. According to Andrews et al. (1996, p. 318), "The basic dispute centers around who has the strongest claim to the child?" The nurse may be involved in focusing the basic dispute on the rights of the child to a normal family life.

ABORTION

Abortion is the premature termination of a pregnancy. The right to have an abortion has been an issue that has drawn impassioned arguments from pro-choice/pro-abortion advocates and pro-life/anti-choice advocates. Ethical issues surrounding abortion are generally related to (1) the legal duties of the nurse, (2) the legal and moral rights and obligations of nurses, (3) the legal rights and obligations of hospitals, (4) the rights of abortion patients (Curtin, 1993, pp. 26–31), and (5) the right of the unborn fetus (Burkhardt & Nathaniel, 1998, pp. 211–212).

The legal duties of the nurse in assisting with an abortion stem from the landmark Supreme Court case *Roe v. Wade* (1973). The decision of the Supreme Court to allow abortion was directly derived from the constitutional right to privacy (Curtin, 1993, p. 26). The right to an abortion is not absolute, and, therefore, is subject to limitations designed to protect the mother's health, the standards of health care, and the life of the fetus (Curtin, 1993, p. 28; *Roe v. Wade*, 1973).

According to the Center for Disease Control and Prevention (CDC), the number of abortions in 1996 increased 0.9 percent over the number in 1995, from 1,210,883 to 1,221,585. The number of abortions had been substantially declining, by 15 percent, from the peak reached in 1990, which was 1,429,577 abortions ("Abortions Up Slightly," 1998).

The reasons for the decrease in the number of abortions, according to the CDC, include (1) reduced access to abortion, (2) changes in attitudes toward abortion, (3) fewer unintended pregnancies, (4) changes in contraceptive methods, for example, contraceptives that are more long lasting. The CDC also reported the following statistics: (1) 9 percent of women who have abortions are white, (2) 80 percent of women who have abortions are unmarried, (3) 20 percent of women who have abortions are younger than age 20, (4) 55 percent of abortions are performed during the first 8 weeks of pregnancy, and (5) 88 percent of abortions are performed in the first 12 weeks of pregnancy ("Abortions Up Slightly," 1998).

Generally, under state law, abortions are allowed during the first and second trimesters of pregnancy. Abortions may be allowed in the third trimester, only (1) to prevent serious risk to the physical and/or mental health of the mother, and/or (2) if the fetus has serious abnormalities, verified by valid diagnostic tests (Murphy, 1995, pp. 174–175).

States may have a difficult time limiting a woman's right to certain types of abortion. The state of Ohio implemented a statute that prohibited abortions performed through dilatation and extraction. This statute failed to exclude the most commonly used type of abortion, dilatation and evacuation. The Sixth U.S. Circuit Court of Appeals held the Ohio statute ". . . imposed an undue burden on a woman's Fourteenth Amendment right to obtain a pre-viability abortion" ("Abortion," 1998, p. 226; *Voinvich v. Women's Med. Professional Corp.*, 1998). The U.S. Supreme Court refused to review the decision of the Sixth U.S. Circuit Court of Appeals. In essence, the Supreme Court supported the 6th Circuit ruling, that women must have access to abortions through dilatation and evacuation, as part of a woman's right to obtain abortions before the fetus is viable ("Abortion," 1998).

According to Curtin (1993, p. 28), the Supreme Court did not create a right to abortion, but protected the decision to have an abortion under the right to privacy. The Supreme Court provided protection for the nurse's legal and moral rights and obligations regarding abortions, making them subject to that health care professional's freedom of conscience. The nurse is free to choose whether or not to assist with abortions. The public is free to choose whether or not to fund abortions. Curtin (1993, p. 28) also wrote, ". . . health-care professionals have no legal obligation to assist with or to perform abortions."

Nurses who are employed by hospitals that perform abortions have legal rights and obligations relative to the performance of this procedure. The nurse's right not to participate in an abortion procedure is not absolute, for the nurse has obligations to both the patient, as health care provider, and the hospital, as employee (Curtin, 1993, p. 28). Nurses who object to abortions must

(1) make these objections known to their supervisor in writing, (2) avoid working in those areas where abortions are performed, and (3) meet the standard of nursing care for those patients who receive an abortion (Curtin, 1993, p. 30).

As noted previously, the right of an abortion patient is specifically limited to the right of privacy to make a decision to have an abortion, not the right to have an abortion. But the abortion patient is also entitled to have informed consent about the procedure from the physician. The law does not specifically provide that the nurse may or may not give the patient information regarding the abortion procedure. The nurse may be obligated to provide information before, during, and after the procedure, under standards set down by their state board of nursing and/or national nursing associations (Curtin, 1993, p. 30).

Ethical dilemmas surrounding the rights of the fetus generally focus on the right of the mother to choose abortion versus the fetus's right to be born. Under the holding in *Roe v. Wade* (1973), the mother's right to choose is protected by law. But issues continue to be raised by pro-choice and anti-choice groups regarding the fetus's rights, including when life begins, the value of life, and the quality of life that can be expected for the unborn, unwanted child (Burkhardt & Nathaniel, 1998, pp. 211–212).

ARTIFICIAL INSEMINATION AND IN VITRO FERTILIZATION

By definition, **artificial insemination** is the insertion of a sperm into the womb of the mother via artificial methods. With **in vitro fertilization,** the sperm is inserted into the egg within the laboratory setting. Either or both the egg and sperm may be donated. Ethical issues related to artificial insemination and/or in vitro fertilization generally raise questions under the following categories: (1) who are the parents of the child; (2) what is the effect of these procedures on the integrity of the family; (3) what is the cut-off age for these procedures; (4) what happens to leftover embryos; (5) what are the effects on child

development; and (6) who should pay for these procedures?

The parentage of the child resulting from either artificial insemination or in vitro fertilization (IVF) is often not well defined under state or federal law. A state may have defined the parentage of a child resulting from artificial insemination but not from IVF. For example, in Texas, if the husband consents in writing to his wife's artificial insemination, then he is considered the father of the resulting child. But no law has been written regarding the parentage of the child that results from in vitro fertilization (Murphy, 1995, p. 174; citing Texas Family Code § 12.03).

Many ethical and religious concerns have been raised regarding the effect of artificial insemination and IVF on the integrity of the family. Arguments have been made that these artificial procedures erode the fabric of family life, by taking pleasure, respect, and love out of the act of procreation (Andrews et al., 1996, p. 316). Some religions view these artificial procedures as morally wrong, a view voiced emphatically by a Vatican speaker, who was of the opinion that "Married couples have no right to children, only the right to perform the procreative act" (Bandman & Bandman, 1995, p. 132; Berger, 1987).

With advances in technology in both artificial insemination and IVF, health care providers are forced to consider what should be the cut-off age for performing these procedures safely, for both the mother and the fetus. Most of these issues regarding age of the mother have been focused on those older than 50 years, labeling artificial conceptions within that age group as "granny pregnancies" (Bandman & Bandman, 1995, pp. 132–133).

Health care providers and the courts have been faced with decisions regarding what happens to leftover embryos. According to Andrews et al. (1996, p. 317), with a single attempt at IVF, as many as 15 to 20 embryos may result, with only three to five implanted in the mother. As the leftover embryos are frozen, the courts have been asked to decide who is responsible for these embryos. For example, in a 1989 divorce in Tennessee, the courts awarded the mother custody of seven fertilized eggs held at an IVF clinic (Andrews et al., 1996, p. 317).

Only future research will be able to determine the effects on children's development of learning they are the product of artificial insemination or IVF. Future nursing research may look to factors related to the child's identity, adjustment, feeling of security as a family member, and perception of the conception (Andrews et al., 1996, p. 317).

Because artificial insemination and IVF are costly procedures, many questions have arisen regarding who should pay for these procedures, raising issues of distributive justice. These questions arise regarding whether public funds should be provided for such costly procedures and research, when the funds benefits what is apparently only a small percentage of the population (Bandman & Bandman, 1995, p. 132). Regardless, some states provide for insurance coverage of IVF under special circumstances (Murphy, 1995, p. 174).

RIGHT TO LIVE OR DIE

Ethical issues centering on patient autonomy arise when those in the nursing profession consider the patient's right to live or die. Ethical dilemmas involving the patient's right to live or die are categorized under the issues of (1) life-saving medical treatment; (2) do not resuscitate, or DNR, orders; (3) rights of the dying patient; (4) euthanasia; and/or (5) assisted suicide.

LIFE-SUSTAINING MEDICAL TREATMENT

Life-sustaining medial treatment (LSMT) is health care used to maintain the patient's life, which may be categorized as ordinary or extraordinary. **Ordinary medical treatment** offers the patient a good prognosis, without excessive pain or expense. For example, for the dying patient in pain, analgesics are an ordinary medical treatment. **Extraordinary medical treatment**, synonymous with the term *heroic measures*, offers the patient little to no hope, with the prospect of a prolonged, expensive, and/or painful life (Andrews et

al., 1996, p. 290). For example, carrying out a DNR order on a dying patient constitutes extraordinary treatment.

According to the 1983 President's Commission for the Study of Ethical Problems in Medicine and Behavioral Research, health care professionals are not obligated to provide extraordinary life-saving medical treatment (Andrews et al., 1996, p. 290). But, Murphy (1995, pp. 175–176) advocates a multidisciplinary treatment team (MDTT) approach when decisions are made regarding the use of ordinary or extraordinary LSMT, using a two-step process. First, decisions regarding LSMT must consider patient autonomy and be based on the patient's informed consent. The patient, family, significant other, and friends should be made part of the decision-making process (Murphy, 1995). Secondly, the MDTT may need to balance the patient's right to refuse treatment against any opposing forces within society at the time, for example, (1) relevant legal issues preventing withdrawal of life support, such as whether or not actions may be viewed as assisted suicide; (2) protection of innocent third parties, such as minor children of the patient; and (3) the ability to provide humane care for the patient during death (Murphy, 1995, p. 176). A patient may wish to withdraw nutrition and hydration as an LSMT. Some states do allow the withdrawal of food and water if specified in an advance directive. But, many states have no laws, nor hospitals have protocols, regarding withholding or withdrawal of these LSMTs.

Decisions when to terminate LSMT are highly subjective and guided by ethical issues involving quality of life. Tools have been developed to guide the MDTT in predicting mortality and assist in deciding when to discontinue LSMT. One such computerized tool is called the Acute Physiology and Chronic Health Evaluation (APACHE) system (Andrews et al., 1996, p. 292).

DO NOT RESUSCITATE ORDERS

No code, do not resuscitate, or DNR orders are well defined in nursing law, standards, and protocols. A **DNR order** is an order written by the patient's physician ordering the withholding of cardiopulmonary resuscitation if the patient goes into cardiac or respiratory arrest. According to Murphy (1995, p. 188), the decision to issue an DNR order should be based on a decision of the MDTT, considering state law and hospital protocol. These protocols generally require that (1) the patient is terminally ill; (2) a written order be in the physician's medical records stating that the decision was made after consultation with the patient; and (3) a periodic review and update of the DNR order be made (Aiken, 1994, p. 111).

A **slow code** is an unwritten agreement between the members of the MDTT to respond slowly to a cardiac or respiratory arrest (Andrews et al., 1996, p. 295). This type of pact occurs when the MDTT is unable to obtain permission for a DNR order from the patient or family. Slow codes create serious ethical and legal dilemmas, as patient autonomy is in conflict with the paternalistic desires of the MDTT. Ethical conflicts regarding DNR orders may be avoided if the code status of the patient is a critical part of the MDTT's treatment plan.

RIGHTS OF THE DYING PATIENT

The rights of the dying patient generally fall into three broad areas, including right to (1) death with dignity, (2) receive the best treatment, and (3) refuse treatment. According to Bandman and Bandman (1995, pp. 278–279), the worth and dignity of the individual is uncompromisable, in life and while dying. This respect is demonstrated by treating patients in order of need, with the sickest receiving priority care. Treating the patient with respect and dignity also encompasses the right to informed consent prior to treatment or nontreatment.

Bandman and Bandman (1995, p. 279) also believe that the dying patient has a right to receive the best available treatment. Thus the patient and/or family have the right to choose extraordinary versus ordinary care, or even more aggressive therapy even in futile situations, if it is available. Regardless of the method of treatment chosen, when necessary, the MDTT must provide and follow a protocol for pain management.

Finally, dying patients have the right to refuse treatment, which does not mean that the patient should be left alone. According to Bandman and Bandman (1995, p. 279), the patient's right to refuse treatment assumes a corresponding duty by the MDTT to provide competent care and support to the patient and family while the patient is dying.

EUTHANASIA

Euthanasia means an action or inaction designed to result in an easy, painless, or good death. E.K. Dvorak (personal communication, November 22, 1998) identifies three subcategories of euthanasia. The first subcategory, **voluntary euthanasia**, occurs when the patient, after informed consent, refuses treatment. The second subcategory, **involuntary euthanasia**, results when treatment is withheld or withdrawn without informed consent. The third subcategory, **nonvoluntary euthanasia**, results when treatment is withheld or withdrawn, without knowledge of what the patient would have wanted.

Ethical dilemmas surrounding euthanasia generally involve issues related to (1) passive euthanasia, (2) active euthanasia, and (3) assisted suicide. According to E.K. Dvorak (personal communication, November 22, 1998), **passive euthanasia**, is facilitation of the patient's death by "withholding life-preserving treatment that would prolong the life of one that is terminally ill and would not survive without it." Dvorak further notes that passive euthanasia is the right to die, as defined by the courts and legislative process.

Active euthanasia is the facilitation of the patient's death by some direct intervention performed by the health care provider. **Assisted suicide** is a form of euthanasia through which another person, usually a physician, provides the patient with a means for the patient to end his or her life. Organizations have been formed that advocate the use of active euthanasia, such as the Hemlock Society (Andrews et al., 1996, p. 296).

In some states, such as Texas, actively assisting with a suicide may result in civil and/or criminal penalties (Murphy, 1995, p. 189). In other states, the right to have assisted suicide is supported and well defined. For example, in the state of Oregon patients have a legal right to assistance with suicide by a physician. But in other states the right to assisted suicide is not so well defined. In an effort to force the state of Michigan to define and provide for laws assisting suicide, Dr. Jack Kervorkian has actively and tirelessly assisted patients to commit suicide (Andrews et al., 1996, p. 296).

When examining ethical issues related to right to life or death, the patient's autonomy in choosing right to life or death is an important consideration. Encouraging the patient to prepare an advance directive may preserve the patient's autonomy.

ASSISTED SUICIDE

In *Washington v. Glucksberg* (1997) and *Vacco v. Quill* (1997), the Supreme Court held that individuals do not have a constitutional right to physician-assisted suicide. The Supreme Court held that the withdrawal of life support was not equivalent to assisted suicide. The Court noted that when withdrawing life support, the patient is passively allowed to die, rather than actively and intentionally administering a substance that would kill the patient, as in assisted suicide (Volker, 1998, p. 40). But the Supreme Court left the door open for states to individually craft appropriate legislation allowing for physician-assisted suicide, as the state of Oregon did in 1998.

The American Nurses Association (1994, p. 1) defined assisted suicide as: "making a means of suicide . . . available . . . with knowledge of the patient's intention. The patient who is physically capable of suicide, subsequently acts to end his or her own life." Volker (1998, p. 43) conducted a review of the nursing literature, identifying (1) empirical studies regarding attitudes and experiences of nurses regarding assisted suicide, and (2) ethical and legal arguments about the appropriateness of assisted suicide in nursing practice (Volker, 1998, p. 43).

One empirical study of oncology nurses revealed they were more likely to assist the suicide of a patient if (1) they had a previous, long-standing relationship, and (2) the patient had experienced prolonged, unrelieved suffering (Volker, 1998, p. 43). Another empirical study of oncology nurses, regarding criteria for participating in assisted suicide, revealed key themes, including (1) a need to know the patient's background and details in-depth, (2) respect for the patient's values and choices, and (3) a desire to stay with the patient while they died (Volker, 1998, p. 44).

A national survey of nurses was conducted regarding attitudes about the legalization of voluntary, active euthanasia. The study revealed that religious belief was the most significant variable related to a nurse's attitudes regarding active euthanasia. Another empirical study revealed that nurses are actually participating in assisted suicide (Volker, 1998, p. 45).

Nurses who opposed assisted suicide cited a variety of reasons for their position, including (1) the sanctity of life, (2) the incompatibility of suicide with traditional nursing values and ethics, (3) potential abuse by health care providers, and (4) the potential extension of the practice to vulnerable patient populations. Opponents also express the concern that, when choosing assisted suicide, the chronically and/or terminally ill patients may be reacting to (1) a treatable depression or unmanageable physical symptoms, and/or (2) a perceived duty to die, to ease family financial and emotional burdens (Volker, 1998, p. 46)

ADVANCE DIRECTIVES

An **advance directive** is a document that includes a **living will,** declaring the person's wishes regarding future health care, specifically right to live and die (see Appendix 4–A), and/or a **durable power of attorney,** which designates a person to make the health care decisions in the event the person is unable to do so (see Appendix 4–B). Issues involving advance directives generally center on implementation of the Patient Self-Determination Act on behalf of the patient, including offering the patient the opportunity to execute a living will and a durable power of attorney.

PATIENT SELF–DETERMINATION ACT

The **Patient Self-Determination Act** (PSDA) was developed to ensure that health care organizations receiving Medicare and/or Medicaid funds were advising patients of their right to refuse treatment and state law regarding advance directive (Aiken, 1994, pp. 108–109). The PSDA provides legal support for the patient's right to autonomy, by providing the patient the right to direct health care after the point the patient is unable to rationally make decisions, through a living will or providing a durable power of attorney.

Badzek, Leslie, and Corbo-Richert (1998) identified four major problems with the utilization of advance directives. The first problem involves the lack of documentation and communication of the advance directive, which results in a wide discrepancy between the patient's wishes and the doctor's end-of-life care (Badzek et al., 1998, p. 52).

The second problem involves accessibility to the patient's previously executed advance directive. This problem may be remedied if the physician has access to the document at the time of the patient's admission (Badzek et al., 1998, pp. 52–53).

A third problem is the level of the patient's knowledge regarding the advance directive. This lack of knowledge ranges from being unaware of ever having been told what an advance directive is to not remembering where the advance directive is actually located (Badzek et al., 1998, p. 53).

The final problem with advance directives is the questionable degree to which it results in patient autonomy (Badzek et al., 1998, p. 53). The suggestion is made that, with educational interventions, the physician may be more inclined to use patient preferences regarding end-of life care.

State legislatures are playing a role in promoting the patient's self-determination, as each state has a right to determine how the PSDA is implemented. State statutes generally provide immunity for health care providers who in good faith follow the patient's directives.

But state statutes do not generally provide for penalties for health care providers who do not follow the patient's directives

(Badzek et al., 1998, p. 54). States such as Alaska and Utah have financial penalties for not following the advance directive, but most courts are hesitant to impose them. Other theories of liability may arise with failure to follow the patient's advance directive, including actions for (1) battery, (2) violation of constitutional rights to privacy and liberty, (3) intentional infliction of emotional distress, (4) failure to follow hospital policies and procedures, and (5) violation of contract and consumer principles (Badzek et al., 1998, p. 54).

Badzek et al. (1998, pp. 61–62) suggest that if advance directives are ignored at great monetary cost and pain to the patient, the courts may begin to impose fines and penalties for the unwanted treatment. Badzek et al. (1998, p. 62) also suggest that advance directives may be encouraged by discounting health care insurance premiums for those with such documents.

LIVING WILL AND DURABLE POWER OF ATTORNEY

As noted previously, a living will provides advance direction for the health care provider in crucial issues related to the patient's wishes regarding health care (see Appendix 4-A). According to Aiken (1994, p. 110), the concept of the living will creates an ethical dilemma, for although it is based on informed consent, in reality, the patient is not capable of giving informed consent at the time the provisions of the living will must be implemented.

Legal and ethical dilemmas arise with or without a living will. Living wills are valid in some states, for example in Texas, under the Natural Death Act (Murphy, 1995, p. 176; citing Natural Death Act, 1992/1999). In some states, a living will must be executed with the same legal requirements as a regular will, including witnesses and a notarized signature. Although very few states do not recognize living wills, they may be used as strong evidence regarding the wishes of the incompetent patient, if the court is forced to intervene (Aiken, 1994, p. 110). Patient's often use a living will to support choices that will be controversial to the family or

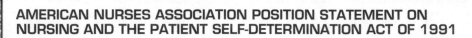

AMERICAN NURSES ASSOCIATION POSITION STATEMENT ON NURSING AND THE PATIENT SELF-DETERMINATION ACT OF 1991

The ANA recommends the following questions be asked in a nursing admission assessment:

1. Do you have basic information about advance care directives including living wills and durable power of attorney?
2. Do you wish to initiate an advance care directive?
3. If you have already prepared an advance care directive, can you provide it now?
4. Have you discussed your end of life choices with your family and/or designated surrogate and health care workers?

Source: American Nurses Association, 1991.

loved ones, such as the desire for a DNR order, organ donation, or passive euthanasia (Burkhardt & Nathaniel, 1998, pp. 210–211). Even with a living will, if families dispute and disagree with the patient's directives, the MDTT may follow the family's versus the patient's wishes.

When a patient is unable to make health care decisions and has not executed a living will, decisions are generally made by (1) referring to the patient's documented directives in the chart; (2) the parents, if the patient is a minor child (the age at which a child is emancipated and can make his or her own health care decisions is generally determined by state law); (3) the physician, alone or in consultation with the family; (4) a legal guardian, who may have been appointed by the court; (5) a person with a durable power of attorney; and/or (6) the MDTT, in collaboration with the previously mentioned parties.

The execution of a durable power of attorney (DPA) allows for a specific surrogate decision maker, appointed by the person rather than a court or selected by a physician, in the event the person is no longer able to direct his or her health care. A DPA is recognized in all 50 states, with not all states allowing the authority of the DPA to extend to health care decisions (Bandman & Bandman, 1995, pp. 284–285; see also, Appendix 4-B).

ISSUES AND TRENDS

Specific ethical issues and trends were identified within the review of the nursing literature, with a great focus on autonomy. The ethical issues and trends to be discussed in this chapter include (1) the Patient Self-Determination Act, (2) recommendations of the National Bioethics Advisory Commission on human cloning and research on the mentally ill, (3) embryonic research, (4) "safe harbor"'" laws, and (5) "whistle-blowing."

PATIENT SELF-DETERMINATION ACT

The trend in health care in general has turned to patient autonomy, because of the Patient Self-Determination Act (PSDA). The PSDA mandates the dissemination of information to patients regarding advance directives, with the idea that the patient provides written directives on health care. Nurses, as members of the MDTT, have a primary responsibility to promote informed decision-making, which includes decisions relative to advance directives (Metzey, Evans, Golub, Murphy, & White, 1994, p. 30).

To facilitate the information process identified in the PSDA, the American Nurses Association (ANA) has developed a Position Statement on Nursing and the Patient Self-Determination Act (American Nurses Association, 1991; Metzey et al., 1994, p. 31). Through this position statement, the ANA instructs the nurse to provide the patient with (1) the knowledge necessary to make treatment decisions, (2) an opportunity to express those decisions, and (3) an opportunity to receive desired treatment (Metzey et al., 1994, p. 31).

But the duties of the physician and the nurse regarding the PSDA may overlap, potentially leaving the nurse's role unclear. As the duties of the nurse are unclear, ethical issues arise regarding the implementation of the PSDA, specifically related to (1) the uncertain role of nurses in discussing advance directives; (2) whether or not the advanced directive accurately states the patient's wishes, (3) whether or not the patient has had informed consent and understands the treatment consequences of the directive, (4) whether or not the surrogate decision-maker is usurping the patient's authority, and ultimately, (5) whether the patient's advance directive is being followed (Metzey et al., 1994, pp. 30–38).

RECOMMENDATIONS OF THE NATIONAL BIOETHICS ADVISORY COMMISSION

The National Bioethics Advisory Commission (NBAC) is an organization that advises the President on bioethical issues. The NBAC has offered advice to President Clinton on the issues of human cloning and research on the mentally ill.

HUMAN CLONING

In response to an urgent request by President Clinton to consider the issue, the Chairman of the NBAC and President of Princeton University, Harold T. Shapiro, stated, "Human cloning will be 'very difficult, if not impossible, to try to stop'." Clinton made the request in response to reports that "human clones had been created by merging human

DNA with donor cow eggs" (McFarling, 1998).

Bioethics may be in a state of crisis, for scientists have not clearly considered (1) whether humans should be cloned, and (2) what the consequences are of "blending" humans with other species. Other advances have occurred that increase the likelihood of human cloning, including the scientific ability to: (1) place the DNA of one human egg into that of another human egg and (2) isolate and grow **embryonic stem cells,** "which have the power to develop into any kind of cell or tissue" (McFarling, 1998).

According to Lee Silver, a professor of genetics at Princeton University, the science of cloning is being driven with lightning speed because of market forces. Silver is of the opinion that humans are willing to spend the money it takes to buy organs that will extend their lifetime. But Silver also believes that, although the technology to clone embryos is developed, it will be years before it happens because of the unknown dangers to the child and potential for a variety of lawsuits, including wrongful birth (McFarling, 1998).

In June 1998, the NBAC recommended that no federal funds be provided to research attempting to clone embryos, and further, that any research related to human cloning be banned. But Congress did not ban cloning, because they feared such a ban may have been an unconstitutional restriction on this type of scientific research. Although federal money cannot be used for research on human cloning, private companies have invested in this research (McFarling, 1998).

RESEARCH ON THE MENTALLY ILL

The NBAC also advised the President that more protection should be provided those mentally ill involved in research. Specifically, the NBAC recommended that family and friends must be given a greater voice in the research decisions made regarding the mentally ill person and that researchers must be cautioned not to exploit persons diagnosed with dementia, schizophrenia, or delirium (McFarling, 1998).

EMBRYONIC RESEARCH

The development of embryonic research has been controlled by principles of distributive justice, because since 1995 the federal government has not financed investigations involving an embryo or fetus. But according to Dr. Harold Varmus, Director of the National Institutes of Health (NIH), who was testifying before the Senate Appropriations Subcommittee on Labor, Health and Human Services:

. . . research with human embryonic cells [is] likely to yield important [health care] benefits and should be supported by the federal government [as] . . . 'this research has the potential to revolutionize the practice of [health care] and improve the quality and length of life . . . ' (Wade, 1998).

NIH researchers also informed the Senate hearing that embryonic stem cells could be cultured and grown into and used to treat any disease of the human body, particularly Parkinson's disease and juvenile diabetes. The stem cell is a "close cousin to the fertilized egg." Although it cannot develop independently into a fetus in the womb, it is the "all-purpose genetic materials from which all of the fetus's tissues are molded" (Wade, 1998).

To date, human embryonic stem cells have been developed by two researchers supported privately by Geron Corporation: Dr. James A. Thomson, of the University of Wisconsin in Madison, and Dr. John Gearhart, of Johns Hopkins University. Most university researchers require federal funding to conduct their investigations and cannot do so without government money. Wade (1998) believes federal lawmakers will have a difficult time ignoring the potential health care cost benefits provided by embryonic stem cell research, as researchers believe that stem cells will provide (1) relief from the need for organ transplants; (2) new treatments for many other diseases, such as diabetes; (3) heart muscle cells, to treat chronic conditions such as congestive heart failure; (4) bone-forming cells, used to replace the cancer patient's bone marrow cells damaged by chemotherapy; (5) blood vessel cells, which will treat atherosclerosis; (6)

insulin-producing cells, used to treat diabetes; and (7) nerve and brain cells, which will be used to treat patients with Parkinson's disease, Alzheimer's disease, and stroke.

Embryonic stem cell therapy is not ready for public use. Researchers are still looking for answers to the following questions: (1) what are the natural signals that control the differentiation of embryonic cells in the human body; and (2) how can the embryonic stem cells be genetically manipulated to prevent stimulating the body's immune system? Treatment for Parkinson's disease by embryonic stem cells, for example, may not be available for 5 to 12 years (Wade, 1998).

Because of the similarity of the stem cell to the fertilized egg, other ethical issues have arisen related to principles of beneficence and nonmaleficence. Richard Doerflinger, of the National Conference of Catholic Bishops, cautioned that stem cells must be obtained only from the fetus that has aborted spontaneously. Doerflinger further objected to research that would either create or destroy embryos for research purposes. Dr. Thomson obtained his embryonic cells from embryos that had been created in a fertility clinic and were scheduled to be discarded. Dr. Gearhart obtained his embryonic cells from aborted fetuses. Doerflinger, who represents the Catholic position, stated that Gerhart's method may be acceptable if only applied to spontaneously aborted fetuses (Wade, 1998).

SAFE HARBOR LAWS

Through the state legislature, the nurse practice act may provide protection for the nurse who refuses to participate in acts or inactions that may potentially be detrimental to a patient. This method of statutory protection for a registered nurse (RN) is called a **safe harbor law,** under which the RN may not be suspended, terminated, disciplined, or discriminated against for refusing acts or inactions believed to be harmful to a patient (Flores, 1998).

Under safe harbor laws, the RN also has a right to request a peer review of either situations or directions that the RN believes would cause a violation of the nurse practice act. At the time the situation occurs or the direction is made, the RN tells the supervisor that the acceptance of the assignment would constitute a violation of the nurse practice act and that the RN is invoking the safe harbor provision of the nurse practice act (Flores, 1998).

The RN, as soon as possible, documents any reservations regarding the acceptance of an assignment on the appropriate safe harbor documentation form. The RN may document any suggestions for methods by which the assignment or situation may be resolved or improved. The safe harbor form then goes to the supervisor, who documents why the assignment was made. The safe harbor form is then sent to the Peer Review Committee for discussion, not as a disciplinary action, but rather for a discussion of the problem and to recommend solutions (Flores, 1998).

The RN may also ask for a determination regarding the medical reasonableness of a physician's order for a patient. In this situation, the safe harbor form goes to the medical director of the health care facility before going to the Peer Review Committee. Regardless of whether the determination concerns a nursing supervisor or physician, during the entire process, the RN is sheltered from any disciplinary action by the Board of Nurse Examiners under the safe harbor statute (Flores, 1998).

THE WHISTLEBLOWER

Whistle-blowing occurs when a nurse reveals unsafe, unethical, illegal, unprofessional, or other behaviors within an organization that may be detrimental to the patient, his or her rights, and/or delivery of health care. According to Polston (1999, p. 29), the ANA supported a variety of legislative initiatives in Congress in 1998 that would have provided legal protection to the nurse whistleblowers. None of the bills passed Congress. Polston (1999, p. 29) further suggests that any nurse considering blowing the

THE PROCESS OF ESTABLISHING A "SAFE HARBOR"

1. The RN tells the supervisor a situation and/or direction will not be accepted and why.
2. The RN tells the supervisor the safe harbor provision of the nurse practice act is being invoked.
3. The RN obtains a safe harbor form and documents the incident, explaining why the situation and/or direction was not accepted, suggesting solutions.
4. The safe harbor form is passed to the nursing supervisor, who completes the section of the form asking why the assignment was made and/or situation occurred.
5. The safe harbor form is sent by the nursing administration to the Peer Review Committee for discussion of the problem and possible solutions. The RN may also need to offer suggestions and solutions to the Peer Review Committee.
6. If the determination involves the reasonableness of a physician's order, the safe harbor form is sent to the medical director for comments on why the physician's order was medically reasonable.
7. The Peer Review Committee decides whether or not acceptance of the situation and/or assignment would have caused a violation of the nurse practice act.
8. The Peer Review Committee forwards their decision to the facility's nurse executive.
9. The nurse executive forwards the decision of the Peer Review Committee to the RN.

Source: Flores, 1998.

whistle on a colleague or organization for denying patient rights, for example under the Patient Self-Determination Act, should first contact the state nurses association to inquire about the protection provided, or lack thereof, under the state's whistleblower's law and nurse practice act.

RECOMMENDATIONS FOR RESEARCH AND MALPRACTICE PREVENTION

The purpose of this section is to identify recommendations for research and malpractice prevention in nursing ethics, by focusing on (1) directions for research in nursing ethics, (2) the Nursing Ethics Network, (3) research on utilization of advance directives, and (4) research on the bioethical change process.

DIRECTIONS FOR RESEARCH IN NURSING ETHICS

Research in the area of nursing ethics should be directed toward (1) describing ethics in nursing practice, (2) monitoring the quality and use of ethics in nursing practice, and (3) measuring the outcome of educating nursing about ethics. Descriptive research may be directed toward clarifying the mechanism for implementation of the models of ethical decision-making within nursing practice, including the previously described models of principled ethics, clinical ethics, casuistry, and feminist ethics.

Further, nurses need to monitor the quality of the ethical education the nurse is receiving, not only in undergraduate and graduate curricula, but also in the clinical area. State boards of nursing need to determine whether education in ethics should be mandatory, and if so, should this begin on the undergraduate level rather than in the clinical area. Finally, nursing needs to measure the outcome benefits of the nurse's participation in (1) ethics courses, (2) ethical case studies, and (3) ethics committees.

In dealing with ethical issues, malpractice prevention must be directed toward patient rights and nursing obligations, by (1) following nursing standards, (2) knowing state and federal laws, (3) following and or developing hospital policy and procedures, and (4) honoring the patient's bill of rights. Initially, nurses must obtain a copy of their nurse practice act and follow the standards of practice identified within the administrative law. Although the American Hospital Association has formulated a Patient Bill of Rights, specific patient rights and nursing obligations are also identified in all nurse practice acts.

In the practice area, the nurse has an obligation to be aware of the state and federal laws affecting nursing practice. If new laws fail to identify specific rights and duties, then the nurse and all members of the MDTT have a duty to initiate policy and procedure that will outline (1) the patient's rights, (2) the health care provider's responsibilities and duties, and (3) a schedule or procedure for implementation.

NURSING ETHICS NETWORK

An Internet ethics service, which is free of charge, has been developed called the Nursing Ethics Network (NEN). The NEN was developed in conjunction with the Boston College School of Nursing, through the Henry R. Luce Professorship in Nursing Ethics. The purposes of the NEN are to provide an Internet online ethical inquiry service for nurses and develop a multistate research study in nursing ethics (Riley, 1998).

ETHICAL INQUIRY SERVICE

The advisory board to NEN responds to ethical inquiries that are asked, not providing answers, but assisting in problem resolution. Thus far, NEN has provided services to a variety of nurses worldwide, practicing in a variety of settings, including (1) undergraduate, graduate, and doctoral students; (2) nurses facing complex ethical issues and decisions in the practice area; (3) nurses looking for the resources to apply ethical decision-making in their practices; and (4) researchers and educators exploring and developing a wide range of ethical principles (Riley, 1998).

ETHICAL RESEARCH

The most frequent use of NEN is for research and education. A 1998 multistate research study described the ethical issues that affect, and resulting educational needs in, nursing practice. The outcome of this ethical study is a specific agenda/curriculum in ethics for nursing education and practice (Riley, 1998).

RESEARCH ON UTILIZATION OF ADVANCE DIRECTIVES

Leslie and Badzek (1996, p. 25) conducted a retrospective chart survey from 1991 to 1994, for the purpose of examining the frequency with which the advance directives of patients were recorded when they entered a tertiary hospital or attended an outpatient clinic. Of the 58,404 admissions, only 850 had advance directives. The forms used to generate the advance directives were standard hospital forms, executed around the time of hospital admission, either the day of, or 1 to 2 days prior to admission (Leslie & Badzek, 1996, p. 28). The advance directives were generated by older populations, who were facing the following life-threatening medical diagnoses: (1) cardiovascular problems, (2) oncology-related problems, and (3) metabolic problems, such as end-stage renal disease (Leslie & Badzek, 1996, p. 32).

The implications of this study for nursing include the need to (1) find methods to both teach and learn about patient preferences in end-of-life care, (2) identify barriers to the use of advance directives, (3) become familiar with the law and trends in end-of-life care, and (4) develop mechanisms by which patient care preferences can be generated and recorded (Leslie & Badzek, 1996, pp. 28–29).

The legal implications of the study reveal that the PSDA is not generating the increase in advance directives that was anticipated. The cost of time and materials to provide patients with information on advance directives is not warranted by the small number of patients who develop an advance directive. Leslie and Badzek (1996, p. 29) suggest research questions related to the PSDA may inquire into whether or not (1) the benefits anticipated by the PSDA are being achieved, and (2) there are other more appropriate mechanisms to provide the public with information on advance directives.

RESEARCH ON THE BIOETHICAL CHANGE PROCESS

Herlik (1996, p. 64) has identified and described an eight-step process through which lawmakers in the courts and legislatures respond to advances in medical technology. Through this **bioethical change process**, clinical concepts or realities become specific ethical and legal standards. For example, through this bioethical change process, the clinical concept of **brain death** evolved into a specific legal standard.

The first step of the bioethical change process is called the bedside or clinical reality (Herlik, 1996, p. 64). For example, in the late 1950s and early 1960s, with the advent of cardiopulmonary resuscitation and technology related to respirators, neurologists and neurosurgeons were faced with the clinical reality that would be called brain death.

During the second step of the bioethical change process, the clinical reality becomes a discrete, well-defined clinical concept (Herlik, 1996, p. 65). Brain death became a discrete, clear-cut, well-defined clinical entity with specific criteria for diagnosis. The third step of the bioethical change process leads to clear implications and dilemmas within clinical practice (Herlik, 1996, p. 65). For example, brain death could be diagnosed within a short time after the initial injury. The implications of brain death are clear—it is irreversible—but ethical dilemmas arose when treatment was continued.

Eventually, the bioethical change process evolves to the fourth step, the period of paradigm clinical cases (Herlik, 1996, p. 65). For example, health care cases occurred and were presented that clearly demonstrated the well-defined clinical concept and result-

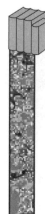

BIOETHICAL CHANGE PROCESS

1. Bedside or clinical reality
2. Discrete well-defined clinical concept
3. Clear implications and dilemmas
4. Paradigm clinical cases
5. Consensus in health care
6. Evolution of case law
7. Endorsement by interdisciplinary organizations
8. Statutory law, uniform law, and social consensus

Source: Herlik, 1996, p. 64.

ing ethical dilemmas of brain death. The case of *Tucker v. Lower* (1972) was the landmark case in which the syndrome of brain death was defined as the legal standard for death (Herlik, 1996, pp. 65–66). Paradigm clinical cases progress into the fifth step, a consensus in medicine (Herlik, 1996, p. 67). A consensus regarding the definition of brain death was rapidly reached and incorporated into standards of medical practice by the end of the 1980s.

The sixth step of the change process, the evolution of case law, overlaps with step five. For example, the medical standard of brain death is still defined and perfected as court decisions continue to evolve, change, and redefine the medical standard (Herlik, 1996, p. 71).

But in order for the bioethical concept to remain viable, under the seventh step, the concept must be endorsed by interdisciplinary organizations (Herlik, 1996, p. 71). The concept of brain death was endorsed and supported by three major organizations, including the American Bar Association, the National Conference of Commissioners on Uniform State Laws, and the President's Commission for the Study of Ethical Problems in Medicine and Biomedical Behavioral Research.

Finally, the bioethical concept evolves to the eighth step, the stage of statutory law and social consensus (Herlik, 1996, p. 71). The clinical reality of brain death evolved for

20 years, until it became the subject of uniform federal legislation, which paralleled the legal definition with the medical syndrome.

To prevent malpractice, the nurse must be aware of what stage of the bioethical change process is occurring, to know who can make the decision to resolve the dilemma. If the nurse is faced with an ethical dilemma, then according to Herlik (1996), the dilemma is at least occurring within the third stage of the bioethical change process, the stage when the implications of the dilemma are clear. For example, nurses are continually faced with ethical dilemmas regarding the implications of **medically futile treatments**, or treatments that will neither result in the patient's survival nor improve quality of life. If the patient has no advance directive, an ethical dilemma regarding medically futile treatments will most likely be resolved by the joint decision-making authority of the ethics committee, working in conjunction with the patient's family.

But if the patient has an advance directive or an assigned surrogate decision-maker, then the nurse is functioning in stage eight of the bioethical change process, a stage when statutory law must be honored. For example, if the patient has identified treatments in the advance directive considered futile and not wanted, then statutory law identified in the PSDA controls, and the patient's decision must be implemented.

SUMMARY

The major ethical principles are (1) autonomy, (2) beneficence, (3) fidelity, (4) justice, (5) nonmaleficence, and (6) veracity. These principles often come into conflict, and nurses must evaluate and weigh clinical situation to determine which principle should be given precedence. Ethical systems have been defined, including utilitarianism, deontology, and virtue ethics, which provide guidelines for making moral determinations. Ethical decisions are made in societal, institutional, and individual contexts. The most frequently used ethical decision-making models include (1) principled ethics, (2) clinical ethics, (3) feminist ethics, and (4) casuistry.

There are many areas of nursing practice in which major ethical issues arise, including (1) organ donation, (2) AIDS, (3) surrogate motherhood, (4) abortion, (5) artificial insemination and in vitro fertilization, (6) right to live or die, and (7) advance directives, including living wills and durable power of attorney. The Patient Self-Determination Act of 1990 has led to increased emphasis on the issue of patient autonomy, which underlies most ethical questions.

Future research and malpractice prevention are crucial to continue to aid nurses when making ethical decisions in clinical practice situations.

POINTS TO REMEMBER

- Key ethical principles are utilized today by nurses in making ethical decisions involving patient care.
- The three most fundamental systems within which the nurse makes bioethical decisions are classified as utilitarianism, deontology, and virtue ethics.
- Typically the nurse's analysis of bioethical dilemmas occurs in all realms, within an ethical system that may be (1) duty based, or a deontological ethical decision-making system; or (2) consequence based, or a utilitarian ethical decision-making system.

- The most common forms of ethical analysis and ethical decision-making are conducted through models called (1) principled ethics, (2) clinical ethics, (3) feminist ethics, and (4) casuistry.
- The Patient Self-Determination Act is designed to promote patient autonomy.
- Safe harbor laws are designed to protect the nurse who refuses to participate in acts considered illegal or unethical.
- Whistle-blowing laws are designed to protect the nurse who reports acts of a coworker or employer considered illegal or unethical.

REFERENCES

Abortion. (1998, April 10). *Health Law Week, 7*(15), 226.

Abortions up slightly after years of decline. (1998, December 4). *Houston Chronicle*, p. 11A.

Aiken, T. (1994). *Legal, ethical, and political issues in nursing.* Philadelphia: F.A. Davis.

American Nurses Association. (1986). *Code for nurses with interpretive statements.* Washington, DC: Author.

American Nurses Association. (1991). *Position statement on nursing and the Patient Self-Determination Act.* Kansas City, MO: Author.

American Nurses Association. (1994). *Position statement on assisted suicide.* Washington, DC: Author.

Andrews, M., Goldberg, K., & Kaplan, H. (Eds.). (1996). *Nurses legal handbook.* (3rd ed). Springhouse, PA: Springhouse Corporation.

Badzek, L., Leslie, N., & Corbo-Richert, B. (1998). An ethical perspective: End-of-life decisions: Are they honored? *Journal of Nursing Law, 5*(2), 51–62.

Bandman, E., & Bandman, B. (1995). *Nursing ethics through the life span* (3rd ed.). Norwalk, CT: Appleton & Lange.

Beauchamp, T., & Childress, J. (1994). *Principles of biomedical ethics* (4th ed.). New York: Oxford University Press.

Berger, J. (1987, October 8). Vatican official assails method of fertilization. *The New York Times*, p. B6.

Burkhardt, M., & Nathaniel, A. (1998). *Ethics and issues in contemporary nursing.* Albany, NY: Delmar Publishers.

Curtin, L. (1993, February). Abortion: A triangle of rights. *Nursing Management, 24*(2), 26–31.

Flores, K. (1998, October). "Safe harbor" offers avenue for protection from disciplinary action. *RN Update, 29*(4), 14–15.

Gilligan, C. (1982). *In a different voice.* Cambridge, MA: Harvard University Press.

Herlik, A. (1996). Medicine at the margins: Our national struggle with medically futile treatments. *Journal of Nursing Law, 3*(2), 63–84.

Jonsen, A., Seigler, M., & Winslade, W. (1986). *Clinical ethics* (2nd ed.). New York: Macmillan.

Jonsen, A., & Toulmin, S. (1989). *The abuse of casuistry: A history of moral reasoning.* Berkeley, CA: University of California Press.

Kant, I. (1959). Foundations of the metaphysics of morals. (J.W. Beck, translator). Indianapolis, IN: Babbs-Merrill.

Kozier, B., & Erb, G. (1988). *Concepts and issues in nursing practice.* Menlo Park, CA: Addison-Wesley.

Leslie, N., & Badzek, L. (1996). Patient utilization of advance directives in a tertiary hospital setting. *Journal of Nursing Law, 3*(2), 23–34.

McFarling, U.L. (1998, November 18). Human cloning called 'difficult, if not impossible to stop.' *Houston Chronicle,* p. 19A.

Metzey, M., Evans, L., Golub, Z., Murphy, E., & White, G. (1994, January/February). The Patient Self-Determination Act: Sources of concern for nurses. *Nursing Outlook, 42*(1), 30–38.

Murphy, S. (1995). *Legal handbook for Texas nurses.* Austin, TX: University of Texas Press.

Natural Death Act, Texas Health and Safety Code § 672. 001 *et seq.* (West 1992/1999).

Noddings, N. (1984). *Caring.* Berkeley, CA: University of California Press.

Polston, M. (1999, January). What's happening at the state level? *American Journal of Nursing, 99*(1), 29.

Riley, J. (1998, Second Quarter). Wired on ethics. *Reflections,* p. 32.

Roe v. Wade, 410 U.S. 113 (1973), 35 L. Ed. 2d 147, 93 S. Ct. 75, rehearing denied, 410 U.S. 959, 35 L. Ed. 2d 694, 93 S. Ct. 1409.

Ross, J., Glaser, J., Rasinski-Gregory, D., Gibson, J., & Bayley, C. (1993). *Health care ethics committees: The next generation.* Chicago: American Hospital Publishing.

R.R. v. M.H., No. SJC-07551 (Mass. Jan. 22, 1998).

Surrogate parenting. (1998, April 17). *Health Law Week, 7*(16), 251.

Tucker v. Lower, No. 831 (Richmond Va., L. & Eq. Ct., May 23, 1972).

Vacco v. Quill, 117 S. Ct. 2293 (1997).

Veatch, R., & Fry, S. (1987). *Case studies in nursing ethics.* Philadelphia: J.B. Lippincott.

Voinvich v. Women's Med. Professional Corp., No. 97-934 (U.S. Mar. 23, 1998).

Volker, D. (1998). Assisted suicide and the domain of nursing practice. *Journal of Nursing Law, 5*(1), 39–50.

Wade, N. (1998, December 3). Scientists implore Senate to support stem-cell research: Embryonic substance raises ethical issues. *Houston Chronicle,* p. 14A.

Washington v. Glucksberg, 117 S. Ct. 2258 (1997).

SUGGESTED READINGS

Broom, K. (1991, November-December). Conflict resolution strategies: When ethical dilemmas evolve into conflict. *Dimensions of Critical Care Nursing, 10*(6), 354–363.

Catalano, J. (1996). *Contemporary professional nursing.* Philadelphia: F.A. Davis.

Donaldson, S. (1998, January 7). Mystery on ward E: Nurse suspected in death of 42 vets. *Prime time live.* New York: American Broadcasting System.

Nightingale, F. (1859). *Notes on nursing: What it is, and what it is not.* London: Harrison & Sons.

INTERNET SITE

http://www. bc. edu/nursing/ethics

APPENDIX 4–A

Living Will

DIRECTIVE TO PHYSICIANS

I [name], being of sound mind, willfully and voluntarily make known my desire that my life shall not be artificially prolonged under the circumstances set forth in this directive.

1. If at any time I should have an incurable or irreversible condition caused by injury, disease, or illness certified to be a terminal condition by two physicians, and if the application of life-sustaining procedures would serve only to artificially postpone the moment of my death, and if my attending physician determines that my death is imminent or will result within a relatively short time without the application of life-sustaining procedures, I direct that those procedures be withheld or withdrawn, and that I be permitted to die naturally.
2. In the absence of my ability to give directions regarding the use of those life-sustaining procedures, it is my intention that this directive be honored by my family and physicians as the final expression of my legal right to refuse medical and surgical treatment and accept the consequences from that refusal.
3. If I have been diagnosed as pregnant and that diagnosis is known to my physician, this directive has no effect during my pregnancy.
4. This directive is in effect until it is revoked.
5. I understand the full import of this directive and am emotionally and mentally competent to make this directive.
6. I understand that I may revoke this directive at any time.
7. I wish to be an organ donor, and have as many organs as possible harvested and donated to only indigent patients. Subsequently, I wish to have my body cremated.

Declarant: _____

   City: _____

   County: _____

   State: _____

STATEMENT OF WITNESSES

I am not related to the declarant by blood or marriage. I would not be entitled to any portion of the declarant's estate on the declarant's death. I am not the attending physician of the declarant or an employee of the attending physician. I am not a patient in the health care facility in which the declarant is a patient. I have no claim against any portion of the declarant's estate on the declarant's death. Furthermore, if I am an employee of a health facility in which the declarant is a patient, I am not involved in providing direct care to the declarant and am not directly involved in the financial affairs of the facility.

   Witness: _____

   City: _____

   County: _____

   State: _____

   Telephone: _____

(continued)

Witness: _____

City: _____

County: _____

State: _____

Telephone: _____

Source: Texas Health and Safety Code §§ 672.001–.021.

APPENDIX 4–B

Durable Power of Attorney

I, [name], APPOINT: [name/address/telephone]
As my agent to make any and all decisions for me, except to the extent I state otherwise in this document. This durable power of attorney takes effect if I become unable to make my own decisions and this fact is certified in writing by my physicians.
LIMITATIONS ON THE DECISION-MAKING AUTHORITY OF MY AGENT ARE AS FOLLOWS:

_____
_____
_____

DURATION:

I understand that this power of attorney exists indefinitely from the date I execute this document unless I establish a shorter time or revoke the power of attorney. If I am unable to make decisions for myself when this power of attorney expires, the authority I have granted my agent continues to exist until the time I become able to make decisions for myself.
(IF APPLICABLE) THIS POWER OF ATTORNEY ENDS ON THE FOLLOWING DATE:
_____
(YOU MUST SIGN AND DATE THIS POWER OF ATTORNEY.)
I sign my name to this durable power of attorney on _____, 2000, at
_____(city and state).
_____
(Signature of Declarant)

STATEMENT OF WITNESSES

I declare under penalty of perjury that the principal has identified himself to me, that the principal signed or acknowledged this durable power of attorney in my presence, that I believe the principal to be of sound mind, that the principal has affirmed that the principal is aware of the nature of the document and is signing it voluntarily and free from duress, that the principal requested that I sign as witness to the principal's execution of this document, and that I am not the person appointed as agent by this document.
I declare that I am not related to the principal by blood, marriage, or adoption and that to the best of my knowledge I am not entitled to any part of the estate of the principal on the death of the principal under a will or any operation of law.
Witness Signature: _____
Print Name: _____
Date: _____
Address: _____
Telephone: _____

(continued)

Witness Signature: _____

Print Name: _____

Date: _____

Address: _____

Telephone: _____

Additional copies to:

1. _____

2. _____

3. _____

4. _____

Source: Texas Civil Practice and Remedies Code § 135.016.

DISCLOSURE STATEMENT FOR DURABLE POWER OF ATTORNEY FOR HEALTH CARE

Information Concerning the Durable Power of Attorney for Health Care

THIS IS AN IMPORTANT LEGAL DOCUMENT. BEFORE SIGNING THIS DOCUMENT, YOU SHOULD KNOW THESE IMPORTANT FACTS.

Except to the extent you state otherwise, this document gives the person you name as your agent the authority to make any and all health care decisions for you in accordance with your wishes, including your religious and moral beliefs, when you are no longer capable of making them yourself. Because "health care" means any treatment, service, or procedure to maintain, diagnose, or treat your physical or mental condition, your agent has the power to make a broad range of health care decisions for you. Your agent may consent, refuse to consent, or withdraw consent to medical treatment and may make decisions about withdrawing or withholding life-sustaining treatment. Your agent may not consent to voluntary inpatient mental health services elctro-convulsive treatment, psychosurgery, or abortion.

Your agent's authority begins when your doctor certifies that you lack the capacity to make health care decisions.

Your agent is obligated to follow your instructions when making decisions on your behalf. Unless you state otherwise, your agent has the same authority to make decisions about your health care as you would have had.

It is important that you discuss this document with your physician or other health care provider before you sign it to make sure that you understand the nature and range of decisions that may be made on your behalf. If you do not have a physician, you should talk with someone else who is knowledgeable about these issues and can answer your questions. You do not need a lawyer's assistance to complete this document, but if there is anything in this document that you do not understand, you should ask a lawyer to explain it to you.

The person you appoint as agent should be someone you know and trust. The person must be 18 years of age or older or a person under 18 years of age who has had the disabilities of minority removed. If you appoint your health or residential care provider (e.g., your physician or an employee of a home health agency, hospital, nursing home, or residential care home, other than a relative), that person has to choose between acting as your agent or as your health or residential care provider; the law does not permit a person to do both at the same time.

You should inform the person you appoint that you want the person to be your health care agent. You should discuss this document with your agent and your physician and give each a signed copy. You should indicate on the document itself the people and institutions that have signed copies. Your agent is not liable for health care decisions made in good faith on your behalf.

(continued)

Even after you have signed this document, you have the right to make health care decisions for yourself as long as you are able to do so, and treatment cannot be given to you or stopped over your objection. You have the right to revoke the authority granted to your agent by informing your agent or your health or resident care provider orally or in writing or by your execution of a subsequent durable power of attorney for health care. Unless you state otherwise, your appointment of a spouse dissolves on divorce.

This document may not be changed or modified. If you want to make changes in the document, you must make an entirely new one.

You may wish to designate an alternate agent in the event that your agent is unwilling or unable or ineligible to act as your agent. Any alternate agent you designate has the same authority to make health care decisions for you.

THIS POWER OF ATTORNEY IS NOT VALID UNLESS IT IS SIGNED IN THE PRESENCE OF TWO OR MORE QUALIFIED WITNESSES. THE FOLLOWING PERSONS MAY NOT ACT AS WITNESSES:

1. The person you have designated as your agent;
2. Your health or residential care provider or an employee of your health or residential care provider;
3. Your spouse;
4. Your lawful heirs or beneficiaries named in your will or a deed; or,
5. Creditors or persons who have a claim against you.

Source: Texas Civil Practice and Remedies Code § 135.015.

APPENDIX 4-C

American Nurses Association Code for Nurses

- The nurse provides services with respect for human dignity and the uniqueness of the client, unrestricted by considerations of social or economic status, personal attributes, or the nature of health problems.
- The nurse safeguards the client's right to privacy by judiciously protecting information of a confidential nature.
- The nurse acts to safeguard the client and the public when health care and safety are affected by the incompetent, unethical, or illegal practice of any person.
- The nurse assumes responsibility and accountability for individual nursing judgments and actions.
- The nurse maintains competence in nursing.
- The nurse exercises informed judgment and uses individual competence and qualifications as criteria in seeking consultation, accepting responsibilities, and delegating nursing activities to others.
- The nurse participates in activities that contribute to the ongoing development of the profession's body of knowledge.
- The nurse participates in the profession's efforts to establish and maintain conditions of employment conducive to high-quality nursing care.
- The nurse participates in the profession's efforts to protect the public from misinformation and misrepresentation and to maintain the integrity of nursing.
- The nurse collaborates with members of the health care profession and other citizens in promoting community and national efforts to meet the health care needs of the public.

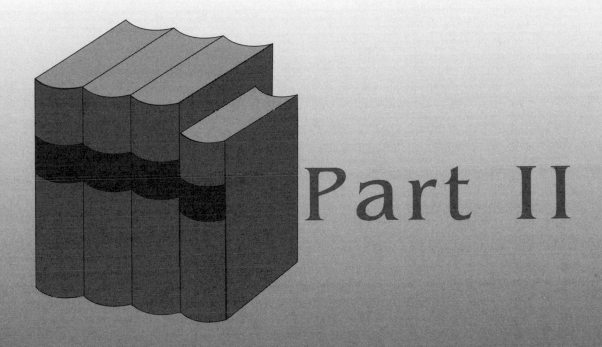

Part II

NURSING PRACTICE AND THE LEGAL SYSTEM

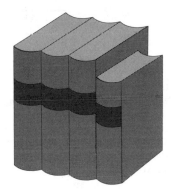

Chapter 5

DEFINING NURSING PRACTICE

Patricia Fedorka
Lenore Kolljeski Resnick

(continued)

LEGAL ISSUES OF ADVANCED PRACTICE
        NURSING
PRESCRIPTIVE AUTHORITY
CONTINUING EDUCATION REQUIREMENTS
**ADDITIONAL ADVANCED PRACTICE NURSING
        ISSUES**
    REIMBURSEMENT
    HOSPITAL (CLINICAL) PRIVILEGES
    CHALLENGES TO SCOPE OF PRACTICE ISSUES
POINTS TO REMEMBER
REFERENCES
SUGGESTED READINGS

KEY WORDS

Advanced Practice Nurse
American Board of
    Nursing Specialties
    (ABNS)
American Nurses
    Credentialing Center
    (ANCC)
Board of Nursing
Certification
Certified Nurse-MidWife
Certified Registered
    Nurse Anesthetist
Clinical Nurse Specialist
Clinical Practice
    Guidelines
Continuing Education
    Requirement
Current Procedural
    Terminology (CPT)
Department of Health
    and Human Services
Healthcare Quality
    Improvement Act of
    1986
Hospital (Clinical)
    Privileges
International
    Classification of
    Diseases, 9th Revision
    (ICD–9)

Interstate Compact for
    the Mutual Recognition
    Model on Nursing
    Regulation
Licensure
Mandatory Licensure
National Council of State
    Boards of Nursing
    (NCSBN)
Nurse Practice Act
Nurse Practitioner
Nursing
Nursing Disciplinary
    Diversion Act
Permissive Licensure
Prescriptive Authority
Primary Care Provider
    (PCP)
Protocols
Provider Number
Reimbursement
Scope of Practice
Unlicensed Assistive
    Personnel (UAP)

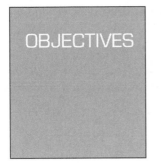

Upon completion of this chapter, the reader will be able to:
- Explain the relationship between the state nurse practice act and state boards of nursing.
- Identify actions for which a nurse could be disciplined by the Board of Nursing.
- Define advanced practice nursing.
- Discuss legal issues that have an impact on the scope of practice of the advanced practice nurse.

HISTORICAL PERSPECTIVE

For more than 90 years, nursing's struggle for recognition as an independent profession has been reflected in the development of the individual states' nurse practice acts (NPAs) and state boards of nursing (SBN). The evolution of nurse practice acts mirrored the profession's progression from the role of handmaiden status to one of an autonomous professional with legal accountability.

Education, licensure, certification, and legal parameters continue to be issues as nursing practice continues to expand reflecting society's needs and the changing health care system. The advent of the advanced practice nurse (APN) has brought to bear a whole new set of regulatory challenges.

NURSE PRACTICE ACTS

"The **nurse practice act** in any state defines nursing practice and establishes standards for nurses in each state. It is the most definitive legal statute or legislative act regulating nursing practice" (Catalano, 1996, p. 306). Each state has laws to protect the health and safety of its constituents (the public). Two national organizations, the American Nurses Association (1996c) and The National Council of State Boards of Nursing (1994), have developed and pub-

lished models to serve as guides for the individual SBN for the development and revision of their respective nurse practice acts as nursing practice expands and evolves. All 50 states, the District of Columbia, and five United States territories have their own nurse practice acts that define nursing for that particular state or jurisdiction. Normally, nurse practice acts discuss the scope of nursing in general, broad concepts that do not provide specific guidelines for nursing practice. This is done intentionally in order not to limit nurses to certain activities. Many states have practice committees or councils that decide whether specific activities are within the scope of the professional nurse.

Although the definitions of nursing and its **scope of practice** are often similar, differences exist from state to state. Therefore, each nurse is responsible for knowing the scope of practice in the state or jurisdiction in which he or she practices. This applies to a variety of nursing roles, e. g., licensed practical nurses, registered nurses, and nurses in advanced practice roles such as nurse midwives, nurse anesthetists, clinical nurse specialists, and nurse practitioners who function under an expanded scope of practice. Recognition of the advanced practice nurse skill level comes from professional certification and statutory nurse practice acts with corresponding rules and regulations (Baker, 1992).

Nursing actions that are within the scope of practice for a registered nurse may be illegal for a licensed practical nurse to perform. The same situation can occur when comparing scope of practice for an APN and a registered nurse. For example, although it is quite acceptable for an APN to have prescriptive writing privileges in many states, it is outside the scope of practice for a registered nurse to prescribe medications.

Neither physician orders nor institutional policy may take precedence over the state's nurse practice act. A nurse who acts outside of or whose actions exceed those allowed under the nurse practice act may actually be violating a state's medical practice act, which ultimately determines the scope of physician practice. The nurse may be infringing on activities that only a physician may legally perform. If this is the case, the nurse could be found in violation of both the state nurse practice act and the state's medical practice act, which is clearly a deviation from the standard of care for nurses.

However, there is a great deal of overlap between licensed professionals. Physicians, registered nurses, and practical nurses all are permitted to administer medications, implement treatments, monitor patient status, and the like under their respective practice acts.

As the nurse's role expands and changes with the health care environment, the nurse practice acts must reflect these expanding roles. Nurses must not only be knowledgeable of their current NPA but must be instrumental in working through their professional organizations to influence the state legislature for revision and updates of the NPAs when needed.

STATE BOARDS OF NURSING

"Nursing, like other professions, is responsible for ensuring that its members act in the public interest in the course of providing the unique service society has entrusted to them" (ANA, 1995, p. 17). In most states, the nursing practice act provides the legal authorization (statutory law) for their respective boards of nursing.

The American Nurses Association (ANA) provides guidelines to each state organization as to structure and functions, but each board has the power to act as an independent body and to accept or reject the recommendations as it sees fit.

The state **board of nursing** is usually given the authority to (1) prescribe regulations setting forth educational requirements and admission standards for licensure of nurses, and in some states, for advanced practice nurses; (2) delineate the tasks that

---

COMMON INFORMATION FOUND IN A NURSE PRACTICE ACT

- Definition of nursing
- Definitions of registered nurse (RN) and licensed practical nurse (LPN)
- Use of the titles RN and LPN
- Functions of boards of nursing
    - Examinations and certifications
    - Fees
    - Education programs, standards
    - Licenses: duration, renewal fee, inactive status
    - Punishments for violations
    - Impaired nurse program (diversion acts)
    - Suspensions and revocation of licenses including appeal process

nurses and advanced practice nurses are permitted to carry out either independently or in collaboration with physicians; and (3) establish criteria and administrative processes for disciplining nurses usually with authority to impose appropriate penalties (Bernzweig, 1996, p. 81).

The ANA (1985) described five models, A through E, that characterize the range of power invested in various boards. In states utilizing Model A, boards of nursing are completely autonomous with final decision-making authority on all substantive matters. However, certain board actions are subject to review and the possibility of being overridden by a central agency. At the other end of the spectrum, in states utilizing model E, the board of nursing serves only in an advisory capacity. The lack of consistency in autonomy and power afforded to boards of nursing leads to confusion among nurses as to the duties and responsibilities of these boards. In 1990 the ANA published *Suggested State Legislation: Nursing Practice Act, Nursing Disciplinary Diversion Act, Prescriptive Authority Act*. This serves as a guide for state legislation for implementation of the above-mentioned topics. Standardization between states' nurse practice acts can be of benefit to the whole nursing profession.

In addition to the ANA, the **National Council of State Boards of Nursing (NCSBN)** was established to "provide an organization through which boards of nursing act and counsel together on matters of common interest and concern affecting the public health, safety and welfare, including the development of licensing examinations in nursing." (National Council of State Boards of Nursing [NCSBN], 1998). The policy-making body of the National Council is composed of two representatives from each member board of nursing. Some of the programs and services offered by the National Council include (1) NCLEX testing for registered nurses (RNs) and licensed practical nurses (LPNs), (2) research functions including licensure and examination statistics, and (3) maintenance of a national disciplinary data bank for nurses who have had disciplinary action taken on their license. In addition, the National Council develops position papers and models addressing the regulation of nursing practice and nursing education (NCSBN, 1998).

Although the ANA recommends that one state board of nursing regulate both practical and registered nurses, there are still five states that have separate boards for registered and practical nurse regulation: California, Georgia, Louisiana, Texas, and West Virginia (NCSBN, 1998).

COMPOSITION

As stated previously, 50 states, the District of Columbia, and five U.S. territories have boards of nursing. Five of the states have two boards of nursing, one for registered nurses and a separate board for LPNs/LVNs.

The composition of the boards of nursing varies, but the majority of states have the members appointed by the governor. Suggestions for members can come from the general public or individual nurses or nursing organizations. The total number of board members ranges from 5 to 19 (Kelly & Joel, 1996). The number of registered nurse members on each board varies from one to nine; the majority of boards have five RN members. Those boards that have jurisdiction over LPNs have one to four LPN members, most having two. Also, most boards have a representative from the general public; both the ANA and the NCSBN support this practice. There can be a variety of other members such as physicians and commissioners. North Carolina is the only state where the board members are elected by other nurses. Qualifications of board members vary greatly, and in many states United States or state residency is not mandatory. Many board members serve for an 8-year term (ANA, 1985).

REGULATION OF EDUCATIONAL INSTITUTIONS

From 1880 to 1910 the number of nursing schools mushroomed from 15 to 1023. Unfortunately, many of the schools provided no formal education for their students. Instruction was inadequate and carried out by utilizing the apprenticeship method of train-

REQUIREMENTS FOR APPLICANTS SEEKING LICENSURE

- The applicant must have completed an educational program in a state-approved school of nursing and successfully completed the requirements resulting in the award of a degree or diploma. The school normally is required to submit an official transcript. (Only North Dakota requires the baccalaureate degree for RN licensure and the associate degree for LPN licensure.)
- The applicant must pass the NCLEX-RN, developed under the auspices of the National Council of State Boards of Nursing for administration in all states. A computerized test is now offered.
- Some states require evidence of good mental and physical health. These requirements vary, and there are some exceptions for some disabilities.
- Most states demand a statement that the applicant be of good moral character, but this requirement is vague and difficult to enforce.
- A fee must be paid prior to admission to the licensing examination. This fee varies from state to state.
- Some states will issue a temporary license to a graduate of an approved program pending the results of the first attempt at the licensure examination.
- Competence in English is a new recommendation in some states (requirements of age, citizenship, and residence have been ruled unconstitutional).

Source: Kelly & Joel, 1995.

ing. Apprenticeship, with its many disadvantages, was being abandoned by other professions in favor of more formalized, standardized curricula. The large numbers of substandard schools with inadequate curricula not only resulted in incompetent practitioners but hindered the development of nursing as a profession. Early on, both the ANA and the National League of Nursing (NLN) fought for state regulation over nursing programs by seeking a formal accreditation process.

Because one of the charges to the boards of nursing is to protect the public from incompetent practitioners, most state boards of nursing regulate, to some degree, the schools of nursing in their respective states. Most boards determine educational standards for all undergraduate programs, graduate programs, and continuing education and re-

fresher courses. In many states, the SBN sets the criteria for advanced practice nurses to function (Pearson, 1998). These include education preparation, practice experience, and certification by a professional organization (ANA, 1994, p. 3). Nurses must apply for approval to practice as an APN. In some states, renewal of license may require that the nurse hold national certification (Pearson, 1998).

In addition to requiring NLN accreditation, 56 boards of nursing approve the basic education programs in their states (NCSBN, 1996). These standards can be broad or specific as to number and content of courses. The criteria that must be met serve to ensure minimum standards for nursing education (Aiken & Catalano, 1994). These standards serve as a basis for consistent, educationally sound, nursing curricula in the attempt to produce competent practitioners as well as assessing minimum competencies based on the state's nurse practice definition of nursing.

The SBN can also set educational requirements for the renewal of license and reentry into practice. *The Journal of Continuing Education in Nursing* conducts a yearly survey of all SBNs and selected national professional nursing organizations and certifying boards. The 1998 survey ("Annual Survey," 1998) reported that 34 of 62 states and territories have no continuing education requirements for renewal of licensure. The remaining 28 states and territories have requirements that range from 15 hours of continuing education in Massachusetts to 45 hours of continuing education in Iowa. Indiana specifies that the topics of AIDS and domestic violence be covered for renewal. The requirements for reentry into practice vary as well. Some states require a certain number of hours of didactic and/or clinical hours and retaking the NCLEX examination. The wide variation in requirements is another example of the autonomy of boards of nursing.

REGULATION OF PRACTICE

The entry of practitioners into the profession is an important regulatory aspect of the boards of nursing. Although variations exist, according to Kelly and Joel (1995) most states have many common requirements for applicants seeking licensure.

PROCESS FOR DISCIPLINARY HEARINGS

Filing of the Sworn Complaint
Individual complaint
Health care agency complaint
Professional organization complaint

Review of the Complaint
Notice of hearing to the involved nurse
Hearing before the board of nursing or state officer
Evidence presented by board and nurse
Witnesses called by board and nurse
Decision by the board of nursing

Disciplinary Action
If found not guilty of misconduct, no action is taken by the board of nursing.
If found guilty of misconduct, the board of nursing may:

Issue a reprimand, public or private
Place the nurse on probation
Deny the renewal of licensure
Suspend the nurse's license
Revoke the nurse's license
Allow the nurse to enter a diversion program

Court Review
Review of the board decision and concur with its finding
Order a new trial
Appeal to a higher court

Source: Guido, 1997, p. 198.

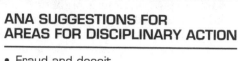

**ANA SUGGESTIONS FOR
AREAS FOR DISCIPLINARY ACTION**

- Fraud and deceit
- Criminal activity
- Negligence, risk to clients, and physical or mental incapacity
- Violation of the nursing practice act or rules
- Disciplinary action by another jurisdiction
- Incompetence
- Unethical conduct
- Drug and alcohol use

Penalties should be commensurate with the infractions, but SBNs are not held to national guidelines for imposing fines or penalties. The most common reasons for license revocation is drug abuse and theft.

Source: ANA, 1990.

ADMINISTRATIVE PROCEEDINGS

Although the SBN has a duty to protect the public from incompetent practitioners, the nurse has rights in the disciplinary proceedings. The process of disciplining nurses is fairly consistent from state to state, although variations can exist.

After a complaint is filed, the board usually investigates the complaint prior to taking any action, unless extreme danger to the public exists. Even where the law permits summary suspension of a nurse's license, the licensee has the right to exercise due process rights.

DISCIPLINARY HEARINGS

The nurse must be notified in advance of the complaint filed against him or her. The time and place of the hearing must also be provided to the nurse well in advance. The disciplinary hearing is held to review the charges of the nurse's unprofessional conduct. This hearing is less formal than the trial process, and the nurse is allowed to present evidence and witnesses and to be presented by legal counsel. The hearing takes place before the authorized group as designated in the state's nurse practice act.

Depending on the severity of the charges, the board of nursing may deny, revoke, suspend, limit, or impose conditions on a license. No action can be taken if the complaint is unsubstantiated.

The nurse has the right to appeal the board's decision. This is done by appeal or judicial review by full board or state court, depending on the state's nurse practice act.

TRADITIONAL DISCIPLINARY PROVISIONS

There have been many changes in state legislation in recent years in regard to disciplining nurses. The ANA recommends that SBNs have the ability to protect the public from incompetent practitioners by having the power to enforce recommended disciplinary acts ranging from public or private reprimands, deny application for a license, suspend, restrict or revoke a license, or require a nurse to submit to care or counseling, participate in a program of education, or practice under supervision (ANA, 1990). According to the ANA (1990), the areas addressed by the nurse practice acts for disciplinary action should include, but are not limited to, those listed in the following box.

DISCIPLINARY DIVERSION ACTS

The ANA has been a proponent of offering addicted nurses an alternative to traditional disciplinary action. In 1990, the ANA published suggested state legislation that included a **Nursing Disciplinary Diversion Act**. This act provides a diversion procedure as a voluntary alternative to traditional disciplinary action, creates a rehabilitative evaluation committee, and defines the powers and duties of that committee. Failure of the nurse to comply with committee recommendations can result in traditional disciplinary procedures such as license revocation. All proceedings and records remain confidential, and barring any relapse, records are destroyed after 5 years. There is immunity for any person providing information related to the nurse's functioning and compliance with the rehabilitation program (Aiken & Catalano, 1994).

NATIONAL PRACTITIONER DATA BANK (NPDB)

As discussed previously, SBNs lack consistency in how the issues of negligence and incompetence issues are handled. This was also an issue for the state boards of medicine. Seldom did incompetent practitioners lose their license, and if a practitioner had his or her license revoked, he or she could simply move to another state and apply for a new license. Most state licensure bodies did not verify whether health care providers had sanctions imposed on them in another state. This lack of regulation resulted in complaints from the public and health care providers that the public was not being protected from incompetent practitioners. To address this void, the U.S. Congress enacted the **Healthcare Quality Improvement Act of 1986**, which was implemented on September 1, 1990. The intent was to provide positive

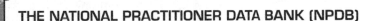

THE NATIONAL PRACTITIONER DATA BANK (NPDB)

The data bank supplies three different types of data:
1. Information relating to medical malpractice payments made on behalf of health care practitioners
2. Information relating to adverse actions taken against clinical privileges of physicians, osteopaths, or dentists
3. Information concerning actions by professional societies that adversely affect membership

The types of information reported:
1. *Required:* Adverse professional review actions against physicians, osteopaths, and dentists
2. *Required:* Medical malpractice payments made on behalf of all health care providers
3. *Optional:* Adverse professional review actions against other health care providers, including nurses

The NCSBN maintains a national disciplinary data bank that contains the names of nurses who have had any type of disciplinary action taken against their licenses. Only a SBN has access to this data to be used in the licensing process.

Source: Aiken & Catalano, 1994.

incentives, participation, and peer review in the form of good faith immunity for those providing information to the data bank. The data bank information is available upon request to hospitals and health care providers engaged in credentialing (Culbertson, 1991). Failure to report mandatory information to the data bank carries fines and penalties.

NURSING LICENSURE

Before **mandatory licensure**, anyone could call himself or herself a "nurse" regardless of what, if any, educational background they possessed. This lack of regulation caused confusion among the public as to the ability and role of the nurse in providing health care.

One of the earliest goals for both the ANA and NLN was to seek mandatory state licensure for regulation of practice. Physicians had early on recognized the importance of regulation, and by 1895 all states had state medical practice acts that defined medical practice. Therefore, when nursing attempted to define its practice, nursing could not assume functions that were already identified by physicians as "independent medical practice."

The first licensure laws were weak because of the lack of a definition of nursing, minimal educational requirements, and adequate nursing representation on nursing boards. By 1946, 10 states had a definition of nursing as part of their licensure statement. In 1955, the ANA presented a definition of nursing that became the basis for many of the nurse practice acts (ANA, 1955).

DEFINITION OF NURSING

The practice of professional **nursing** means the performance for compensation of any acts involving:

- The observation, care, and counsel of the ill, injured, or infirm, or
- The maintenance of health or prevention of illness of others, or

- The supervision and teaching of other personnel, or
- The administration of medication and treatments as prescribed by a licensed physician or dentist;
- Requiring substantial specialized judgment and skill and
- Knowledge and application of principles of biological, physical, and social science
- But not acts of diagnosis or prescription of therapeutic or corrective measures.

This definition served as the basis for the role of nursing for more than two decades. However, by 1970, the definition was too restrictive because of the expanded roles and increased responsibilities that nurses were assuming. Therefore, in 1981, the ANA published an updated definition, which was much less restrictive, to serve as the basis for amending state nurse practice acts (ANA, 1981). In 1990, the ANA published a revised model nursing practice act, which again updated the definition of nursing, which includes "the performance of services for compensation in the provision of diagnosis and treatment of human responses, the health or illness. This practice includes, but is not limited to:

- Assessment, diagnosis, planning, intervention, and evaluation of human responses to health or illness
- The provision of direct nursing care to individuals to restore optimum function or achieve a dignified death
- The procurement, coordination, and management of essential client resources
- The provision of health counseling and education
- The establishment of standards of practice for nursing care in all settings, including the development of nursing policies, procedures, and protocols for specific settings
- The direction of nursing practice, including delegation to those practicing technical nursing
- The supervision of those who assist in the practice of nursing
- Collaboration with those who assist in the practice of nursing
- The administration of medication and treatments as prescribed by those profes-

EVOLUTION OF NURSING LICENSURE

1889 U.S. Supreme Court decision held that occupational licensing laws were valid for states to regulate (Dent v. West Virginia, 1888).

1895 All states had state medical practice acts.

1903 North Carolina enacted the first permissive licensure act. Earliest registration laws lacked consistency from state to state. Nonregistered nurses were not prohibited from practicing nursing, only from identifying themselves with the term *registered nurse*. Nursing practice was not defined.

1915 *ANA drafted its first model nurse practice act.*

1923 Forty-eight states along with Hawaii and the District of Columbia enacted permissive licensure laws. One did not have to register, and one could not use RN unless one had registered.

1938 New York established mandatory licensing. Now in addition to not using RN, one could not call oneself a nurse or practice as a nurse without being licensed.

1946 Ten states had definitions of nursing in the licensing act.

1950 First year the same national examination was used for licensure purposes.

1987 First year that North Dakota mandated a BSN for RN licensure and AD for LPN licensure.

1994 Computer testing initiated.

1998 Utah became the first state to sign into law the Nursing Regulation Interstate Compact Act (implemented on January 1, 2000).

sionals qualified to prescribe under the provision of applicable state statute." (ANA, 1990, pp. 8–9)

NURSING REGULATION INTERSTATE COMPACT ACT

In 1997, the NCSBN developed the **Interstate Compact for the Mutual Recognition Model on Nursing Regulation** to address the problems encountered with individual state licensing. Under this act, nurses receive their license in their state of residence; however, they would be permitted to practice nursing in any state that has adopted the Compact as long as nurses adhere to the applicable NPA in the state in which they practice. This permission to practice in states outside the state in which the nurse received his or her license allows nursing practice to cross state lines through technology such as video conferencing and telenursing. On March 14, 1998, Utah was the first state to adopt the Nursing Regulation Interstate Compact Act as law, implemented on January 1, 2000. Many states were expected to introduce this mutual recognition of licenses in their respective legislatures in 1999 (Romig, 1998).

Over the years, through use of the legislative process, nursing gained recognition as an independent profession with its own practice and standards, with responsibility and accountability for its own actions. Several states issue a second license that statutorily defines the scope of practice of the APN (Pearson, 1998). The debate over second licensure versus certification as the means to standardize the regulatory aspect of the APN has not been resolved (Andreoli & Dvorak, 1993; Havens, 1992; Kraus, 1992; Smreina, 1993).

UNLICENSED ASSISTIVE PERSONNEL

As discussed previously, nursing's scope of practice is outlined in general terms in the state's nurse practice act, which contains a definition of nursing. With this in mind, the question arises as to how nurses can effectively utilize **unlicensed assistive personnel (UAP)**. Nurses are very aware of the effects of managed care on the health care delivery system. As a result of economic constraints, health care systems are utilizing more and more UAP in an attempt to contain costs. According to the Bureau of Labor Statistics, in 1994, there were 1,259,100 UAP in the United States, with approximately 306,000 in hospital settings and 643,080 in nursing homes. These figures were projected to increase 33 percent by the year 2000, with an even greater increase in the home health field. Because of the close working relationship and the ultimate responsibility of the nurse for patients' outcomes, the registered nurse is the most logical person to supervise these workers (ANA, 1996a).

When considering which task to delegate, the ANA (1996a) encourages nurses to be well acquainted with their state's nurse practice act because no nursing activity can be delegated if the task requires nursing knowledge, judgment, and skill. Some of these activities would include the initial nursing assessment and any subsequent assessment or intervention that requires professional nursing knowledge. Some factors a RN should consider before delegation to an UAP are:

- An assessment of patient condition
- Capabilities of the UAP

- Complexity of the nursing task
- The amount of supervision the RN will be able to provide
- The available staff assigned to accomplish the unit workload

Nurses must be able to differentiate between appropriate and inappropriate delegation of tasks. The nurse must use his or her professional judgment when delegating, and the ANA (1996a) encourages nurses to be educated in the art of delegation. This is in recognition of the fact that many nurses are not exposed to delegation procedures in their basic nursing curriculum and are unfamiliar with the process. Appropriate delegation is a learned activity.

In addition to the ANA, the NCSBN have also published several publications that address the use of UAP and appropriate delegation of tasks (NCSBN, 1998).

ADVANCED PRACTICE NURSING

ADVANCED PRACTICE NURSE

According to the ANA, "Advanced practice registered nurses manifest a high level of expertise in the assessment, diagnosis, and treatment of complex responses of individuals, families, or communities to actual or potential health problems, prevention of illness and injury, maintenance of wellness, and provision of comfort" (ANA, 1996b, p. 2). The American Association of Colleges of Nursing (AACN) gives the following definition: "**Advanced Practice Nurse** is an umbrella term appropriate for a licensed registered nurse prepared at the graduate degree level as either a Clinical Specialist, Nurse Anesthetist, Nurse-Midwife, or Nurse Practitioner" (AACN, 1994).

The advanced practice nurse is prepared at the master's or doctoral level of education with concentration in a specialized area of nursing practice and clinical practice supervision during the graduate program of studies (ANA, 1996b; AACN, 1994). In addition, "advanced practice registered nurses who have completed an accredited or approved educational program to prepare them for their advanced role prior to the implementation of graduate level education in their specific area of advanced practice are considered to have met the educational requirements for advanced practice" (ANA, 1996b, p. 2).

Although the advanced practice nurse performs many of the interventions that are basic to nursing practice, the advanced practice role involves a "greater depth and breadth of knowledge, a greater degree of synthesis of data, and complexity of skills and intervention" (ANA, 1996b, p. 2). Boundaries and intersections that define scope of practice for the advanced practice nurse include state licensure, regulations in regard to specialized practice, and educational requirements mandated by the professional organization (Baker, 1992). Development of national standards for the advanced practice role presents a challenge because of differences between states in scope of practice legislation for advanced practice nurses. Some states have no requirement for advanced practice nurses to work with, or have supervision or collaboration with, a physician, whereas other states require the advanced practice nurse to work in collaboration with a physician, or work according to protocols that have been developed by a committee of physicians and nurses (Pearson, 1998). In several states, both nursing and medicine have joint regulation of advanced practice nurses (Pearson, 1998). Three states have no reference to the advanced practice nurse role (Pearson, 1998, p. 16). Other states require that advanced practice nurses attain national certification in their specialty area. An estimated 162,000 registered nurses are prepared as advanced practice nurses (Division of Nursing, 1997, p. 18).

CLINICAL NURSE SPECIALIST

As an expert clinician in a specialty nursing area, the **clinical nurse specialist** (CNS) may work in a variety of settings and function in a variety of roles that may include direct client care, education, research, consultation, and client advocacy (ANA, 1996b). Roles may include the coordination of care for a specific client population (such as the care of clients with diabetes or cardiovascular disease), client teaching, psychotherapy, and conducting support groups (Elder & Bullough, 1990). In the role of providing direct client care, the clinical nurse specialist is involved in assessing, diagnosing, planning, and managing care that may include the prescribing of nonpharmacological and pharmacological treatment of health problems in addition to providing health promotion and disease prevention interventions (ANA, 1996b). Historically, the role of the clinical nurse specialist has included that of change agent and advocate for quality of care improvement (Baer, 1999).

NURSE PRACTITIONER

"The **nurse practitioner** is a skilled health care provider who utilizes critical judgement in the performance of comprehensive health assessments, differential diagnosis, and the prescribing of pharmacologic and non-pharmacologic treatments in the direct management of acute and chronic illness and disease" (ANA, 1996b, pp. 3–4). The role of the nurse practitioner includes health promotion and the prevention of injury and illness. Nurse practitioners are prepared with specializations in such areas as family health, women's health, adult health, gerontology, pediatrics, neonatology, school health, mental health, home care, and acute care nursing (American Academy of Nurse Practitioners, 1993). In addition to being responsible for direct health care management of clients, the nurse practitioner may also be involved in research, education, and influencing public policy (American Academy of Nurse Practitioners, 1993; ANA, 1996b).

Nurse practitioners may work autonomously or as a resource to interdisciplinary health care teams (American Academy of Nurse Practitioners, 1993; ANA, 1996b). With changes in health care, boundaries between the role of nurse practitioner and clinical specialist are becoming less obvious (Schroer, 1991; Soehren & Schumann, 1994). Educational preparation of the nurse practitioner and clinical specialist is similar, yet practice settings may differ (Forbes, Rafson, Spross, & Kozlowski, 1990). A major function of the role of the nurse practitioner is to increase primary care access. Although nurse practitioners tend to deliver primary care to communities, families, and individuals (American Academy of Nurse Practitioners, 1993), changes in health care along with increased levels of acuity in hospitals have extended the nurse practitioner's role into tertiary care settings (Richmond & Kean, 1992).

NURSE ANESTHETIST

The **certified registered nurse anesthetist** (CRNA) is responsible to administer anesthesia and to provide "anesthesia-related care, including performance of preanesthetic preparation and evaluation; anesthesia induction, maintenance, and emergence" (ANA, 1996b, p. 3). In addition, the CRNA may assist with acute and chronic pain management; acute and chronic ventilation problems, and emergency resuscitation (American Association of Nurse Anesthetists, 1998). The scope of practice for the CRNA is outlined in the American Association of Nurse Anesthetists (AANA) Scope and Standards for Nurse Anesthesia Practice (AANA, 1998). "The practice of anesthesia is recognized as a specialty in both nursing and medicine" (AANA, 1998). Currently, all states have legal recognition for CRNA, and most states recognize the nurse anesthetist as an APN (Mannino, 1996). Nurse anesthetists work independently or with physicians in ambulatory outpatient surgical centers, in hospital operating rooms, and in dentists' offices (Moore, 1993). Although nurses have administered anesthesia for nearly a century, controversy as to APN role and the illegal practice of medicine continues (Mannino, 1996). Approximately 80 percent of CRNAs collaborate with anesthesiologists, and approximately 20 percent collaborate with surgeons and work alone as anesthesia providers (AANA, 1998). In addition to the clinical role of client care, a CRNA may be involved in administrative, educational, and research activities. Some CRNAs become specialized in such areas as pediatric, obstetrical, dental,

neurosurgical, and cardiovascular anesthesia (AANA, 1998). The AANA acts as a certifying body and accredits nurse anesthesia education programs (Mannino, 1996).

CERTIFIED NURSE-MIDWIFE

The **certified nurse-midwife** (CNM) is an advanced practice nurse who "is prepared with the judgement and skills necessary for the management of care of women and newborns" (ANA, 1996b, p. 3). According to the American College of Nurse-Midwives (ACNM), the certified nurse-midwife is "educated in the two disciplines of nursing and midwifery" (ACNM, 1997a). The certified nurse-midwife practices according to the professional standards of the ACNM. In addition to the autonomous management of the care of healthy newborns and women throughout childbearing, the certified nurse-midwife manages the primary care of healthy women seeking contraception and well gynecological care throughout the life span (ACNM, 1997a). Although autonomous, the nurse-midwife practices with medical collaboration and consultation and referral as indicated (ACNM, 1997c). CNMs work in a variety of settings, including the hospital, home, and birthing centers (ACNM, 1997b).

Most states require that CNMs work under physician supervision in the management of uncomplicated pregnancies and childbirth (Moore, 1993). Although statutory laws vary greatly regarding licensing and practice (Suarez, 1993), the practice of nurse-midwifery is legal in all 50 states and the District of Columbia (ACNM, 1998). Maryland, Ohio, West Virginia, and Wisconsin are the only four states to statutorily define midwifery as a function of nursing, making the practice of midwifery by nonnurses illegal (Suarez, 1993).

Standards for practice have been the responsibility of the two largest midwifery organizations in the country, the American College of Nurse-Midwives and the Midwives Alliance of North America (Suarez, 1993). Standards for certified nurse-midwife education programs at both the certificate and degree level have been set by the ACNM since 1962. As of June 1999, the American College of Nurse-Midwives Division of Accreditation (ACNM DOA) requires that for all ACNM DOA–accredited programs of studies a baccalaureate degree either is an admission prerequisite or is granted at the completion of the program of studies (ACNM, 1998).

PROTOCOLS

Not all states require nurse practitioners to have written protocols for practice (Pearson, 1998). Because **protocols** tend to contain medical diagnoses and treatment aspects of care, they are a way for physicians to delegate certain medical tasks, place limits on the scope of practice of the advanced practice nurse, and define responsibilities of the advanced practice nurse and the physician (Courtney, 1997). These required protocols are distinguished from **clinical practice guidelines** or guidelines for practice that are not mandated by the state for the advanced practice nurse to function. Advanced practice nurses must be aware of what parts of their practice, if any, are required by their state law to have written protocols. Protocols that are required by state legislation to be developed and implemented jointly with a collaborating physician may impede the autonomous practice of the advanced practice nurse (Courtney, 1997).

Only identified steps in the protocol can be followed when working within an established relationship with a physician. For example, if protocols are required by the state in which an advanced practice nurse functions, the advanced practice nurse must follow them and be very clear in the documentation if she or he does not choose to follow the criteria as written in the protocol. Protocols should contain medical aspects of care and not decisions that are independent nursing functions (Courtney, 1997). In addition, protocols should reflect the minimal standard of care, so that the protocol can be implemented with all clients (Courtney, 1997). This is especially important in the event of a malpractice suit in which the standard of care is challenged.

CERTIFICATION AND REGULATION OF ADVANCED PRACTICE NURSING

Advanced practice is not a requirement to attain certification, and certification is not always required for a nurse to practice as an advanced practice nurse. For example, a registered nurse who is not an advanced practice nurse may seek certification in a specialty area such as critical care nursing. Although professional **certification** is a way to validate and standardize the competencies of the advanced practice nurse (AACN, 1994), neither educational preparation nor the process of certification has been standardized. For example, educational preparation for the nurse practitioner role has ranged from short-term continuing education programs of several weeks' duration to a master's degree program consisting of 2 years or more of education. The educational backgrounds of advanced practice nurses vary from diploma level to master's level preparation. As a result, nurses without master's degrees may be functioning as advanced practice nurses, and not all advanced practice nurses with advanced degrees are certified (Journal of Continuing Education in Nursing, 1998).

One example of an agency that provides advanced practice nurses with certification is the **American Nurses Credentialing Center (ANCC),** which originated in 1973. Examinations can be taken in the following areas: acute care nurse practitioner, clinical specialist in community health nursing, clinical specialist in home health nursing, school nurse practitioner, clinical specialist in gerontological nursing, gerontological nurse pactitioner, pediatric nurse practitioner, clinical specialist in medical-surgical nursing, advanced nursing administration, adult nurse practitioner, family nurse practitioner, clinical specialist in adult psychiatric and mental health nursing, and clinical specialist in child and adolescent psychiatric and mental health nursing (ANCC, 1998).

The ANCC requires a master's degree and successful completion of an 8-hour written examination. Examination questions are written and reviewed by advanced practice nurses. The advanced practice nurse applicant for certification provides evidence of specific clinical practice for a set amount of hours prior to the examination. Once certification criteria have been met, the advanced practice nurse is certified for 5 years. At the end of 5 years, the advanced practice nurse must reapply for recertification by taking the examination or by demonstrating continuing education credits and a required amount of hours of clinical practice (ANCC, 1998).

The **American Board of Nursing Specialties (ABNS)**, established in 1991, serves as the umbrella organization that sets standards and requirements that certifying bodies for APN must meet, such as the level of educational preparation (AACN, 1994).

LEGAL ISSUES OF ADVANCED PRACTICE NURSING

The advanced practice nurse's role and the scope of practice continue to evolve as a result of the profession, society, culture, reimbursement laws, and health-related policies (ANA, 1994, p. 4). Each January, *The Nurse Practitioner: The American Journal of Primary Health Care* publishes an update of the legal issues affecting the advanced practice nurse. Areas addressed include legal authority, prescriptive authority, and third-party reimbursement.

Each state independently defines the advanced practice nurse and the scope of practice. Barriers to independent practice include limitations in legal authority, the authority to prescribe, reimbursement for services, and hospital privileges (Pearson, 1998). The inability to receive reimbursement and the lack of prescriptive authority limit the autonomy of the advanced practice nurse and his or her ability to practice independently. In a 1997 study, most nurse practitioners practiced in states in which they receive prescriptive authority (Pan, Geller, Gullicks, Muus, & Larson, 1997).

Establishing a uniform scope of practice for the APN is a challenge because the scope of practice is designated at the state level rather than at the federal level. In several states the state board of nursing and the state

board of medicine have joint regulation of advanced practice nursing.

Independent practice becomes more of a reality as advanced practice nurses assume expanded legal authority, prescriptive authority, third-party reimbursement, and hospital privileges. With independent practice, the likelihood for being named as a defendant in a malpractice suit increases. Advanced practice nurses are responsible for being familiar with legal issues involved in their expanded role.

PRESCRIPTIVE AUTHORITY

Often questions arise as to what is meant by **prescriptive authority**. Exactly what the law allows is unclear. Prescriptive authority may mean an approved formulary by the state board of medicine or the state board of nursing (Pearson, 1998). It may mean that the advanced practice nurse may order only certain categories of drugs from a formulary (Pearson, 1998). In some states, the advanced practice nurse can even prescribe controlled substances independent of any physician involvement (Pearson, 1998). Other states require a degree of physician collaboration (Pearson, 1998). Yet, in several states, there is no provision for the advanced practice nurse to have prescriptive authority (Pearson, 1998, p. 19)

Some states limit the classification of drugs that an APN can prescribe. The federal government passed the Controlled Substances Act in 1971, which classified drugs into schedules I through V depending on the potential for abuse and usefulness. Schedule I drugs have no known medical usefulness and are high in their potential for abuse. Schedule II drugs have high potential for abuse but are useful medically. Schedules III, IV, and V drugs are those with less potential for abuse (Pearson, 1994).

CONTINUING EDUCATION REQUIREMENTS

States vary in their **continuing education requirements** for advanced practice nurses, often according to the type of advanced practice. For example, Alabama requires that for license renewal the CNS must complete 34 hours of continuing education over a 2-year period, whereas the CRNP, CRNA, and CNM must complete the continuing education requirement of their specific certifying agency ("Annual Survey," 1998, p. 6).

Also, requirements vary for APNs to have prescriptive authority. For example, for initial licensure the requirement may range from no continuing education requirement up to 45 contact hours, or three credits of pharmacology within a period of 2 years before the application date (ANA, 1997). In regard to renewal of licensure, there may be no continuing education requirement for renewal, or a specified number of hours may be required before renewal of licensure is approved (ANA, 1997).

National professional nursing associations that are also certifying boards require continuing education for initial certification and renewal of certification. For example, the American College of Nurse-Midwives requires 50 hours over a 5-year period; the continuing education requirements of the American Nurses Credentialing Center vary according to the specific certification ("Annual Survey," 1998, p. 8).

ADDITIONAL ADVANCED PRACTICE NURSING ISSUES

REIMBURSEMENT

In addition to increasing the ability of the advanced practice nurse to provide care and improve access to care, direct **reimbursement** provides the advanced practice nurse recognition and visibility as a primary care provider (Mittelstadt, 1993). Reimbursement determines whether the advanced practice nurse will be able to survive financially as a health care provider.

Reimbursement by Medicare, Medicaid, managed care organizations (MCOs), businesses, and indemnity insurers depends on individual fee schedules, laws, and policies of each third-party payer (Buppert, 1998). Currently, pediatric nurse practition-

ers (PNPs) and family nurse practitioners (FNPs) are directly reimbursed under Medicaid. The state determines the reimbursement rate of the nurse practitioner. Each state may decide to reimburse other types of nurse practitioners (ACNP, 1996).

Some third-party payers have begun to directly reimburse APNs. In the spring of 1998, the Health Care Financing Administration (HCFA) in the **Department of Health and Human Services** ([DHHS] the federal agency in charge of the Medicaid and Medicare programs) issued a statement that nurse practitioners and clinical nurse specialists would receive direct Medicare reimbursement under their own provider number. In addition, the geographic location restriction was eliminated (ACNP, 1998; DHHS, 1998).

Advanced practice nursing services are reimbursed at 80 percent of the actual cost or 85 percent of the physician fee schedule, whichever amount is smaller. An employer of a nurse practitioner may receive 100 percent reimbursement if the service is rendered under a physician's direct supervision (Buppert, 1998, p. 67).

Advanced practice nurses must apply for a **provider number** in order to provide service to patients with Medicare coverage. If the client is a Medicare or Medicaid patient enrolled in a managed care organization (MCO), the advanced practice nurse must also apply to the MCO to become an approved **primary care provider (PCP)**. To receive reimbursement under Medicaid, the advanced practice nurse must be designated as a state Medicaid provider (Buppert, 1998).

For reimbursement, advanced practice nurses must be careful that documentation in the chart reflects the client encounter that is being billed. In addition, to maintain accurate public health statistics, advanced practice nurses must be familiar with **current procedural terminology (CPT)** codes and the **International Classification of Diseases, 9th Revision (ICD-9)** codes as published by the federal government as a classification for morbidity and cause-of-death coding. These codes are based on categories developed by the World Health Organization (WHO), which serves as a liaison between nations for comparable classifications of morbidity and mortality (U.S. Department of Health and

Human Services, 1997). Failure to document correctly can result in charges of a fraudulent claim (Buppert, 1998, p. 81). The advanced practice nurse must be careful to code at the appropriate level. A code higher than what is reflected by the documentation could be considered a false claim (Buppert, 1998).

HOSPITAL (CLINICAL) PRIVILEGES

Standards of the Joint Commission on Accreditation of Healthcare Organizations (JCAHO) currently permit independent and dependent nonphysician practitioners to be included on the medical staff of a hospital (Bissonette, 1989). The American Hospital Association has developed recommendations for nonphysician practitioners who provide care within a hospital setting. **Hospital (clinical) privileges** are usually extended by a hospital committee after review of the applicant's credentials. The committee may be the medical staff or hospital management. This practice originates from the principle that the hospital is ultimately responsible for the safety and quality of care of the patients and is liable for incompetent care providers who are agents of the hospital (Warren, 1984, p. 277). There is neither federal nor state legislation involved (Guido, 1995). The designated committee is responsible for periodic review of credentials and recommending clinical privileges based on the individual's credentials and competence (Bissonette, 1989). Hospital or clinical privileges may range from visiting the patient to admission and entry into hospital records (Guido, 1995). Because hospital privileges are essential for the advanced practice nurse to function to his or her full capability and to manage the health care of clients throughout the full health care continuum, it is essential for the APN to maintain an active role in the formation of policies regarding clinical privileges within the health care community (Kerr, Tenaud-Tessier Smellie-Decker, Stockwell, & Warren, 1996).

CHALLENGES TO SCOPE OF PRACTICE ISSUES

A review of the law literature suggests that most court cases involving advanced prac-

tice nurses have focused on issues related to scope of practice and the unauthorized practice of medicine. Two frequently quoted cases that have influenced APN scope of practice and legalized the APN role are *Sermchief v. Gonzales* (1983) and *Bellegie v. Texas Board of Nurse Examiners* (1985) (Guido, 1995; Rhodes, 1996).

Sermchief v. Gonzales was the first significant case challenging the role of advanced practice nurses who were charged with practicing medicine (Rhodes, 1996). The case involved advanced practice nurses who had postgraduate education in women's health. The decision was that the advanced practice nurses were found to be practicing within the scope of professional nursing standards. Their actions did not involve the unlawful practice of medicine, but were within the limits of their respective knowledge "and nurses referred patients to physicians upon reaching limits of their knowledge" (*Sermchief v. Gonzales*, 1983, p. 1). The implications of the final decision were that the courts recognized the role of the advanced practice nurse and ruled that the nurses' actions were consistent with the Nurse Practice Act.

In the case *Bellegie v. Texas Board of Nurse Examiners*, "various individuals and medical associations" challenged the authority of the Texas Board of Nursing to regulate the title, education, and activities of the advanced practice nurse. The court upheld the authority of the Texas Board of Nursing to issue rules related to the regulation of activities and education of advanced practice nurses under its jurisdiction (*Bellegie v. Texas Board of Nurse Examiners*, 1985).

Nursing practice has gone through monumental changes since 1899 when the U.S. Supreme Court upheld the states' authority to license various occupations. From permissive licensure in the early twentieth century, the profession progressed to mandatory licensure, with the development of state nurse practice acts and state boards of nursing to regulate the profession. To meet the challenge of the changing health care system, the definition of nursing evolved and expanded to include the advanced practice nurse role. Although the progress and development of the nursing profession has been profound, there is still much to be accomplished as nursing strives to become a cohesive profession with the responsibility and power to regulate itself.

POINTS TO REMEMBER

- Nurse practice acts define nursing practice and establish standards for nurses in each state.
- State boards of nursing have authority to carry out many functions involved in the regulation of nursing practice within their state.
- The Nursing Disciplinary Diversion Act provides a voluntary alternative to traditional disciplinary action for addicted nurses.
- The national practitioner data bank provides data on physicians, osteopaths, and dentists.
- Nursing licensure issues have continued to evolve for almost 200 years.
- The definition of *nursing* is continually evolving and expanding to meet the increased responsibilities that nurses are assuming.
- Both the ANA and the NCSBN have published guidelines for the use of unlicensed assistive personnel in health care settings.
- The advanced practice nurse is prepared at the master's or doctoral level of education with concentration in a specialized area of nursing practice and clinical practice supervision during the graduate program of studies.
- Development of national standards for the advanced practice role presents a challenge because of differences between states in scope of practice legislation for advanced practice nurses.
- Written protocols define responsibilities of the advanced practice nurse and the physician.
- Although professional certification is one way to validate and standardize the competencies of the advanced practice nurse, neither educational preparation nor the process of certification has been standardized.
- Independent practice becomes more of a reality as advanced practice nurses assume expanded legal authority, prescriptive authority, third-party reimbursement, and hospital privileges.

REFERENCES

Aiken, T., & Catalano, J. (1994). *Legal, ethical, and political issues in nursing.* Philadelphia: F.A. Davis.

American Academy of Nurse Practitioners. (1993). *Scope of practice for nurse practitioners.* Austin, TX: Author.

American Association of Nurse Anesthetists. (1998). *Qualifications and capabilities of the certified registered nurse anesthetist* [On-line]. Available: http://www. aana.com/documents/qualifications.htm

American Association of Colleges of Nursing. (1994, December 23). *Position statement certification and regulation of advanced practice nurses.* Washington, DC: Author.

American College of Nurse-Midwives. (1997a, August). *Definition of a certified nurse-midwife.* [On-line]. Available: http://www.acnm.org/prof/defcnm.htm

American College of Nurse-Midwives. (1997b, August). *Certified nurse-midwives and certified midwives as primary care providers/case managers.* [On-line]. Available: http://www. acnm. org/prof/primary. htm

American College of Nurse-Midwives. (1997c). *Standards for the practice of nurse-midwifery.* [On-line]. Available: http://www. acnm. org/prof/standard. htm

American College of Nurse-Midwives. (1998, November). *Mandatory degree requirements for midwives.* [On-line]. Available: http://www.acnm.org/prof/mandator.htm

American College of Nurse Practitioners. (1996). *Reimbursement for NPs: Fact sheet.* Washington, DC: Author.

American College of Nurse Practitioners. (1998, March 30). *Summary of HCFA program memorandum.* Washington, DC: Author.

American Nurses Association. (1955, December). ANA board approves a definition of nursing practice. *American Journal of Nursing, 55,* 1474.

American Nurses Association. (1990). *Suggested state legislation: Nursing practice act, nursing disciplinary diversion act, prescriptive authority act.* Washington, DC: Author.

American Nurses Association. (1995). *Nursing's social policy statement.* Washington, DC: American Nurses Publishing.

American Nurses Association. (1996a). *Registered professional nurses & unlicensed assistive personnel.* Washington, DC: American Nurses Publishing.

American Nurses Association. (1996b). *Scope and standards of advanced practice registered nursing.* Washington, DC: Author.

American Nurses Association. (1996c). *Model practice act.* Washington, DC: Author.

American Nurses Association. (1997, October 29). *Continuing education requirements for prescriptive authority.* [On-line] Available: http://www.ana.org/gova/rxce.htm

American Nurses Association Center for Research. (1985). *Boards of nursing: Composition, member qualifications, and statutory authority.* Kansas City, MO: Author.

American Nurses Association Council of Primary Health Care Nurse Practitioners. (1994). *The scope of practice of the primary health care nurse practitioner.* Washington, DC: American Nurses Publishing.

American Nurses Credentialing Center. (1998). *Advanced practice board certification catalogue.* Washington, DC: Author.

Andreoli, K. G., & Dvorak, E. (1993). Regulation—when is it appropriate and when is it not. *Journal of Professional Nursing, 9*(6), 310.

Annual survey. (1998). *The Journal of Continuing Education in Nursing, 29*(1), 2-9.

Baer, E. A. (1999). Philosophical and historical bases of advanced practice nursing roles. In M. D. Mezey & D. O. McGivern (Eds.), *Nurses, nurse practitioners* (3rd ed., pp. 72–91). New York: Springer Publishing.

Baker, S. E. (1992, Summer). The nurse practitioner in malpractice actions: Standards of care and theory of liability. *Health Matrix: Journal of Law-Medicine* p. 325.

Bellegie v. Texas Board of Nurse Examiners, 685 S.W.2d 431 (Tex. App. 3rd Dist., 1985).

Bernzweig, E. P. (1996). *The nurse's liability for malpractice* (6th ed.). St. Louis: Mosby.

Bissonette, D. (1989). Hospital privileges and PAs: Principles and practices. *Journal of the American Academy of Physician Assistants, 2*(2),132-135.

Buppert, C. (1998). Reimbursement for nurse practitioner services. *The Nurse Practitioner, 23*(1), 67-81.

Commonwealth of Pennsylvania, State Board of Nurse Examiners v. Rafferty, 508 Pa. 566, 499 A. 2d 289 (Sup. Ct. Pa. 1984).

Courtney, R. (1997). Working with protocols. *American Journal of Nursing, 97*(2), 16E-16H.

Culbertson, R. A. (1991). National practitioner data bank has implications for nursing. *Nursing Outlook, 39*(3),102-103, 142.

Dent v. West Virginia, 129 U.D. 114 (West Virginia, 1888).

Department of Health and Human Services Health Care Financing Administration. (1998, April). *Transmittal No. AB-98-15 Program memorandum intermediaries/carriers.* [On-line]. Available: http://www.hcfa.gov/pubforms/transmit/AB981560.htm

Division of Nursing. (1997). *The registered nurse population: Findings from the national sample survey of registered nurses, March 1996.* Washington, DC: Department of Health and Human Services.

Elder, R. G., & Bullough, B. (1990). Nurse practitioners and clinical nurse specialists: Are the roles merging? *Clinical Nurse Specialist, 4*(2), 78-84.

Forbes, K. E., Rafson, J., Spross, J. A., & Kozlowski, D. (1990). The clinical nurse specialist and nurse practitioner: Core curriculum survey results. *Clinical Nurse Specialist, 4*(2), 63-66.

Guido, G. W. (1995). Advanced nursing practice: Legal concerns. *AACN Clinical Issues, 6*(1), 98-104.

Guido, G. W. (1997). *Legal issues in nursing.* Prentice Hall, NJ: Appleton and Lange.

Havens, D. H. (1992). Licensure of advanced practice nurses. *Journal of Pediatric Health Care, 6*(60), 378–380.

Kelly, L. Y., & Joel, L. A. (1995). *Dimensions of professional nursing* (7th ed.). New York: McGraw-Hill.

Kelly, L. Y., & Joel, L. A. (1996). *The nursing experience: Trends, challenges, and transitions* (3rd ed.). New York: McGraw-Hill.

Kerr, K. L., Renaud-Tessier, A., Smellie-Decker, M., Stockwell, C. J., & Warren, W. (1996). Clinical privileging for advanced practice nurses. *The Nurse Practitioner, 21*(12), 94-98.

Kraus, J. (1992). Regulation of advanced practice nursing—the cog in the health policy engine. *Journal of Professional Nursing, 8*(4), 200.

Mannino, M. J. (1996). Legal aspects of nurse anesthesia practice. *Nursing Clinics of North America, 31*(3), 581-589.

Mittelstadt, P. C. (1993). Federal reimbursement of advanced practice nurses' services empowers the profession. *Nurse Practitioner, 18*(1), 43-49.

Moore, S. (1993). Promoting advanced practice nursing. *Advanced Practice Nursing, 4*(4), 603- 608.

National Council of State Boards of Nursing. (1994). *Model nursing practice act.* Chicago: Author.

National Council of State Boards of Nursing. (1996). *Profiles of member boards.* Chicago: Author.

National Council of State Boards of Nursing. (1998). *Basic facts about the council.* [On-line]. Available: http://www.ncsbn.org/files/aboutmb.html

Pan, S., Geller, J. M., Gullicks, J. N., Muus, K. J., & Larson, A. C. (1997). A comparative analysis of primary care nurse practitioners and physician assistants. *The Nurse Practitioner, 22*(1), 14-17.

Pearson, L. J. (1994). Annual update on how each state stands on legislative issues affecting advanced nursing practice: Key to abbreviations and terminology used in the table. *The Nurse Practitioner, 19*(1), 21.

People of the State of Illinois v. Stults, 291 Ill. App. 3d 71, 683 N.E.2d 521, 225 (Ill. December, 1997).

Rhodes, A. M. (1996). Litigation on advanced nursing practice. *Maternal Child Nursing, 21*, 271.

Richmond, T. S., & Keane, A. (1992). The nurse practitioner in tertiary care. *Journal of Nursing Administration, 22*(11), 11-12.

Romig, C. L. (1998). Interstate compact for the mutual recognition model on nursing regulation. *Association of Operating Room Nurses Journal, 68*(2), 292-294.

Schroer, K. (1991). Case management: Clinical nurse specialist and nurse practitioner, converging roles. *Clinical Nurse Specialist, 5*(4), 189-194.

Sermchief v. Gonzales, 660 S.W.2d 683 (Mo banc 1983).

Smreina, C. (1993). Licensure of advanced practice nursing. *Orthopedic Nursing, 12*(1), 13.

Soehren, P. M., & Schumann, L. L. (1994). Enhanced role opportunities available to the CNS/Nurse practitioner. *Clinical Nurse Specialist, 9*(3), 123-127.

Suarez, S. H. (1993, Spring). Midwifery is not the practice of medicine. *Yale Journal of Law and Feminism, 5*, 1–45.

United States Department of Health and Human Services. (1997). *The international classification of diseases, 9th revision. Clinical modifications* (6th ed.). Washington, DC: Author.

Warren, J. D. (1984). Legal perspectives on hospital privileges. In R. D. Carter & H. B. Perry (Eds.), *Alternatives in health delivery: Emerging roles for physician assistants* (pp. 277-294). St. Louis: Warren H. Green.

SUGGESTED READINGS

Alabama Board of Nursing v. Herrick, 454 So. 2d 1041 (Alabama, 1984).

American Academy of Nursing. (1987). *The evolution of nursing professional organizations: Alternatives models for the future.* Kansas City, MO: American Nurses Association.

American College of Nurse-Midwives. (1998, August). *Basic facts about certified nurse-midwives.* [On-line]. Available: http://www.acnm.org/prof/basicfct. htm

American Nurses Association. (1975). *A plan for implementation of the standard of nursing practice.* Kansas City, MO: Author.

American Nurses Association. (1980). *Nursing: A social policy statement.* Washington, DC: Author.

American Nurses Association. (1981). *The nursing practice act: Suggested state legislation.* Kansas City, MO: Author.

American Nurses Association. (1984). *Standards for professional nursing education.* Washington, DC: Author.

American Nurses Association. (1985). *Code for nurses with interpretive statements.* Washington, DC: Author.

American Nurses Association. (1986). *Enforcement of the nursing practice act.* Kansas City, MO: Author.

American Nurses Association. (1990). *Liability prevention & you: What nurses & employers need to know.* Kansas City, MO: Author.

American Nurses Association. (1991). *Standards of clinical nursing practice.* Washington, DC: American Nurses Publishing.

American Nurses Association. (1995). *Nursing's social policy statement.* Washington, DC: American Nurses Publishing.

American Nurses Association. (1998). *Catalog of publications.* Washington, DC: Author.

Catalano, J. T. (1996). *Contemporary professional nursing.* Philadelphia: F.A. Davis.

Gonzales v. State of Missouri, 660 S.W.2d 683 (1983).

Joint Commission for Accreditation of Healthcare Organizations. (1997). *Comprehensive accreditation for hospitals: The official handbook.* Oakbrook Terrace, IL: Author.

Nicholson v. Ambach, as Commissioner of Education, 80 A.D.2d 690, 436 N.Y.D2d 46.

Pearson, L. J. (1998). Annual update on how each state stands on legislative issues affecting advanced nursing practice. *The Nurse Practitioner, 23*(1), 14–66.

Shoenhair v. Commonwealth of Pennsylvania, Department of State, Bureau of Professional and Occupational Affairs and the State Board of Nurse Examiners, 74 Pa. Cmwlth., 217, 459 A. 2d 877 (Pa. 1983).

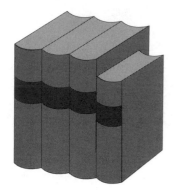

Chapter 6

ELEMENTS OF NURSING NEGLIGENCE

Elizabeth L. Higginbotham
Rosemary Conlon McCarthy

(continued)

KEY WORDS

Actual Agents
Agency
Apparent Agency
Borrowed Servant
  Doctrine
Captain of the Ship
  Doctrine
Cause in Fact
Collateral Source
Comparative Negligence
Concurrent Causes of
  Injury
Contributory Negligence
Damage
Defense of Fact
Discovery Rule
Duty
Expert Testimony
Foreseeability
Foreseeable
Governmental Functions
Immunity
Joint and Several Liability
Joint Tortfeasors

Limitations Period
Mitigate
Modified Responsibility
Negligence
Negligence Per Se
Nurse Practice Acts
Nursing Malpractice
Nursing Negligence
Ostensible Agency
Proprietary Functions
Proximate Cause
Pure Responsibility
Release
Respondeat Superior
Satisfaction
Sovereign Immunity
"So What" Defense
Standard of Care
Statutes of Repose
Subrogation
Substantial Factor
Unavoidable Accident
Vicarious Liability

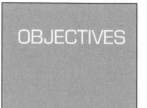

Upon completion of this chapter, the reader will be able to:
- Identify the various elements of the negligence cause of action and analyze fact patterns or scenarios in which the elements are present.
- Identify defenses to the negligence cause of action.
- Recognize sources of nursing standards.

INTRODUCTION

Negligence refers to the broad basis for which civil liability may be imposed without a showing of intent to harm or cause damages. Notwithstanding, there must be proof of fault arising from violation of some duty that is required under a particular set of circumstances. This means that the nurse's conduct must fall below the level of an accepted standard, which causes harm or damages to a patient, in order for liability to attach.

Nursing negligence is defined as a nurse's failure to use the degree of care that a reasonable and prudent nurse would use under the same or similar circumstances. The negligent act can be by commission or by omission, either doing something that a reasonable and prudent nurse would or would *not* have done. This necessarily means that the "reasonable and prudent nurse" standard may fluctuate, depending on the nurse's practice area, education, and experience. For example, the conduct of an advanced practice nurse (such as a certified registered nurse anesthetist [CRNA]) would be evaluated by comparing his or her conduct with that of another CRNA, as opposed to comparing the conduct with that of an entry-level nurse.

THE FOUR ELEMENTS OF NEGLIGENCE

In order for a plaintiff to prevail in a suit for negligence, he or she must prove all four elements of the cause of action: duty, breach, causation, and damages.

EXISTENCE OF A DUTY OR STANDARD

The first element is duty, which triggers the nurse's action and requires that the action conform to the standard of care. The standard is static—to act or not act as a reasonable and prudent nurse would under the same or similar circumstances. The "trigger" for action is the commencement of the nurse-patient relationship. If there is no relationship present, there is generally no duty to act on the nurse's part. In most jurisdictions, nurses have no duty to act or care for persons involved in accidents, unless the nurse caused the accident (Restatement (Second) of Torts § 324A). If a nurse chooses to take action to assist a victim in an emergency, liability for civil damages could result if the victim is injured owing to the nurse's willful or wanton negligence (Hernandez v. Lukefahr, 1994). For example, if a nurse decides to assist victims at the scene of a car accident and drags a victim from a car without justification, resulting in injury to the patient, liability may attach if the nurse's actions are found to be wantonly or willfully negligent.

BREACH OF DUTY OR STANDARD OF CARE

The second element to be proven is breach of the nurse's duty. To determine whether or not a duty was violated, it is necessary to delineate the **standard of care** for that particular circumstance, i. e., what a reasonable and prudent nurse would have done or not done. A common breach of duty involves medication errors. It is well established that a nurse must adhere to the "five rights" of medication administration—administering the right medicine to the right patient, in the right amount, in the right route, at the right time. If the nurse violates one of the five rights, he or she has breached the duty to act as a reasonable and prudent nurse.

In a nursing malpractice case, the standard of care is established by **expert testimony.** A nurse who is familiar with the standard of care may be qualified to testify about what a reasonable and prudent nurse would have done, then render an opinion as to whether or not the nurse defendant acted accordingly.

CAUSATION

In relation to a negligence action, causation is the most difficult concept to grasp. It is difficult for nurses to understand that proof of the first two elements of negligence does not necessarily entitle a patient to recovery of damages, especially if more than one reason or cause contributed to the patient's injuries.

CAUSE IN FACT

The causation element requires proof of two components: cause in fact and proximate cause. **Cause in fact** is also known as actual cause, or "but for" causation. Simply put, this means but for the nurse's negligence, the patient would not have sustained injuries. This is significant in that if the determination is made that the same injury would have occurred without regard to the nurse's act or omission, the act or omission may not be the actual cause of the injury. An example of this would be the scenario where the nurse gives the wrong medicine (ephedrine, as opposed to epinephrine) in a code situation and the patient dies. There is no doubt that the nurse made a medication error that can be fatal. In this case, it is later (on autopsy) discovered that the patient died of massive pulmonary

emboli. Obviously, the patient would have sustained the same injury (death) notwithstanding the obvious medication error. Therefore, the nurse's action, although obviously negligent, was not the proximate cause of the patient's injuries. Defense attorneys sometimes call this the **"so what" defense**; so what if the nurse was negligent, she did not cause the injury. This may protect the nurse from civil liability; however, he or she may not fare as well if the licensing board decides to investigate the medication error.

Other scenarios also arise, such as **concurrent causes of injury** or harm. In the situation where multiple persons are involved in causing harm by their separate acts of negligence and the patient would not have been harmed but for *both* acts, both parties are liable. Imagine the situation in which a doctor leaves a sponge inside the patient's abdomen and the nurses count the sponges incorrectly. The actions of both parties took place at the same time and would not have caused harm but for the fact that they happened together.

Contrast the situation in which a medication is transcribed on a Medication Administration Record without comparison to a patient's allergy profile. The medication is then administered several times and an overdose is also given. The patient has a serious allergic reaction and is injured, but it cannot be determined which action caused the injury (the allergy or the overdose). In this case, since the conduct of either party could have caused the injury, all parties will be liable if each person's conduct was a **substantial factor** in causing the injury (Corey v. Havener, 1902).

PROXIMATE CAUSE

Proximate cause means next cause or legal cause. In addition to proving that the nurse's conduct actually caused injuries to a patient, in order for the nurse to be legally responsible for all of the consequences of his or her actions, the plaintiff must prove that the consequences were **foreseeable.** This is an analysis that concerns occurrences or consequences following the nurse's action. The emphasis in the proximate cause analysis is on **foreseeability.** Generally speaking, it is the fact of injury as opposed to the extent of injury that the patient sustains that should be foreseen. An example of this would be the intravenous administration of undiluted potassium chloride; it is foreseeable that this can cause injury to a vein, but the extent of injury (loss of a limb) does not have to be foreseen in order for the nurse to be liable for improper administration of the medication and all consequences that result.

At times, other forces come into play that may have nothing to do with the original negligent act but still may expose the nurse to liability if it was foreseeable that such forces could occur. For example, as a general rule, one is not liable for the intentional or criminal act of a third party, unless the action of that third party was foreseeable. If a nurse administers narcotics to a patient, he or she should be aware of the fact that the patient might be susceptible to injury as a result of sedative effects. For example, if persons enter the patient room and the nurse is aware of their presence, the nurse must ensure that no harm befalls the patient, as it is foreseeable that patients under the influence of narcotics are less capable of protecting themselves.

DAMAGES AND INJURIES

Even if the patient proves the first three elements of the negligence cause of action, he or she must prove that **damage** or injury occurred as a result of the negligent act in order to prevail. Without this proof of actual damage to person or property, there is no basis for recovery, as the purpose of an award of money damages is to restore the patient as nearly as possible to his or her original position or condition. There are several types of injuries that are compensated by an award of money damages. A patient may recover for pain and suffering in the past and future, for disfigurement, for disability, for past and future medical expenses, for past lost wages, and for future loss of earning capacity.

In analyzing damages, it is generally accepted that the patient has a duty to **mitigate,** or minimize, the amount of damages or

further injury, if able to do so. An example of a patient's failure to mitigate is identifiable in the case of a patient who falls out of bed as a result of the nurse's negligent act of leaving the side rails down on the bed. During the patient's rehabilitation, the patient fails to attend physical therapy as prescribed and sustains a permanent disability as a result. In this instance, the disability would not have occurred or been as severe if the patient would have complied with the treatment regimen. The nurse will not be responsible for that disability percentage or portion attributed to the patient's failure to mitigate (noncompliance) after the injury occurred.

When calculating damages, most states allow plaintiffs to recover damages without regard to amounts already received from another or **collateral source**, such as insurance coverage. Notwithstanding, the opposing view is that this allows for a double recovery, because the same amount of damages is paid by two sources. To remedy this, most private insurance companies have a right of **subrogation** with regard to a plaintiff's claim against a third party. This means that if an insurance company pays a patient's medical bills for injuries arising out of a nurse's malpractice, the insurance company will have a right to recover the amount from the patient when the patient recovers it from the nurse.

THEORIES OF NEGLIGENCE

There are several theories or doctrines of negligence. This simply means that there are several ways to establish the negligence cause of action. The theories or doctrines may also be referred to as different types of negligence.

MALPRACTICE

Nursing malpractice is the term that subsumes professional negligence or deviation from the standard of care. The term is interchanged with *negligence* or *professional negligence*. Without regard to the label, the fundamental issue is still the same: whether or not the nurse acted or failed to act as a reasonable and prudent nurse would under the same or similar circumstances.

NEGLIGENCE PER SE

Negligence per se involves breach of a duty imposed by a civil or criminal statute. Some statutes provide a civil remedy for violation, whereas others specifically do not. An example of a statute with no civil remedy is the Texas Nursing Practice Act, which specifically negates a private cause of action under the act (Tex. Rev. Civ. Stat. Ann. art 4513–4528, 1998). Other statutes may give rise to a claim or allegation for the purpose of a civil negligence action if the statute in question clearly specifies the duty of care required and has as its purpose prevention of the type of injury suffered by the class of people of which the plaintiff/patient is a member. In a jury trial litigated by one of the authors of this chapter, the plaintiff alleged negligence per se arising out of violation of Medicare standards for long-term care facilities. The standard required that a nursing care plan be formulated in writing within a certain number of days of patient admission. A negligence per se jury instruction was allowed and was based on the facility's failure to complete a care plan within a prescribed time period. The instruction was allowed because of the statute's prefatory language, which proclaimed the purpose of the statute to be the protection of the public. The resident was considered to be in the class of persons (the public) meant to be protected by the statute (*Perez et al. v. Del Rio Nursing Home*, 1993). In that case, the duty and breach were assumed in the jury instruction; notwithstanding, the jury still had to decide whether that breach was a proximate cause of patient's injuries. The question was answered in the affirmative.

VICARIOUS LIABILITY

RESPONDEAT SUPERIOR

Vicarious liability refers to liability incurred by one person by virtue of another person's bad acts, based on the relationship between them. This is different from the imposition of liability based on someone's own fault. A common relationship that gives rise to this kind of liability is the employer-employee relationship. An employer may be vicariously liable for the acts of its employees under the doctrine of **respondeat superior**, "let the master answer." Thus, a hospital or health care facility can be legally responsible for its nurse employee's negligence. A hospital or facility has a duty of reasonable care to its patients and is generally liable for any and all injuries negligently inflicted upon its patients by nurse employees of the hospital or facility. There is no question that the individual nurses are accountable and personally liable for nursing actions performed on nursing judgments made. In the legal arena, those actions and judgments could place the nurse's employer at risk to pay money damages to the injured patient who files a malpractice lawsuit. As a practical matter, hospitals and other health care facilities have much more money available to pay claims than nurses have and thus are named as defendants in lawsuits arising from nursing negligence.

AGENCY

Another relationship that gives rise to vicarious liability is the agency relationship. **Agency** simply means that one person has the authority to act on behalf of another. There are various theories of agency, including actual agency, **apparent agency**, and **ostensible agency**. Nurses are **actual agents** of the hospital as the hospital controls the details of their work. Many cases have been decided based on the theories of apparent and ostensible agency and generally involve physicians or other independent contractors, with the issue being the hospital's liability for their actions. The Texas Supreme Court has held that hospitals were not liable for the acts of an emergency room physician when the physician was acting as an independent contractor of the hospital (*Sampson v. Baptist Memorial Hospital System*, 1998). That case also illustrates the general rule that a hospital is not liable for the acts of its independent contractor physician unless (1) there is a reasonable belief that the doctor was an employee or agent, (2) the belief was generated by some conduct on the part of the hospital, and (3) there is a justifiable reliance by the patient that a doctor was an agent or employee. Also, a health care facility may be liable for the negligence of an independent contractor if the patient had no choice in the provider's selection of the particular contractor, such as a radiologist, who then commits malpractice (*Merrick v. Professional Health Services*, 1981). An employer may be liable in that instance for negligently selecting the contractor. In the nursing realm, this would apply to entities such as nursing agencies providing temporary staff who fail to properly check credentials of the nurses before making assignments.

BORROWED SERVANTS

Another theory of vicarious liability is the **borrowed servant doctrine**, which involves an employee of one party who is temporarily controlled by another person. Essentially, this doctrine means that a person who "borrows" the use of someone else's employee is legally responsible for the employee's actions. In this case, if a nurse is truly the "borrowed servant" of a physician, the physician may be liable for the nurse's negligence if she or he had a right to control the nurse's actions. This is not a popular theory in most jurisdictions today.

CAPTAIN OF THE SHIP

Another form of vicarious liability is the **captain of the ship doctrine**, which makes a party responsible for the acts of everyone that he or she controls. A common scenario involving this claim arises in the surgical setting where allegations are made that a physician is the captain of the ship because he or she controls the acts of all nonphysician personnel in the operating suite. This doctrine has been limited in several states. In Texas, this doctrine offers no protection for nurses, because the registered nurse has a duty to his or her patient independent of

physician orders or hospital policies by virtue of the Texas nursing license (*Lunsford v. Board of Nurse Examiners*, 1993).

DEFENSES TO A NEGLIGENCE CLAIM

STATUTE OF LIMITATIONS

The time period in which a lawsuit must be brought is called the **limitations period**. Each state specifies by statute the period in which the suit must be brought or it is forever barred. The period of limitations is based on the particular type of complaint that is being lodged. For example, in most states the limitations period for breach of contract is 4 (or more) years. A suit for negligence or medical malpractice must be brought within a 2- or 3-year period after the malpractice is committed.

In some jurisdictions the limitations period is not absolute, but can vary based on the facts. If a practitioner actively and fraudulently conceals his or her malpractice to prevent a patient from discovering it until after the limitations period has expired, the law allows for the period to commence upon discovery of the fraud. In other circumstances, the **discovery rule** applies and the limitations period does not begin to run until the malpractice victim knew or should have known that he or she was injured. Statutes that do not allow for the discovery rule to toll limitations are called **statutes of repose** (*Crier v. White Cloud*, 1986).

UNAVOIDABLE ACCIDENT

Unavoidable accident is a defense to a negligence cause of action. The defense of unavoidable accident is appropriate when the evidence shows that neither party proximately caused the incident in question; for example, if the evidence showed that the plaintiff's skin deterioration was caused by a number of factors, none of which the defendants could have prevented (*Wisenbarger v. Gonzales Warm Springs Rehabilitation Hospital*,

1990). Another example of unavoidable accident is the inability to know of a child's allergy to ether prior to surgery, resulting in death of the child (*Swartout v. Holt*, 1954). In that case, physicians were not aware of the child's previous reaction to ether, as they had not been informed. The child was taken to surgery, was given ether, and died. The court held that because they were not informed of the allergy, they could not be liable for the result that occurred when the ether was administered and the child died.

CONTRIBUTORY NEGLIGENCE

Contributory negligence refers to the amount of fault contributed to the injury by the patient. The patient's negligence is evaluated by analyzing the four elements of negligence: duty, breach, causation, and damages. **Duty** is interpreted as the duty to exercise care in avoiding one's own injury, or the duty to protect oneself from harm. The **standard of care** is an objective one, based on what a reasonable person would have done under the same or similar circumstances. This is different from a patient's failure to mitigate or reduce his or her damages, because mitigation has nothing to do with the amount of plaintiff's fault in causing the original accident but is related only to reducing the amount of resulting damages. The failure to mitigate serves to reduce the amount of damages the plaintiff can recover, whereas contributory negligence may even eliminate a plaintiff's claim if the amount of fault attributable to the plaintiff is high enough. In comparison to the earlier example of mitigation, where the nurse left the side rails down, if the nurse had put the rails up and the patient climbed over them and the patient was injured, contributory negligence would be assessed with regard to the patient's actions in causing the original injury—climbing over the side rails when they were up and he was warned not to.

COMPARATIVE NEGLIGENCE

Comparative negligence is the apportionment or distribution of fault or negligence among the various parties responsible for a plaintiff's injury, to include the plaintiff. There are two forms of comparative negligence or responsibility: modified and pure. In the case of **modified responsibility**, the plaintiff can recover if his or her negligence does not exceed that of the defendant or if the plaintiff's negligence is less than that of the defendant. This necessarily means that a plaintiff's negligence cannot be more than 50 percent of the total. For example, if the plaintiff is found to be 51 percent responsible, he or she cannot recover any damages, because his or her fault in causing the damages or injury exceeds that of the defendant(s) (*McIntyre v. Balentine*, 1992). Ninety-nine percent of the jurisdictions in this country embrace the doctrine of modified responsibility. In the case of **pure responsibility**, a plaintiff's damages will be reduced or decreased in relation to his or her portion of fault. If a plaintiff is 80 percent responsible, he or she can still collect 20 percent of the damages awarded. Only 1 percent of all jurisdictions subscribe to the pure comparative responsibility theory (Laben & Rudolph, 1996).

DEFENSE OF FACT

Defense of fact is defined literally. This simply means that the plaintiff and defendant(s) disagree as to how an event actually happened or who caused an injury, i. e., the facts of the case. An example of this type of defense would be the situation where a patient had three abdominal surgeries within a period of 10 years. Two years after the last surgery it is discovered that a surgical sponge was retained in the patient's abdomen. Due to the fact that the three surgeries involved the same surgical site (the entire abdomen), the plaintiff will have to prove where (which surgery/which hospital) the sponge actually came from. Obviously, only one of the surgeons will be responsible for leaving the sponge in, notwithstanding the fact that the others may be responsible for not discovering it. The "innocent" surgeons will defend on the facts of the case, which will likely be decided on the brand of sponge discovered and/or sponge count information contained within the medical records.

IMMUNITIES

Immunity affords protection to a defendant based on the category or classification of the defendant as opposed as to the nature of the defendant's conduct. To put this another way, the defendant's conduct may be negligent, but his or her status, such as that of a public servant, limits the ways in which to hold the defendant accountable for the negligent conduct.

GOVERNMENTAL IMMUNITY

Governmental immunity is based on the doctrine of **sovereign immunity** or "the king can do no wrong" (*Russell v. Men of Devon*, 1798). Based on this doctrine, state and federal governments as well as various state and federal facilities such as hospitals and schools are generally immune from tort liability. A distinction is drawn between governmental versus private or proprietary functions. **Governmental functions** are those that can be performed adequately only by a governmental unit; examples would be police protection and judicial administration. **Proprietary functions**, or private functions, are those functions that are provided by a governmental unit but could also be provided by private corporations, such as provision of utilities like water, gas, or electricity.

Governmental immunity may be limited by statute commensurate with the extent that liability is actually allowed for by the statute. For example, in Texas, liability of a governmental entity is created (or allowed) in two instances by the Texas Tort Claims Act: "(1) the condition or use of tangible personal or real property; and (2) property damages, personal injury and death proximately caused by an employee active within the scope of his employment if it arises from the operation or use of a motor driven vehicle or motor driven equipment" (Charitable Immunity and Liability Texas Civil Practice and Remedies Code Chapter 84, 1998). The Act also provides specific limits on recovery depending on the nature of the public entity and the status of the defendant. The state and cities enjoy protection from damage awards (once liability is proved in accordance with the Act) above $250,000, and other governmental entities are protected from damages above $100,000.

CHARITABLE IMMUNITY

In general, volunteers of charitable organizations such as parish nurses are immune from civil liability unless their actions are intentional, willful, or wantonly negligent. Under the Texas Charitable Immunities Act, liability of employees of charitable organizations is limited to damages in a maximum amount of $500,000 per person or $1,000,000 for each single occurrence of bodily injury or death, with a $100,000 limit for each single occurrence for injury to or destruction of property (Charitable Immunity and Liability Texas Civil Practice and Remedies Code Chapter 84, 1998). These limitations do not apply to health care providers in general and do not apply to charitable organizations that do not carry insurance for its employees and volunteers.

NURSING STANDARDS

STANDARD OF CARE

The **standard of care** is generally defined as that degree of care, expertise, and judgment exercised by a reasonable and prudent nurse under the same or similar circumstances. In a nursing malpractice case, the standard of care is established by expert testimony. Both parties to the controversy will retain a nursing expert who gives an opinion about the standard of care or what a reasonable and prudent nurse would have done under the same or similar circumstances. The nursing experts use a variety of sources to formulate and/or bolster their opinions. No single source contains the standard of care, and not all the sources contain the same information. Likewise, the various sources are subject to the interpretation of the expert, which may be skewed or incorrect. Hence, both sides of the case retain experts, and the jury is left to decide the credibility of the experts and the weight to be afforded to their testimony.

SOURCES OF NURSING STANDARDS

HOSPITAL POLICIES AND PROCEDURES

The policies and procedures for the hospital or facility where a defendant nurse is employed are frequently used as evidence of the standard of care. For this reason, it is imperative that the nurse be familiar with policies and procedures, and even more critical that they reflect actual practice. It is a favored technique of plaintiff's counsel to grill the defendant nurse on policies and procedures, after learning that they are either out of date or no longer in use. Not all facilities are JCAHO accredited, and Medicare surveys do not occur regularly; the result is that outdated policies are found more often than expected in facilities without these external mechanisms in place that force review and updating of policy and procedure manuals.

PHYSICIAN ORDERS

It can be argued that doctor's orders also mandate what the nurse's behavior is or should have been. This can be tricky depending on the propriety of the order in the first place. If a nurse fails to comply with the physician's order, he or she must have some justification for doing so, such as the exercise of the duty to question unsafe or inappropriate orders. In that instance, the nurse must utilize and access the chain of command for his or her facility. This is in keeping with the nurse's independent duty to the patient (*N.K.C. Hospitals Inc. v. Anthony*, 1993).

JCAHO STANDARDS AND ANA STANDARDS

Standards of professional organizations are often used to delineate or benchmark the standard of care, especially when the hospital that the nurse works in embraces the standards. For example, in a case involving a CRNA, the hospital's decision to adopt more stringent standards (such as JCAHO standards) than the law required was used to establish the standard of care (*Denton Regional Medical Center v. LaCroix*, 1997). Specifically, hospital policy required that an anesthesiologist provide or supervise all of anesthesia care. The court noted that to determine the standard of care, the court could look to the JCAHO standards as well as the hospital's internal policies and bylaws. In this case, a CRNA provided the anesthesia care, and no anesthesiologist was present to supervise care despite the hospital's policy that supervision be direct and in person. Even though the jury did not find negligence on the part of the doctors or the nurse, this did not preclude a finding of negligence by the hospital for breach of its duty to the patient in violating policies and procedures.

NURSING LITERATURE AND TREATISES

Nursing literature is also a favorite source for plaintiff's attorneys to establish the standard of care. In deposition, the attorney often asks the nurse what he or she learned in nursing school and thereafter with regard to nursing diagnoses and procedures. Attorneys will also attempt to get the nurse to agree that a particular treatise or source is authoritative. Once the nurse does that, the attorney will point out instances where the nurse's actions did not conform to the treatise he or she relies on as authoritative. For this reason, it is imperative that nurses stay current, at least with regard to their practice area. The authors of this chapter recommend that mandatory continuing education be directed to a nurse's particular practice area as a tool for malpractice prevention.

NURSE PRACTICE ACTS

The legislatures of every state have passed laws regulating and defining nursing practice, which are commonly referred to as **nurse practice acts**. These statutes are designed to protect the health care consumer of nursing services, by defining the legal scope of nursing practice. In addition, each nurse practice act creates a state board of nursing, which promulgates and enforces established rules and regulations concerning the practice of nursing. Thus, each state licenses and sanctions its professional nurses as authorized by that state's nurse practice act and accompanying rules and regulations. Professional nurses who violate these statutes or rules and regulations are deemed to be practicing below the acceptable professional standard of care. Depending on the violation, they face not only disciplinary action by their respective state board of nursing but also civil or criminal liability. Nursing experts often cite the nurse practice act as evidence of the standard of care, *whether or not* the nurse involved has been disciplined by the state board.

Moreover, evidence gained during the peer review process by a state board may be used against the nurse in a subsequent negligence suit. In one case, the Kansas Supreme Court held that the peer review privilege did not protect material obtained from the Kansas State Board of Nursing from use in a malpractice case. In that case, plaintiffs alleged that their daughter suffered injury and died from a ruptured ectopic pregnancy because the emergency room nurse who initially assessed the patient failed to recognize the seriousness of her condition and did not alert a physician to the need for immediate attention. The hospital and doctor were both sued. The nurse was also subjected to a disciplinary proceeding before the State Board (*Adams v. St. Francis Regional Medical Center*, 1998). In that case, the court allowed forms and documents containing factual accounts and witness statements into evidence. Because the documents were generated by the Board (as opposed to the hospital) as part of the investigation, the court held that they were not privileged.

Even though nurse practice acts do not generally create a private cause of action, violation of rules and regulations promulgated to implement them can be used as evidence of negligence.

MULTIPLE DEFENDANT ISSUES

JOINT AND SEVERAL LIABILITY

When more than one defendant is involved in a malpractice action, the defendants may be jointly and severally liable for damages. **Joint tortfeasors** are defendants who act in concert or by agreement and cause an injury, or who act independently with their acts causing a single indivisible injury. These defendants are also subject to the comparative negligence rules discussed previously. The comparative responsibility rules are applied to determine whether one of the joint tortfeasors may be responsible for paying an entire judgment. In Texas, the rules have changed to require that a joint tortfeasor will be required to pay an entire judgment only in the event that his or her negligence exceeds 50 percent. Otherwise, a defendant will be responsible to pay only the amount of damages equivalent to that percentage of negligence attributed to him or her.

SATISFACTION AND RELEASE

In general, **satisfaction** or payment of a judgment extinguishes a cause of action and bars a later suit for more or additional monies against other parties. A **release** or settlement is generally applicable only to the party actually released. In malpractice actions when multiple defendants are sued, many times the plaintiff will settle with one or more defendants, leaving one or more defendants for trial. In that instance, the remaining defendants will get a credit for either the percentage of money or actual dollars previously contributed by the settling defendants, but the suit can still go forward. After a trial and judgment, no further suits can be brought based on the same set of facts and circumstances because the matter has been disposed of completely.

ISSUES AND TRENDS

NURSING ISSUES AND TRENDS

The scope of nursing practice has expanded dramatically. This provides more opportunities for RNs who are now providing subsequent dosing of epidural analgesia, acting as first assistants in surgery, and performing procedures at the bedside that were traditionally reserved for physicians, such as removing Swan-Ganz catheters.

In addition, nurses have moved into hospital management positions and are now responsible for a variety of hospital operations, including complete budgetary control over nursing services. In the field, advanced practice nurses are providing primary health care in their communities in rural health clinics and other nontraditional sites. Physician supervision is now broadly defined and no longer requires physical presence of the doctor for the nurse to have authority to act.

LEGAL ISSUES AND TRENDS

With the increase in responsibility comes a commensurate increase in exposure to liability. Many nurses are now carrying their own malpractice insurance. Some nurses feel that the purchase of such insurance increases their chances of being named as the defendant in a malpractice lawsuit. Nurses are named as defendants in malpractice lawsuits based on the facts of the particular situation. Ordinarily, the presence or absence of insurance coverage is not ascertained until after some initial investigation is conducted and after a lawsuit has been filed. The more important consideration for the nurse in deciding to purchase professional insurance is the nature of the nurse's practice. Although the nurse may feel reasonably comfortable that the employer has coverage for his or her actions, the employer is the named insured and for the most part can and will

control the defense of the malpractice case.

Under an employer's policy, the nurse-employee is not entitled to representation by an attorney solely on his or her behalf unless there is a conflict in interest (usually a disagreement about the facts or the potential for personal or criminal liability). If more than one employee of the defendant hospital is named as a defendant in a malpractice lawsuit, one attorney usually represents the employer and all named employees. There have been instances where the employer has settled a malpractice lawsuit in which the individual nurse is also a defendant and the employer failed to get a release of any further liability arising from the incident on behalf of the nurse. Also, the nurse may still be liable. Consider the case where both hospital-employer and nurse-employee were named defendants. The employer settled the case and then looked to the nurse to recoup the damages paid out in settlement on the nurse's behalf under an indemnification clause of the insurance policy. Although the purchase of professional liability insurance is a professional decision to be made by the practicing nurse, careful consideration should be given to all factors surrounding an individual nurse's practice. It is the official position of the American Association of Nurse Attorneys that nurses should carry their own malpractice insurance.

ETHICAL CONSIDERATIONS AND CONFLICTS

There is no question that licensed professional nurses are accountable to the public for nursing judgment and for the actions that naturally flow from that judgment. Nurse practice acts and hospital and facility policies and protocols are effective tools to use in formulation of nursing decisions. However, nurse practice acts and hospital policies do not always agree. For example, nurses are professionally and legally bound to follow a lawful, medically appropriate doctor's order. If the nurse believes that the order is potentially harmful to a patient, the nurse is obligated to prevent injury to that patient. Hopefully, the facility has an official chain of command policy in place, which will support the nurse's duty to the patient. In this situation, that duty requires the nurse to communicate concerns about patient safety to the physician giving the order. Should that process fail to accommodate patients' safety, the nurse should bring those concerns to nursing management, the chief of the medical staff, or the facility risk manager. Should the nurse decide not to follow the order, documentation of that fact with the reason for not following the order is mandatory. Further, the nurse should document which facility personnel were contacted and the outcome of each contact.

There are times when the nurse is forced to make decisions and take actions that risk violating facility policies, creating a conflict between professional practice and employee status. Although the nurse is an employee of the facility and as an employee should follow facility policies, the nurse must balance the duty owed to the patient with the obligations owed to the employer. Staffing shortages and use of float personnel often present such dilemmas. Nurses confronted with "the license or the job" dilemma are generally better served by adhering to the requirements of their state nurse practice act while attempting to resolve the issues with their employer.

RECOMMENDATIONS FOR RESEARCH AND MALPRACTICE PREVENTION

Nursing judgment involves the analysis of facts and circumstances on a case-by-case basis. To prevent malpractice, it is essential that the nurse undertake this evaluation with regard to everything that he or she does in the clinical setting. The ultimate duty that a nurse has is to care for his or her patient without exceeding the bounds of professional licensure. Malpractice prevention starts with the individual nurse recognizing his or her own limitations and seeking to expand his or her knowledge base as it pertains to the practice area. A good working knowledge of licensing board rules and regulations as well as the state nurse practice

act is critical to safe and ethical practice. Especially important are rules pertaining to unprofessional conduct, delegation of nursing tasks to unlicensed personnel, and scope of practice.

SUMMARY

Nursing negligence is defined as a nurse's failure to use that degree of care that a reasonable and prudent nurse would use under the same or similar circumstances. This includes acts of omission as well as commission. To prevail in a negligence case against a nurse, the patient/plaintiff must prove all four elements of the negligence cause of action. The patient must prove that a nurse-patient relationship existed that gave rise to a nurse's duty to care for the patient. The second element involves proof of the breach of that duty by the nurse, which is demonstrated by expert opinion as to what the nurse should have or should not have done on the occasion in question. The third element to be proved is causation, which requires proof of two aspects. First, the patient must prove that the nurse's breach of duty to the patient was the actual cause, or cause in fact, of his or her injury and that the consequence of the nurse's breach of his or her duty was foreseeable. There are occasions when a nurse may be guilty of breaching a duty to a patient, but that breach is not the cause of the patient's injury. An example would be administration of the wrong medication to a patient, with the end result being the patient's death due to a completely unrelated cause. In that example, despite the fact that the nurse made an error, the medication did not harm the patient and would not have saved the patient if given correctly. The final element of a cause of action for negligence requires proof of injury or damages. In the situation just described, the plaintiff is unable to prove causation or damages. In other words, even though the nurse's conduct was below the standard of care, the patient suffered no harm as a result.

There are numerous defenses to an action for nursing negligence, including limitations, immunity, unavoidable accident, and defense of fact. If a case is not successfully defended and defendants are adjudicated or found liable, there are several methods of apportioning damages among or between those persons at fault.

The increase in the responsibility that a nurse takes on is accompanied by an increase in liability exposure. Knowledge of the standards governing nursing practice and scope of licensure is critical to malpractice prevention as well as preservation of a nursing license.

POINTS TO REMEMBER

- A plaintiff must prove all elements of the negligence cause of action to prevail.
- Negligence involves errors of both omission and commission.
- Nurse practice acts, hospital policies, nursing treatises, and organizational standards all may be sources of the standard of care.
- Nursing negligence may give rise to a civil lawsuit, criminal charges, and discipline by licensing authorities.
- A nurse's primary obligation is to care for his or her patient, despite hospital policies or doctor's orders.

REFERENCES

Adams v. St. Francis Regional Medical Center, Original Action No. 77,848 (Kan. 1998).

Charitable Immunity and Liability Texas Civil Practice and Remedies Code Chapter 84, 1998).

Corey v. Havener, 65 N.E. 69 (Mass. 1962).

Crier v. White Cloud, 496 So. 2d 305 (La. 1986).

Denton Regional Medical Center v. LaCroix, 947 S.W.2d 941 (Tex. App.–Ft. Worth 1997).

Hernandez v. Lukefahr, 879 S.W.2d 137 (Tex. App.–Houston [14th Dist.] 1994, no writ).

Laben, J., & Rudolph, E. (1996). The doctrine of comparative negligence. *American Journal of Nursing Law, 3,* 62.

Lunsford v. Board of Nurse Examiners, 648 S.W.2d 391 (Tex. App.– Austin 1993, no writ).

McIntyre v. Balentine, 833 S.W.2d 52 (Tenn. 1992).

Merrick v. Professional Health Services, 432 A. 2d, 538 (New Jersey, 1981).

N.K.C. Hospitals Inc. v. Anthony, 849 S.W.2d 564 (Ky. App., 1993).

Nurse Practice Act Tex. Rev. Civ. Stat. Ann. art 4513–4528 (Vernon Supp. 1998).

Perez et al. v. Del Rio Nursing Home, No. 19653 original proceeding (1993).

Restatement (Second) of Torts § 324(A).

Russell v. Men of Devon, 100 Eng. Rep. 359 (1798).

Sampson v. Baptist Memorial Hospital System, 41 Tex. S. Ct. J. (1998).

Swartout v. Holt, 272 S.W. 2d 756 (Tex. Civ. App.–Waco 1954, writ refused, n.r.e.).

Wisenbarger v. Gonzales Warm Springs Rehabilitation Hospital, 789 S.W.2d 688 (Tex. App.–Corpus Christi 1990, writ denied).

SUGGESTED READINGS

American Nurses Association. (1985). *Code for nurses.* Kansas City, MO: Author.

Cushing. M. (1988). *Nursing jurisprudence.* Norwalk, CT/San Mateo, CA: Appleton & Lange.

Murphy, S. (1995). *Legal handbook for Texas nurses.* Austin, TX: University of Texas Press.

Tammelleo, A.D. (1992, July). Court upholds nurse's refusal to float. *The Reagan Report on Nursing Law, 33*(2), 1.

Tammelleo, A.D. (1994, October). Vicarious liability for nurses: "Borrowed servant" doctrine. *The Reagan Report on Nursing Law, 35*(5), 1.

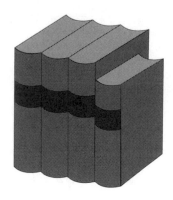

Chapter 7

NEGLIGENCE SPECIFIC TO NURSING

Jacquelyn K. Hall
Daniel Hall

Failure to Evaluate—Observe, Monitor,
Communicate, Follow Up
ISSUES AND TRENDS
  TRENDS IN NURSING PRACTICE
  TRENDS IN ADVANCED NURSING PRACTICE
    LIABILITY
  LEGAL TRENDS
  ETHICAL CONSIDERATIONS AND CONFLICTS
**RECOMMENDATIONS FOR RESEARCH AND
MALPRACTICE PREVENTION**
  RESEARCH IN NURSING LIABILITY
  MALPRACTICE PREVENTION
SUMMARY
POINTS TO REMEMBER
REFERENCES
SUGGESTED READINGS

KEY WORDS

Beneficence	Medication Errors
Civil Law	Nursing Care Plan
Crime	Omnibus Budget
Criminal Law	Reconciliation Act of
Employment Retirement	1987 (OBRA)
Income Security Act	Ordinary Negligence
(ERISA)	Outcome Standards
Least Restrictive	Per se Standard of Care
Environment Standard	Vicarious Liability
Malpractice	

Upon completion of this chapter, the reader will be able to:

- Explain malpractice law as a minimum enforcement of a higher standard.
- Recognize common situations that give rise to nursing malpractice cases.
- Respond to situations in nursing practice that have potential legal liability.

INTRODUCTION

This chapter elaborates on negligence specific to professional nursing practice. The legal term for negligence committed by professionals is **malpractice**. Malpractice law holds nurses responsible as individuals, independent of employer or doctor liability.

Nurses need to know the areas of their practice with the greatest legal danger. In this chapter, the malpractice liability incurred in nursing is categorized under the headings of assessment, planning, implementation, and evaluation.

Nurses can avoid excessive worry about the specifics of the law, by remembering one concept: Good practice is ethical and legal (Hall, 1996a). Both law and morals are on a continuum of conflict resolution. Good practice is a higher standard than the minimum behavior mandated by the law. If nurses practice as they were taught to practice in their educational program, and keep competent through continuing education and experience, their practice will be "good." They may only avoid liability for malpractice—a lower standard of behavior than good nursing practice.

As shown in Figure 7–1, good nursing practice is above the minimum enforced by negligence law. If nurses fail to practice as reasonable prudent nurses—a lower level than good nursing practice—the law will punish them by holding them liable in malpractice or disciplining their licenses.

At the end of this chapter under the section Malpractice Prevention, a simple way to avoid liability in malpractice is discussed fully. Patients who sue usually are angry about something. One study found that fewer than 10 percent of obstetricians sued accounted for a majority of the lawsuits, and patient satisfaction with those obstetricians was lower (Hickson, Clayton, & Entman, 1994). To recover for malpractice, the patient must have been harmed by a negligent act. Through the cases reviewed in this chapter, watch for methods by which the nurse could have avoided harming the patient by avoiding a breach of the standard of care (Hall, 1996a).

Nursing malpractice law enforces at a minimum level the value of beneficence for the patient. An Anglo-Saxon word, **beneficence** simply means doing good, to benefit the health of the patient. This value above all others characterizes nursing. The value of beneficence, of caring for the patient, underlies all of nursing law. The most important area of law enforcing the ethical value of beneficence is malpractice law, a subdivision of tort law. Tort law can be classified according to how accidental the act is.

At the unintentional end of the intent scale in Figure 7–2, wrongs that are not caused by intentional acts are described as being caused by negligence. Some association with

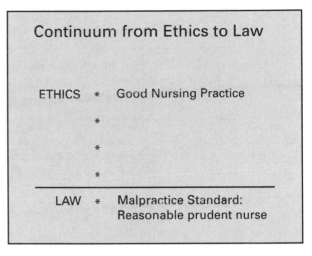

FIG. 7-1. Continuum from ethics to law. (Adapted with permission from Hall, J. K. (1996). *Nursing ethics and law.* Philadelphia: W.B. Saunders.)

accident is implied. Negligence law covers such occurrences as car wrecks and falls in supermarkets. A subdivision of negligence law is malpractice law—the negligence of professionals like doctors, nurses, and lawyers that causes injury to their patients or clients.

The scale of intent shown in Figure 7–2 pertains to civil cases, not criminal law. **Civil law** deals with wrongs against individuals. **Criminal law** deals with acts that are considered to be against the people as a whole. A **crime** usually is considered to be the result of an intent to harm or a reckless disregard of whether harm will occur as a result of the action.

Malpractice is not the worst event that the law can visit on the nurse. Under malpractice law, at worst the nurse loses money; under criminal law, nurses might lose their liberty. Some acts that are negligent also might be crimes. For example, nurses in Denver gave penicillin to a newborn in the wrong dosage and by the wrong route. When the baby died, they were charged with the crime of negligent homicide (Nornhold, 1997). Also, people who are managers in health care corporations are at risk of indictment for crimes associated with fraud and abuse of Medicare law ("Columbia HCA Employees," 1997).

HISTORICAL PERSPECTIVE

For thousands of years, the law has held professionals personally responsible for their actions. Even the ancient Greeks wrote about right treatments and how to judge professional practice (Amundson, 1977). As nurses gain more independence, more money, and more insurance, they increasingly are held responsible for their actions under nursing malpractice law. Nursing law was developed from the law that was applied in malpractice suits against doctors.

In the past, patients sued for negligent acts by nurses, using four different legal theories: *respondeat superior*, captain of the ship, borrowed servant, and ordinary negligence. The first three are forms of **vicarious liability**, in which someone other than the nurse was held responsible for the nurse's actions. Nurses were sued personally only under ordinary negligence.

Ordinary negligence uses as a reference that standard of conduct required of reasonable prudent people, conduct that would cause laypeople to be held liable for their acts (*Black's Law Dictionary*, 1990). When a nurse was sued using the ordinary negligence standard, the allegedly negligent conduct was compared with the reasonable

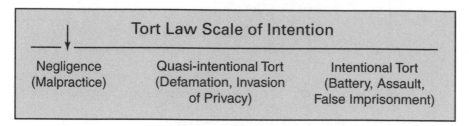

FIG. 7-2. Tort law scale of intention. (With permission from Hall, J. K. (1996). *Nursing ethics and law.* Philadelphia: W.B. Saunders.)

prudent person—not the reasonable prudent nurse.

The theory of ordinary negligence now has fallen into disuse in cases against nurses. In contrast to ordinary negligence, **malpractice** is defined as the "failure of one rendering professional services to exercise that degree of skill and learning commonly applied under all the circumstances in the community by the average prudent reputable member of the profession with the result of injury, loss or damage to the recipient of those services or to those entitled to rely on them" (*Black's Law Dictionary*, 1990). Professionals are held to a higher standard than the lay public.

Nurses were sued under the theory of ordinary negligence because they were seen as doctor's helpers, merely carrying out doctor's orders without independent judgment. Courts did not view nurses as professionals, so they applied the ordinary negligence standard to nurses as they did to other nonprofessionals. Nurses now take on more responsibility and are said to work within a much enlarged practice scope (Makar, 1996; Salatka, 1992).

Under the borrowed servant theory, the nurse's employer is assumed to allow or direct the nurse to work for another employer. During the time this work is being done, the nurse is considered to be borrowed by, or the employee of, the subsequent employer.

Courts increasingly have held nurses liable for malpractice or professional negligence, in part because of their heightened responsibility, and in part because some have malpractice insurance, which makes them financially attractive to plaintiffs (*Fraijo*

v. Hartland Hospital, 1979; Makar, 1996). The terms *negligence* and *malpractice* often are used interchangeably.

RECURRING CAUSES OF NURSE LIABILITY

Accurate data about malpractice suits are not readily available. It surprises the layperson that no organized central repository of legal cases exists. Research studies about lawsuits vary in design, and the information obtained is not arranged in consistent categories. Specifics of studies about the subject vary (Faherty, 1998). Despite these problems, some common trends can be identified regarding areas of greatest risk for nursing malpractice.

Miller-Slade (1997) cited a study of malpractice claims in which nursing negligence led to a settlement or verdict for the patient. Of 747 such cases, there were 219 deaths. Inadequate communication to the doctor led to 76 of the deaths; inadequate assessment, 46; medication errors, 42; inadequate nursing intervention, 17; inadequate care, 21; unsafe environment, 7; inadequate infection control, 3; and improper use of equipment and products, 7 deaths. The causes of these suits are not unpredictable. They are failures to adhere to the standard of care.

Another listing of most likely negligence in nurse lawsuits, by the Doctor Insurers Association of America (1993), found the most common causes of lawsuits were (1) medication and treatment errors, (2) lack of observation and timely reporting on the patient, (3) defective technology or equipment, (4) infections caused or worsened by poor nursing care, (5) poor communication of important information, and (6) failure to intervene to protect the patient from poor medical care. These lawsuits can be avoided by good practice, the way a reasonable prudent nurse would practice.

The causes of all these suits were failures to maintain a standard of practice. These suits prove the thesis: good practice is moral and legal. Next, specifics of the failures of the standard of care are discussed—assessment, planning, implementation, and evaluation.

FAILURE TO ASSESS

Nurses, theorists, and lawyers alike agree that assessment and observation of the patient is a fundamental nursing duty (Sweeney, 1997). This standard is established by practice and formalized in the various sources of standards, including most nurse practice acts. Round-the-clock care primarily is left to nurses. In this role, the nurse acts as an adjunct to the absent doctor or other prescriber. The duty of the nurse is to assess, monitor, and/or observe the patient and report any abnormalities to the doctor (Miller-Slade, 1997). Implicit in this duty to assess are four separate requirements.

1. The nurse must possess the knowledge and skill required to properly assess and/or monitor the patient, including making a nursing diagnosis. Interestingly, the courts have not been sensitive to the word diagnosis. As early as 1955, a California court held an occupational health nurse liable for the failure to timely "diagnose" a patient's skin cancer and to refer him to a doctor (*Cooper v. National Motor Bearing Co.*, 1955).
2. The assessment and monitoring of the patient actually must be carried out.
3. If the assessment and monitoring reveal a condition that should be reported, the nurse must notify the doctor or other prescriber. The nurse must carry out appropriate nursing and ordered medical interventions, in an effort to correct the problem.
4. The nurse must continue to assess and

monitor, to evaluate the effectiveness of the interventions until the patient is stable.

Each of these requirements must be met, or the standard of care is breached. If harm comes to the patient as a result of the breach, the nurse could be held liable. In the New Jersey case of *Adams v. Cooper Hospital* (1996), the hospital and nurse were held jointly liable for $1.5 million for failing to monitor the patient. The nurse left the patient, who needed frequent suctioning, for 30 minutes or more. The patient's fall out of bed resulted in head injury, a broken hip and nursing liability.

To avoid harm to patients, and to avoid the related legal liability, nurses should incorporate a real or mental checklist of the requirements of every patient in their care. For most experienced nurses, this checklist is second nature. For the new nurse, the process must be consciously applied and even written down. Such a checklist, if dated and signed, might be admissible as evidence of meeting the standard of care.

FAILURE TO PLAN

Clinical decision-making through care planning is an integral part of nursing care. Plans of care are said to be the best way to apply the nursing process to actual patient care. Many states and the federal government have enacted specific statutes and regulations that require nurses to write patient plans of care, and to evaluate them periodically for effectiveness. The term **nursing care plan** is used less than formerly, being replaced in some organizations by protocols, critical pathways, or other tools. Regardless of the name, some formal planning of nursing care is required by the standard of practice.

The plan of nursing care theoretically could be unwritten, in earlier days when patients paid their own bills and insurance companies did not need written proof that the nurse had done the care. A nurse can assess, plan, care and evaluate without writing it down. But the nurse is unlikely to be able to communicate that plan to others on the care team without writing. Without a written tool, the insurer or regulator who audits the care could not know what the plan was or whether a plan was made.

Some state nurse practice acts require plans of care—Texas and Illinois are examples. Federal regulations in almost every area of health care require plans of care (for example, home health and hospice). A federal regulation issued in 1998 as part of patient rights legislation requires nursing plans of care for all patients of health maintenance organizations (HMOs). Federal law requires nurses working in nursing homes to formulate and institute a written plan of care for their patients on the day of admission (Public Health Welfare, 1997).

Additionally, the American Nurses Association (ANA), starting in 1973, established standards that provide all nurses are expected to assess, document health data, and assign nursing diagnoses to their patients. Nurses then are expected to use this information to develop a nursing plan of care according to their assessment and diagnosis.

FAILURE TO CREATE A PLAN OF CARE BASED ON THE PATIENT'S CONDITION

Failure to complete and then follow a plan of care may result in malpractice. In *Smith v. Juneau* (1997) the court found nurses negligent for failing to develop a plan of care to protect the skin of an orthopedic patient in traction. Evidence was presented that nurses had not moved the patient, assessed the patient's skin under the traction sling, written a plan of care addressing skin integrity, or instituted such care. Those failures caused the patient serious injury. The court held that if a plan of care had been made, the patient would not have developed serious ulcers.

Another case found that failure to complete a plan of care was a breach of the standard of care. In *Green v. Berrien General Hosp. Auxiliary, Inc.* (1990) the court found that, among other breaches of the standard, not completing a plan of care for a child whose endotracheal tube failed was malpractice. The court reasoned, failure to write

a plan of care usually means failure to do the care that would be called for in the plan. The court further noted, if the nurses actually had done the care, the failure to write the plan probably would not have resulted in liability, because the patient would not have suffered harm.

FAILURE TO IMPLEMENT THE PLAN OF CARE BASED ON THE PATIENT'S CONDITION

Even if a plan is made, failure to implement the plan of care can result in malpractice. The areas of potential failure encompass all implementation that can be planned and written. In the Texas case of *Nix Medical Hospital v. Slazer* (1995), the elderly patient's plan of care identified his problems as confusion and getting out of bed without help. The planned intervention was to help the patient up to the commode when necessary, with constant nursing assistance. A nursing student who was not assigned to the patient helped the patient to a bedside commode and left him there while she notified the patient's nurse. The patient fell and suffered serious injuries. The case demonstrated that a negligence verdict can result from failure to follow the plan of care. The plan of care itself set the standard by which the nurse's action was measured.

In *St. Germain v. Pfeifer* (1994) the nurse was held to have a duty to know the patient's plan of care, which addressed the danger of the patient's moving. The patient's movement caused injury that required further surgery. If the nurse had known about the plan and the danger, the nurse would have noted the inconsistency of the orders for movement, between the resident and the doctor.

These cases demonstrate that nurses have a duty to use the nursing process to develop plans for the care of their patients. The making and writing of a plan itself is evidence that the nurse assessed the patient, thought about the patient's care, and had an intent to implement the plan. After being made, plans of care must be implemented and evaluated on an ongoing basis. Plans of care that are standardized, computerized, packaged, and preprinted must be individualized to the particular patient.

FAILURE TO FOLLOW ORGANIZATION POLICY AND PROCEDURE

To recover for malpractice, the patient must show that the nurse had a duty that was breached and caused damage. Nursing duties can be established with organization policies and the procedures written in manuals and in unit-specific guidelines. Nurses can be held liable in malpractice law for not following organization policies and procedures.

Procedure documents have a long history. Some of Nightingale's writings actually are early hospital procedure manuals—about cleaning the patient's room, opening windows, making rounds, and so on. Many health care organizations seek Joint Commission on Accreditation of Healthcare Organizations (JCAHO) accreditation, and the JCAHO standards require that nursing departments develop policies and procedures for nursing practice. The resulting documents can be used to establish the standard of care (Sweeney, 1997).

Quality assurance theory and quality improvement language have changed the terms used here. What were called "policies" before are now known as "process standards," and what were before "procedures" may now be the "structure standards." **Outcome standards**, sometimes called critical pathways and protocols, also may be used to establish standards of care.

Many cases from several states have used written organization policies in determining a nurse's duty. The Arizona case of *Peacock v. Samaritan Health Service* (1989) found that a failure to follow written organization policy could be used as evidence of negligence. In that case, a suicidal patient was admitted to a room in which the windows did not have safety mechanisms, which was counter to organization policy. The patient opened the window, fell out, and suffered serious injury. The court held the jury could conclude that the policy was the standard of care, and that the failure to follow that standard was negligence.

The lesson from that case: If a nurse fails to follow a written organization protocol and such failure results in patient injury, the nurse can be found to have breached a nursing duty to the patient. The organization policy need not be specifically related to nursing, only to patient care. In the *Peacock* (1989) case, the policy was said to be not directly related to nursing care, but the court inferred that the nurses should not have allowed the suicidal patient to be admitted into a room without window safety mechanisms.

The nurse can be found negligent for failing to follow the organization protocol that provides for periodic review of doctor and other prescriber medication orders if that failure injures the patient. Some other examples of liability for failure to follow procedures: not following organization policy in conducting a surgical sponge count (*Sullivan v. Methodist Hospitals of Dallas*, 1985) and failing to call the doctor when hospital protocol dictates that a call be made (*Holster v. Sisters of the Third Order of St. Francis*, 1995).

However, following hospital policy rigidly when the situation calls for a different response may be wrong. In a well-publicized case, emergency department policy prohibited staff from leaving the premises to assist in an emergency. A boy was shot and brought to the hospital, just off the hospital property. The ambulance called to bring the boy onto the property did not come. The staff followed the letter of the policy and left the boy outside bleeding. When the boy died as a result, nationwide censure of the staff and the policy resulted (Gray, 1998).

FAILURE TO IMPLEMENT A PLAN OF CARE

THE DUTY TO INTERVENE

Nurses, theorists, and lawyers can agree that the essence of nursing practice consists of appropriate interventions. The nurse's duty extends beyond actions taken personally by the nurse. The nurse has a duty to intervene when someone causes or might cause harm to the patient.

The failure of the nurse to intervene is examined from three perspectives: (1) when a nurse harms the patient, (2) when a doctor or other prescriber harms the patient, and (3) when a family member or significant other harms the patient.

When a Nurse Harms the Patient

Nurses have a duty to safeguard the patient from harm caused by their own care. When a nurse fails to intervene, or the intervention is improper, and harm comes to the patient as a result, the nurse may be liable.

The nurse has a duty to safeguard the patient from harm by other nurses. If a nurse reasonably can foresee harm to the patient at the hands of another nurse, then the nurse has a duty to try to prevent the harm. Failure to act for the patient's safety, with resultant harm to the patient, may result in liability for the negligence that another nurse commits.

In most states, the nursing practice act or other statute specifically requires the nurse to report another nurse who harms a patient.

When the Doctor or Other Prescriber Harms the Patient

As a general rule, people are held liable for their own acts. When the doctor or other prescriber is the wrongdoer, it is that person, not the nurse, who is held responsible. But nurses may be liable also, especially when the doctor or other prescriber writes an erroneous order. Nurses have a duty to implement valid medical orders, and nursing liability will result if the nurse who is responsible fails to do so. The nurse must ascertain the validity of that order.

The nurse has a duty to be knowledgeable about the medical orders to be carried out. If a nurse knows or should know that a medical order will cause harm to the patient, then the nurse could be held liable for resulting damages from carrying out the erroneous medical order.

In *Wingo v. Rockford Memorial Hospital* (1997), a pregnant patient whose membranes

apparently had ruptured came to the hospital. The nurse observed the patient leaking fluid but did not remember reporting that fact to the patient's doctor, who ordered the patient to be discharged. There were no nursing notes about the conversation. The patient returned the next morning, giving birth to a septic infant with several problems, including cerebral palsy and mental retardation. The court upheld damages of more than $10 million against the hospital. The standard of care was (1) to recognize that the discharge of the patient was inappropriate in those circumstances and (2) to protect the patient from the harm an inappropriate order might cause.

When a Family Member or Significant Other Harms the Patient

The nurse has a duty to safeguard the patient from physical harm, even at the hands of a family member. Failure to act for the patient's safety, with resultant harm to the patient, may result in nursing liability. Problems in this area include intentional and even negligent injuries, for example, contraindicated administration of home remedies, assistance to ambulate a patient on total bed rest, and providing a steak dinner for a patient on NPO (nothing by mouth) status. However, if the nurse did not know and could not have known that the family member or other caregiver would harm the patient, then the nurse will not be held liable (*Morgan v. Cohen*, 1986).

Statutes in every state require nurses to report neglect or abuse of dependent persons such as children, the aged, or the disabled. Those statutes could be used to establish a *per se* **standard of care.** The breach of the standard of care would result in liability, without the need for expert testimony to prove the breach.

FAILURE TO ADVOCATE FOR THE PATIENT THROUGH THE ORGANIZATION HIERARCHY

Related to the general duty to intervene, is a duty to advocate for the patient, through the organization hierarchy chain of command. In *Wingo v. Rockford Memorial Hospital* (1997), the failure to advocate for the patient according to organization guidelines, when the patient was being discharged with ruptured membranes, resulted in malpractice.

The nurse must advocate for the patient through the hierarchy or face liability—even if there is no set organization protocol for the situation. In the North Carolina case of *Campbell v. Pitt County Memorial Hospital* (1987), nurses were liable for failure to advocate for the patient, through the organization hierarchy, about a hypoxic fetus. The nurse recognized that the fetus was hypoxic, reported to the doctor, and the doctor did nothing. The nurse did nothing more. The baby subsequently was born seriously injured. The nurse defended on grounds that there was no policy for advocating for the patient through the organization hierarchy. The hospital defended itself on the ground that the nurse merely followed the "do nothing" orders of the doctor. The appellate court decided against both the nurse and the hospital.

The hospital was liable under the theory of corporate negligence. In this case, the hospital was held liable for its negligent administrators, who did not have a policy in place for advocating for patients. The court found the nurse's duty was to advocate for the patient through the organization hierarchy. The specific duty was to contact the immediate supervisor when faced with a dangerous situation that the doctor ignored. When the nurse knows or should know that a doctor's or other prescriber's course of action or inaction will result in patient harm, the nurse's duty is to advocate for the patient.

In *NKC Hospitals Inc. v. Anthony* (1993), the doctor had discharged a patient who was in pain and had not been examined by any doctor. The court held that the hospital's nurses had an independent duty to the patient, so the hospital was not relieved of its liability under the theory of *respondeat superior*. Nurses were not merely following a "chain of command" by doing what the doctor ordered. The nurse's duty does not end with the doctor's or other prescriber's order. If the nurse is not satisfied with the action taken by the doctor or other prescriber, then the nurse must proceed to advocate for the patient through the organization hierarchy until there is an appropriate resolution.

Obviously, the nurse must stand on firm factual ground when making these contacts. A solid base of clinical knowledge and experience is essential. This requirement to advocate for the patient is not related to minor issues such as disagreeing with the doctor or other prescriber about the choice of antibiotics. Only in the most obvious and dangerous of circumstances, when the patient's life or health clearly is at stake, does the law expect the nurse to continue to advocate for the patient through the hierarchy, including the doctor or other prescriber, the supervisor, and perhaps even the chief of medical staff.

Nurses in one case were liable when they did not question the medical standard of care. *Thompson v. Nason Hosp.* (1991) held that the hospital and nurse may be jointly liable with the doctor for damages to a patient who was paralyzed because the doctor failed to monitor treatment of her heart disease. The court said that nurses and other hospital employees have a duty to question a doctor's order that is not in accord with standard medical practice. This decision could be interpreted as meaning that nurses not only must know and practice standard nursing practice but also must know at least minimum standard medical practice and enforce it by advocacy. A good reference for this duty to advocate can be found in the article by Hardy (1986).

MEDICATION ERRORS—FAILURE TO FOLLOW THE FIVE RIGHTS

Medication errors are said by some authorities to be the most common source of nursing negligence (Cavico & Cavico, 1995). The most useful technique for preventing errors in the administration of medication ordered by the prescriber is to use the "five rights" of medication administration. These rights are included as minimum practice standards in some nursing practice acts: Give the right drug, give the right dose, to the right patient, by the right route, at the right time. The prosecution for negligent homicide discussed earlier (see Wornhold, 1997) was for error in dose and route of penicillin. The wrong dose was sent by the pharmacist, but the nurses, including a pediatric nurse practitioner, did not catch the error.

Failure to follow any one of these procedural safeguards, with consequent harm to the patient, can result in liability. Because the five rights are so easy to follow and so effective, medication error suits are difficult to defend (Salatka, 1992).

In addition to adhering to the five rights, nurses have an independent duty to be knowledgeable about all the drugs they administer. The nurse's medication knowledge should include an understanding of drug names and therapeutic categories, adverse drug reactions and interactions, dosage, timing, technique of administration, expected therapeutic response, duration of drug use, and procedures to minimize the incidence or severity of adverse drug effects (Salatka, 1992).

Once the medication is given correctly, it must be documented. The phrase "not documented, not done" legally is wrong. Verbal testimony about what was done always is admissible. But law favors written evidence because (1) it is permanent, (2) it was made concurrent with the event, and (3) it is not subject to the vagaries of the memory—time and wishful thinking.

Document the five rights—which medication, to whom, in what dose, through which route, and at what time. Document fully any suspected adverse drug reaction by time and character of the reaction. Document interventions undertaken and their results.

Laws have changed to allow practitioners other than doctors to prescribe medications, including nurse practitioners, clinical nurse specialists, and physician assistants. The duty to administer medications safely has not changed, regardless of who writes the orders. Doctors or other prescribers must be sure that their own education and experience is adequate to make them competent to prescribe drugs safely. Advanced practice nurses have a duty to be certain that their medication orders are appropriate.

The trend toward legalizing assisted suicide concerns nurses who might be asked to administer medications to patients who will use them to commit suicide. Physician-assisted suicide is legal in Oregon. Nurses may be asked to deliver an overdose to the patient because suicide can be assisted in the hospital or nursing home in that state. As part of the medication administration protocol for suicide, it is advised to put a plastic bag over the patient's head to ensure suffocation in case the drugs fail and the patient wakes up. Home health and hospice nurses may be asked to put the bag in place or to hold the patient's hands to keep him or her from tearing off the bag (Hall, 1996b).

A 1997 decision by the U.S. Supreme Court upheld the right of state government to keep assisted suicide criminal (*Vacco v. Quill*, 1997; *Washington v. Glucksberg*, 1997). The decision did not prohibit states from making assisted suicide legal, and Oregon has done so.

FAILURE TO IMPLEMENT SPECIFIC ACTIONS

Failure to Respond to the Patient

Failure to respond to the patient results in liability when the nurse actually hears the patient's complaint and does nothing about it. The nurse either fails to assess, or assesses and then fails to intervene. The patients who sue usually are angry.

For example, in *Manning v. Twin Falls Clinic & Hosp., Inc.* (1992), the patient's family pleaded with the nurse not to disconnect the patient's oxygen during a move to another room. They asserted that the patient could not survive without oxygen, and that the patient should have portable oxygen during the move. The nurse moved the patient without oxygen. The patient turned blue and died. The patient was on DNR (do not resuscitate) status and was not resuscitated. An award of punitive damages was upheld by the court, because the nurse's action was characterized as extreme deviation from the standard of care.

Patients who are harmed by a negligent act can sue; angry patients and families will. Take all patient complaints seriously. According to Werner (1998), patients who are ill are those who have (1) an organic illness that might be dangerous, like heart disease, (2) a nonorganic illness that is not dangerous, like chest wall syndrome, or (3) both. Werner (1998) also notes if the nurse ignores patients in category 1 or 3—meaning any patient—the nurse is at risk for a lawsuit.

Nurses who work in conditions that endanger patient safety may be liable for malpractice that results, because no one is forced to work in such conditions. If inadequate staffing prevents nurses from giving patients care according to the standards of nursing practice, the nurse may be liable for the failure. In *Merritt v. Karcioglu* (1996), the nurse, doctor, and hospital were held liable for the injury and subsequent death of an elderly woman who fell during the time her private duty nurse left the room to participate in a code blue. The nurse was required to participate in the code blue by hospital policy.

In *Adams v. Cooper Hospital* (1996), a nurse left a patient who needed frequent suctioning, for 30 minutes or more. Choking, trying to reach the call bell, the patient fell out of bed and suffered a head injury and broken hip. The nurse and hospital were held liable for a verdict in excess of $1.5 million. In this case, it was not clear that poor staffing caused the failure; but that is a common complaint of nurses who say they "don't have time" to monitor such patients.

In *Fincke v. Peeples* (1985), while a recovery room nurse cared for another patient, her 17-year-old patient stopped breathing and sustained brain damage. The nurse was found personally liable for the injury to the young patient because she was not constantly monitoring him.

The nurse may not be liable for inadequate staffing if the management has been informed. Always document this situation for legal protection. If a licensure complaint arises from a situation where there was inadequate staffing, the nurse can use that documentation in defense. The lawyer for the nursing board will ask (1) whether the nurse informed the management, (2) what the management's response was, and (3) what the nurse did if the management's response was inadequate. The hospital itself may be responsible for inadequate staffing under the legal theory of corporate negligence.

Failure to Educate the Patient

Nurses and theorists agree that one of the nurse's most important duties is that of teacher. As teacher, the nurse answers questions, explains procedures, and instructs the family and patient in home care and self-care, including the proper use of medical equipment (Breau & Dracup, 1982). Failure to properly educate a patient, with resulting harm to that patient, can result in liability.

A Texas court held the hospital grossly negligent under the theory of *respondeat superior*, for $3.5 million, for failure of its home health nurse (an employee) to provide teaching. A patient sent home with intravenous (IV) antibiotics failed to mix the antibiotic into the bag of saline. The diabetic patient was described as noncompliant, in denial of her illness because of her desire for a normal life. The patient told the jury that she self-administered the IV, which was saline without antibiotic, and her infection worsened, requiring amputation of her left leg and damage to her right foot. A lawyer for the hospital said the patient told the nurse she knew how to medicate herself, and that the patient ignored instructions printed in red on the bag that said to pull the bag's inner stopper to mix the drug with the saline. Unfortunately, the attorney also said: "We made a mistake. We made an error. We should have insisted on a return demonstration." ("Hospital Held Liable," 1996).

Failure to Perform Care
According to the Standard of Care

The first duty in performing procedures according to the standard of care is to make sure the patient has given informed consent to the procedure. Failure to provide informed consent is a source of legal liability. Consent for usual treatment such as injections and catheters can be implied in the patient's coming to the organization to receive health care. In addition, the patient often gives express consent in a consent signed on admission.

In *Ritter v. Delaney* (1990) a patient sought to hold a hospital and doctor liable for failing to obtain informed consent to surgery. The court found that obtaining consent was the doctor's responsibility. Delegating the responsibility for obtaining a signature on the consent form to the nurse did not make the nurse and the employer liable.

But another Texas court found the nurses personally liable, and their employer liable under the theory of *respondeat superior*, for negligence in obtaining informed consent. The patient had signed a consent for procedures including a hemorrhoidectomy; but several times prior to surgery she had insisted to staff that she would not have the hemorrhoidectomy. The court said the nurses should at least inquire about the validity of the consent, when the patient had made direct, unambiguous, verbal objections to having the procedure (*Urban v. Spohn Hospital*, 1993).

After inferred consent, the nurse's duty is to perform treatments safely and according to the accepted standard of care. Nurses should know and follow hospital policy, but not if the policy is inappropriate. Nurses should work hard to change policies that reflect poor standards of care.

In performing care, equipment must be used safely. This is a dangerous area, not only for the personal safety of the nurse and patient, but for legal liability. Nurses must know how to operate the equipment they use. This may require reading both the organization policy and the instruction manual for the equipment. There is no defense to wrongly using equipment when the patent is harmed.

Failure to Adequately Supervise Care

Nurses have a duty to perform care for which they are competent, as well as a duty to supervise activities of others under their direction. Nurses are not automatically liable for whatever the subordinate does—only liable for negligently supervising that subordinate. For example, the supervisor may be liable for negligently assigning a practical nurse to care for a patient on a ventilator, if the supervisor knows or should know that the practical nurse has never had training or experience with such patients. Sufficient staff must be assigned to do the job; the staff should be competent to care for those particular patients; and adequate time must be allowed for patient care.

When alerted to a problem, supervisors must respond. The supervisor must (1) teach and inform appropriately; (2) ascertain that staff complied generally with policies and procedures; (3) verify that the staff's training was adequate; (4) report conditions that could injure patients, including staffing levels, to senior management; and (5) provide for student supervision.

Neither staff nurses nor supervisors are held liable legally for poor staffing if the harm to the patient is not due to the nurse's own negligence or the supervisor's decision to assign inadequate staff. The staff nurse and supervisor are liable for any malpractice they themselves commit, regardless of availability of staff. Staff nurses have a duty to tell supervisors that staffing is inadequate—every time it happens, in writing. The supervisor must act on that information. They must investigate, assess, and if needed supply more staffing if it is within their authority, or inform the next level of management.

Failure to Adhere to the Standard of Care in Specific Instances

Patient falls are often a result of breach of the standard of care, provoking lawsuits. Falls are more worrisome to nurses because of tightened restrictions on patient restraints. The JCAHO, the federal, state, and local governments, and individual organization policies all caution against using restraints inappropriately. Restrictions on the use of restraints were included in the **Omnibus Budget Reconciliation Act of 1987 (OBRA)**, which govern healthcare practice in long-term care. The various restrictions on restraints are specific, for example to amount of time restraints can be used, who must order them and how often, and so on.

Realistically, all the nurse can do is try to protect the patient from falls, without overusing restraints. The duty is to allow the patient as much freedom as possible, but restrain if necessary for safety, checking frequently and getting reorders as needed i.e. **least restrictive environment standard.**

Another specific instance of a breach of the nursing standard is negligence concerning bed rails. Lawsuits are common if patients are harmed in a fall from bed, and also if patients are harmed by the bed rails themselves. Regulations on restraints prohibit the general use of bed rails at night for all patients. When nurses do not have a rule to guide them, they must use their own independent judgment in the situation. Rules and policies are made for the average situation, the usual encounter. Nurses need education because they must use judgment in situations that do not fit the general rule.

Lawsuits in the operating suite demonstrate another specific instance of failure to adhere to the standard of care. Foreign objects may be retained after surgery, resulting in a lawsuit for nurses who work in the surgical department. The statute of limitations cuts off most medical malpractice lawsuits after 2 or 3 years, depending on the state's law. But if the patient could not discover the negligence, the patient can sue years later, after the discovery. That discovery may come when the patient has surgery again, a decade later, and a sponge is found.

Techniques to avoid the problems of retained sponges and surgical instruments include computerized counts and standard sets of instruments. Such cases rarely go to trial because liability is practically automatic. Nurses do the counts, so they are liable. The employer too is liable under the legal theory of *respondeat superior*. Doctors are also liable if they participated or signed off on the count or sometimes just because they are present on the case. The legal standard allows no human error in surgical counts in the operating suite.

FAILURE TO EVALUATE—OBSERVE, MONITOR, COMMUNICATE, FOLLOW UP

Nurses have a duty to observe and monitor their patients, and communicate the observations to the appropriate provider. The reason for patient stays in the hospital, and for employment of nurses around the clock, is to observe, monitor, and communicate change. The duty is to observe changes, recognize when they are significant, report them to the appropriate person, and follow up if that response is not sufficient.

Failure to Observe a Significant Change or Condition

Most nursing practice acts require the nurse to observe the patient for change in condition (Miller-Slade, 1997). The duty is to know what the patient's condition has been, what it is now, and what it should be, according to the natural history or progression of the patient's condition.

Failure to Appreciate the Significance of a Change or Condition

The duty to the patient is not met merely by observing a change or condition. The nurse must know the significance of the observation. Much of nursing education is aimed towards this nursing process. Merely noting an increase in the pulse rate is not enough, even if it also is documented. An increase in pulse might mean hemorrhage, even if there is no visible hemorrhage. For example, in a malpractice case on which the author contributed, a nurse observed a patient in an intensive care unit (ICU) all night, recording blood pressures averaging 40 systolic and 20 diastolic. But, she did not recognize the significance of the readings, or report them to the nurse in charge. The patient's hypoxia led to death and a large settlement for plaintiff from the resulting lawsuit.

Failure to Report or Document a Significant Change or Condition

There are two components to this failure— failure to report and failure to document. Failure to report is the most serious breach of duty. The nurse has a duty to assess change and decide whether it is significant. If it is, the nurse must report the change to the appropriate provider.

In advance of needing it, the nurse should

be familiar with the organization policy on reporting changes in patient condition. If such a policy does not exist, nurses should write one. Nurses have a duty to develop their own procedure for getting help for the patient. A lawsuit is not the worst result of failure to report a change in the patient. The worst result is that the patient will be harmed.

In *Convalescent Services, Inc. v. Schultz* (1996), a nursing home patient progressed from a stage 1 to a stage 4 decubitus ulcer. The evidence showed failure to turn the patient, failure to notify the doctor of the skin deterioration, failure to give daily whirl-pool baths as ordered, failure to provide proper nutrition and appropriate mattress, and failure to document the patient's progress on the "skin assessment flow chart." Punitive damages were awarded against the nursing home. Failure to document was an inherent of the negligence, but not the only ground for liability.

Poor documentation of even good care may be breach of the standard of patient care. In a lawsuit, failure to document may be presented as evidence of poor care in other areas. Further, poor documentation may result in a charge of failure to document, brought by the nursing board. Disciplinary action by the nursing board may follow failure to document, even if no harm comes to the patient.

Based on statutory regulation, a plaintiff might bring a malpractice action under the theory of liability of negligence per se. No expert witness would need to testify to the standard of care. For example, a regulation used by plaintiffs in malpractice cases is the Texas Nursing Practice Act § 217.117(1999).

[The RN shall] accurately report and document the client's symptoms, responses, and status (adopted 1992).

The regulations written by boards of nursing are often used against nurses in malpractice suits, as well as in licensure discipline. Merely failing to document occasionally, if good nursing practice was done otherwise, is unlikely to be reported to the board and even more unlikely to result in sanctions.

Failure to Follow Up or Document Follow-up

The duty to observe, monitor, and report changes is enforced by lawsuits requiring nurses to advocate for the patient through the organization hierarchy. Advanced practice nurses (APNs), especially nurse practitioners (NPs), may have a special liability in this area. Patient follow-up is part of accurate diagnosis; the patient's anticipated response to care confirms the diagnosis originally made. If the follow-up does not confirm the initial assessment or diagnosis, the nurse must look for the reason or else risk liability for incorrect diagnosis.

The failure to recognize adverse medication reactions or complications is an integral part of observing, monitoring, and reporting. Nurses must know the expected natural history of diseases or conditions and be ready to act when the patient's condition warrants. Because of the duty to recognize adverse drug reactions, nurses must know the expected effects and any side or toxic effects of medications the patient is prescribed.

ISSUES AND TRENDS

TRENDS IN NURSING PRACTICE

Some authorities have reported there is more personal liability now for nurses, but the data are difficult to obtain (Faherty, 1998). More research is recommended. If personal liability of nurses is increasing, it is important to know why.

The increase in managed care has led to downsizing of hospitals, with more care being given outside the hospital. In addition, patients are paying increasingly out of their own pockets for their care. This trend will continue, because Medical Savings Accounts will dominate the payment for care.

This downsizing and direct pay by the patient will have two results. More care will be given in the patient's home; and nurses will be paid directly by the patient. The legal standards of care are different in the home because the nurse has less equipment and fewer resources. Assessment becomes more important because the short visit is the only professional contact. The patient's ability to pay directly probably means a return to the prior morals, law, and economics that existed when the relationship was between nurse and patient, not between nurse and insurance company and patient.

TRENDS IN ADVANCED PRACTICE LIABILITY

The standard of care for APNs is different from that for other nurses. Nurses are held to that action that a reasonable prudent nurse in a similar circumstance would do. The standard of care for nurses who prescribe medicine in addition to practicing nursing is different; that standard is "that action which a reasonable prudent doctor or other prescriber of medicine in similar circumstance would do" (Hirsh, 1991). Several cases that have provided legal parameters for nurse prescribers have been reported, among the first being *Flickenger v. United States* (1981). The standard of care for the NP giving primary care is the same standard of care as a doctor. For example, the public's expectation that the health care standard should be the equivalent to that given by a doctor, even if the care is given by a nurse.

LEGAL TRENDS

The law holds nurses individually liable, and that trend may increase. If HMOs are successful in protecting themselves from lawsuit under the **Employment Retirement Income Security Act (ERISA)** preemption, one outcome might be more liability for nurses. Attorneys have a duty to get compensation for the client's injury and want a contingency fee for themselves. Lawyers will seek plaintiff's damages and their attorney's fees from someone. If nurses have insurance, they may be seen as one source.

The trend for the twenty-first century is toward individual responsibility. As the government pays less for care, and cares for fewer people, charity care will be a backup. Immunity from lawsuit will persuade chari-

table organizations to give such care. The patient will seek someone else to pay for money damages, and the nurse, seen as an independent decision–maker equal to the doctor, may be a target for liability.

ETHICAL CONSIDERATIONS AND CONFLICTS

Malpractice is amoral. Good practice is moral and legal. Through malpractice law, the minimum standard of nursing behavior is designed to enforce the moral value of doing good for the patient. The standard of good nursing practice requires the nurses to assess, plan, implement, and evaluate. Under Christian values, the standard of moral practice is: "Do unto others as you would have them do unto you" (Luke 6:31).

RECOMMENDATIONS FOR RESEARCH AND MALPRACTICE PREVENTION

RESEARCH IN NURSING LIABILITY

Although widely believed, there is little hard evidence that more nurse malpractice suits are being filed, or that nursing malpractice judgment awards are increasing any more than the population or general inflation would explain (Faherty, 1998). If true, the purchase of malpractice insurance by increasing numbers of nurses may increase liability for nurses overall, as they are perceived as being resources for many damages. Research is needed in all these areas.

Another question for research: Does the absence of responsibility for malpractice affect the level of health care of someone who has that status? As an example, nurses and doctors who work for the federal government cannot be sued for malpractice. The government may be liable, but not the employee. This situation is similar to what is envisioned under the system of enterprise liability advocated by government health reformers. Further, under decreased liability status are there more patient injuries or fewer; better nursing and medical care or worse?

MALPRACTICE PREVENTION

Malpractice may be avoided by the following proactive nursing actions:

1. Responding to the patient
2. Educating the patient
3. Complying with the standard of care
4. Supervising care
5. Adhering to the nursing process
6. Documentation
7. Follow-up

SUMMARY

Good nursing practice is both moral and legal. Malpractice law enforces the moral value to "do good" for the patient. The law represents the minimum standard of nursing practice. The standard of good nursing practice includes assessment, planning, implementation, and evaluation.

POINTS TO REMEMBER

- Patients/plaintiffs sue for negligent acts committed by nurses under three legal theories: *respondeat superior*, borrowed servant, and ordinary negligence.
- *Respondeat superior* is a theory of liability that makes the employer responsible for the negligent acts of the employee.
- In ordinary negligence, the conduct is compared with what a reasonable prudent person—not a professional—would do in the same or similar circumstances.
- Malpractice is failure of one rendering professional services to exercise that degree of skill and learning commonly applied in the community by the average prudent reputable member of the nursing profession.
- All commonly recurring areas of liability for nursing can be characterized as failures to assess, plan, implement, or evaluate.

- Nursing duties arise from a number of sources, including the nursing practice act, organization policies and procedures.
- Failure to follow any of the procedural safeguards of right drug, right dose, right patient, right route, and right time, with consequent harm to the patient, can result in liability.
- Nurses may be liable for not knowing how to use equipment, or for using faulty equipment.
- The nurse has a duty to supervise what others do under his or her direction.
- Failure to document may be viewed as failure of care generally. The nurse whose documentation is poor may be assumed to be poor at other components of care.

REFERENCES

Adams v. Cooper Hospital, 684 A. 2d 506 (1996).

Amundson, R. (1977). Liability in the physician in classical Greek legal theory and practice. *Journal of History and Medicine, 32*, 172–203.

Black's law dictionary. (1990). St. Paul, MN: West Publishing.

Breau, C., & Dracup, K. (1982). Survey of critical care nursing practice, part III: Responsibilities of intensive care unit staff. *Heart & Lung, 11*, 157.

Campbell v. Pitt County Memorial Hospital, 352 S.E.2d 902 (1987).

Cavico, F. J., & Cavico, N. M. (1995). The nursing profession in the 1990's: Negligence and malpractice liability. *Cleveland State Law Review, 43*, 557.

Columbia HCA employees subpoenaed to testify before a Florida grand jury. (1997, July 22). Nashville AP Amarillo Globe News, Business Section.

Convalescent Services, Inc. v. Schultz, 921 S.W.2d 731 (1996).

Cooper v. National Motor Bearing Co., 288 P. 2d 581 (1955).

Faherty, B. (1998). Medical malpractice and adverse actions against nurses: Five years of information from the national doctor or other prescriber data bank. *Journal of Nursing Law, 51*, 17-27.

Fincke v. Peeples, 476 So. 2d 1319 (1985).

Flickenger v. United States, 523 F. Supp. 1372 (W.D. Pa. 1981).

Fraijo v. Hartland Hospital, 160 Cal. Rptr. 246 (1979).

Gray, B. B. (1998). Use your head: When to bend the rules instead of following them. *Healthweek, 314*, 4.

Green v. Berrien General Hosp. Auxiliary, Inc., 464 N.W.2d 703 (1990).

Hall, J. K. (1996a). *Nursing ethics and law*. Philadelphia: W.B. Saunders.

Hall, J. K. (1996b). Assisted suicide: Nurse practitioners as providers? *Nurse Practitioner, 21*(10), 63-71.

Hardy, I. T. (1986). When doctrines collide: Corporation negligence and respondeat superior when hospital employees fail to speak up. *Tulane Law Review, 61*, 85.

Hickson, G. B., Clayton, E. W., & Entman, S. S. (1994). Obstetricians' prior malpractice experience and patient satisfaction with care. *Journal of the American Medical Association, 272*(20), 1583-1587.

Hirsh, H. L. (1991). Medico-legal considerations in the use of doctor extenders. *Legal Medicine*, 127-205.

Holster v. Sisters of the Third Order of St. Francis, 650 N.E.2d 985 (1995).

Hospital held liable for woman who lost leg during care at home. (1996, September 22). *Houston Chronicle*, p. 4D.

Makar, M. C. (1996, March). Nursing in Florida: The path to professional liability. *Florida Bar Journal, 70*, 18.

Manning v. Twin Falls Clinic & Hosp., Inc. 830 P.2d 1185 (Idaho 1992).

Merritt v. Karcioglu, 668 So. 2d 469 (1996).

Miller-Slade, D. (1997, May). Liability theories in nursing negligence cases. *Trial*, pp. 52–57.

Morgan v. Cohen, 523 A. 2d 1003 (1986).

Nix Medical Hospital v. Slazer, WL 611880 (1995).

NKC Hospitals Inc. v. Anthony, 849 S.W.2d 564 (1993).

Nornhold, P. (1997, July). Nursing on trial. *Nursing 97*, p. 33.

Peacock v. Samaritan Health Service, 765 P.2d 525 (1989).

Physician Insurers Association of America. (1993, June). *Medication Error Study*. The Association.

Ritter v. Delaney, 790 S.W.2d 29 (1990).

Salatka, M. A. (1992). Professional liability in critical care nursing. *Ohio North University Law Review, 19*, 85.

Smith v. Juneau, 692 So. 2d 1365 (1997).

St. Germain v. Pfeifer, 637 N.E.2d 848 (1994).

St. Luke. The new testament: The gospel according to St. Luke (6:31). Holy Bible (Masonic Ed., p. 64). Chicago: The Masonic History Company.

Sullivan v. Methodist Hospitals of Dallas, 699 S.W.2d 265 (1985).

Sweeney, P. F. (1997). *How to prove nursing negligence*. Annual Medical Malpractice Conference, San Antonio, Texas.

Texas Board of Nurse Examines Rules (BNE) § 217.117 (1999).

Thompson v. Nason Hosp., 5 91 A. 2d 783 (Pa. 1991).

Urban v. Spohn Hospital, 869 S.W.2d 450 (1993).

Vacco v. Quill, 521 U.S. 1858 (1997).

Washington v. Glucksberg, 521 U.S. 110 (1997).

Werner, H. V. (1998). *Diagnosis for the 21st century*. Ohio: Bookmasters.

Wingo v. Rockford Memorial Hospital, No. 2-96-1268 (Ill. App. 2d Dist. 1997).

SUGGESTED READINGS

Lundberg v. State, 255 N.E.2d 177 (1969).

Synnott v. Midway Hosp., 178 N.W.2d 211 (1970).

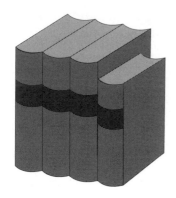

Chapter 8

VICARIOUS LIABILITY FOR NURSING NEGLIGENCE

Jacquelyn K. Hall

STRICT LIABILITY AS THEORY OF VICARIOUS
        LIABILITY
ERISA IMMUNITY FOR HMOS
ISSUES AND TRENDS
ISSUES AND TRENDS IN VICARIOUS LIABILITY
        IN NURSING PRACTICE
ISSUES AND TRENDS IN VICARIOUS LIABILITY
        LAW
MORAL CONSIDERATIONS AND CONFLICTS IN
        VICARIOUS LIABILITY
**RECOMMENDATIONS FOR RESEARCH AND
        MALPRACTICE PREVENTION**
RESEARCH IN VICARIOUS LIABILITY
MALPRACTICE PREVENTION IN VICARIOUS
        LIABILITY
SUMMARY
POINTS TO REMEMBER
REFERENCES
SUGGESTED READINGS

KEY WORDS

Abrogated	Disabled Nurse
Actual Knowledge	Discrimination
Affirmative Defense	Employee Retirement
Agency	Income Security Act
Agent	(ERISA)
Americans with	Failure to Fire
Disabilities Act (ADA)	Gross Negligence
Apparent Agency	Health Maintenance
Assumption of the Risk	Organizations (HMOs)
At-Will Employment	Immunity
Borrowed-Servant	Impaired Nurse
Doctrine	Imputed Negligence
Cap of Damages	Inadequate Staffing
Captain-of-the-Ship	Independent Contractor
Doctrine	Informed Consent
Charitable Immunity	Joint Commission on
Compensatory Damages	Accreditation of
Corporate Liability	Healthcare
Corporation	Organizations (JCAHO)
"Deep Pocket"	Legal Entity
Defamation	Libel

(continued)

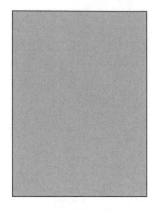

Medical Savings Accounts (MSAs)	Standard of Employment
Negligent Hiring	Stipulated
Ostensible Agency	Strict Liability
Punitive Damages	Termination for Cause
Qui tam	Texas Peer Assistance Program for Nurses (TPAPN)
Respondeat superior	
Scope of Employment	Vicarious Liability
Slander	Wergild
Sovereign Immunity	Wrongful Termination

OBJECTIVES

Upon completion of this chapter, the reader will be able to:
- Identify the major categories of vicarious liability.
- Assess actions that would give rise to a lawsuit for vicarious liability.

INTRODUCTION

The origin of the word *vicarious* is from the Latin word *vicarius*, which means to change, or to substitute something or someone in place of another. Through the principle of **vicarious liability**, another provider or corporation may be substituted in place of the actual defendant. Although the doctor or corporation may be vicariously liable for the acts of another, the actual defendant may also be sued personally.

Vicarious liability is another way of saying that those who benefit bear responsibility—meaning the superior responds and pays, or those with the money are those sued. In cases of nursing negligence, either the doctor or the employer organization is more likely to have assets and thus to be the target for liability for the actions of the nurse (Hall, 1996).

Almost all organizations that employ nurses are corporations. A **corporation** is a legal structure formed to avoid individual liability. By incorporating, liability is transferred from the individual to the corpora-

tion. In essence, **corporate liability** extends to the corporation's assets and not to the individual corporate shareholder.

If an injury occurs in the course of the business of the corporation through negligent acts of its employee, the organization is vicariously responsible. In general, through the legal principle of vicarious liability, the corporation is held liable for any injury to the patient by its employees.

The subject of this chapter is vital to nursing managers for a variety of reasons. Firstly, the legal health of the corporation affects its financial ability to compensate the nurse. Secondly, the presence of an entity that is legally responsible for any damages that the nurse-employee causes in practice indemnifies the employee financially. Finally, the principle saves nurses money on malpractice insurance because the plaintiff will usually seek to sue the corporation, which has the **"deep pocket"** or more money, rather than the individual nurse.

The principle of vicarious liability is also important to nurses, because lawsuits against the hospital corporation are more numerous under this legal theory than any other type of lawsuit against individual nurses. Case law derived from this theory has defined the legal standard of care applied to nurses sued on an individual basis. Most of nursing malpractice law has been written via vicarious liability case law. Finally, the individual nurse may be interested in the principle of vicarious liability because sometimes the corporation is liable to the nurse. For example, the nurse may sue the corporation for damage done to the nurse by the corporation. This was not always so, as the theory of vicarious liability has a long history.

HISTORICAL PERSPECTIVE

Throughout the history of law, individuals have been held liable not only for their own actions but, in specific circumstances, for the acts of others—for their children, families, and slaves. For example, members of a family could be held liable for damages or harm caused by another family member—a form of **wergild**. This principle of law holds true today, for example, as one partner can be held vicariously liable for damage caused by another partner.

At the turn of the twentieth century, doctors and nurses practiced independently and were paid directly by the patient. Hospitals could not be held vicariously liable for the acts of their employees, because the hospital was not considered a **legal entity**, a thing that could be sued. The hospital was simply considered a physical place consisting of bricks, mortar, beds, and equipment, where doctors and nurses happened to provide care (*Schloendorff v. Society of New York Hospital*, 1914). In *Schloendorff*, Justice Cardozo laid the groundwork for informed consent, holding that people have a "right control" over their own body. The right of control is the basis for requiring **informed consent** from the patient for health care procedures.

For centuries and continuing today, businesses have been considered responsible for the acts of their agents. An **agent** is either an employee or **independent contractor** of the organization, who works on behalf of the organization. **Agency** is a legal term for a relationship in which one person acts with authority for or represents another. Principals are responsible for the acts of actual agents, and may be responsible for the acts of apparent or ostensible agents. Likewise, hospitals have also become responsible for the acts of their employees and agents.

The idea of hospital liability is not new. This legal theory is sometimes called **corporate liability**. Corporate liability is merely an application of existing legal theories of vicarious liability to hospital corporations, including laws related to agency and *respondeat superior*.

CATEGORIES OF VICARIOUS LIABILITY

VICARIOUS LIABILITY FOR THE ACTS OF ANOTHER

The most common legal theory of vicarious liability the corporation may be subjected to is *respondeat superior*. Doctors who are employers, like hospitals who are employers, may also be held liable for their employees under the theory of *respondeat superior*. If the doctor hires and pays the salary of the nurse, the doctor's liability is like any other employer under this doctrine. However, if the nurse is actually an employee of the doctor, the doctor may also be held liable for acts of the nurse under the captain-of-the-ship and/or borrowed-servant doctrines.

DOCTOR LIABILITY FOR NURSES' ACTS

CAPTAIN-OF-THE-SHIP DOCTRINE

The doctrines of captain-of-the-ship and borrowed servant are legal theories that have the same result. In both doctrines, the doctor, not the actual employer, is held liable for damage negligently caused by the nurse.

The captain-of-the-ship doctrine developed in response to the principle of charitable immunity. **Immunity** is a legal theory designed to protect specific persons and/or legal entities from liability. The doctrine of **charitable immunity** protects organizations that perform charity work from a lawsuit that could potentially bankrupt a charitable, not-for-profit organization. Charitable immunity has been eliminated—in legal terms, **abrogated**—in a majority of states. Many of the functions the charities were responsible for, now are conducted by the government, which has reduced the need to protect charitable institutions. Also, not-for-profit corporations in general have assets and insurance, just like the for-profit organizations, so they have resources sufficient to pay damages to plaintiff.

Immunity of charitable organizations to lawsuit meant the injured patient had to find someone else to pay their damages. Under the **captain-of-the-ship doctrine,** doctors can also be held liable for the negligence of providers under their supervision. A plaintiff could recover from the doctor for the negligence of a nurse, even though the nurse was not the doctor's employee (*McConnell v. Williams*, 1949). However, in most states, plaintiffs can now sue not-for-profit organizations, and consequently the utilization of the captain-of-the-ship doctrine has declined.

Lawsuits that result in defendants claiming governmental or **sovereign immunity** have also prompted the same attempt by plaintiffs to vicariously hold liable the doctor and/or the nurse, who has malpractice insurance. Government organizations, which are state or local tax supported, often either are immune from suit or have a low **cap of damages** on the monetary amount that patients can recover—for example, $100,000 limit per incident. Federal organizations that are health care providers have limited liability for damages under federal law, whereas federal employees have sovereign immunity from lawsuit. Further, some **health maintenance organizations (HMOs)** also have immunity from lawsuit under federal law, for example, under the **Employee Retirement Income Security Act (ERISA)**.

BORROWED-SERVANT DOCTRINE

Under the **borrowed-servant doctrine**, again, someone other than the nurse is held liable for the nurse's negligence. According to this legal theory, the actual employer allows or directs the nurse to work for another person, who is considered the controlling employer. Thus, the nurse has been "borrowed" by, and now is the employee and under the control of, the second employer.

The second employer then becomes liable for the negligent acts of the borrowed employee that are performed while under the second employer's control, via the umbrella doctrine of *respondeat superior*. Simply stated, the actual employer has surrendered direction and control of the employee nurse to a second employer. Consequently, the actual employer is not liable for the nurse's acts of negligence while under the control and supervision of that doctor or other entity, or second employer (*Synnott v. Midway Hosp.*, 1970).

An employment setting within which the need to use the borrowed-servant doctrine may arise is an operating room setting. For liability to attach, the facts must show that the doctor has control over the nurse's acts; then the doctor will be considered the employer and liability will attach. For example, in *Spager v. Worley Hospital, Inc.* (1977), the hospital and surgeon were sued for negligence because of a retained sponge. Testimony of the scrub nurse revealed that the doctor had no control over the nurse's actions for (1) the doctor did not direct the sponge count, (2) the nurses knew how to make the sponge count, and (3) they did so according to hospital procedure (see also *Rogers v. Duke*, 1989).

Case law based on the borrowed-servant doctrine has defined specific legal duties that, if breached, will establish liability. Further, the borrowed-servant doctrine can be the theoretical framework within which the plaintiff establishes liability on the part of the borrowing employer.

CORPORATE LIABILITY FOR NURSES' ACTS

The theoretical basis of corporation liability for nursing acts is not new. The liability of the corporation may be framed within a number of legal theories, including the doctrine of *respondeat superior*.

RESPONDEAT SUPERIOR

Darling v. Charleston Community Memorial Hospital (1965) set the standard for corporation liability. In *Darling* (1965), nurses monitored the worsening condition of a college football player, whose casted leg demonstrated toes that were swelling, growing darker, becoming cold, losing feeling; and generating a foul odor. The nurses assessed, documented, and reported these symptoms to the doctor on numerous occasions. The patient eventually lost his leg from gangrene, after days of inaction by the doctor. The corporation was held liable under the doctrine of *respondeat superior* for the nurses' failure to advocate for the patient through the organizational hierarchy when there was negligent care by the doctor (Hardy, 1986).

In most cases, the status of the nurse as employee will be **stipulated** to by the employer—that is, agreed to without dispute. This step is necessary to ensure that the employer's malpractice insurer will defend the nurse. But in other instances, the corporation may deny that the provider was an employee, as in instances of negligence by a temporary nurse who has been assigned to the hospital, or when the doctor or nurse clearly may be independent contractors and not employees. Even if the nurse is an independent contractor, the organization might still be held liable under the doctrines of *respondeat superior* or agency for **negligent hiring** of the employee. Specifically, the employer may be held liable for negligently selecting this particular nurse to perform this particular procedure. Another theory that might be used to establish employer liability for a nonemployee is agency theory, when the nurse is acting as an agent of this employer.

In *Drennan v. Community Health Investment Corporation* (1995), the issue was whether the nurse anesthetist was an employee of the hospital or an independent contractor. The court held that as the doctor, who was also an independent contractor and not an employee, had arranged for the employment of the nurse anesthetist, the doctor and the nurse were both independent contractors; therefore, the hospital was not liable.

The status of a nurse as employee or independent contractor is also important under tax law. Employers are not liable for payment of taxes for independent contractors (see also Kemper, 1996, for other cases regarding this issue).

GROSS NEGLIGENCE AND PUNITIVE DAMAGES

If the nurse is held to have been guilty of **gross negligence**, punitive damages may be awarded. **Compensatory damages** are used to reimburse the plaintiff for actual harm done, for example, medical costs. **Punitive damages** are used to punish the wrongdoer. Punitive damages usually require evidence that the defendant had actual, subjective awareness of the risk of the action to be taken and acted in conscious disregard of the risk. For example, a court held that sufficient evidence of knowledge of risk existed to justify a punitive damage award when nurses knew of a nursing home patient's worsening decubitus ulcer and did nothing to intervene (*Convalescent Services, Inc. v. Schultz*, 1996).

Under the doctrine of *respondeat superior*, a hospital was held liable for gross negligence when a practical nurse and nursing aide left an actively suicidal patient unattended. The hospital's defense was that it was liable only for gross negligence of employees who were at least a **vice-principal** of the hospital. That would mean they were liable only for nurses who at least were "in charge"—a charge nurse or RN. The appeals court disagreed, holding the hospital could be liable for the gross negligence of a practical nurse and nursing aide (*Texarkana Memorial Hospital v. Firth*, 1988).

In yet another example of gross negligence, a home health nurse's failure to teach home health care resulted in an award against the nursing home of $1.5 million in actual damages and $2 million in punitive damages, because the patient unknowingly self-administered saline without antibiotic and lost a leg ("Hospital held liable," 1996). Under the doctrine of *respondeat superior*, this type of negligence can also be classified as **imputed negligence**, which occurs when the negligence of one person is attributed to another.

AGENCY—ACTUAL, APPARENT, AND OSTENSIBLE

As mentioned previously, agency is a legal term for a relationship in which one person has the authority to act for or represent another (*Black's Law Dictionary*, 1990). Under the basic rule of agency, "An employer, master, or principal is [held] liable for the negligent acts of his employees, servants or agents when those acts arise in the course and scope of their employment, service, or agency" (Restatement [Second] of Agency, 1957). Within the context of health care lawsuits, the principal is usually the hospital, and the agent is usually the nurse or doctor.

When a plaintiff claims the defendant was an **apparent or ostensible agent** of the principal, the hospital has either intentionally or by want of ordinary care induced the plaintiff to believe that the defendant is in fact an agent of the principal. The principal may not have conferred authority on the "agent" either expressly or by implication (*Black's Law Dictionary*, 1990). **Apparent agency** and **ostensible agency** are two terms used interchangeably.

If a nurse appears to act on behalf of the organization, the organization may be liable for the nurse's acts, whether or not the nurse actually has authority to act or is an agent of the principal. The nurse may be held to have ostensible or apparent authority. Consequently, the principal—the organization—may be held liable for damages, because the nurse was permitted to appear to have authority, whether the authority was actual or not. For example, the corporation may be held liable for acts of a temporary nurse, who was not in fact an actual employee of the organization.

CORPORATE LIABILITY FOR NEGLIGENT STAFFING

The consequences of negligent staffing are numerous, and may include (1) malpractice suits, for resulting patient injuries; (2) a report to the nursing licensure board, for violations of the state's nursing practice act; (3) potential deficiencies on inspections for licensure; and/or (4) a *qui tam* (whistleblower) lawsuit, for overcharging Medicare for nursing services, such as those charged and not given.

The principal or health care organization is responsible for any damage to patients caused by the malpractice or negligence of an employee secondary to unsafe staffing. Liability may be levied against the principal because the organization represented and warranted to patients that safe nursing care will be provided in return for payment.

In *Darling v. Charleston Community Memorial Hospital* (1965), the issue of **inadequate staffing** was addressed. But the plaintiff was unable to provide evidence that nurses were unable to care for the patient for lack of staffing, as the nurses had time to assess, report to the doctor, and document their findings repeatedly. Instead, the nurses breached the duty to advocate for the patient when the doctor failed to treat the patient's worsening symptoms.

To prove inadequate and/or unsafe staffing practices, plaintiff's counsel may introduce evidence of the employer's own staffing standards, the actual staffing, and consequential failure of the corporation to meet its own staffing guidelines.

In addition, the standards of the **Joint Commission on Accreditation of Healthcare Organizations (JCAHO)** may be introduced to provide evidence of the standard of staffing. If the organization is accredited by JCAHO, failure to adhere to its standards can also be used to provide evidence of a breach of the standard of staffing.

Finally, some corporations must adhere to state or federal regulations for staffing of nursing home and convalescent centers. These statutory regulations can be used by state licensing agencies to discipline the health care corporation, under administrative law, for inadequate staffing. Again, these statutory regulations can be introduced as evidence by plaintiff's attorney to show another standard of staffing that the principal or corporation failed to meet.

CORPORATE LIABILITY FOR NEGLIGENCE IN EMPLOYEE RELATIONS

Under the theory of negligent hiring, the principal or health care organization is held liable for failing to ascertain the skills, references, licenses, and other attributes of the potential employee or medical staff person at the time of employment or admission to the staff. The employer has the responsibility and thus the legal mandate to protect patients from employees and medical staff that might harm them, either negligently or deliberately. Not only the employer corporations, but also solo doctors or partnerships, can be held liable for negligent hiring and/or negligent admission to the medical staff. These cases usually arise when the employer cannot be sued under the theory of *respondeat superior* for an employee's act of malpractice.

Even if the wrongdoer is an employee, the employer is liable under the doctrine of *respondeat superior* only if the employee's act is considered within the **scope of employment,** that is, within the job description. Often in such cases, the employee has not been negligent, but instead has committed an intentional tort like assault and battery. With that set of facts, the employer will usually assert that the employee's job description does not include assaulting a patient or other person.

This duty of the employer to protect patients may conflict with the moral responsibility and legal mandates to treat prospective employees and medical staff fairly. Numerous laws enforce the responsibility to be fair to employees and medical staff.

Obtaining information about an employee's work record from former employers may be difficult, because employers are sensitive to lawsuits by employees. However, at a minimum, information that can be obtained about the employee's term of service may include whether discharge was voluntary or not and whether the employee is eligible for rehire. Further, employers who give out information that is true cannot be held liable for defamation.

In *Deerings West Nursing Center v. Scott* (1990), the court held that a nursing home was liable for hiring an unlicensed employee who assaulted a visitor. The court held the standard of care or duty of the nursing home was to exercise reasonable care in selection of its staff. Although the employee had six prior criminal convictions, no effort was made to ascertain whether the person was licensed as a practical nurse, nor was a local criminal record check done. The court held there was a duty to hire competent persons, especially in a business where the employee must be skilled or specialized.

However, if the nurse has not committed a negligent or intentional harmful act in the first place, negligently hiring him or her will not result in corporate liability. In *Clark v. Harris Hospital* (1976), evidence that the nurses were foreign and unlicensed by the state was held not to be important, because the jury found they had not committed malpractice in the first place.

NEGLIGENT SUPERVISION AND ASSIGNMENTS

Supervisors or staff nurses are not automatically held liable for the negligent acts of all the people under their supervision. The employer, not the nursing supervisor, is held liable under the doctrine of *respondeat superior* for acts of negligent supervision committed by their employee. If the supervisor is held liable for negligently assigning a practical nurse to care for a patient on a ventilator, the employer will automatically be held liable for the negligent acts of the practical nurse and supervisor. The nursing supervisor may also be held liable for negligent supervision, but not under the doctrine of *respondeat superior*. The supervisor is unlikely to be held liable under a theory of negligence or malpractice, but is accountable to the state board of nursing for negligent supervision.

The employer can be held liable, under the doctrine of *respondeat superior*, for the actions of nursing supervisors who make assignments negligently. Supervisors must (1) assign enough staff to provide standardized patient care, (2) assign staff competent to provide the type of patient care prescribed for the patients, and (3) allow staff adequate time to provide standardized patient care.

The employer may be held liable under the doctrine of *respondeat superior* if the nursing supervisor is alerted to a problem and does not respond to it. For example, a prompt response to allegations of sexual harassment is very important, because the employer will be held liable for what the supervisor knew and failed to do, even if the employer did not know about the allegations. In summary, the principal or organization is assumed to have **actual knowledge** of a problem if its supervisors or agents have knowledge of the problem.

FAILURE TO FIRE

Lawsuits are usually filed under a claim of **failure to fire** when the employer cannot be sued for negligence under the legal theory of *respondeat superior*. Again, the employer is held liable under the doctrine of *respondeat superior* only if the employee's act is considered one that is within the scope of employment or within the job description. If the employee has not been negligent, but instead has committed an intentional tort like assault and battery, the employer defends against any claims of liability under the doctrine of *respondeat superior*, by affirming that the employee's job description does not include assault or other intentional tort.

A claim under failure to fire may give rise to employer liability if the nurse's performance, documented in the personnel record, warranted such a claim. The **standard of employment** at trial will be: Would a reasonable, prudent employer have fired such a nurse, before the nurse committed the tort that now is alleged, under the same or similar circumstances? The nursing negligence that warrants firing could encompass any number of breaches of the standard of nursing practice.

Nurses and supervisors should realize that the patient chart and personnel files are among the first documents requested by plaintiffs in a lawsuit, and by investigators by the board of nursing. The information in the personnel file can make or break both malpractice and licensure cases, so the file should be as accurate and complete as the patient record. In particular, suits by the

employee for wrongful discharge depend on whether the personnel file is complete and accurate.

CORPORATE LIABILITY FOR DEFAMATION IN THE PROCESS OF FIRING—LIBEL AND SLANDER

Organizations can be held vicariously liable for the acts of their agents, if the agent defames a patient, nurse, or doctor. A nurse and doctor can also be held individually liable for their own acts of defamation. Liability for **defamation** will result from an untrue statement, communicated to a third person, that injures the reputation of the person spoken about. **Libel** is written defamation—nurses can defame in a chart. **Slander** is spoken defamation. Truth is an absolute defense to defamation.

Management nurses should take care not to defame employees and not repeat information they do not know to be true. The organization may be vicariously liable for defamation of an employee that is committed by managers in the process of firing. In summary, nurse managers should say or write about employees only what is true, provable, and documented—and only to the person who needs to know the information.

CORPORATE LIABILITY FOR AND TO IMPAIRED NURSES

A nurse abusing or addicted to alcohol or drugs is termed an **impaired nurse**. The problem for employers is that impaired nurses may endanger patients. The manager's concern for the employee must be subordinated to the safety of the patient.

The management can seek recovery programs to help employees with addiction, once patient safety is ensured. Many states have assistance programs for impaired nurses; for example, there is the **Texas Peer Assistance Program for Nurses (TPAPN)**.

A nurse in recovery is now classified as a **disabled nurse** and is protected by the **Americans with Disabilities Act (ADA).** For example, nurses with past addictions to legal drugs, such as meperidine, or illegal drugs, such as crack cocaine, are disabled and protected by the ADA. Employees who are currently addicted to illegal drugs are not covered by the ADA. Advice from the corporation attorney should be sought to protect not only the rights of the patients but also the rights of the disabled nurse.

CORPORATE LIABILITY FOR WRONGFUL TERMINATION

Employees may sue corporations for **wrongful termination**, alleging discrimination in the course of firing. This liability of the corporation is grounded in the doctrine of *respondeat superior* and/or agency law, because agents or employees of the corporation have acted wrongfully in terminating the employee. The staff must understand that **termination for cause** of an employee can be accomplished only through documented and provable reasons. Basing termination on allegations that are not true opens the supervisor to lawsuit under a claim of defamation.

In many jurisdictions or states, nurses and most other employees work without contracts, as employees in an **at-will employment** situation. These nurses may be terminated at will, or for no reason at all. However, the employee may claim **discrimination** if termination is based on (1) sex, (2) race, (3) disability, or (4) other conditions prohibited by discrimination law.

STRICT LIABILITY AS THEORY OF VICARIOUS LIABILITY

Under the captain-of-the-ship doctrine, a doctor may be held liable without fault under a claim of **strict liability.** Strict liability torts, a subdivision of vicarious liability, are not often encountered in medical or nursing law. One of the defenses to strict liability, **assumption of the risk**, is relevant to nursing law. This is an **affirmative defense**, or one that must be pled by the defendant. Assumption of the risk, which may be affirmed as a defense to a malpractice claim, can be expressed, implied, or imputed to the plaintiff by misconduct (Farrell, 1997). According to this

affirmative defense, the patient is said to have assumed the risk of the procedure or treatment that he or she willingly consented to have.

ERISA IMMUNITY FOR HMOS

One kind of immunity from lawsuits, which is important for Health Maintenance Organization (HMOs) and other health insurance plans, is that provided under the Employment Retirement Income Security Act of 1974 (ERISA). **ERISA** is a federal law that governs employee benefit plans, such as pension plans and health insurance for employees. One of the law's provisions preempts any state law with which any of its provisions may be in conflict or may contradict. Quite simply, state laws that allow malpractice suits against insurance plans are not allowed under federal law. HMOs may qualify for this protection. Once federal law preempts state law, the state law remedies of malpractice lawsuits are not available. This is a hardship to the plaintiff, as the federal remedies under ERISA are minuscule, compared with damages available under state malpractice law.

In effect, the ERISA exemption makes HMOs virtually immune from lawsuit, under the doctrine of *respondeat superior*, for any negligence of their employees or agents. Several states have passed legislation to try to change this situation, to allow patients to sue insurers, HMOs, and other ERISA plans (Relating to Review of Liability for Certain Health Care Treatment Decisions, 1997). These laws are now being challenged in court by the insurers and HMOs.

The American Medical Association (AMA) and other providers are working to have the ERISA preemption removed by Congress. In the meantime, and in the search for money to compensate the victim for damages, nurses may become more likely targets if the American Medical Association (AMA) is unsuccessful and the insurers and HMOs are able to maintain their immunity (Shaloub & Kratner, 1997).

ISSUES AND TRENDS

ISSUES AND TRENDS IN VICARIOUS LIABILITY IN NURSING PRACTICE

The concept of **medical savings accounts (MSAs)** is in its infancy, but is proving very popular with the public. For example, patients pay for the first $3000 of the health care yearly out of money that the employer has put in an account for that purpose. When the whole $3000 is spent, a catastrophic insurance policy with a $3000 deductible begins to pay for health care. If the employee does not spend the whole $3000 during the year, he or she keeps the rest. Another $3000 is then put into the MSA for the next year.

In the future, the advanced practice nurse (APN) will likely be paid by the patient, not the insurer—reducing hassles over payment, excess paperwork, claims denied, and so on. With this trend in out-of-pocket payments, the control of health care may be reverting to the patient, who can now be a true partner in care, newly empowered with cash.

These payment out of pocket by the individual patient is likely to increase in general, reversing a trend in third-party payments that started in 1965 with the passage of Medicare. The perception that care was "free" when paid for by insurance or by taxpayers caused great inflation in the cost of care. Out-of-pocket payments will make patients more cost conscious, because they will be spending their own money for the first time since insurance became popular.

As nursing practice is becoming more independent of doctor and employer control, the incidence of personal suits against nurses will increase. The effect of the increased utilization of nursing malpractice insurance may have an impact, by increasing numbers of suits and amount of awards against nurses.

ISSUES AND TRENDS IN VICARIOUS LIABILITY LAW

Managed care liability is a current issue. The ERISA exemption is used by insurers and HMOs to escape liability. Insurers also argue that they are not the providers of care—the doctors and nurses are. Watch for legislative efforts to counter the ERISA exemption, so that patients can sue HMOs directly.

MORAL CONSIDERATIONS AND CONFLICTS IN VICARIOUS LIABILITY

Throughout this chapter and in the preceding chapter, the truism is repeated: "Law is inseparable from ethics." Even JCAHO now mandates that provider organizations, which it accredits, have a set of business ethics to which they adhere. Hall (1996) states that the essence of the business ethic recommended by JCAHO is: Do unto others as you would have them do unto you.

RECOMMENDATIONS FOR RESEARCH AND MALPRACTICE PREVENTION

RESEARCH IN VICARIOUS LIABILITY

A continuing trend is to find the "system," instead of individuals, vicariously responsible for error that harms patients. This is the base of no-fault compensation in automobile accidents and workers' compensation. Research could reveal whether these ideas would work in health care. As discussed in Chapter 7, research is needed on the effect of reducing or eliminating liability for professionals. For example, doctors and nurses employed by the Veterans Administration have no liability for negligence. Additional issues that need to be addressed include: Is the trend toward increased vicarious liability for the principal, and decreased personal liability for the individual provider, reducing (1) awards of money damages to plaintiffs, (2) the practice of defensive medicine by providers, (3) overall medical costs, (4) professional image of health care and the provider, (5) autonomy of the health care provider, (6) concern about the patient, and/or (7) the number of malpractice lawsuits that are filed?

Alternatively, another issue needs to be addressed: Does personal liability by the health care provider have a role in decreasing acts of malpractice? If not, then why are professionals liable for negligence?

MALPRACTICE PREVENTION IN VICARIOUS LIABILITY

Vicarious liability law defines the legal standard of care or duties that will be imposed on individual nurses. However, the presence of an entity that is legally responsible for damages the employee causes in practice relieves the nurse of any liability or financial responsibility. Generally, the nurse is "shielded" from malpractice lawsuits by the corporate health care provider. Further, the organization or corporation is also held responsible for damage to patients that results from the unsafe staffing practices of the nursing supervisor.

SUMMARY

Vicarious liability law is important to nurse employees as well as nurse managers. The potential for vicarious liability puts responsibility on the organization and thus its management. The trend always has been to hold organizations or corporations liable. The organization, in turn, will most likely attempt to hold the individual nurse and/or the nursing manager responsible, even if the court does not hold the nurse or executive liable. For example, the nurse and managers must know the liability that can arise from negligent staffing. The nurse or manager may not be a party to the lawsuit, but may lose a job because of "malpractice" in management. Nurse managers walk a fine line between controlling and reducing the cost of staff, equipment, and supplies and yet maintaining a safe level of care.

POINTS TO REMEMBER

- All liability of a corporation or organization is vicarious liability.

- If the nurse is held to be grossly negligent, punitive damages may be awarded.
- Agency is a legal term for a relationship in which one person acts for or represents another, with authority. Principals are responsible for the acts of actual agents, and may be responsible for the acts of apparent or ostensible agents.
- Defamation is any untrue statement communicated to a third party. Libel is written defamation. Slander is spoken defamation. Truth is an absolute defense to defamation.
- Strict liability is a theory of recovery that is not based on negligence. Even if the defendant was not negligent, he or she can still be found liable for damages.
- Assumption of the risk is an affirmative defense to strict liability. More pertinent to nursing practice, this theory is a largely unacknowledged but potential defense to a suit for malpractice.

REFERENCES

Black's law dictionary. (1990). St. Paul, MN: West Publishing Co.

Clark v. Harris Hospital, 543 S.W.2d 743 (1976).

Convalescent Services, Inc. v. Schultz, 921 S.W.2d 731 (1996).

Darling v. Charleston Community Memorial Hospital, 211 N.E.2d 253 (1965).

Deerings West Nursing Center v. Scott, 787 S.W.2d 494 (1990).

Drennan v. Community Health Investment Corporation, 905 S.W.2d 811 (1995).

Employment Retirement Income Security Act of 1974 (ERISA), 29 U.S.C. § 1002(5).

Farrell, M. J. (1997). Resurrecting the dormant defenses: Assumption of risk, patient negligence, avoidable consequences and winning the medical malpractice case. *Defense Research Institute in Modern Health Care Defense Issues*, pp. 8–25.

Hall, J. K. (1996). *Nursing ethics and law*. Philadelphia: WB Saunders.

Hardy, I. T. (1986). When doctrines collide: Corporation negligence and respondeat superior when hospital employees fail to speak up. *Tulane Law Review*, 61, 85.

Hospital held liable for woman who lost leg during care at home. (1996, September 22). *Houston Chronicle*, p. 4D.

Kemper, J. R. (1996). Hospital liability for nurse assisting surgeon. *American Law Review (3rd ed.), 29,* 1065.

McConnell v. Williams, 65 A. 2d 243 (1949).

Relating to Review of Liability for Certain Health Care Treatment Decisions SB386, Texas Legislature (1997).

Restatement (Second) of Agency § 220(1) (1957).

Rogers v. Duke, 766 S.W.2d 547 (1989).

Schloendorff v. Society of New York Hospital, 105 N.E. 92 (N.Y. 1914).

Shaloub, M. D., & Kratner, D. S. (1997). Managed care liability for medical malpractice and the preemptive effect of ERISA. *Defense Research Institute 1997 in Modern Health Care Defense Issues,* pp. 1–8.

Spager v. Worley Hospital, Inc., 547 S.W.2d 582 (1977).

Synnott v. Midway Hosp., 178 N.W.2d 211 (1970).

Texarkana Memorial Hospital v. Firth, 746 S.W.2d 494 (1988).

SUGGESTED READINGS

Gray, B. B. (1998). Use your head: When to bend the rules instead of following them. *Healthweek, 3*(14), 4.

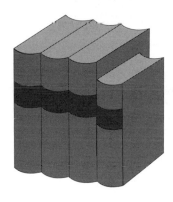

Chapter 9

DOCUMENTATION

Elizabeth L. Higginbotham

KEY WORDS

Business Records	Medical Record
Care Map	Narrative Charting
Charting by Exception	PIE
Defamation	Quality Assurance
Incident Reports	SOAP

OBJECTIVES

Upon completion of this chapter, the reader will be able to:
- Identify the purposes for compilation of medical records.
- Recognize statutory and regulatory requirements for documentation.
- Recognize appropriate documentation practices and improve documentation skills.
- Identify advantages and disadvantages of computerized medical records.

INTRODUCTION

The **medical record** serves as a summary of all observations made and the care and treatment rendered to a patient during hospitalization. The manner and form of documentation by nurses in the medical record has metamorphosed over time. Past practice entailed documenting patient observations in the narrative form, with records of vitals signs and medications administered on separate and distinct forms. Today, narrative "normal" is documented. In many facilities, the use of checklists or flow sheets is the norm. In addition, there is a definite trend toward use of computer-based patient records and nursing information systems. Without regard to the form that documentation exists, juries often believe that "if it wasn't documented, it wasn't done."

MEDICAL RECORDS

The purpose of the medical record is to provide a summary of all observations made regarding nursing and medical diagnoses and to accurately reflect measures taken to alleviate identified problems as well as patient response to intervention.

The medical record is a legal document and is admissible in a court of law as evidence. Unfortunately, patients in general have a very naive view of hospital operations. They are shocked to learn that minute-by-minute observations are not documented; therefore, the "if it wasn't documented, it wasn't done" myth is perpetuated. What is missing from the medical record is often more important than what is written down.

STATUTORY AND REGULATORY REQUIREMENTS

The reasons for compilation and retention of medical records are varied: (1) to ensure continuity of patient care, (2) to aid in medical decision making in the future, (3) to use for teaching and statistical purposes, (4) to establish proof for reimbursement, and finally (5) to preserve evidence with regard to any issue involving liability or professional negligence (Texas Health Information Management Association, 1994). Various federal and state standards of accreditation prescribe time requirements for retention of medical records. It is generally accepted that when state and federal time requirements conflict, the longer time requirement will control. For example, the Medicare/Medicaid interpreted guidelines of the conditions of participation for hospitals state that "medical records must be retained in their original and legally reproduced form in hard copy, microfilm, or computer memory banks." Conditions of Participation for Hospitals (1995). The requirement also provides that "medical records must be retained in their original or legally reproduced form for a period of at least five years." Notwithstanding, Texas law provides that hospitals may dispose of medical records 10 years after the date on which the patient, who is the subject of the record, was last treated in the hospital. Likewise, medical records of persons, who are minors at the time of treatment, may be destroyed on or after the date of the patient's 20th birthday or 10 years after the date on which the patient was last treated, whichever date is latest (Texas Health and Safety Code § 241.103). As this is an example of one state's regulation compared with federal requirement, it may be different in other states. Obviously, records that are the subject of litigation should not be destroyed until the litigation has ended.

The Medicare conditions of participation for hospitals require hospitals to have a system of record identification and maintenance to preserve the integrity of authentication and to protect the security of patient record entries. Providers must safeguard medical records against destruction, loss, and unauthorized use. Accordingly, written policies and procedures that govern the use of medical records, the removal of records, and conditions for release of information must be in place. Accreditation by the Joint Commission on Accreditation of Healthcare Organizations (JCAHO) is a voluntary process. Notwithstanding, these standards are incorporated in hospital licensing standards for various states. JCAHO's standards measure a hospital's method of promoting and ensuring security, confidentiality, and integrity of medical records. The standards require that records be accurate and complete and prescribe a period for record completion.

In addition to state, federal, and accreditation guidelines, legal requirements pertaining to privacy and the confidentiality of patient information are contained within the Constitution of the United States and constitutions of various states as well as the common law. The American Nurses Association's Code for Nurses (American Nurses Association, 1985) provides guidance to nurses on this subject as well, by charging the nurse with safeguarding the patient's right to privacy by "judiciously protecting information of a confidential nature."

OWNERSHIP AND ACCESS

In general, the physical medical record is the property of the health care facility that compiles it. Notwithstanding, the information contained within the record belongs to the patient who is entitled to confidentiality of information. Because of the requirements for retention, patients may receive copies of records but are not entitled to keep original medical records.

NURSE'S ROLE IN PROTECTION OF CONFIDENTIALITY

Hospitals and their employees have a duty to protect the patient medical record on the patient's behalf (*Cannel v. Medical and Surgical Clinic*, 1974). It follows then that the nurse must safeguard patient information, whether in written form or not. Unfortunately, this effort is not made consistently, in that nurses and other health care providers are frequently guilty of casual conversation among themselves about patient events, thereby inadvertently breaching confidentiality. This seemingly innocent breach of confidentiality violates patient rights and may subject the nurse to discipline or civil liability as some jurisdictions provide for a private cause of action for unauthorized release of medical information (Texas Health and Safety Code, Chapter 241).

The patient may pursue other causes of action related to unauthorized disclosure of medical information. For example, a patient may file an action for negligent disclosure (*Prince v. St. Francis–St. George Hospital*, 1985) (patient's diagnosis of acute and chronic alcohol detoxification disclosed). A patient may sue for invasion of privacy (*Urbaniak v. Newton*, 1991) or for tortious breach of confidence (*Anderson v. Strong Memorial Hospital*, 1988). The tortious-breach-of-confidence action was based on the patient's picture in a news article on acquired immunodeficiency syndrome (AIDS) research. The patient, who was positive for the human immunodeficiency virus (HIV), was photographed while in the hospital's infectious disease unit. The implication of this type of mistake is obvious.

In addition to these actions, a patient may sue for **defamation**, which is defined as an intentional false communication made verbally or in writing that injures another's reputation. In one case, a physician was sued by his male patient for defamation when he advised his patient's fiancé "to run as fast and as far as she could in any direction away from him" after learning private information during his examination of the patient (*Berry v. Moench*, 1958). Patients may also sue for public disclosure of private facts or for breach of contract (*Clark v. Geraci*, 1960; *Doe v. Roe*, 1977). An action for public disclosure of private facts or for breach of contract could be brought if a true but confidential fact was revealed, such as statements made to one's psychiatrist. The *Doe* court reasoned that anytime a health care provider treats a patient, a contract is made and one of the terms of the contract is secrecy.

Many health care providers embrace the theory that without a disclosure of a patient's name, there can be no cause of action. This is simply not true, as a cause of action for breach of contract or defamation requires only that enough information be supplied to allow third parties to identify the person who is the subject of the communication (*Hammonds v. Aetna Casualty & Surety Co.*, 1965).

A companion cause of action to an allegation of breach of confidentiality is a claim for negligent or intentional infliction of severe emotional distress. Not all jurisdictions recognize a cause of action for negligent infliction of emotional distress, with Texas being one of those that does not (*Boyles v. Kerr*, 1993).

Even a seemingly innocent undertaking in the ordinary course of business may subject a health care provider to liability for breach of patient confidentiality. In one case, a hospital's chief financial officer hired a law firm to review patient registration forms to identify patients who were eligible for additional reimbursement of medical expenses through Supplemental Security Income (SSI). The forms contained patient names, dates of birth, and admitting diagnoses. A law firm employee who was responsible for contacting patients learned that she was about to be fired and photocopied several registrations, sent them to a local television station, and waited in the wings while the station did an investigative report on alleged breach of confidentiality at the hospital. Many of the patients whose names were released sued the hospital and the law firm for unauthorized disclosure of confidential information. Although the suit was dismissed by the trial court, it was reinstated by the court of appeals (*Biddle v. Warren Gen. Hosp.*, 1998). The hospital claimed that the patients had expressly authorized release of information at the time of admission. When the court reinstated the charges against the hospital, it observed that the consent signed by the patients authorized release of information only to the patients' insurance company or third-party payer, not the law firm. Therefore, it is critical that health care providers be aware of the *scope* of a release of information as opposed to the mere fact that a patient has consented to disclose information.

HOSPITAL VERSUS PATIENT RECORDS

Hospital records encompass much more than medical records. Medical records are only one element of hospital record keeping. The various types of records include records relating to purchasing and financing, cost reports, employee health records, medical records, committee minutes, and incident reports.

INCIDENT REPORTS

In general, **incident reports** should be kept in accordance with the hospital's record retention policy. For example, Medicare conditions of participation require records to be kept for 5 years, and state law dictates separate retention requirements. As stated earlier, the longest retention period should be followed. Records that are the subject of potential litigation as well as all records requested by an attorney or administrative agency should be retained until the matter is fully resolved. In the event that no litigation results, the records should be maintained at least until the limitations period expires. In Texas, the statute of limitations for a minor to bring a medical malpractice claim is 2 years after the date of majority, which is the 20th birthday (Medical Liability & Insurance Improvement Act, 1998). In contrast, Maryland law provides that medical or laboratory records of minors may not be destroyed until 3 years after the age of majority or 5 years after the record or report is made, whichever is later, unless the parent or guardian of the child is notified or the minor patient was able to give consent to the care and is notified (Maryland Health General Article § 4-403(c)).

COMMITTEE MINUTES

Committee minutes are also retained in accordance with hospital policy. State statutes address confidentiality of committee records and meetings. In Texas, these protections have been subject to attack in the civil arena. Attorneys have attempted to "prove up" the records as **business records** to gain access to them. Generally, records kept in the ordinary and usual course of business (like the medical record) can be obtained, or "discovered." Records that are generally considered to be privileged have also been obtained by attacking the method by which the records were originally generated or provided to the committee. For example, medical staff applications have been requested based on the theory that such records were "gratuitously provided" to the committee as opposed to actually compiled by the committee and were, therefore, not privileged. The Texas Supreme Court disposed of any doubt with regard to the privilege attached to these records and committee records in back-to-back opinions, which held that the records were definitely privileged (*Irving Healthcare System v. Brooks*, 1996; *Memorial Hospital–The Woodlands v. McCown*, 1996). Courts in other states have reached different conclusions. For example, the Illinois Supreme Court held that information that was not actually generated by the medical staff committee prior to the granting of privileges was not protected (*May v. Wood River TP Hosp.*, 1994).

QUALITY ASSURANCE, PEER REVIEW, AND RISK MANAGEMENT RECORDS

Quality assurance, peer review, and risk management records are generally privileged and exempt from discovery inasmuch as they fulfill the purpose of allowing hospitals to recognize and correct their mistakes beyond the purview of the general public who could use such information against them. This is akin to the confidentiality of subsequent remedial measures taken by a manufacturer in a products liability action. The public policy reason behind affording such protections is to promote safety by encouraging progress. In addition, many risk management records created in anticipation of litigation are privileged under the attorney work-product and investigative privileges.

AREAS OF EXPOSURE

ASSESSMENT

Several common mistakes are worthy of mention. The first is the failure to do a thorough admission assessment and record all observations. It is difficult to convince many nurses that they are responsible for all of the patient's problems without regard to the reason for admission. In addition, failure to pay attention to basic instinct or personal observations when doing an assessment can have disastrous consequences. In one case followed by the author, a patient was admitted to a rural hospital accompanied by her daughter, a licensed vocational nurse (LVN). During the initial assessment and nursing history, the patient's daughter provided most of the information and vigorously denied any history of diabetes. In light of this information, the nurse ignored indurations on the patient's body (from years of insulin administration). Because this happened in a rural hospital, the admitting laboratory work was sent off site and results were not received until the next morning, by which time the patient was in a diabetic coma. The reason that neither the patient nor her daughter revealed her diabetes was that they had been to a faith healer who told them that even mention of the word *diabetes* would cause the disease to return. A claim was made without suit being brought; the case was settled in the face of obvious liability.

RECORD OF NURSING ACTIONS

Another major mistake is the failure to record all nursing actions. Consider the scenario of an actively suicidal patient brought to the emergency room by the police. The patient ran away, and the chart contained no nursing assessment, no suicide assessment, and no indication of one-on-one observation. To this day, no one can verify what happened to the patient. If a suit were brought, the hospital and nurses would have nothing to support their contentions regarding assessments done or care given.

Another mistake is failing to record changes in the patient's condition (*and* notify the doctor of the same). This author once reviewed a medical record that contained a textbook description of the evolution of stroke in an elderly male. The nurses failed to notify the doctor of the changes in the patient's condition until the patient became completely nonresponsive. Their meticulous documentation served as evidence to support an allegation of gross negligence. Note that this is not a criticism of the nurses' documentation, but rather an indictment of the nurses' failure to follow through and report changes in the patient's condition to the physician.

COMPLETE DOCUMENTATION

Failure to document completely is a charting error that can make a malpractice case indefensible. As stated earlier, the assumption, although mythical, is that all observations, interventions, and evaluations should document or one may assume they are not done. Nurses often claim that inadequate documentation is tangible proof of the fact that they are overworked and understaffed or that charting is less important than caring for the patient. This is an especially dangerous position to take when combined with failure to remedy the situation. The result is a poor record that subjects the nurse to disciplinary action before the Board of Nurse Examiners *and* a failed defense in a civil suit.

CHARTING IN ADVANCE

Another common charting error is charting in advance on flow records or check-off forms. This is not only unethical and dishonest but also dangerous, because it is impossible to predict what will happen to the patient. This author has reviewed and defended several cases in which the nurse charted in advance only to have the patient expire prior to the time of recorded treatments and interventions. Unfortunately, in many cases, the nurse attempted to cover her mistake by circling the treatment or intervention, indicating that the patient refused it. Juries have difficulty believing that the dead are able to exercise that choice. The great danger here is that the entire record and everything that the nurse says will be tainted, as the jury will likely question his or her truthfulness.

IMPROPER TRANSCRIPTION

Another common charting error that can cause major problems is the improper transcription of orders. This type of charting error frequently leads to medication errors. By now, it is well known by nurses across the country that medication errors and resulting patient injuries may culminate in criminal indictment. In Colorado, three nurses were indicted for negligent homicide for their involvement with a medication error. An infant was to receive an intramuscular dose of penicillin. The pharmacist inadvertently prepared 10 times the dose in a syringe and sent it up. Considering the amount of medication to be delivered, the nurses elected to administer the medicine via the intravenous route after doing some independent research, without questioning the amount or calling the physician. The baby later died (Plum, 1997).

FALSIFICATION

Criminal charges may also result if a provider violates state or federal law by falsifying a patient record. In North Carolina, the director of nursing for a long-term care facility was charged with a felony count of falsifying an admission record of a resident (*State v. Whittle*, 1995). She falsified the medical record by documenting that the resident was admitted with stage IV decubitus ulcers on his heels and feet; the ulcers did not actually develop until after the patient was admitted. She was also charged with two misdemeanor counts for failing to establish and institute skin care protocols for the patient and failing to institute procedures related to daily recording of the status of the patient's skin.

TYPES OF CHARTING

Much attention has been given to the literal form in which records are compiled. In a move to streamline and simplify the process, many facilities have created various forms and checklists for nursing personnel to use in documenting assessments and treatments. As discussed previously, documentation using check sheets or forms is sometimes more difficult to utilize and is subject to a greater incidence of mistakes, such as stray marks and charting in advance.

NARRATIVE

The traditional form of charting, **narrative charting**, is still used today and is the preferred method of this author for several reasons. First, the record is actually written in the nurse's own handwriting, which makes it appear more authentic. In addition, if the record is complete, there is little question as to when the information was compiled. Using forms sometimes creates the appearance that missing or incomplete information can be added after the fact, which is never advisable.

PIE

Narrative charting may be accomplished by using a variety of formats. The most common forms of narrative charting are PIE and SOAP charting. The **PIE** charting system provides a format for documenting the *p*lanning, *i*mplementation, and *e*valuation of the nursing process for each patient. The problem list is formulated after patient assessment and is recorded as nursing diagnoses.

SOAP

The **SOAP** format also centers on the nursing process, with the assessment documented in terms of both *s*ubjective and *o*bjective problems, followed by the *a*ssessment recorded as a nursing diagnosis and *p*lanning interventions specific to the nursing diagnoses.

CARE MAP

Another format for charting is the **care map**, "an integrated treatment plan for a specific procedure or treatment over a projected length of stay that identifies services, patient outcomes and length of stay" (Fitzgerald, Bennet, Gillette, & McDermott, 1996). Charting by exception using a care map involves charting only the variances and exceptions in patient outcomes.

CHARTING BY EXCEPTION

A trend related to narrative charting is to chart only abnormal findings. This is known as **charting by exception**. In fact, this is the standard form of documentation used by many long-term care facilities and has been considered in other settings (Davis, Gray, Caldwell, & Bernardo, 1997). In general, day-to-day assessments and interventions are not documented in narrative form; because documentation is not required on a daily basis, only abnormalities are documented. This can be very misleading when records are shown to a jury because of the often naive view of what should be documented. Again, plaintiffs' attorneys often capitalize on this type of charting by dragging out that old myth: "if it wasn't documented, it wasn't done."

PHOTOGRAPHY

"A picture is worth a thousand words," especially when documenting wound assessment (Halpin-Landry, 1994). This type of documentation provides an accurate and objective description of a wound or interruption in skin integrity; it is the best means available to evaluate the effectiveness of intervention because wound progression or healing can be objectively analyzed by comparison of photographs. From the liability standpoint, a dated and timed photograph of a patient's bedsore at the time of admission, together with accurately staging a detailed skin care plan, serves several purposes. If the patient is suspected of being a victim of abuse or neglect, the photographs will provide objective evidence to support a mandatory report to law enforcement authorities. Likewise, if the patient is admitted from the care of another facility, the photograph will serve to substantiate a defense that the patient's problem predated any care given by the admitting facility, as well as accurately portray either wound healing or progression. As part of a nursing assessment and evaluation, photographs of the patient are part of the permanent medical record and should be labeled with the patient's name, dated, timed, and placed in the chart. The patient's consent must be obtained to photograph, because the patient can be identified by virtue of the label and/or identifying features.

ENTRIES AND CORRECTIONS

It is generally accepted that all entries in a medical record should be dated, timed, and properly authenticated. Notwithstanding, there are times when an entry simply does not make it into the record as a result of an accident or mistake. The question is how to make the entry, authenticate the entry, and preserve the integrity of the record. It is acceptable to add entries after the fact, but only if the author is personally able to recall the events that are the subject of the entry to properly authenticate the entry. This means that the date and time that the entry is actually being made should be evident on the face of the record, as well as the date and time that the entry should have originally been recorded.

There are times, however, when late entries should not be made. One common misconception is that a late entry is to be made when the nurse loses the "race to the charts." This occurs when care is provided by more than one nurse and the nurse who provided the earlier treatment (or assessment) does not have the opportunity to document in due order. This is not a late entry. The nurse should simply document the time that she is making the entry and indicate when the assessment and/or intervention was actually done. Other situations occur when a late entry could have been made but it is no longer prudent to do so. Examples of situations would include (1) adding entries to the records after they have been copied and sent to a third party, (2) adding to the records after an adverse patient result, and (3) adding to or deleting from the records after a patient complaint. It is obvious why these situations dictate

against amending the record. It will certainly be argued by opposing counsel that the entries were made in an effort to put the health care provider in a better light, or to commit fraud by stating facts. Keep in mind that additional information may still be elicited during the investigation of the case. If the nurse has malpractice insurance that provides a defense (either through the employer's policy or his or her own private insurance), the attorney will assist in presenting those facts that the nurse failed to include in the original records with a reasonable explanation of why such facts were not included. This is a much more credible method of supplementing information and will not give rise to allegations of falsification of the records.

It is imperative that records not be falsified or destroyed. Not only is this a violation of statutes and regulations concerning retention and security of medical records, it may subject the nurse to professional discipline or even license revocation by his or her state board of nursing. In addition, in the civil context, evidence of intentional or reckless destruction of records or evidence may entitle the patient/plaintiff to a jury instruction stating that missing evidence is presumed to be detrimental to the party or person who destroyed it or allowed it to be destroyed. Furthermore, it is well known that the federal government's challenge of health care costs is ultimately resolved by review of documentation to determine whether care was actually rendered. In 1996, HCFA overpaid $23.2 billion in Medicare payments. Forty-seven percent of all overcharges were discovered by OIG's review of medical records that revealed insufficient or no documentation to support the charges (*Health Lawyers News*, 1997).

RECOMMENDATIONS FOR IMPROVED DOCUMENTATION

ASSESSMENT AND CARE PLAN

Documentation begins with a thorough assessment and appropriate plan of care. The plan of care should include nursing diagnoses based on patient history and presenting complaints. Nursing interventions will be based on medical interventions and nursing judgment. Goals relate to resolution of patient problems. The care plan should be used to improve documentation and communication about patient problems and progress. The care plan can be used to streamline documentation, in that all patient contacts originate with the three elements of the care plan: problems, interventions, and evaluation. Each time a nurse has a patient encounter, it is for assessment, intervention, or evaluation, and all these elements should be contained within a care plan. Obviously, if new problems arise, they should be added to the plan.

OTHER PURPOSES OF THE CARE PLAN

In addition to streamlining documentation, the care plan can communicate end-of-shift report in a very efficient fashion. Obviously, the patient still has problems by virtue of the fact that he or she is still hospitalized; shift reports communicate current patient status to other caregivers without requiring them to read the medical record. Using the care plan to document and give a report ensures that all patient problems are addressed. Chart information should be stated in objective terms. The rationale behind the conclusions should be presented instead of making statements that may be interpreted as judgment-laden. For example, instead of using a word like "filthy" to describe a patient's hygiene, state what led to that conclusion: "patient has dried feces/mud on skin and under nails."

COMPUTERIZED RECORDS

Many hospitals and health care facilities have adopted computerized patient records. Computerized records are created, authenticated, and stored on a computer. The most pressing concerns related to the compilation of medical information in this medium are legal and security issues.

As a threshold issue, it must be determined whether federal and state regulations and voluntary accreditation standards allow medical records to be created and stored on computer. Medicare requirements for participation allow records to be created and retained in this medium; however, many state statutes specifically delimit or prohibit the creation and/or retention of computerized records. This is obviously a concern, because the medical record is the cornerstone of the hospital's data management system.

Security issues are prevalent, with major concerns being confidentiality, access, alteration, and falsification. The system should be secure to prevent unauthorized access and prevent authorized users from accessing the system beyond their need to know. Other issues concern computer viruses and sabotage, which endanger the integrity of the entire system (Waller, 1991).

The benefits of automated records are tangible. In addition to freeing up physical space in the hospital for other purposes, computerized records provide physicians and other practitioners ready access to complete patient history that is essential for medical decision making. In addition, some studies indicate that computerized charting may save both time and money and increase the quality of patient care by giving nurses more time to spend with their clients (Lower & Nauert, 1992).

ISSUES AND TRENDS

NURSING AND LEGAL ISSUES

The trend is obviously moving toward a paperless hospital environment. Not only are patient records computerized, but hospital records—such as financial records—are tied into the same system. Moreover, as hospitals move toward integrated network delivery systems, the flow of information between facilities and providers will become smoother and more efficient.

At the same time, the issues of confidentiality and security will become more important, in that easier access to records by a greater number of people creates a risk for breach of even the most sophisticated system.

ETHICAL ISSUES AND CONSIDERATIONS

The ethical issues also revolve around security and confidentiality. If a private insurer has access to information that could influence a coverage decision, the issue of need to know is a critical consideration. Suppose that the patient/client had genetic testing done and the insurer decides to deny coverage for that condition in advance by exclusion in the policy, is this ethical? Many states have already addressed this concern by making it illegal for insurers to deny coverage based on genetic testing.

Other need-to-know issues relate to broad access of hospital records by any employee with a password to the system. This has been a problem with many facilities when employees find out that their coworker was admitted to the facility and are unable to resist the temptation to snoop and tell. Audit trails are utilized to track access, and employee discipline (such as termination) has been a successful deterrent to such actions in many facilities.

RECOMMENDATIONS FOR RESEARCH AND MALPRACTICE PREVENTION

Document, document, document, and keep your eyes to yourself are the rules to live by. Without regard to the particular charting format used, if a nurse makes sure that his or her charting reflects the assessment, analysis of problems, planning, and implementation of nursing care with ongoing evaluation of care, then the documentation will be acceptable. Systems are continuously being developed and improved to combat the confidentiality and security issues inherent in computerized patient record systems. Additional research should be conducted to improve the accuracy of nursing information

systems as well as their ease of use in a variety of environments. Nurses are utilizing computers in many settings, and uniformity is lacking. Research is needed to determine the impact of computerized medical records on patient care.

Will the future hold something akin to video-recorded patient care? The same issues will arise with the addition of the constitutional privacy issues. Additional research continues to find the most cost-effective, efficient way to record patient care without compromising the quality of care being delivered. Nurses' input and participation in this process is crucial because nurses will be affected by the systems ultimately utilized.

SUMMARY

The medical record is a legal document. Because of the time that elapses between the delivery of patient care and legal proceedings, the record may be the only evidence of the delivered care. It is, therefore, critical that the medical record accurately reflect the nursing process, with documented evidence of nursing assessment, planning for nursing intervention, implementation, and evaluation of planned interventions and patient response. There are many forms or types of charting that may be utilized; without regard to the particular format, the basic elements of the nursing process should be evident in order that the care given be accurately summarized.

Inadequate documentation may give rise to a civil lawsuit and, in addition, can be the basis for a disciplinary action before a nurse's licensing board. Falsified records have merited felony and misdemeanor criminal charges in some jurisdictions and can give rise to allegations of Medicare fraud.

A court in at least one state views the relationship between a health care provider, whether it is a hospital, doctor, or nurse as a contract, with an obligation of secrecy or confidentiality. Violation of the confidentiality requirement is actionable as a breach of contract. Unauthorized disclosure of patient information can give rise to actions for invasion of privacy, breach of confidence, and even defamation.

POINTS TO REMEMBER

- The purpose of the medical record is to provide a summary of a patient's hospitalization, condition, all treatment rendered, and evaluation of effectiveness of treatment.
- The medical record is a legal document and is admissible in a court of law as evidence.
- In general, the hospital owns the physical medical record and the patient owns the information contained within it.
- Nurses have an independent duty to safeguard patient confidentiality.
- Failure to document completely can make a malpractice case indefensible.
- Without regard to the format for charting, the most important elements to be included are patient assessment, to include problems; plan for nursing or medical intervention as well as implementation; and evaluation of treatments and interventions.

REFERENCES

American Nurses Association. (1985). *Code for nurses with interpretive statements*. Washington, DC: Author.

Anderson v. Strong Memorial Hospital, 531 N.Y.S. 735 (1988).

Berry v. Moench, 8 Utah 191, 331 P. 2d. 814 (1958).

Biddle v. Warren Gen. Hosp., No. 96-7-5582 (Ohio Ct. App. Mar. 27, 1998).

Boyles v. Kerr, 855 S.W.2d 593 (Tex. 1993).

Cannel v. Medical and Surgical Clinic, 315 N.E.2d 278 (1974).

Clark v. Geraci, 29 Misc. 2d. 791, 208 N.Y.S. 2d 564 (1960).

Conditions of Participation for Hospitals, 42 CFR § 482.24 (1995).

Davis, M., Gray, L., Caldwell, D., & Bernardo, L. M. (1997). Children's Hospital Pittsburgh, new charting for ER documentation by exception. *Journal of Emergency Nursing, 23*(5), 481-486.

Doe v. Roe, 400 N.Y.S. 2d 668 (1977).

Effects of Accreditation, 42 U.S.C. § 1395(bb) (1995).

Fitzgerald, A., Bennet, M., Gillette, J., & McDermott, K. (1996). Development of a multidisciplinary care map: Documenting by exception. *Oncology Nursing Forum, 23*(2), 356.

Halpin-Landry, J. (1994). Documenting wounds through the camera's eye. *Nursing 94*, pp. 58-60.

Hammonds v. Aetna Casualty & Surety Co., 243 F. Supp. 793 (W.D. Ohio 1965).

Health Lawyers News, *OIG faults HCFA's controls on spending, estimates $23.2 billion over paid in FY 1996 1*(9), 24–25.

Hospital Licensing Texas Health and Safety Code § 241.103.

Irving Healthcare System v. Brooks, 927 S.W.2d 12 (Tex. 1996).

Lower, M., & Nauert, L. (1992). Charting: The impact of bedside computers. *Nursing Management, 23*(7), 40-43.

May v. Wood River TP Hosp., 629 N.E.2d 170 (Ill. 1994).

Medical Liability and Insurance Improvement Act, Texas Revised Civil Statutes Annotated, Article 4590i (Vernon's Supp. 1998).

Memorial Hospital–The Woodlands v. McCown, 927 S.W.2d 1 (Tex. 1996).

Prince v. St. Francis–St. George Hospital, 20 Ohio App. 3d 4 (1985).

Plum, S. (1997). Nurses indicted. *Nursing 97, 27*(7), 34.

Pyramid Life Insurance Co. v. Masonic Hospital Association, 191 F. Supp. 51 (W.D. Okla 1961).

State v. Whittle, 454 S.E.2d 688 (N.C.Ct. App. 1995).

Texas Health Information Management Association, Retention and Storage. (1994). *Health record information manual*. Austin, TX: Author.

Urbaniak v. Newton, 226 Cal. App. 3d 1128, 277 Cal. Rptr. 354 (1991).

Waller, A. (1991). Legal aspects of based patient records and records systems. In R.S. Dick & E.B. Sleen (Eds.) The computer based patient record: An essential technology for health care (a report of the Institute of Medicine) (App. B. p. 156). Washington, D.C.: National Academy Press.

SUGGESTED READINGS

American Bar Association. (1995, May 11). *Maintenance, release and retention of medical records*. American Bar Association Forum on Health Law, Hospital and Health Care Facility Records: Maintenance, Release and Retention.

NHLA/AAHA Practice Guide Series. (1997). *Health information systems and electronic medical records practice guide*.

NHLA/AAHA. (1994). *Health records information manual: Practice guide series* (Vol. V).

Texas Health Information Management Association. (1994). Health record information manual.

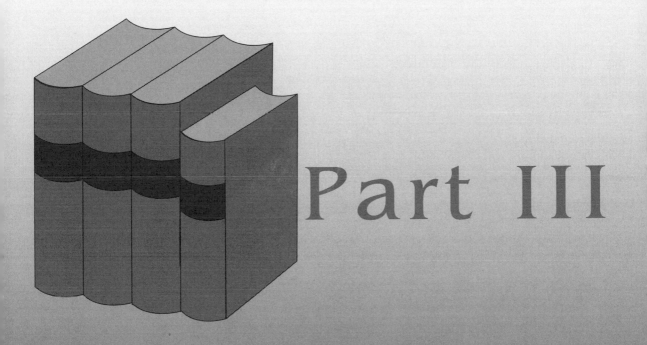

Part III

NURSING LAW
AND THE
PATIENT

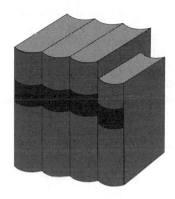

Chapter 10

THE NURSE-PATIENT RELATIONSHIP

Anne Marie K. Catalano

Abandonment
Assault and Battery
Authorization For
   Release of Information
Charting by Exception
Confidentiality
Continuity of Care
Derivative Privilege
Disclosure
Documentation
Duty to Warn
Evaluation
Float

Good Samaritan Act
Implied Contract
Narrative Charting
Nursing Assessment
Nursing Interventions
Privileged
   Communications
Reliance
Reportable Situation
Scope of Employment
Statutory Law
Tarasoff Duty
Team Nursing

Upon completion of this chapter, the reader will be able to:
- Identify when the nurse becomes legally responsible for the care of patients.
- State the provisions and limits of the Good Samaritan Law.
- List the necessary components of adequate patient documentation.
- Identify the difference between confidential and privileged communications.
- Summarize the responsibility of the nurse in maintaining patient confidentiality.
- Identify the reportable situations required by state statutes.
- Explore some of the ethical considerations involving confidentiality in the nurse's own practice situation.

INTRODUCTION

The nurse-patient relationship has evolved from that of the nurse providing care in the patient's home only when a family member was not available to do so, to that of hospital-based nursing care, to one where nurses can now be independent practitioners and autonomous in providing highly skilled health care. Laws and statutes are modified more slowly, resulting from the changes in nursing practice and the resulting conflicts that arise.

STAGES OF THE NURSE-PATIENT RELATIONSHIP

In nursing literature, the nurse-client relationship is described by several names, such as an interpersonal relationship or a therapeutic relationship. Peplau (1980) describes the development of the nurse-patient relationship as consisting of four phases: (1) orientation, (2) identification, (3) exploitation, and (4) resolution. Regarding the legal aspect of the nurse-client relationship, a different set of criteria is used to identify the various moments in time when a relationship is initiated and when it is terminated.

INITIATION

Most state nurse practice acts agree that the "licensed nurse-patient relationship begins when the nurse accepts the assignment for patient care" (Fletcher, 1997, p. 12). If the occurrence of malpractice or negligence by a nurse is to be proven, then four elements need to be established. The first of these elements is that the nurse had a *duty* toward the client. If the client was hospitalized during the incident under question, then duty becomes easier to prove. The client is considered a "captive audience," and the nurse is an employee of the hospital; therefore, duty exists. The legal concept of **reliance** applies; the client has a right to expect or rely on the fact that the nursing staff has a clear duty to act in his or her best interests. This concept is clear when speaking of models of delivery of nursing care such as private duty or primary nursing. However, the concept of reliance also applies to the team nursing model of delivery. In **team nursing**, designed to eliminate the fragmentation of care resulting from a task-oriented approach to the delivery of nursing care, a professional nurse leads a nursing team in delivering client-centered care. This team would consist of both licensed and unlicensed nursing personnel. If a client requests assistance from a nurse (or staff member) that is not a member of his or her "team," and the rendering of such assistance is

immediately required to preserve the client's health and/or safety, then the nurse has a duty to provide aid as needed. Stating that this client was not an assigned patient of the nurse is not a defense. As a client of the hospital, the nursing staff is required to respond to his or her needs. The client is entitled to the level of care indicated by his or her age and mental or physical condition. It would be expected that the disabled, very young, and elderly would require a higher duty of care (Hemelt & Mackert, 1982).

The contract for the nurse-patient relationship is an implied one in many cases. "An **implied contract** is one that has not been explicitly agreed to by the parties but that the law nevertheless considers to exist" (Kozier, Erb, Blais, & Wilkinson, 1995, p. 222). The client has the right to expect competent nurses caring for his or her needs. On the other hand, the nurse also has the right to expect that the client will provide complete and accurate health information on which to base nursing care.

The delivery model for health care is changing. An expanding number of clients are receiving care in their homes. This home care model may be in place of the client's admission to a hospital, or to facilitate a discharge from the hospital when the client no longer needs the services of an acute care facility. In these cases, when is the relationship between nurse and client established? Often, there are several nurses involved in the care of a home-based client. Examples would include a nurse case manager from the hospital or insurance company, a staff nurse from the hospital calling the client at home to evaluate how the client is progressing, and a nurse from a home health care or public health or visiting nurse agency coming to the home to provide care for the client. The time at which clients are discharged from acute care facilities to home often leaves the client arriving home late in the evening. A home care agency may not have staff available to visit the home to admit the client until the next day. Needed assessments and treatments may be missed. If harm is caused to the client, the courts will have to decide who failed in the duty of care in this situation.

LIMITATIONS

Nurses continue to think and function as nurses beyond the scope of employment. A different set of rules determines when the nurse-client relationship is established outside of an employer-employee situation. These rules are often covered under a state **Good Samaritan Act**. For example, if the nurse is attending a county fair with family and friends and suddenly an elderly woman unknown to the nurse clutches her chest and falls to the ground, the nurse now has several options from which to choose her next action. If the nurse were at work, she would have an absolute duty of care to her clients as she is within the **scope of employment** (Ashley, 1997, p. 46). Outside of her employment agency, the nurse does not have a nurse-patient relationship with the public at large unless she voluntarily takes up that relationship. She may feel an ethical or professional obligation but, in most states, is not under a legal duty to provide nursing care. A few states do obligate health care professionals to assist at scenes requiring medical intervention. Minnesota requires all persons, not just health care professionals, to render assistance. If she identified herself as a nurse to those in the crowd that gathered around the elderly woman, or if she simply commenced performing cardiopulmonary resuscitation without identifying herself, she would then have acted affirmatively as a professional nurse and thus volunteered her professional services. If a neighbor of the nurse announced to the crowd that this was a nurse, the nurse is not legally obligated to respond. The nurse must identify herself or perform nursing actions; another person cannot volunteer her services (Ashley, 1997).

The nurse must consider that the client has a right to refuse health care measures, regardless of the outcome to the client. **Assault and battery** charges may be brought against a nurse who performs treatments the client has indicated are not acceptable (Catalano, 1995). An example would be administering a blood transfusion to a client who has refused one based on a religious conviction. The basis for the refusal is not important; the client has a right to refuse treatment as long as he or she is legally competent.

TERMINATION

The termination or resolution phase of the nurse-client relationship occurs when the client is well enough to meet his or her health care needs on his or her own or when the care of the client needs to be assigned or referred to another agency. It is expected that this phase is reached by a consensus of the client and care providers. However, with the recent changes in the economy of health care delivery, clients many times feel they are discharged from professional care prior to being ready. Nurses must follow the standards of care in these situations and document completely and appropriately.

Nurses must be aware of their state's definition of patient **abandonment**. It generally is defined as "leaving the nursing assignment without transferring responsibilities to appropriate personnel or care giver when continued nursing care is required by the condition of the client(s)" or "abandoning or neglecting a client who is in need of nursing care, without making reasonable arrangements for the continuation of care" (North Carolina Board of Nursing, 1995, 21NCAC 36.0217 (b)(10); Washington RN Nursing Regulations, 1998, WAC 246-839-710(4)c). A supported charge of abandonment is cause for disciplinary action by the state board of nursing. Many times the main issue involved when a nurse is charged with abandonment is the refusal to work overtime. This is usually an employer-employee issue and not a cause for board disciplinary action. Overtime policies should be addressed by an employee contract, or if one does not exist, then in the employee handbook. In many cases, if a licensed nurse is asked to work beyond the regularly scheduled shift, he or she may simply reply no. As long as the nurse can transfer the care of patients to an appropriate individual, the nurse is performing his or her duties according to the standards of care. A problem arises when there is no appropriate personnel available to take over the care of the patients. In this case, the nurse should immediately notify the supervisor to make the appropriate arrangements. The nurse must realize that if he or she is too fatigued to work, the patients may be placed in danger. Although tiredness may be considered in a disciplinary hearing or malpractice case against the nurse, it is not a defense.

Charges of abandonment may also be brought against a nurse for refusal to accept an assignment. The nurse's reasons for rejecting an assignment must be based on competent nursing judgment. An example would be when the risk of harm to the patient is greater by accepting the assignment than by rejecting it (American Nurses Association, 1995). If a registered nurse (RN) from the postpartum unit is temporarily assigned to the birthing unit to monitor patients in early labor, the RN must be knowledgeable and competent to provide the required nursing care, such as interpreting fetal monitor strips and assessing the laboring woman. If he or she cannot, then the assignment must be rejected. However, if the nurse has been cross–trained to work in the birthing unit, and that training is documented, then he or she may be subject to the abandonment charge by refusing the assignment.

Another situation in which a nurse may face a charge of abandonment is caring for a client who decides to pursue a course of action the nurse finds morally or ethically objectionable. Examples would include a client who has decided on assisted suicide or a therapeutic abortion. In regard to assisted suicide, the Oregon Nurses Association Assisted Suicide Guidelines (1995) state the nurse "may conscientiously object to being involved in delivering care. You are obliged to provide for the patient's safety, to avoid abandonment, and withdraw only when assured that alternative sources of care are available to the patient." The licensed nurse is responsible for limiting his or her own scope of practice, by both educational and ethical considerations. The nurse should be aware of the scope-of-practice situations that routinely occur in his or her employment and refuse those positions in which conflicts are likely to arise (Catalano, 1995).

DOCUMENTATION

Documentation is the written record of nursing care. It is a record of important information about the patient and should be presented clearly and concisely. From a legal point of view, if it is not documented, it did not happen (Creighton, 1987). In a review of 200 case summaries directly involving nurses in litigation found in professional nursing journals, consumer-oriented insurance information packets, and medical malpractice journals and newsletters, Mayberry and Croke (1996, p. 16) found that the majority of cases could be divided into four categories: failure to monitor, failure to document, failure to follow standards of care, and failure to notify a physician. A large component of the failure to-document subset involved a failure to record discharge instructions.

Health care facilities and agencies have used a variety of documentation styles. **Narrative charting** was once the sole method available for documentation. Now it is usually incorporated as a portion of another form when unusual clinical situations occur (White, 1992). When well done, written narrative notes were an excellent record of what transpired during the client's time under the nurse's care. However, the narrative style was tedious and time consuming. Another form of documentation was sought; one that expedited charting. Flow sheets and charts came into common practice, particularly in areas where much of the basic care was predictable. This allowed forms to be developed where a check mark or nurse's initials would indicate the completion of a routine task or intervention. **Charting by exception** is a style that has gained popularity. Nursing care is delineated in care plans, and only unexpected outcomes are documented (Behrend, 1994). However, it becomes more difficult to prove in a court of law that certain aspects of nursing care were in fact rendered, when they are not specifically documented.

Notes, charts, flow sheets, in fact, any documentation tool that ends up in the patient's chart, becomes a part of the medical record and is considered a legal document. It is the record of what transpired during the patient's care and treatment and should be the nurse's best defense against legal action. Callahan (1989) delineated documentation policies for the emergency department nursing staff. On review of these policies, one can appreciate their relevance to other areas of nursing practice: (1) documentation of vital signs, (2) nursing procedures, (3) discharge instructions, (4) maintenance of patient confidentiality, (5) incident reporting, (6) news media release policy, and (7) continuous nursing chart audit (Callahan, 1989, p. 37).

Documentation of nursing care should be completed as soon as feasible. In this manner, it is easier for the nurse to recall the details of the nursing care or patient experience without time or subsequent factors confounding the recording. If entries are made out of sequence (i.e., detailing an event of 9 A.M. after an 11 A.M. entry), the nurse should clearly identify the late entry according to agency policy. If the nurse makes an error in documentation, a single line being drawn through it should indicate the error. The error should remain legible; plaintiffs' attorneys are very skeptical of a nurse's explanation of sections of the record that have been obliterated by multiple cross-outs. It is also necessary to record the date and time of the discovery and correction of an error in the medical chart.

"Nurses have a duty to communicate accurate and clear information to other health care workers" (Killion, 1993, p. 131). This is critical when communicating with physicians regarding the care, treatments, and medications they wish their patients to receive. Institutions and agencies should have clear policies on how verbal or telephone orders are to be recorded and verified by the nurse. Usually orders such as these need to be confirmed by receipt of written communications or signature of the physician within a specified time frame.

Nurses should strive to document only the relevant facts of patient care and leave out personal opinions of other health care professionals' actions. It is more legally sound to record the patient's response to another's actions (providing the nurse is not negligent or derelict in his or her duty to the patient) than to risk facing a defamation of character suit by stating in the record that the other health care worker was incompetent or mishandled the care of the patient.

PATIENT TEACHING

Patient education has increasingly been recognized as one method of decreasing length of stay (Creighton, 1986). This is true in both inpatient and outpatient settings. However, documentation of teaching is often the exception rather than the rule (Whitman, Graham, Gleit, & Boyd, 1992). Some studies have found that nurses documented patient teaching only 15 percent of the time (Porter, 1990, p. 135). Nurses have cited several reasons for not documenting patient teaching. These reasons include a lack of time related to heavy patient assignments and shorter lengths of stay.

Many nurses, particularly home health nurses, provide a great deal of teaching that they deem informal and almost conversational (Killion, 1993). Such teaching is often overlooked when it comes to documenting the interaction with the patient. However, to cover himself or herself legally, the nurse should include a formal teaching plan with specific objectives, nursing interventions, and evaluation criteria. It is recommended that patients (or responsible family members) sign "receipts" for important information and these receipts should be added to the client's record (Killion, 1993, p. 132).

In documenting patient teaching, including discharge instructions, specific actions such as "identified fetal movements in a ten minute window with 100% accuracy" rather than relying on terms with vague meanings such as "understands counting fetal movements" are preferred. Charting as soon as the teaching session or patient interaction is completed also ensures that an accurate accounting is recorded. It is suggested that the following information be included when documenting patient teaching:

- **Nursing assessment**—The patient's diagnosis and condition, current level of understanding regarding his or her diagnosis and care, learning needs.
- **Nursing interventions**—The teaching provided by the nurse.
- **Evaluation**—The assessment of the patient response to intervention, either by verbalization or actions such as a return demon-

stration. This would apply to the relevant family members in cases in which the patient either cannot or will not be a party to the teaching session.

Discharge instructions require a great deal of detail. Oral instructions should be followed up with written instructions, with any exceptions to routine care clearly identified. Signs and symptoms of disease progression as well as of medication or treatment side effects should be outlined. It is particularly important to review with the patient when it is necessary to call the physician or to seek emergency care services. The documentation of the discharge instructions not only needs the content covered and the patient's response to the teaching intervention, but an accounting of any written materials or audiovisual aids given to the patient (Eggland, 1997).

THE CONFIDENTIAL RELATIONSHIP BETWEEN NURSE AND CLIENT

The patient's right to privacy and **confidentiality** is a key concept in both the American Nurses Association Code for Nurses (American Nurses Association, 1985) and the Canadian Nurses Association Code of Ethics for Nursing (Canadian Nurses Association, 1991), as well as the nurse practice acts for each state. Patients have a right to expect that nurses, and indeed all health care workers, will not divulge information to those not directly involved in their care. "Insurance companies have no legal right to demand access to medical records, even though they may be determining compensation to the client" (Kozier et al., 1995, p. 176). The patient must sign an **authorization for release of information** clearly indicating what information is to be released, to whom, and for what purpose. Nurses need to be familiar with what information their agency considers confidential, and in what manner and by whom it may be revealed.

In the United States, there is no explicit federal legislation or constitutional right to medical privacy or confidentiality. There are several cases, including *Roe v. Wade,* 1973, in which the U.S. Supreme Court has cited several amendments that imply that right. Each state has laws addressing confidentiality, but many are unclear and limited in their scope. All states do recognize a legal duty of confidentiality in certain situations, but they also address exceptions to the duty (Dellinger, 1997).

Most health care agencies allow students and those involved in research access to patient records with the understanding that the records will be held in strict confidence. If that trust is violated, that is, the patient can be identified by those not involved in his or her care, the health care or educational institution usually has policies in place to punish the violators. It may be as simple as a verbal reprimand—or as severe as termination of privileges as a student or researcher, demand for expulsion from the school, or termination of employment.

PRIVILEGED COMMUNICATIONS

Privileged communications are communications that include "information given to a professional person who is forbidden by law from disclosing the information in a court without the consent of the person who provided it" (Kozier et al., 1995, p. 220). In their statutes regarding privileged communications, most states identify professional person(s) as physicians, priests, lawyers, and newspeople. Communications between a married couple are also considered privileged. Nurses are generally not included in these groups unless covered by separate legislation. For example, in 1995 the Georgia General Assembly passed a bill granting exclusion from discovery for communications between clients and psychiatric/mental health clinical nurse specialists (Mazacoufa, Teahan, Bryant, & Hawkins, 1995, p. 1). However, in North Carolina the courts have included nurses within the physician privilege, even though nurses are not specifically mentioned. This is a **derivative privilege** and may be interpreted differently in different cases. Nurses need to be aware of this possibility.

The privileged relationship can be waived under certain circumstances. For example, medical records may be used to prove a claim and thus used in a court of law. Even so, the clients must waive that privilege and do so in writing. Also, a privileged communication should be made in a "private setting where confidentiality could reasonably be expected" (Loecker, 1998, p. 14). If the information is shared with a third party, the privilege is lost.

EXCEPTIONS TO CONFIDENTIALITY

Most states recognize the need for **disclosure** of what is otherwise considered confidential information under certain circumstances. For example, all 50 states require disclosure in cases of child abuse when certain professionals suspect the abuse. The list of professionals varies from state to state, but usually includes nurses, physicians, school teachers, and child care workers. In fact, the Massachusetts Board of Registration in Nursing requires applicants for renewal to attest by signature to a statement affirming they have reported all suspected cases of child abuse. Other types of abuse may be required to be reported, such as elder abuse or abuse of the disabled. The states are more varied in regard to these types of mandated reporting.

If a client is dangerous to himself or herself or to others, certain case law may be used to guide the actions of those involved. Three California court cases—*Tarasoff v. Regents of the University of California* (1976), *Bellah v. Greenson* (1978), and *Gross v. Allen* (1994)—have been cited by others involved in similar circumstances. In the first of these cases, *Tarasoff v. Regents of the University of California*, 1976, a decision was rendered in 1976 that resulted in what became known as the **Tarasoff duty,** or the **duty to warn.** This meant that if a health care provider was treating a client, and that client revealed an intent to harm another person, the health care provider had a legal obligation to notify the intended victim. The second case, *Bellah v. Greenson* (1978) did not expand the duty to warn to include threats of suicide or

self-harm. However, the decision in *Gross v. Allen* (1994) notified mental health professionals that they must communicate to their patients' subsequent caregivers any known intent of suicide or intent to harm other identifiable victims. In summary, the three cases inform mental health professionals that "they have a duty to communicate serious threats and known dangers not only to their patients' readily identifiable victims but also to their patients' subsequent caregivers" and that duty "can be extended to threats of suicide" (Meyers, 1997, p. 365). The professionals involved in the cases were psychiatrists and psychologists, but the relevance to advanced practice nurses is clear.

REPORTABLE SITUATIONS REQUIRED BY STATUTE

In order to protect the well-being of society, federal and state legislators establish **statutory law.** The purpose of these laws is to "help maintain a government's right to uphold the social order and to protect the rights of individuals" (Catalano, 1995, p. 48). Some statutes dictate that specific occurrences of a certain nature are reportable to an identified agency. Again, these statutes regarding a **reportable situation** vary from state to state, but generally include the following: gunshot or stabbing wounds, rapes or sexual assaults, some sexually transmitted diseases, and abuse of children, the elderly, and the disabled (Catalano, 1995, p. 68). Burns that cover more than a specified area of the body (e. g., more than 5 percent) often are reportable to the local fire marshal.

ISSUES AND TRENDS

NURSING ISSUES AND TRENDS

The nurse-client relationship is an active and continually evolving relationship. Employment trends of professional nurses demonstrate a shift in the place of employment from in-hospital settings to community agencies. Issues that previously had been clear now need redefinition and reassignment of responsibility.

The staffing numbers at most health care agencies have been diminished to the smallest complement of staff to meet the needs of the client population. If an employee is absent from work, this often creates a situation requiring another nurse to **float** from his or her usually assigned floor. The nurse who is assigned to cover the shortage needs to be sure he or she is competent to meet the standards of care for the unit to which he or she is temporarily assigned. Does the nurse have the necessary skills and education? Those factors will be scrutinized in court or by the state board of nursing should a complaint regarding the nurse's care arise. A desire to "help out" in one's place of employment is not a defense, as it might be in a situation outside of work. The nurse also needs to understand that if he or she is indeed competent in the care required on the other unit, then he or she must go, or otherwise be liable for patient abandonment.

The lengths of stay patients are allowed for various admissions are much shorter than those allowed as recently as 1995. This necessitates that staff nurses (along with the attending physicians) oversee that **continuity of care** is maintained. When a patient is transferred to another agency or sent home, arrangements for specialized care often need to be made. Nurses need to ascertain that patients receive required medications or treatments as detailed in the plan of care, regardless of the timing of their discharge from the admitting facility.

Documentation standards have changed, as have documentation styles, from narrative notes to charting by exception. All nurses need to take the time to document patient assessments and care completely and accurately. Materials distributed to the patient and their family members need to be documented, as well as the teaching plan.

LEGAL TRENDS AND ISSUES

Issues of confidentiality, and breaches thereof, are the basis for many legal actions involving nurses. Nurses must be aware of their state's nursing practice act in this regard, as well as specific guidelines for the agencies in which they are employed. In addition, nurses must be knowledgeable of mandated reportable situations, in which the state or federal statutes mandate a breach of confidentiality. Many of these statutes are still evolving, especially those involved with domestic abuse. Advanced practice nurses, particularly those in the mental health field, need to be aware of the duty to warn as well as the duty to inform in cases where a patient may be a danger to himself or herself or others.

The legal response to many of these issues has yet to be determined. For example, in Texas, adolescents who have not reached the age of majority are requesting and being tested for human immunodeficiency virus (HIV) status (Richardson, 1996). Legally speaking, they should not be tested without their parents' or guardians' knowledge and consent. Likewise, the results of these tests should be available to the parents prior to the child's receiving them. However, many of the clinics in Texas are performing the tests based on the adolescent's request alone. Results are first given to the patient, and then, only if the patient signs a release, given to the parents. Currently, parents are not aware of their child's seeking such testing until they receive the medical billing in the mail. And sometimes that does not occur, if the testing has been performed at a free or reduced-cost clinic. These cases must first wind their way through the court system before becoming case law or statutes.

ETHICAL CONSIDERATIONS AND CONFLICTS

The subject of the nurse-patient relationship, with its relevant areas such as patient confidentiality and mandated reporting, is ripe for many ethical considerations and conflicts. Many have already been addressed in this chapter. Others will be explored here.

Many patients who are HIV positive or have acquired immunodeficiency syndrome (AIDS) do not wish to be identified to others as having this disease. If the others are not sexual or drug partners, they do not have a right to be so informed, under the present law. Consider the following two scenarios. Abe, who is approaching the terminal stage of AIDS, desires to return to his parents' home for care. He does not want to reveal his true diagnosis, but speaks to the home care workers about telling his parents he has cancer, rather than AIDS. If his parents do not know the true nature of his illness, they may not follow the appropriate measures to protect themselves from the transmission of the HIV virus. But they do not fall into the category of notification. How can the nurse respect the confidentiality of the patient and, at the same time, protect his parents and other caregivers from exposure?

A second scenario involves a 7-year-old child who is HIV positive. The school nurse and teacher are informed by the parents, with the directive not to inform any other parents or children, as they fear their child may be shunned by his classmates. A fall occurs on the playground, resulting in a bloody nose. A best friend tries to help. Again, how can you protect the friend and follow the parents' wishes?

Sometimes confidential matters must be allowed to stand, no matter how uncomfortable to the nurse. Consider the following scenario. A couple is undergoing genetic testing and counseling after the death of their infant from genetic causes. The gene typing reveals that the male partner was not the father of the baby. When confronted with this information alone, the female partner enjoined the health care team not to reveal the true parentage. "What's the point," she argued, "the lethal gene combination won't occur again." Can't the truth be padded so as not to reveal her actions? How should the nurse respond?

RECOMMENDATIONS FOR RESEARCH AND MALPRACTICE PREVENTION

All these issues—initiation of the nurse-patient relationship, documentation, confidentiality, and mandated reportable situations—are rapidly being modified. Nurses and other health care providers need to remain aware of how these issues evolve and how their actions need to change accordingly.

RESEARCH IN NATIONWIDE LICENSURE

An area that certainly will need study and clarification involves nurses who are employed across state lines. Certainly, nurses have worked for years for agencies that have assigned them to temporary positions outside of the nurses' home state. It is clear the nurses are now under the jurisdiction of the state in which they are employed. What happens when the state lines are crossed via telephone line or electronically? Many health insurance companies require notification and authorization of certain treatments and therapies that are prescribed by calling a toll-free number, often not in the caller's state. Are nurses legally able to assess if they are not licensed in that state? The same issue applies in cases of the nurse information help lines. Several professional nurse organizations are beginning to address this issue by calling for a nationwide licensure of professional nurses that would be valid in all 50 states.

MALPRACTICE PREVENTION

As always, the best defense against malpractice is to be aware of the statutes affecting professional nursing practice in your state. Specifically, in regard to the content covered in this chapter, nurses must be clear regarding their agency's policy (or their own guidelines, if they are in private practice or self-employed) on acceptance of patients or clients for care. Does the nurse have the necessary knowledge and skills to provide competent care? The plan of care should be available, with adequate documentation of patient assessment, teaching, and discharge instructions.

The nurse should be aware of what is considered confidential in the care of the patient, what may be disclosed, and under what circumstances. If the nurse has been granted the status of being able to hold privileged communications (as in the case of advanced practice mental health care nurses), how he or she should handle documenting these conversations should be discussed. In a similar vein, the avenues for properly reporting circumstances that must be reported should be known by every nurse. It is important to observe time frames for reporting; otherwise, the nurse may be implicated in the matter.

POINTS TO REMEMBER

- The nurse should accept a patient care assignment only if he or she is educated and skilled in providing all aspects of the care required.
- Each state has a governing body for the practice of nursing in that state, and nurses need to observe the guidelines.
- The nurse must refrain from performing treatments or administering medications that the legally competent patient refuses; otherwise, the nurse may be liable for assault and battery.
- Patient abandonment occurs when the nurse leaves his or her patients without appropriately transferring their care to another nurse or specified person.
- Documentation of the nursing process (assessment, plan, implementation, and evaluation), regardless of the documentation style used, is critical in providing evidence that safe and competent nursing care was delivered.
- Although patient education occupies a large proportion of the time nurses spend with patients, it often is not adequately documented. This would include a list of the written and visual information given to the patients and other family members, and how they demonstrated understanding of the material.
- All health care received by patients is considered confidential; that is, it should remain private and should be discussed only with those directly involved with the care of the patient. However, it may not be privileged information, and the nurse may

have to testify in court regarding such conversations.
- Each state has identified several mandated reportable situations, such as child abuse, that the nurse is mandated to report to the appropriate agency if he or she has knowledge that they exist.

REFERENCES

American Nurses Association. (1985). *Code for nurses with interpretive statements*. Washington, DC: Author.

American Nurses Association. (1995). *Position statement on the right to accept or reject an assignment*. Washington, DC: Author.

Ashley, R. C. (1997). Avoiding malpractice—Beyond the scope of employment. *Journal of Nursing Law, 4*(4), 45–49.

Behrend, S. W. (1994). Documentation in the ambulatory setting. *Seminars in Oncology Nursing, 10*(4), 264–280.

Bellah v. Greenson, 81 Cal. App. 3d 614 (1978).

Callahan, F. (1989). Emergency department nursing risk management. *Journal of Ambulatory Care Management, 12*(1), 31–39.

Canadian Nurses Association. (1991). *Code of ethics for nursing*. Ottawa, Ontario: Canadian Nurses' Association (CNA).

Catalano, J. T. (1995). *Ethical and legal aspects of nursing* (2nd ed.). Springhouse, PA: Springhouse.

Creighton, H. (1986). *Law every nurse should know* (5th ed.). Philadelphia: WB Saunders.

Creighton, H. (1987). Legal significance of charting. *Nursing Management, 18*(17), 20–22.

Dellinger, A. M. (1997). Legal requirements for confidentiality in hospice care. *The Hospice Journal, 12*(2), 43–48.

Eggland, E. T. (1997). Charting tips. Documenting discharge teaching. *Nursing, 27*(3), 25.

Fletcher, V. (1997). Nursing Commission update: Patient abandonment policy. *The Washington Nurse, 27*(1), 12–13.

Gross v. Allen, 22 Cal. App. 4th 354 (1994).

Hemelt, M. D., and Mackert, M. D. (1982). *Dynamics of law in nursing and health care* (2nd ed.). Reston, VA: Reston Publishing.

Killion, S. W. (1993). Case commentary—Bass v. Barksdale: Implications for public and home care nurses. *Public Health Nursing, 10*(2), 129–133.

Kozier, B., Erb, G., Blais, K., & Wilkinson, J. M. (1995). *Fundamentals of nursing: Concepts, process, and practice* (5th ed.). Redwood City, CA: Addison-Wesley.

Loecker, B. L. (1998). Attorney-client privilege and confidentiality. *Journal of Legal Nurse Consulting, 9*(1), 14–15.

Mayberry, A., & Croke, E. (1996). Issues leading to malpractice show little change: A review of the literature. *Journal of Legal Nurse Consultants, 7*(2), 16–19.

Mazacoufa, D., Teahan, C., Bryant, M., & Hawkins, J. (1995). P.A.'s win prescriptive rights; psych nurses win privileged communication; school health loses in 1995 legislative session. *Georgia Nursing, 55*(2), 1–2.

Meyers, C. J. (1997). Expanding Tarasoff: Protecting patients and the public by keeping subsequent caregivers informed. *The Journal of Psychiatry & Law,* 25(3), 365–375.

North Carolina Board of Nursing. (1995). *North Carolina nursing regulations: Revocation, suspension, or denial of license.* Raleigh, NC: The Division.

Oregon Nurses Association. (1995). *Assisted suicide guidelines.* Portland, OR: Author.

Peplau, H. E. (1980). The Peplau developmental model for nursing practice. In J. P. Riehl & C. Roy (Eds.), *Conceptual models for nursing practice* (2nd ed., pp. 53–73). New York: Appleton-Century-Crofts.

Porter, Y. (1990). Brief: Evaluation of nurses' documentation of patient teaching. *The Journal of Continuing Education in Nursing, 21*(3), 134–137.

Richardson, J. I. (1996). Legal issues for nurses. Minors and the ability to consent to HIV testing. *Texas Nursing, 70*(4), 12–13.

Roe v. Wade, 410 US 113, (1973).

Tarasoff v. Regents of the University of California, 17 Cal. 3d 425, 444 (1976).

Washington RN Nursing Regulations. (1998). *Standards of practice: Violations of standards of nursing conduct or practice.* Olympia, WA: Board of Nursing.

White, C. L. (1992). Symptom assessment and management of outpatients receiving biotherapy: The application of a symptom report form. *Seminars in Oncology Nursing, 8*(5), 23–28.

Whitman, N. I., Graham, B. A., Gleit, C. J., & Boyd, M. D. (1992). *Teaching in nursing practice. A professional model* (2nd ed.). Norwalk, CT: Appleton & Lange.

SUGGESTED READINGS

Aiken, T. D., & Catalano, J. T. (1994). *Legal, ethical, and political issues in nursing.* Philadelphia: F.A. Davis.

Catalano, J. T. (1996). *Contemporary professional nursing.* Philadelphia: F.A. Davis.

Lacombe, D. C. (1990). Avoiding a malpractice nightmare. *Nursing 90, 19,* 42–43.

Powers, J. L. (1993). Accepting and refusing assignments. *Nursing Management, 24*(9), 64–68.

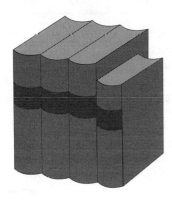

Chapter 11

PATIENT RIGHTS

Roselyn Holloway

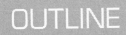

OUTLINE

Advance Directive
Empower
Ethic of Care
Informed Consent
Living Will

Medical Durable Power
    of Attorney
Patient Rights
Patient Self–Determination
    Act of 1990

OBJECTIVES

Upon completion of this chapter, the reader will be able to:
- Identify trends in patient rights.
- Describe the nurse's responsibilities in advance directives, living wills, and informed consent.
- Discuss how a living will can be used.
- Discuss patient rights from the consumer standpoint.
- List the elements of informed consent.

INTRODUCTION

To say that we as a profession are indebted to Florence Nightingale for her vision of nursing and **patient rights** is an understatement. History tells us that the notion of the rights of patients so needed in Nightingale's time remains the beacon of today's times also. Society has not always been concerned with the individual rights of ill persons. Throughout history, patients have been deprived of personal rights, freedom of choice, and dignity. Nursing students are encouraged to appreciate the focus for the humane care and legal protection of the vulnerable, very old, and very young of our society.

The basic rights of every human being for independence of thought, decision-making, action, and concern for personal dignity and human relationships are of great importance. During illness, however, the presence or absence of human rights becomes a necessary deciding factor in survival, recovery, and restoration. A prime responsibility for hospitals is to strive to ensure that these rights are preserved for patients.

Until recently, consumers felt helpless in the patient role. Stripped of individuality as well as belongings, they are placed in an environment where they have no control and are surrounded by unknown persons asking very private questions. Their dignity is lost. The consumer hesitates to complain or ask questions, thinking their nurse either will be too busy to answer or will criticize the patient. Most rights about which patients are concerned are those President Kennedy presented to Congress in 1962:

- The right to safety
- The right to be informed
- The right to choose
- The right to be heard

From these beginning rights, patient care has moved forward to **empower** the patient to make decisions concerning care. Now, an increasing number of consumers are not willing to accept the traditional role of the passive patient—the one who does as he or she is told and asks no questions. The frequent denial of fundamental rights of courtesy, privacy, and, most of all, information has brought about the ultimate form of patient rebellion—malpractice suits.

THE NURSE-PATIENT RELATIONSHIP

The nurse-patient relationship is the building block for all professional nursing. The nurse's obligation to the patient has assumed increasing importance through the years. This relationship has always been a part of the professional code for nurses. An examination of the historical perspective of patient rights brings to light the notion that the traditional nursing process, based on a linear problem-solving model, is inadequate for nursing practice in the twenty-first century. The belief is that the ambiguity of today's nursing practice demands more complex thinking skills than the nursing process accommodates. Changes in the discipline of nursing and the health care system require nurses with expert outcome-oriented clinical reasoning skills. The current health care system demands accountability in minimizing client costs and maximizing care outcomes.

The first official code for nurses, published in 1950, emphasized the nurse's primary obligation to the physician. In later versions, the emphasis shifted the loyalty to the employing institution. Until the 1960s, the primary source of patients' rights was the legislative controls of nursing practice (Carroll & Humphrey, 1979). In fact, many times patients were denied basic human rights. In 1985, the American Nurses Association (ANA) revised and published *A Code for Nurses* with Interpretive Statements (ANA, 1985). The National League for Nursing (NLN), the American Hospital Association (AHA), and many states have passed a Bill of Rights for Patients. The latest Code for Nurses (ANA, 1985) and the Bill of Rights for Patients (ANA, 1992) provide an avenue to steer both the nurse and the patient to a path of ethical sensitivity through general principles that result in the formation of conscious and critical judgment, for empowering the patients' lives.

EFFECT OF THE CONSUMER MOVEMENT ON THE NURSE-PATIENT RELATIONSHIP

There has been a movement by consumers to make the health care system more accountable for its actions. The American public, fueled by the principles of consumerism, criticized the dehumanization of health care. This criticism led to the development in 1972 of the AHA's document A Patient's Bill of Rights, which guaranteed certain rights and privileges to every hospitalized patient. It was revised by the AHA in 1992.

Even though the public believed this document to be the first formal one of its kind, actually, in 1952, the NLN produced a statement about patients' rights. Until the publication of the AHA's Bill, the prevailing attitude in health care was that providers knew best (Marquis & Hutson, 1996). The nurse must play a leadership role in helping to inform consumers about their rights. This paradigm shift of the consumer to a proactive role means the development of personal accountability for one's health and medical choices.

In the 1976 edition of the Code for Nurses, all 11 principles of the code emphasized the primacy of duties to patients (Carroll & Humphrey, 1979). In general, the nurse's obligation to patients as outlined in the code involves putting the patient's interests before one's own. Today, patients are more assertive and involved in their health care. They demand more information when deciding on treatment options and have more participation in decisions concerning their own care. The right to information and to participate in decisions regarding medical care has led to conflicts in the areas of **informed consent** and access to medical records. It is the nurse manager's responsibility to ensure that all patient rights are met. Particularly sensitive areas of human rights involve the right to privacy and personal liberty, both guaranteed by the U.S. Constitution.

At this juncture a new language emerged: the language of the patient as consumer. The image of the healthy, immunized, bran-eating purchaser of health care replaced that of the needy ill person as the object of the health care consumer. Until the "consumer" is struck by illness or an accident, no conflicts occur. Then, as a vulnerable person—a patient and not a consumer—his or her needs must be fully and truthfully met by the system that he or she has in essence supported, or a violation of an essential promise of health care will have been made. It is a promise made not only by the physician but by every nurse who works in the system, whose wages are paid in advance, by the patient in "trust" for a future time when he or she will need health care.

PATIENT CARE QUALITY AND SAFETY

True nursing goes beyond a skillful performance of isolated tasks under a physician's orders. Often, nurses in the past have not successfully identified done a good job of identifying patients' rights. It is an intuitive, deep perception of the entire patient with an anticipation and meeting of all his or her needs. Anyone can physically count a pulse or make a bed or see to the patient's comfort. An expert nurse assesses the needs of the patient and makes sure that the patient's autonomy remains intact. By providing a means by which the patient knows that the nurse will advocate for the patient's rights, the patient is assured that his or her rights will be protected, and health care and restoration becomes a trend and not an exception.

The work of nurses in health care today is much different than that of nursing only a few years ago. Our health care system is undergoing a dramatic restructuring that amounts to nothing short of a major revolution. People in health care have much different expectations and values than they had in years past. Diversity has brought many changes to the workplace and affects the rights of patients. Changes occur in the workplace when cultural differences arise and when the role of the nurse demands understanding of these various cultures. The nurse becomes cognizant of the needs of various cultures and the rights of these individual patients. When the nurse is knowledgeable regarding diverse cultures, he or she can enter a nurse-patient relationship

that is full of available options presented in a clear and consistent fashion. Furthermore, the patient becomes aware of his or her ability to participate freely and is able to proclaim his or her values. As the patient realizes that his or her rights are acknowledged, safety and quality of health care are provided with reassurance by a nurse steeped in culturally congruent care (M. Leininger, personal communication, 1998).

A PATIENT'S BILL OF RIGHTS

In 1992, The American Hospital Association revised the document A Patient's Bill of Rights, which guarantees certain rights and privileges to every patient.

The time is ripe for transformation to a health care system that will bring consumers into the mainstream as equals in the delivery of health care and leaders in the promotion of their own care. Nurses must couple health promotion efforts and traditional public health messages with a campaign to empower consumers within the delivery system. Nurses must also expose the mythology of enforced passivity that many Americans believe is endemic to receipt of health services. Nurses can be proud that nursing is pushing forward to promote such changes in the delivery of health care.

SUSPENSION OF RIGHTS

In providing health care, hospitals have the right to expect behavior on the part of patients, relatives, and friends that, considering the nature of their illness, is reasonable and responsible (JCAHO, 1987). Occasionally, it is necessary to suspend rights for the protection of patients or of others. Suspension of a patient's rights requires the nurse to clearly document that allowing the patient to continue to exercise the specific right could result in harm to the patient or to others. For example, a suicidal patient's right to access personal belongings may be suspended because he might attempt to harm himself with those personal objects. The nurse must

BILL OF RIGHTS*

1. The patient has the right to considerate and respectful care.
2. The patient has the right to and is encouraged to obtain from physicians and other direct caregivers relevant, current, and understandable information concerning diagnosis, treatment, and prognosis. Patients have the right to know the identity of physicians, nurses, and others involved in their care.
3. The patient has the right to make decisions about the plan of care prior to and during the course of treatment and refuse a recommended treatment or plan of care to the extent permitted by law and hospital policy and to be informed of the medical consequences of this action. In case of such refusal, the patient is entitled to other appropriate care and services that the hospital provided or transferred to another hospital. The hospital should notify patients of any policy that might affect patient choice within the institution.
4. The patient has the right to have an advance directive (such as a living will, health care proxy or durable power of attorney for health care) concerning treatment or designating a surrogate decision maker with the expectation that the hospital will honor the intent of that directive to the extent permitted by law and hospital policy. Health care institutions must advise patients of their rights under state law and hospital policy to make informed medical choices, ask if the patient has an advance directive. and include that information in patient records. The patient has the right to timely information about hospital policy that may limit its ability to implement fully a legally valid advance directive.
5. The patient has the right to every consideration of privacy. Case discussion, consultation, examination, and treatment should be conducted so as to protect each patient's privacy.
6. The patient has the right to expect that all communications and records pertaining to his/her care will be treated as confidential by the hospital, except in cases such as suspected abuse and public health hazards when reporting is permitted or required by law. The patient has the right to expect that the hospital will emphasize the confidentiality of this information when it releases it to any other parties entitled to review information in these records.
7. The patient has the right to review the records pertaining to his/her medical care and to have the information explained or interpreted as necessary, except when restricted by law.
8. The patient has the right to expect that, within its capacity and policies, a hospital will make reasonable response to the request of a patient for appropriate and medically indicated care and services. The hospital must provide evaluation, service, and/or referral as indicated by the urgency of the case. When medically appropriate and legally permissible, or when a patient has so requested, a patient may be transferred to another facility. The institution to which the patient is to be transferred must first have accepted the patient for transfer. The patient must also have the benefit of complete information and explanation concerning the need for, risks, benefits, and alternatives to such a transfer.

(Continued)

BILL OF RIGHTS* *(Continued)*

9. A patient has the right to ask and be informed of the existence of business relationships among the hospital, educational institutions, other health care providers, or payers that may influence the patient's treatment and care.

10. The patient has the right to consent to or decline to participate in proposed research studies or human experimentation affecting care and treatment or requiring direct patient involvement, and to have those studies fully explained prior to consent. A patient who declines to participate in research or experimentation is entitled to the most effective care that the hospital can otherwise provide.

11. The patient has the right to expect reasonable continuity of care when appropriate and be informed by physicians and other caregivers of available and realistic patient care options when hospital care is no longer appropriate.

12. The patient has the right to be informed of hospital policies and practices that relate to patient care, treatment, and responsibilities. The patient has the right to be informed of available resources for resolving disputes, grievances, and conflicts, such as ethics committees, patient representatives, or other mechanisms available in the institution. The patient has the right to be informed of the hospital's charges for services and available payment methods.

A Patient's Bill of Rights was first adopted by the American Hospital Association in 1973. This revision was approved by the AHA Board of Trustees on October 21, 1992.

*These rights can be exercised on the patient's behalf by a designated surrogate or proxy decision maker if the patient lacks decision-making capacity, is legally incompetent, or is a minor.

Source: Copyright 1992 by the American Hospital Association, 840 North Lake Shore Drive, Chicago, IL 60611. All rights reserved. Catalogue No. 157759.

document the concern and suspension of the patient's right in the nurses' notes.

PATIENT RIGHTS LEGISLATION

A Bill of Rights that becomes law or state regulation has the most legal authority because it provides the patient with legal recourse. A Bill of Rights issued by health care organizations and professional associations is not legally binding, but may influence funding and certainly should be considered professionally binding (Marquis & Hutson, 1996).

The legal obligation of the registered nurse is to respect the patient's right to exercise personal autonomy by allowing him or her to take part in decision-making, respecting the privacy and dignity of patients, maintaining professional competence, and engaging in activities that establish and maintain quality patient care. The Code for Nurses serves as a public statement of nursing's commitment to individual patients and to the community at large (ANA, 1985).

Many rulings have influenced the current legal view of patient rights. Those presented here, although not an exhaustive list of major court decisions, reflect decisions that have shaped the health system in our country today and are part of an ongoing process to accomplish the following legislative objectives:

• To guarantee and protect public safety
• To safeguard individual rights through judicial review
• To provide prompt evaluation and treatment

- To provide individualized treatment supervision and services throughout a conservatorship or guardianship program for gravely disabled persons
- To encourage the full use of existing agencies, professional personnel, and public funds to accomplish these objectives and to prevent duplication of services and unnecessary expenditures

A Patient Bill of Rights is a rights list that patients should be guaranteed even if being treated involuntarily. The specific rights vary somewhat from state to state, but are derived from a bill of rights established in 1980 by the federal Health Systems Act. This congressional action recommended to state governing bodies a set of basic patient rights that most states either fully or partially support. JACHO (1987) mandates that a list of patient rights be prominently displayed for all to see and should be given to each patient on admission to the facility.

LANDMARK RULINGS AFFECTING PATIENT RIGHTS

The following landmark rulings have had a significant influence on our health system and the actualization of patients' rights:

- *Rouse v. Cameron* (1966) was the case in which a man, who pled not guilty by reason of insanity to the charge of illegally carrying a dangerous weapon, was committed to a mental hospital. After a few years in the hospital, the man argued he was not receiving treatment (and therefore could not improve enough to be discharged). The court ruled that he had the *right to receive treatment.*
- *Griswold v. Connecticut* (1965) was a case in which the U.S. Supreme Court first recognized a right of personal privacy exists under the Constitution of the United States. The case addressed the issue of the state of Connecticut's right to prohibit the giving of birth control information to married couples. A majority of the Court held the Ninth Amendment supports the creation of peripheral rights not expressly mentioned in the Bill of Rights, including the *right of privacy.*

These two cited federal rulings have had the greatest effect on the legal rights of patients (Kelter, Schwecke, & Bostrom, 1995).

THE PATIENTS' BILL OF RIGHTS ACT OF 1998

The Patients' Bill of Rights Act was introduced in the House and Senate in April 1998. If enacted, this Act would offer a variety of rights and protections to consumers, including provisions for the choice of health plans for consumers, access to specialty care, antidiscrimination protection, access to emergency services, and the right to appeal decisions. Although 44 states have already passed laws providing for at least one of these patient protections recommended by the President's Advisory Commission on Consumer Protection and Actuality, these laws do not cover more than 122 million Americans with health plans under the Employee Retirement Income Security Act of 1974 (ERISA). A federal law is the only approach to the provision of basic consumer protections for these persons covered under ERISA (ANA, 1998). Unfortunately, the Bill was not passed before the session ended, despite the intense pressure from constituents to provide some sort of legislation limiting the power of managed care organizations.

PATIENT SELF-DETERMINATION ACT

The **Patient Self-Determination Act of 1990 (PSDA)** is a federal law that mandates that hospitals and other health care facilities inform a patient of the right to have a living will and durable powers of attorney for health care. The PSCA (1990) also provides the impetus for nursing involvement with the patient's right to a living will and durable power of attorney. Although it is useful for incoming patients to be informed of these rights, the time of admission is generally not the most fruitful time for development of this document. It is important to raise awareness of the importance of these documents to patients, families, and society and assess the effect of the attitudinal change facilitated in the patient. Every human being has as a benchmark individual freedom to make choices such as where to live, what one does with one's property, and in terms of health care, what one will allow to be done with one's body. The Bill of Rights of the U.S. Constitution ensures Americans the freedom to speak their mind, the freedom to associate with persons and groups as desired, the right to practice their own religion, and the right to privacy.

The concept of informed consent has become widely accepted in health care and legal groups as the standard for entering into a patient–health care provider contract for services. The importance of raising the subject in advance provides the patient a way to articulate his or her wishes to the health care agency. This gives the nurse a method in which to empower the patient, by providing information about services to be given so that the patient is able to make a more meaningful choice from the available options.

A corollary of the right to consent to treatment is the right to refuse treatment. An **advance directive** in the health care context usually outlines what the patient does not want done and, in effect, refuses to have done. Nurses are influencing patients and their significant others in the use of advance directives and are encouraging patients to use this form of empowerment.

LIVING WILL

The **living will** is a document that states under what circumstances, such as terminal illness, an individual prefers to have certain choices exercised on his or her behalf. In 1976, California became the first state to enact legislation that allowed advanced decision-making for end-of-life situations (Fade, 1995). The typical direction of the living will is that life-sustaining treatment, such as food, fluid, and cardiopulmonary respiration are to be withheld so that the person may die a dignified, peaceful death. Without this directive, a health care professional may feel obliged to maintain life for fear of a lawsuit alleging wrongful death. The living will puts the patient in charge by

promoting the patient's wishes rather than the wishes of a person who is likely to benefit directly from the estate of the patient. Laws differ somewhat from state to state, but in general, a patient's expressed wishes will be honored. In 1990, the U.S. Supreme Court held, in the case of Nancy Cruzan, that the state of Missouri could require "clear and convincing" evidence of a patient's wishes in order to remove life supports (AHA, 1998; Annas, 1990). Requirements for execution of a living will vary from state to state. But generally, a living will should be signed, dated, and witnessed by two people, preferably individuals who (1) know the patient's desires (2) are not related to him or her and (3) are not potential heirs or health care providers.

MEDICAL DURABLE POWER OF ATTORNEY

The **medical durable power of attorney** for health care enables an individual to name another person to be a substitute decision-maker under the circumstances of impaired functioning on the part of the person executing the document. If the person is impaired to the point of being unable to make decisions, then the substitute decision-maker can do so. Most states have enacted laws that provide for a living will and durable power of attorney for health care (Cate & Gill, 1991). All states except Massachusetts, Michigan, and New York have laws governing living wills, and all states but Alaska and Alabama have statutes that allow appointment of a durable power of attorney for health care (Fade, 1995).

The usefulness of these advance directives in assisting clinical decision-making is not yet clear. One team of researchers concluded that advance directives were irrelevant to decision-making regarding resuscitation of seriously ill patients.

THE NURSE'S ROLE TODAY

The nurse can evaluate the patient when the use of advance directives is considered. As part of the assessment of the patient's goals in relation to health care status, the nurse can discuss provisions of the patient's living will or durable power of attorney for health care with the multidisciplinary treatment team (MDTT). Because members of the MDTT need to implement provisions of the living will, they must appreciate the meaning of the document to the patient as well as legal requirements for the document to be valid. In a much publicized 1992 case in Texas, the patient and his family were distraught when the patient's living will was not followed by the health care facility. Texas state law requires that two physicians certify the patient terminally ill and only one physician had done so (Gamino, 1992). Working closely with the attorney to make the legal requirements clear to staff and administrators is essential. For example, the patient may mention something about organ donation to the nurse. If the patient has no advance directive, discussion of personal values may assist the patient in making a choice to execute a living will. Knowing the patient's understanding and beliefs about artificial extension of life, the nurse can plan and implement care that is respectful of the patient.

Advance directives also act as preventive measures. Just as primary prevention in health care means the practice of health-promotion and disease-prevention behaviors, risk management means preventing litigious difficulties. Advance directives prevent legal problems when the prognosis of the patient may be at issue. Economically, respecting the patient's health care choices may reduce escalating health care costs by ruling out a number of expensive procedures. The encouragement of advance directives may also provide an opportunity for nurses to extend a relational **ethic of care**. Parker (1990) describes this ethic as a process of sharing relational stories of caregiving. The process focuses on reciprocity and interconnectedness among human beings. To converse with patients about their beliefs of the meaning of life and death assists them in making decisions about advance directives. Self-disclosure by the nurse enriches the process and contributes to mutual concern and understanding.

An important basis on which the realization of the care ethic and the legal goal of self-determination are founded is the relationship between the nurse and patient. The nurse comes to realize that there is no single right or wrong answer for how life should be lived. Health care providers, as well as, patients have vulnerabilities, conflicting motivations, interests, and expectations. Like interest cannot be presumed. Human behavior contains both rational and irrational elements that must be accepted in health care providers and patients. Naomi Judd, a noted country singer, in her speech to the ANA delegate assembly of 1998, related her history of contracting hepatitis C while working as a nurse. A nurse who took care of Ms. Judd recognized the variety of answers to the coping mechanisms she embraced while facing her problems and how mutual understanding was effective as the healing process became a realization. Today Ms. Judd, who is empowered by her "complementary therapies," using both medical as well as alternative treatments, is in remission (N. Judd, 1998).

SUMMARY

Nurses play a key role in the planning and implementation of advance directives and the Patient's Bill of Rights. Nursing values of mutuality, open belief systems, caring, and health promotion and prevention support the use of advance directives in health care. In this new era of managed care, nurses will be further involved with the advocacy of the needs of patients. Ultimately, responsibility in the system of today's caregiving rests where it has always rested—in the heart and hands of the nurse planning and giving the care.

Patient rights are the hallmark for advocacy of nursing care. Nurses are compelled to strive for excellent care of patients and the inclusion of their rights in today's health care system.

POINTS TO REMEMBER

• The nurse-patient relationship is the building block for all professional nurses.

NURSING QUOTE

The following is an anonymous saying from nursing history:

We help our patients speak.
We help them look deep within
For truth, conflict and decision.
Then we accept their paths
As we accept our own.

- A medical durable power of attorney for health care enables the person to name a substitute decision-maker under the circumstances of impaired functioning on the part of the person executing the document.
- A living will is a document that states that under what (medical) circumstances, such as terminal illness, an individual prefers to have certain choices exercised on his or her behalf.
- The Patient's Bill of Rights guarantees certain rights and privileges to every patient in a hospital.

REFERENCES

American Hospital Association. (1998). *A patient's bill of rights.* Chicago: Author.

American Nurses Association. (1985). *A code for nurses.* Kansas City, MO: Author.

American Nurses Association. (1998). *Capitol update: Clinton and Gore rally in support of consumer rights and protection.* Washington, DC: Author.

Annas, G. (1990, September 6). Nancy Cruzan and the right to die. *New England Journal of Medicine, 323,* 670-672.

Carroll, M., & Humphrey, R. (1979). *The nurses professional code of ethics: Its history and improvements in moral problems in nursing: Case studies.* New York: University Press of America.

Cate, F., & Gill, B. (1991). *The Patient Self-Determination Act: Implementation issues and opportunities.* Washington, D C: Annenberg Washington Program of Northwestern University.

ERISA (1974). Employee Retirement Income Security Act (ERISA) 1994.

Fade, A. (1995, March). Advance directives: An overview of changing right-to-die laws. *Journal of Nursing Law, 2,* 27-38.

Gamino, D. (1992). A living will fails to ensure dignified death. *Austin American Statesman,* pp. A-1, A-12.

Griswold v. Connecticut 382 U.S. 479 (1965).

Joint Commission American Hospital Organizations. (1987). Washington, DC: Author.

Judd, N (1998). Personal Communication American Nurse Association Convention. San Diego, CA.

Kelter, N., Schwecke, L., & Bostrom, C. (1995). *Psychiatric Nursing* (2nd ed.). St. Louis: Mosby.

Leininger, M (1998). Personal Communication, Transcultural Nursing Society Annual Meeting. Sacacus, NJ.

Marquis, B., & Hutson, C. (1996). *Leadership roles and management functions in nursing: Theory and application* (2nd ed.). Philadelphia: Lippincott-Raven.

Mental Health Systems Act 1980, PUBL. 96-398, 94 STAT. 1564 (Oct 7, 1980).

Parker, R. (1990, January). Nurse's stories: The search for rational ethic of care. *Advances in Nurses Science, 13,* 31–40.

Patient Self-Determination Act of 1990, 42 USCA. & 1395 cc (f) (l) (A) (I) (1991 Supp. Pam.).

Patients' Bill of Rights Act of 1998 (HR 3605 and S. 1890).

Rouse v. Cameron, 373 F2d 451 (D.C. Cir. 1966).

SUGGESTED READINGS

Benjamin, M., & Curtis, J. (1992). *Ethics in nursing* (2nd ed.). New York: Oxford University Press.

Hastings Center. (1998). *Advance directives.* New York: Author.

Quinn, C., & Smith, M. (1987). *The professional commitment: Issues and ethics in nursing.* Philadelphia: WB Saunders.

Sheehan, J. (1996, January). Advice of counsel: Putting advocacy for patients' rights against job security. *RN, 59,* 55–56.

Silverman, H., Fry, S., & Armistead, N. (1994, January). Nurses' perspectives on implementation of the Patient Self-Determination Act. *The Journal of Clinical Ethics, 5,* 30–37.

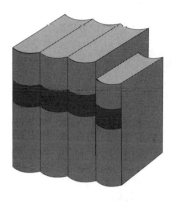

Chapter 12

INFORMED CONSENT

Taralynn R. Mackay

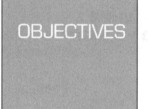

KEY WORDS

Assault	Patient Self-Determination Act (PSDA)
Battery	Prisoners
Competency	Prudent Patient Standard
Consent	Reasonable Person Standard
Emancipated Minor	Reasonable Physician Standard
Emergency	Right to Refuse Treatment
Expressed Consent	Therapeutic Privilege
Implied Consent	Treatment
Informed Consent	Waiver
Liability	
Mature Minor	
Mentally Incompetent	
Minor	
Negligence	
Omnibus Budget Reconciliation Act (OBRA)	

OBJECTIVES

Upon completion of this chapter, the reader will be able to:
- Identify the elements of informed consent.
- Discuss the variations and exceptions involved with informed consent.
- Discuss the nurse's role in informed consent and the consequences of inadequate informed consent.

HISTORICAL PERSPECTIVE

A long-standing legal standard holds that "every human being of adult years and sound mind has a right to determine what should be done with his own body" (*Scholendorf v. Society of New York Hospitals*, 1914). However, the concept of informed consent did not appear until the late 1950s and early 1960s (Faden, Beauchamp, & King, 1986). Prior to the twentieth century, physicians were instructed to reveal as little as possible to a patient, and there were even suggestions on how to distract the patient from knowledge of their health care procedures or **treatment**. However, a lawsuit in 1957 established the importance of providing sufficient information to a patient to allow the patient to make an informed decision about medical treatment and care. In *Salgo v. Leland Stanford, Junior University Board of Trustees* (1957), the physician failed to provide sufficient information about an aortography that a patient underwent. The patient's legs became permanently paralyzed. The court held that the physician had a duty to provide the facts necessary to the patient so that the patient could provide informed consent (*Salgo v. Leland Stanford, Junior University Board of Trustees*, 1957). Health care providers now accept the patient's right to know all relevant facts prior to consenting to a procedure or a treatment. Therefore, a health care provider's duty is to provide informed consent, but the provider cannot make the decision for the patient. Even if the patient's decision is detrimental to the patient, the decision remains the patient's.

Not all states require the same standards for informed consent. In Georgia, for example, "a physician does not have an affirmative duty to disclose risks, but if a patient inquires about risks or complications, the physician must respond" (Rozovsky, 1990). Therefore, informed consent is a complex issue for nurses because of the differences in the laws between states, the variations of what constitutes valid informed consent, the exceptions involving informed consent, and the liability involved with the nurse's role in informed consent.

ELEMENTS OF INFORMED CONSENT

CONSENT

Expressed consent is the explicit acknowledgment of a health care provider's request to provide treatment. **Implied consent** is a nonverbal acknowledgment of a health care provider's request to provide treatment. For example, a nurse has an order to give an injection. The nurse tells the patient, "I have a tetanus shot for you, which is a vaccination ordered by the doctor because you were cut with that piece of metal." If the patient states, "Okay, go ahead," the patient has given expressed consent. If the patient offers the nurse his arm, that is implied consent.

INFORMED CONSENT

Informed consent involves more than just an acknowledgment of a health care provider's request to provide treatment. Informed consent requires that the health care provider meet certain elements before the acknowledgment by the patient is considered informed consent. Generally, adequate **informed consent** contains the following information:

1. The patient's diagnosis or suspected diagnosis
2. The nature and purpose of the proposed treatment or procedure
3. The expected outcome
4. The expected benefits
5. Who will perform the proposed treatment or procedure
6. The complications, risks, or side effects of the treatment or procedure
7. Any reasonable alternatives
8. If applicable, possible prognoses, if the treatment or procedure is not performed (Brent, 1993)

Informed consent may be verbal or written. A written informed consent is preferable, but a completed, signed consent form does not necessarily prove that informed consent was provided. For example, a court found that the provider did not meet the imposed duty of obtaining consent just by having the patient sign the consent form (*Keomaka v. Zakaib*, 1991). As many nurses are aware, some patients will sign anything given to them regardless of whether they understand the document's contents or not. Thus, informed consent includes the process of informing the patient, not simply the process of completing a form.

Many states have a **reasonable person standard** or **prudent patient standard** when applying the law to informed consent. This means that the situation in question is analyzed depending on what a reasonable person or a prudent patient would have done if placed in the same situation. Or, additionally, what information should a reasonable person or a prudent patient have received to make an informed decision about the treatment being offered by the health care provider. Pennsylvania uses this standard by requiring the provider to inform the patient of the proposed treatment, the risks involved, and the alternatives and to do so in light of what a reasonable patient

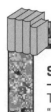

SUFFICIENCY OF CONSENT IN IDAHO

The State of Idaho addresses the sufficiency of consent as follows: "Any such consent shall be deemed valid and so informed if the physician or dentist to whom it is given or by whom it is secured has made such disclosures and given such advice respecting pertinent facts and considerations as would ordinarily be made and given under the same or similar circumstances, by a like physician or dentist of good standing practicing in the same community."

Source: Idaho Health and Safety Code, § 39-4304.

would consider material for the decision of whether to grant consent (Health Care Services Malpractice Act, 1996).

Some states use a **reasonable physician standard** when applying the law to informed consent, and this appears to be the standard used by courts. In this standard, the situation is analyzed depending on what a reasonable health care provider in the local community would disclose during informed consent under the same or similar circumstances. This standard was utilized in *Natanson v. Kline* (1960), a case involving a provider who failed to disclose the risks of cobalt radiation therapy to a patient. The court held that the duty imposed on the provider was to inform the patient of risks that a "reasonable medical practitioner would disclose under the same or similar circumstances" (*Natanson v. Kline*, 1960).

Because of the nature of health care today and the use of referrals for treatment, a question arises whether a referring provider is held responsible for informed consent. In a case in Hawaii, a patient sued a provider who advised a patient on a procedure and another provider who gave a second opinion about the proposed procedure. The patient alleged that both health care providers failed to disclose risks of the procedure and that the patient suffered from pain and disfigurement due to the procedure. The Hawaii court held that both providers were responsible for disclosing the risks of the surgery (*O'Neal v. Hammer*, 1998). However, the Supreme Court also pointed out that if a subsequent health

care provider fully discloses the risks to the patient prior to the institution of the procedure or treatment, the initial health care provider would not be held liable (*O'Neal v. Hammer*, 1998).

COMPETENCY

Competency is a necessary component of informed consent. A patient is competent to give informed consent if the patient is an adult or an emancipated minor or mature minor, conscious, and uncoerced. Each of these components will be addressed further.

If a patient is mentally incompetent as determined by a court, intoxicated, under the influence of drugs, in shock, or unconscious, the patient is not capable of consenting. If a health care provider believes a patient to be incompetent, the policies of the facility and the laws of the state will specify who can give consent for that patient and what steps need to be taken to ensure legal consent.

For example, a patient who has been declared **mentally incompetent** by a court will have a court-appointed guardian who has the legal authority to provide consent for treatment (Brent, 1993). The health care provider has a right to request that the guardian provide proof of the court-appointed guardianship of the patient. The health care provider should note that there are some types of procedures that may be injurious to a patient and, thus, are not allowed to be made by a legal guardian. An example of a potentially injurious procedure is sterilization of a mentally retarded or mentally incompetent individual. It is important to note that commitment to a mental facility does not automatically render a patient incompetent (Rozovsky, 1990).

SPECIAL AREAS OF CONCERN WHEN PROVIDING INFORMED CONSENT

MINORS

Generally, minors are not capable of providing valid consent for treatment. A **minor** is an individual whose age is below the age of majority, as determined in the specific state. In the past, all consent for medical treatment, testing, and procedures had to be obtained from the minor child's parents. Many states now are attempting to reconcile the right of the parents to determine their child's medical care to that of the minor child's right to obtain medical care. Included in this controversy is the question of who has the right to privileged medical records.

Some states allow minors to consent to certain types of medical treatment without requiring parental consent or the consent of a legal guardian. The medical treatment in these instances usually involves treatment for sexually transmitted diseases, medical care during a pregnancy, treatment for phys-

ical abuse, and treatment or counseling for substance abuse. The states that allow the consent of minors in these instances have also enacted legislation that addresses the issue of whether or not health care providers may disclose information about treatment of the minor to the parent or guardian.

Usually a parent's or legal guardian's consent is required for a minor's medical care and treatment; however, the minor's consent should also be obtained if the minor is able to provide consent. An exception to obtaining parental consent occurs when the medical situation is an emergency. The courts have supported the premise that if the parents or legal guardian had been aware of the emergency situation, then they would have given consent for the treatment in order to save the minor's health or life (Rozovsky, 1990).

Another exception to the requirement of parental consent involves a mature minor or an emancipated minor. A **mature minor** is an individual "judicially recognized as possessing sufficient understanding and appreciation of the nature and consequences of treatment despite their chronological age" and, thus, can give consent for treatment (Rozovsky, 1990). An **emancipated minor** is defined as a minor who is financially independent, who lives apart from his or her parents, who is married, or who is in the military service of the United States and is considered to have the same legal capacity as an adult. Some states recognize mature minors, other states recognize emancipated minors, and some states have established statutory ages of consent (Rozovsky, 1990).

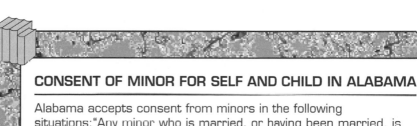

CONSENT OF MINOR FOR SELF AND CHILD IN ALABAMA

Alabama accepts consent from minors in the following situations:"Any minor who is married, or having been married, is divorced or has borne a child may give effective consent to any legally authorized medical, dental, health or mental health services for himself or his child or for herself or her child."

Source: Consent of Minor for Self and Child, 1971.

It is accepted that if a minor meets the mature minor or emancipated minor exception and is able to give consent for treatment, then the confidentiality of the treatment should be respected and not disclosed to parents or guardians (Rozovsky, 1990). However, there are some states that permit the health care provider to notify the parents or guardians in certain instances. Therefore, health care providers should be aware of the confidentiality provisions of their state's laws before releasing medical records to anyone other than the patient.

Another area of concern that arises when caring for minors involves other family members who are recognized as able to give consent for a minor. Because of the various family compositions (divorced parents, stepfamilies, single parents, guardians, and so forth), it is important that the health care provider ensure that the person giving consent is legally capable of providing the consent. Many states have legislation that establishes who is allowed to give consent and under what conditions. For example, after a divorce, both parents may not retain the legal authority to grant consent because the capability would depend on the terms of the divorce and custody agreement.

The laws involving minors and consent is constantly changing. Therefore, the health care provider should monitor the laws regarding minors in the health care provider's state. Likewise, because of the nature of the issues between minors and parents, health care providers should be certain that the law supports any decision made concerning a minor's informed consent.

CONSENT FOR A MINOR IN TEXAS

"(a) The following persons may consent to medical, dental, psychological, and surgical treatment of a child when the person having the right to consent as otherwise provided by law cannot be contacted and that person has not given actual notice to the contrary:

(1) a grandparent of the child;

(2) an adult brother or sister of the child;

(3) an adult aunt or uncle of the child;

(4) an educational institution in which the child is enrolled that has received written authorization to consent from a person having the right to consent;

(5) an adult who has actual care, control, and possession of the child and has written authorization to consent from a person having the right to consent;

(6) a court having jurisdiction over a suit affecting the parent-child relationship of which the child is the subject;

(7) an adult responsible for the actual care, control, and possession of a child under the jurisdiction of a juvenile court or committed by a juvenile court to the care of an agency of the state or county; or

(8) a peace officer who has lawfully taken custody of a minor, if the peace officer has reasonable grounds to believe the minor is in need of immediate medical treatment."

Source: Consent to Treatment of Child by Non-parent or Child, 1995.

HIV/AIDS TESTING

Acquired immunodeficiency syndrome (AIDS) is a disease that strikes all ages, sexes, races, professions, and ethnic backgrounds. There has been considerable legislation and court cases involving testing for human immunodeficiency virus (HIV) and AIDS. Generally, most states require consent prior to performing HIV/AIDS testing.

However, many states have exceptions that allow testing without consent. Some examples are autopsies, donated tissues and fluids, qualification for an occupation, and as protection for caregivers (Rozovsky, 1990). "The laws reflect a social attitude that the need to test far outweighs the individual's interest in refusing such intrusions: that in certain, well-delineated circumstances, society's need to know should prevail" (Rozovsky, 1990). Thus, if a health care provider is exposed to a patient's body fluids, the need to know whether the patient is HIV positive in order to treat the health care provider outweighs the patient's consent to HIV/AIDS testing. Some facilities inform patients of this waiver of consent in case of exposure to body fluids, prior to the provision of any treatment by the facility. Because of the differences between the states, a nurse should be aware of what procedures are required and allowed when obtaining or providing consent for testing in that nurse's state.

An area of concern for nurses is whether they have a duty to warn the spouse or significant other of a patient's positive HIV/AIDS test result. This is a constantly changing area of legislation and judicial action. Some states have addressed the issue of to whom a positive test result may be disclosed. However, the legislation and the supporting case law do not generally impose a duty to warn on the health care provider, instead the provider is permitted to disclose the information.

PRISONERS

There have been various discussions concerning whether **prisoners** can truly give informed consent because of the nature of their confinement. Some argue that prisoners, who are attempting to be model prisoners to increase their chances of parole, will agree to any treatment or procedure proposed to them (Rozovsky, 1998). However, a health care provider should not be held accountable for the motivation behind a patient's decision to provide consent or to withhold consent. Therefore, the requirements for informed consent in the prison population are the same as for the average nonincarcerated patient (Rozovsky, 1998). Issues regarding prisoners are discussed in more detail in Chapter 26, Correctional Nursing.

PATIENT'S RIGHT TO SELF–DETERMINATION

The **Patient Self-Determination Act (PSDA)** was passed in 1990 by the U.S. Congress, and it became effective in 1992 as part of the **Omnibus Budget Reconciliation Act (OBRA).** The Act requires any health care provider (hospital, long-term care center, or home care agency) to inform patients of their right to execute advance directives, to determine which lifesaving or life-prolonging actions they want to be carried out on their behalf. (Advance directives are discussed in more detail in Chapter 11, Patient Rights.)

NEGLIGENCE OR BATTERY

If the health care provider fails to disclose or to adequately disclose the risks and complications involved in the medical or surgical treatment that is being proposed to the patient, negligence could result. The theory of negligence in this situation is based on the premise that the patient deciding whether to give or not to give consent to a treatment (1) was influenced by the health care provider's failure to disclose or the failure to adequately disclose the risks and complications, and (2) may not have made the same decision if the patient had received information or disclosure.

In actual practice, a failure of informed consent is not usually the basis for a lawsuit, but it is often contained within a lawsuit alleging negligence of the health care provider. For example, a nurse administers an injection of pain medication to a patient without informing the patient of the medication side effects or getting the patient's expressed or implied consent to the injection. The patient is allergic to the pain medication, and if the patient had been informed of the side effects of the injection, the patient would have refused the injection. Therefore, the failure of the nurse to obtain consent from this patient prior to administering the injection would most likely be included in a lawsuit alleging that the nurse administered medication that was contra-indicated, rather than prompting a lawsuit on its own.

Assault is the attempt or threat to inflict injury on the person of another, and **battery** is the unlawful application of force to the person of another (*Black's Law Dictionary*, 1990). In other words, assault is an attempt or a threat to hurt someone by a person who has the capability to carry out the threat, and battery is the intentional touching of someone without the person's consent. Assault and battery can occur with inadequate informed consent (*Fox v. Smith*, 1992). To prove that medical assault or battery occurred, a patient would have to provide evidence that an examination or procedure took place for which the patient did not give expressed or implied consent (Rozovsky, 1990).

Battery can also occur if the treatment performed is beyond the scope of the informed consent given to the patient. In *Guin v. Sison* (1989), a claim arose when a physician performed a procedure that was beyond what was disclosed in the patient's informed consent.

In *Lounsbury v. Capel* (1992), a suit claiming battery, the patient alleged that he had refused to provide consent to back surgery, but that when he was under the influence of preoperative medication, consent for the surgery was obtained from his wife. The court held, "the mere temporary incapacity of the patient will not serve as justification for obtaining consent from the patient's spouse, if there was a reasonable opportunity to obtain the patient's own consent" (McCafferty & Meyer, 1985).

In *Winters v. Miller* (1971), a patient who was a Christian Scientist was given medica-

tion against her will. She was awarded damages in her lawsuit for assault and battery because it was determined by the court that she was not incompetent and consent was not obtained (*Winters v. Miller*, 1971). Likewise, an Ohio court case suggests that cardiopulmonary resuscitation (CPR) on a patient who had a No CPR/No Code Blue status may constitute battery (*Anderson v. Saint Francis–St. George Hospital*, 1992).

There are some states that still permit a claim based on medical assault and battery; however, many states do not. For example, in Texas, the ability to bring a claim based on medical assault and battery was removed by the legislature as part of tort reform (Rozovsky, 1990). Thus, in those states that do not allow claims based on medical assault and battery, a failure to provide informed consent or to provide adequate informed consent would give rise to a claim of negligence.

EXCEPTIONS TO INFORMED CONSENT

EMERGENCIES

Consent is not required in a life-threatening emergency. In order for a situation to be deemed an **emergency**, the following factors must be present: (1) the patient is unable to make an informed choice; (2) the situation does not allow time for another person, who is authorized, to give consent; and (3) the situation is life- or health-threatening (Rozovsky, 1990).

If the patient is incompetent to give consent and the situation is not an emergency, consent will have to be obtained by an individual who is given authority to grant consent by state law. If the state legislature has not enacted a law determining who can give consent on behalf of the patient, a court will have to appoint a guardian to provide consent (Rozovsky, 1990).

RIGHT TO REFUSE TREATMENT

If a patient has the right to determine the course of treatment and to consent to treat-

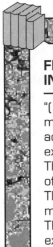

FLORIDA'S EMERGENCY EXAMINATION AND TREATMENT OF INCAPACITATED PERSONS

"(1) No recovery shall be allowed in any court in this state against any emergency medical technician, paramedic, or physician as defined in this chapter, or any person acting under the direct medical supervision of a physician, in an action brought for examining or treating a patient without his or her informed consent if:
The patient at the time of examination or treatment is intoxicated, under the influence of drugs, or otherwise incapable of providing informed consent . . .
The patient at the time of examination or treatment is experiencing an emergency medical condition; and
The patient would reasonably, under all the surrounding circumstances, undergo such examination, treatment, or procedure if he or she were advised by the emergency medical technician, paramedic, or physician."

Source: Emergency Examination and Treatment of Incapacitated Person, 1997.

ment, then it follows that the patient also has the **right to refuse treatment**. For example, if a patient had advance directives or had predetermined a refusal of medical care, then consent is not implied. Likewise, if a patient had identification or documents indicating that the patient did not want cardiac or respiratory resuscitation, then consent for CPR is not implied, and the patient's refusal of consent should be respected. Moreover, if a patient is competent and refuses medical care, even if the situation is health- or life-threatening, the patient's choice supersedes the opinion of the health care provider, and if medical treatment occurs even though the patient refused treatment, a battery will result (*Anderson v. Saint Francis–Saint George Hospital*, 1992).

Another example of patients' right to refuse treatment is seen in conjunction with religious beliefs. Members of certain religious groups, such as Jehovah's Witnesses and Christian Scientists, are opposed to some types of medical or surgical treatments. The problem arises when the health care provider believes that treatment is necessary, but the patient refuses to consent to the treatment because of religious beliefs. Courts are then petitioned to order treatment for the patient based on the precedent set in an 1879 U.S. Supreme Court case in which

the Court stated, "When the state can demonstrate a compelling interest in the preservation or promotion of health, life, safety, or welfare, religious practices may be curtailed." (Rozovsky, 1990).

Another area where refusal of treatment can occur involves patients with terminal illnesses. Court cases have upheld the terminal patient's right to refuse care and treatment and, in addition, the patient's right to withdraw life-sustaining treatment (Rozovsky, 1990). However, the law is not clear regarding cases involving incompetent, terminal patients. In the absence of advance directives, health care providers who find themselves faced with the withdrawal of life-sustaining treatment from an incompetent, terminal patient should seek legal advice.

Some health care providers choose to avoid the constraints and difficulties placed on care and treatment by the patient's refusal to consent by declaring the situation an emergency or by waiting until the situation becomes an emergency. The health care provider then improperly proceeds under the emergency waiver for informed consent. It is important to know that a "refusal of care, if properly made, survives the patient's lapsing into a state in which she is incapable of giving or declining consent to care"

PATIENTS' RIGHTS

A selection of the American Hospital Association's Patient's Bill of Rights:
"2. The patient has the right to obtain from his doctor complete current information about his diagnosis, treatment, and prognosis in terms the patient can be reasonably expected to understand. When it is not medically advisable to give such information to the patient, it should be made available to an appropriate person in his behalf. . .
The patient has the right to receive from his doctor information necessary to give informed consent prior to the start of any procedure or treatment. Except in emergencies, such information for informed consent should include but not necessarily be limited to the specific procedure or treatment, the medically significant risks involved, and the probable duration of incapacitation.
Where medically significant alternatives for care or treatment exist, or when the patient requests information concerning medical alternatives, the patient has the right to such information. . .
The patient has the right to refuse treatment to the extent permitted by law and to be informed of the medical consequences of his action." (American Hospital Association, 1973)

A selection from the National League of Nursing, Patient Bill of Rights:

"Patients have the right to information about their diagnosis, prognosis, and treatment—including alternatives to care and risks involved—in terms they and their families can readily understand, so that they can give their informed consent.
Patients have the legal right to informed participation in all decisions concerning their health care. . .
Patients have the right to refuse treatments, medications, or participation in research and experimentation, without punitive action being taken against them."
(National League of Nursing, Patient Bill of Rights)

(Rozovsky, 1990). An ethical concern also arises if a health care provider uses the emergency waiver to circumvent informed consent.

Therefore, the prudent health care provider should never impose the health care provider's own opinion, beliefs, or will on a patient. Likewise, the health care provider must keep current on the law regarding the refusal of treatment.

WAIVER OF INFORMED CONSENT

A competent adult patient can waive informed consent, and the patient's decision must be followed by the health care provider (Brent, 1993). **Waiver** of informed consent occurs when a patient tells the health care

provider that the patient does not want to hear the information that is the basis of informed consent. Although a health care provider may proceed with the treatment, the health care provider may wish to attempt to proceed with informed consent on the pretext that "I am required by law to tell you these things." However, if the health care provider decides to honor the waiver of informed consent, the health care provider should carefully document the patient's request for no information.

THERAPEUTIC PRIVILEGE

Therapeutic privilege occurs when a health care provider decides, in his or her opinion and based on medical judgment, that it would be harmful to a patient to provide complete disclosure regarding the proposed treatment or procedure. Early court cases held there was a therapeutic privilege to withhold information if in the physician's medical judgment "a frank discussion would actually complicate or interfere with treatment because of the patient's physical or emotional state, or where the patient is likely to become so ill or emotionally distraught on disclosure that rational choice on his part would be foreclosed" (Palmisano & Mang, 1987).

Most courts today do not accept therapeutic privilege as an exception to providing consent. A patient's medical condition is

TEXAS STATE BOARD OF MEDICAL EXAMINERS ETHICAL ISSUES STATEMENT ON INFORMED CONSENT: ENSURING PATIENT AUTONOMY

Understanding and implementing informed consent and avoiding paternalism first requires the physician to understand and respect the concepts of patient autonomy, freedom, and mental competence. The Board believes that it is a physician's duty to determine to the best of the physician's ability, under any given set of circumstances, if a patient is mentally competent and able to deliberate rationally. In other words, it is the physician's duty to ensure that decisions made by the patient are made with basis in fact (i.e., that factual errors which influence decisions are not present and that valuative errors are not present so that no inappropriate values are given to certain facts). It is the physician's duty to present the patient with all of the facts necessary for the patient to deliberate rationally.

The physician must also determine if the patient is truly autonomous so as to be able to act freely without internal or external constraints (i.e., mental illness, under the influence of drugs or physical coercion). If a physician determines that a patient is mentally competent and deliberating rationally, is truly autonomous and acting freely and, in addition, is not harming others, then on an ethical basis the physician has no choice but to honor the patient's decisions for his own life plan even if that decision appears to be to the patient's detriment or even death. If these criteria are not met, then it is a physician's duty to provide the patient's family, legal guardians or the courts with all of the pertinent information required for them to make a rational and informed decision regarding the patient's medical care. Under either of the two scenarios described above, the physician will have met his obligation of informed consent and avoided the pitfalls of paternalism.

Because of the nature of the doctor-patient relationship and the patient's position of dependence upon the physician, the physician frequently assumes the role of a benevolent authority or "pater." It is in this position of "father" that the doctor-patient relationship can be abused in so far as the physician could disregard a patient's own will either by omission of informed consent or through other undue influence. Informed consent and avoidance of paternalism are principles that the Texas State Board of Medical Examiners believes in, adheres to, and will uphold in deliberating related complaints against physicians (Texas State Board of Medical Examiners, 1994).

Sources: Childress, J. (1989). Autonomy. In R. M. Veatch (Ed.), *Cross cultural perspectives in medical ethics & readings* (pp. 233–240). Boston: Jones and Bartlett.

Dworkin, G. (1972). Paternalism. *The Monist, 56*, 1. Reprinted in: J. Arras & R. Hunt (Eds.) (1983), *Ethical issues in modern medicine* (2nd ed., pp 74–84). Palo Alto, CA: Mayfield Publishing Co.

usually not a valid excuse for failing to give or deciding not to give the patient complete information regarding the proposed treatment or procedure. Many states do not allow the therapeutic privilege waiver because there is a potential for abuse in that the health care provider may impose his or her own will and neglect the patient's freedom to determine his or her own course of medical care. Some state medical boards have even adopted statements against such paternalism. Therefore, the health care provider must be aware that, although the therapeutic privilege exception may have been a justified exception to informed consent in the past, today's courts have questioned the use of the practice and the chance of finding that the health care provider failed to provide informed consent has increased.

NURSE'S VERSUS PHYSICIAN'S RESPONSIBILITIES

In most states it is the duty of the physician to obtain informed consent. Some states recognize that advance practice nurses provide medical treatment and procedures, and those states have revised their informed consent laws to reflect the *health care provider*, rather than the *physician*, performing the treatment or procedure has the nondelegatable duty of obtaining informed consent. The reasoning behind holding the health care provider performing the treatment or procedure responsible for obtaining informed consent is that usually only the health care provider has complete background information about the patient and the medical knowledge to provide the information necessary to fulfill the elements of adequate informed consent specific for that patient. Thus, nurses, with the exception of advanced practice nurses, are generally not required to obtain informed consent, because nurses do not routinely perform treatments or procedures requiring documented informed consent.

However, nurses frequently are requested to witness the provision of informed consent and to obtain the patient's signature on informed consent forms. Remember that informed consent is the provision of information to the patient and not the administrative function of signing a form. Thus, the action by the nurse of obtaining the patient's signature or witnessing the signing of the document does not then transfer the legal liability for obtaining and providing informed consent to the nurse.

Although the nurse is not usually held legally accountable for ensuring informed consent, the nurse has an ethical obligation to the patient to ensure that the patient exercises his or her patient rights regarding the right to determine what is being done to the patient's body (Health Care Services Malpractice Act, 1996). Therefore, if a nurse believes that informed consent has not occurred, the nurse should notify the health care provider responsible for providing the informed consent of the patient's apparent lack of knowledge. However, if a competent patient waives consent and is aware of his or her right to informed consent, then the nurse is under no ethical or legal requirement to ensure that the patient is well informed.

ISSUES AND TRENDS

Advanced practice nurses are increasingly involved with obtaining informed consent in response to their expanding scope of practice, which includes the performance of procedures and treatment. Therefore, advanced practice nurses should be informed about the components of informed consent, and they should diligently follow their state's laws regarding informed consent because they would be held liable if adequate informed consent is not obtained.

Nurses are increasingly being named in lawsuits. Therefore, nurses should also be aware of their state's laws, because they are often involved in informed consent, even if they are not responsible for obtaining informed consent. Furthermore, as patient advocates, nurses have an ethical duty to understand informed consent laws to ensure that informed consent occurs.

DELEGATION OF INFORMED CONSENT

In *Butler v. South Fulton Medical Center, Inc.* (1994), the physician delegated the process of obtaining the patient's signature on the consent form to the nurses in the hospital. The consent form filled out by the nursing staff listed a different procedure than that which the physician performed. The patient received an injection into her back that was administered too close to the spinal cord, resulting in the patient's becoming a ventilator-supported C-1 quadriplegic. The patient had testified that she did not read the consent form, nor did she understand the differences between the procedure on the form and the procedure actually performed. The Court held that in obtaining the signature on the consent form, the nurses were performing an administrative act and not utilizing their professional skill or judgment.

Thus, the nurses in this case were not obtaining informed consent, rather they were involved in the administrative act of having a form filled out by a patient and were not held liable in this case.

ETHICAL CONSIDERATIONS AND CONFLICTS

As discussed earlier in this chapter, the most common ethical consideration or conflict facing health care providers is imposition of their will, opinions, and decisions on patients. Because of the relationship between a health care provider and a patient, it is easy for a health care provider to slip into the role of parent and dictate what will or will not happen to the patient.

A way to avoid being placed in the parental role is for the health care provider to communicate and inform patients regarding their situation. This tends to create a more independent, informed patient who is able to make decisions on his or her own.

RECOMMENDATIONS FOR RESEARCH AND MALPRACTICE PREVENTION

RESEARCH

Because of the variations between the states and the ever-changing law regarding in-

formed consent, the local law library should prove helpful to the health care provider seeking to clarify informed consent issues specific to a patient, facility, or situation. Another source of information is the local nursing library. A search under "informed consent" at either the law or nursing library should leave the health care provider with adequate background information on the basics of informed consent. However, for current information or for an analysis of the application of the law to a specific situation, the health care provider should consult an attorney who specializes in health care and in issues involving health care providers.

MALPRACTICE PREVENTION

Unless the nurse wants to increase the chances for a lawsuit based on negligence or battery, the nurse should always obtain consent prior to performing nursing interventions. As discussed earlier in this chapter, consent may be expressed or implied, but consent must be obtained. Likewise, a nurse must respect a patient's refusal of nursing procedures or the administration of medical procedures. If a patient refuses an ordered medical procedure, the nurse should contact the physician regarding the patient's refusal, and the nurse should document the refusal.

Malpractice prevention in the area of informed consent for the most part revolves around knowing the state's laws and respecting the patient's decisions. Communication with the patient can prevent a lawsuit, and the health care provider should be diligent about ensuring that the patient has been properly informed. Documentation is always important and can help establish the health care provider's defense to a liability lawsuit. Being aware of informed consent and its requirements is the first step in preventing malpractice in this area.

SUMMARY

Informed consent is not completing a consent form. Informed consent is the process of informing a patient about a proposed treatment or procedure. To have adequate informed consent, the patient must be competent and an adult. However, if an exception is applicable, informed consent can be waived or obtained in a different manner. Some exceptions involve mature or emancipated minors, emergencies, and HIV/AIDS testing.

If a health care provider proceeds to perform a treatment or procedure without informed consent or an exception to informed consent, the health care provider could be held liable for assault and battery and/or negligence. A health care provider could also be held liable if the treatment or procedure occurs after a patient's refusal to consent to treatment.

POINTS TO REMEMBER

- Informed consent involves the process of informing the patient, not just completing a form.
- The laws regarding informed consent vary from state to state.
- A competent adult's decisions about health care should be respected.
- A health care provider should not impose

his or her own opinions or decisions on a patient.

REFERENCES

American Hospital Association. (1973). *Patient bill of rights*. Washington, DC: Author.

Anderson v. Saint Francis–Saint George Hospital, 83 Ohio App. 3d 221, 614 N.E.2d 841, motion overruled 66 Ohio St. 3d 1459, 610 N.E.2d 423 (Ohio 1992).

Black's law dictionary. (1990). St. Paul, MN: West Publishing.

Brent, N. J. (1993, July). Nurses Service Organization *Risk Advisor* [online]. Available at http://www.nso.com/informed.html.

Butler v. South Fulton Medical Center, Inc, 452 S.E.2d 768 (Georgia 1994).

Childress, J. (1989). Autonomy. In R. M. Veatch (Ed.), *Cross cultural perspectives in medical ethics & readings* (pp. 233–240). Boston: Jones and Bartlett.

Consent of minor for self and child. Code of Alabama, No 2281, § 22-8-5 (1971).

Consent to treatment of child by a non-parent or child, Texas Family Code, Title 2, Chapter 32, § 32.001 (1995).

Conservatorship of Drabick, 200 Cal. App. 3d 185, 245 Cal. Rptr. 840 (6th District 1988).

Dworkin, G. (1972). Paternalism. *The Monist*, 56,1. Reprinted in: J. Arras & R. Hunt (Eds.) (1983), *Ethical issues in modern medicine* (2nd ed., pp. 74–84). Palo Alto, CA: Mayfield Publishing Co.

Emergency examination and treatment of incapacitated person. Sufficiency of Consent, Florida Statutes, §401.445 (1997).

Ethical Issue Statement on Informed Consent: Ensuring Patient Autonomy. Texas State Board of Medical Examiners Newsletter.

Faden, R. R., & Beauchamp, T. L., & King, N. M. (1986). *A history and theory of informed consent*. Oxford University Press, New York.

Fox v. Smith, 594 So. 2d 596 (Miss. 1992).

Guin v. Sison, 552 So. 2d 60 (La. Ct. App. 1989).

Health Care Services Malpractice Act. Pennsylvania Constitutional Statutes, 40 P.S. § 1301.103 (amended 1996).

Idaho Health and Safety Code, Title 39, Chapter 43, § 39-4304.

Keomaka v. Zakaib, 811 P. 2d 478 (Haw. Ct. App. 1991).

Living wills and life prolonging procedures 1993. Indiana Code, IC 16-36-4-6 (1977).

Lounsbury v. Capel, 191 Utah 40, 836 P. 2d 188, certiorari denied, 843 P. 2d 1042 (Utah 1992).

McCafferty, M. D., & Meyer, S. M. (1985). *Medical*

malpractice basis of liability. McGraw-Hill, Colorado Springs, Co.

Natanson v. Kline, 186 Kan. 393, 350 P. 2d 1093 (1960).

National League for Nursing. *Patient bill of rights.* New York: Author.

O'Neal v. Hammer, 953 P. 2d 561 (Haw. 1998).

Palmisano, D. J., & Mang, H. J., Jr. (1987). *Informed consent: A survival guide.*

Rozovsky, F. A. (1990). *Consent to treatment: A practical guide* (2nd ed.). Boston, Toronto, London: Little, Brown.

Rozovsky, F. A. (1998). *Consent to treatment: A practical guide* (2nd ed., 1998 Supplement). Gaithersburg MD: Aspen Publishers, Inc.

Salgo v. Leland Stanford, Junior University Board of Trustees, 154 Cal. App. 2d 560, 317 P. 2d 170 (1957).

Scholendorf v. Society of New York Hospitals, 105 N.E.2d 93 (1914).

Texas State Board of Medical Examiners. (1994, Fall/Winter). *Texas State Board of Medical Examiners Newsletter, 16*(2), 10.

Winters v. Miller, 446 F. 2d 65 (1971).

SUGGESTED READINGS

Appelbaum, P. S., Lidz, C. W., & Meisel, A. (1987). *Informed consent, legal theory and clinical practice.* Oxford New York: University Press.

Morrissey, J. M., Hofmann, A. D., & Thrope, Jeffrey C. (1986). *Consent and confidentiality in the health care of children and adolescents: A legal guide.* New York: The Free Press.

Rosoff, A. J. (1981). *Informed consent: A guide for health care providers.* Rockville, MD: Aspen Systems Corporation.

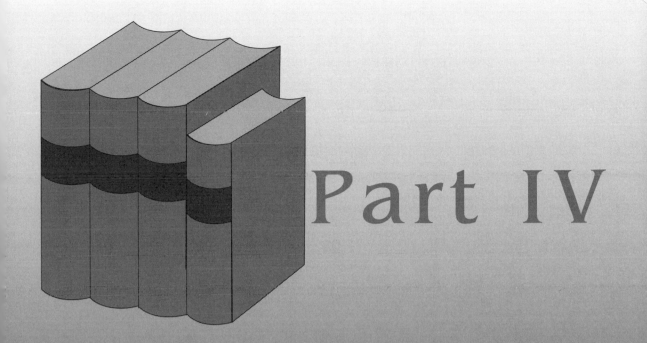

Part IV

NURSING LAW
AND
MANAGEMENT

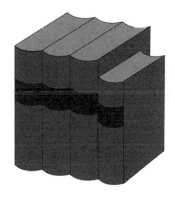

Chapter 13

NURSING LAW AND EMPLOYMENT ISSUES IN NURSING

Victoria Berry

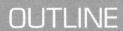

OUTLINE

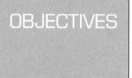
Age Discrimination in Employment Act (ADEA)	Family and Medical Leave Act of 1993 (FMLA)
Americans with Disabilities Act of 1990 (ADA)	Handicap
	Harassment
	Hostile Working Environment
At Will Employment	Impairment
Bona Fide Occupational Qualification (BFOQ)	Independent Contractor
	Major Life Activity
Constructive Discharge	Mental Impairment
Contingent Workers	Quid Pro Quo
Contract	Reasonable Accommodation
Disability	
Discrimination	Religion
Employer	Resignation At Will
Employment Law	Severe Obesity
Equal Employment Opportunity Commission (EEOC)	Sexual Harassment
	Undue Hardship
	Unwelcome Conduct
Fair Labor Standards Act of 1938 (FLSA)	Whistleblower Laws
	Wrongful Termination

Upon completion of this chapter, the reader will be able to:
- Identify the employment laws affecting the nurse as an employee and as a manager.
- Identify the major areas of employment liability and the associated laws affecting the nurse employee.
- List the major areas of employment discrimination.

INTRODUCTION— HISTORICAL PERSPECTIVE

Historically, employment relationships were not a matter of law. Employers could indiscriminately choose the employees they wanted to hire and could decide the employee's compensation and tenure as they wished. Employees had little or no recourse when their civil rights were violated by employers. In the mid-1800s, laws began to be established that eventually influenced the employee and workplace (New York Employment Law Forum Web Site, 1998). Table 13–1 provides a historical summary of the progression of statutory enactments influencing the employer-employee relationship.

TABLE 13–1. HISTORICAL SUMMARY OF THE PROGRESSION OF STATUTORY ENACTMENT'S INFLUENCING THE EMPLOYER/EMPLOYEE RELATIONSHIP

Date	Act	Provisions
1866	Civil Rights Act of 1866	Declared that all persons shall have the same rights; and prohibited discrimination based on race, lineage, and national origin.
1868	14th Amendment of 1868	Stated that all persons born or naturalized in the United States shall have equal protection under the law.
1934	13th Amendment	Supreme Court upheld the 13th Amendment prohibiting involuntary servitude.
1938	The Fair Labor Standards Act of 1938	Allowed states to set minimum wage laws.
1963	Equal Pay Act of 1963	Prohibited sex-based pay differential in employment.
1964	Title VII of the Civil Rights Act of 1964	Was probably the most sweeping law ever enacted to address discriminating practices by employers and supervisors in the workplace.
1967/1986	Age Discrimination in Employment Act of 1967	Prohibited age discrimination for employees older than the age of 40. It was amended in 1986 to remove mandatory retirement at age 65.
1972	Title IX of the Education Amendment of 1972	Prohibited sex discrimination in education facilities that receive federal funds.
1973	Section 504 of the Rehabilitation Act of 1973	Barred federal employers from employment discrimination on the basis of disability.
1990	Americans with Disabilities Act	Prohibited disability discrimination by all employers with 15 or more employees.
1991	Civil Rights Act of 1991	Substantially expanded compensation available to persons injured by discrimination.
1993	Civil Rights Act, amended	Ensured that all persons have equal rights under the law and outlined damages available to complainants in actions brought against employers under Title VII of the Civil Rights Act of 1964, the Americans with Disabilities Act of 1990, and the Rehabilitation Act of 1973.

EMPLOYMENT LAW

Nurse managers know that a large percentage of their time is spent in managing personnel issues. Today's nurse must not only have excellent interpersonal skills and clinical expertise but must also possess a comprehensive understanding of certain aspects of the law governing employment. **Employment law** is a specialty area of the law requiring knowledge of hundreds of complicated federal and state statutes. Employment law addresses the broad aspects of the employer-employee relationship with the exclusion of the negotiation process. Negotiation is covered by collective bargaining and the labor laws.

Nurses must have a working knowledge of the basic employment laws and their application to health care to avoid both personal and institutional liability. All nurse managers who supervise others, and are in a position of hiring, terminating, promoting, and demoting staff, have potential liability under certain employment laws. This chapter will present the employment laws that nurses must know to safeguard their rights, the rights of the employee, and help prevent liability.

TITLE VII OF THE CIVIL RIGHTS ACT OF 1964

An important area of employment law for nurse managers is employment discrimination. In 1964, Congress passed Title VII of the Civil Rights Act of 1964. This law protects the employee from discrimination based on race, color, national origin, sex (including pregnancy), or religion. Employment discrimination laws were enacted to prevent discrimination of the employee in the practices of hiring, promotion, compensation, benefits, assignment, and termination (Title VII of the Civil Rights Act of 1964).

The Bureau of Labor Statistics lists the number of U.S. workers at 131 million (U.S. Department of Labor, Bureau of Labor Statistics, 1998). Lawsuits against employers and individual supervisors have shown staggering growth with monetary awards in the millions of dollars. A large percentage of these cases were based on discrimination (U.S. Equal Employment Opportunity Commission, 1995).

As the labor force becomes more and more diverse, nurse managers are employing and supervising more foreign nurse graduates and nurses with diverse cultural backgrounds. The U.S. Bureau of Labor Statistics predicts that one third of the work force in the United States will be minorities by the year 2010 (Blouin & Brent, 1994).

According to a 1993 survey, minority employees increased as follows: women, by 69 percent; African Americans, 59 percent; Hispanics, 49 percent; Asians, 44 percent; older workers, 43 percent; workers with disabilities, 33 percent; gays and lesbians, 15 percent; and European-American males, 10 percent (Swart, 1996). The nurse manager's personnel management of minority staff will undoubtedly be held to more intense scrutiny than ever before.

Title VII also makes it illegal to retaliate against former employees. Section 704(a) of Title VII states it is unlawful "for an employer to discriminate against any of his employees or applicants for employment" who have sought Title VII protection.

The **Equal Employment Opportunity Commission (EEOC)** interprets and enforces certain employment laws. These include the Equal Pay Act, the Age Discrimination in Employment Act, Title VII of the Civil Rights Act of 1964, Americans with Disabilities Act (ADA), and sections of the Rehabilitation Act. The EEOC was established by Title VII. Section 2000(e)(5) of Title 42 contains the enforcement provisions, and the guidelines and regulations are contained in Title 29 of the Code of Federal Regulations.

RACIAL DISCRIMINATION

Title VII prohibits employer **discrimination** against job applicants or employees because of their race, skin color, hair texture, or certain facial features. Employers also may not discriminate against employees because of the employee's marriage or association with an individual of a different race or association with minority groups (U.S. Equal Employment Opportunity Commission, 1997d). Employment decisions may not be made based on employer assumption about traits, stereotypes or characteristics attributable to a certain race (U.S. Equal Employment Opportunity Commission, 1997d). Employers may not segregate or classify a group of employees because of race. This federal law prohibits the isolation or assignment of groups of employees to certain assignments or geographical locations based on their race. **Harassment** based on race or color also violates Title VII. This includes racial slurs, ethnic jokes, or offensive remarks based on the employee's race or color that create a hostile or offensive work environment. Title VII requires that employers and supervisors deal with the employee based on individuality, that is, skills, training, expertise, and knowledge. To do otherwise is a violation of the law (U.S. Equal Employment Opportunity Commission, 1997d).

ETHNIC DISCRIMINATION

Persons may not be denied employment, promotion, or compensation because of their birthplace, ancestry, culture, or ethnicity. A "speak English only" rule may also violate Title VII. The employer must show that speaking English only is necessary to conduct business, and the employer must have informed the employee of the rule (U.S. Equal Employment Opportunity Commission, 1997b). One employer was ordered by the court to change its English-only rule and require the employees to speak English only when "dealing directly with the customer" (*Kim v. The Southland Corp.*, 1995).

However, Title VII does not protect an employee's right to speak his or her native language while performing job duties. The privilege to converse on the job in non-English is given at the employer's discretion. The employer may define where and when non-English may be spoken. In one court case, four employees sued their employer because of a English-only rule. However, other employees had complained that the four employees would talk about them and make fun of them in Spanish, which created a hostile environment. The court ruled that just as the employer has the right to prohibit foul language in the workplace, "Speaking one's native tongue at any time on the job is not a privilege of employment" (*Long v. First Union Corp. of Virginia*, 1996). EEOC statistics indicate that 32 complaints regarding the English-only rule were filed in 1996; 14 were filed the first quarter in 1997 (U.S. Equal Employment Opportunity Commission, 1997b). Court decisions regarding these complaints will affect the interpretations made by employers when employees claim that an English-only rule causes a hostile environment or is discriminatory.

Title VII also protects the employee from discrimination against the employee's accent or manner of speaking. The employer would have the burden of proof that the employee's accent or manner of speaking was detrimental to the job and job performance. In *Odima v. Westin Tucson Hotel* (1995), an employee from Nigeria was turned down for several promotions because, in part, of his heavy accent, which employers stated would "inhibit communications." The court ruled against the employer, stating that the employee's speech was clear and understandable.

Employers may not discriminate against the employee because of associations the employee has with persons or affiliations of others of specific national origin. As with harassment based on race or color, harassment based on ethnicity is also a violation of Title VII. Employers and supervisors may be held responsible for on-the-job harassment even if the offenses were strictly prohibited (U.S. Equal Employment Opportunity Commission, 1997b).

RELIGIOUS DISCRIMINATION

Religion is defined as organized faith. Title VII also prohibits employment discrimination based on the person's religious preference. Employers are required to make reasonable accommodations for the employee's religious practice unless it creates a hardship for the employer. Employers may not schedule work activities that conflict with the employee's religious activities unless the employer can prove that not doing so would create an undue hardship (U.S. Equal Employment Opportunity Commission, 1997e). The employer may not force the employee to participate in training programs or activities that the employee feels are inconsistent with his or her religious beliefs. Employees may not be discriminated against because of their affiliations with others of a specific religious preference. Restrictive dress codes and refusal of observance of a religious holiday may not be instituted unless the employer can show that not doing so would cause an undue hardship (U.S. Equal Employment Opportunity Commission, 1997e).

Employers may have the right to insist on the employee's performing the job when the job is accepted with full knowledge of requirements that conflict with the employee's religious beliefs. For example, if a nurse accepts a position in surgery knowing that therapeutic abortions are performed in the facility, the nurse has little ground for objection to performing the job based on religious objections. Some states, such as Texas, do protect the nurse's right to refuse to indirectly or directly participate in an abortion procedure if the nurse objects to participating (Murphy, 1995). However, if the nurse accepted the job with full knowledge of the abortion participation requirement, the nurse entered into a contract with the employer fully informed and agreed to fulfill the job requirement. However, if at the time of hire, the nurse was told she or he would not have to participate in therapeutic abortions, the nurse cannot be forced to participate at a later date.

In *Chalmers v. Talon* (1996), the court stated that for an employee to establish religious discrimination under Title VII, he or she must prove that he or she had a bona fide religious belief that conflicted with the employer's requirement, that he or she informed the employer of this belief and was disciplined for failure to comply with the conflicting employer requirement. Atheists are also protected from discrimination under Title VII (*EEOC v. Townley Manufacturing*, 1988).

SEXUAL DISCRIMINATION

Sexual discrimination refers to discrimination based on gender, not sexual practices or sexuality. Prohibition of sexual discrimination applies to both males and females. Employers are violating the law if they treat employees differently based on the sex of the individual. Discrimination is not an issue in cases where treatment is based on a **bona fide occupational qualification** (BFOQ). However, with societal changes allowing women in previously male-dominated roles,

it is more difficult for the employer to prove a legitimate BFOQ need for deferential preference.

In *Little Forest Medical Center of Akron v. Ohio Civil Rights Commission* (1993), an applicant successfully sued a skilled nursing facility for refusing to hire him because he was male. Male nurses are the minority in the nursing profession. Nurse managers must be aware of their hiring and management behavior toward male nurses to ensure nondiscriminatory practices.

For some employers, there may still be an issue of male nurses performing certain nursing functions. This is especially true in obstetrics and gynecological environments. The numbers of male nurse continues to climb. In 1972, the rate of male graduate nurses was 1 percent. In 1996, the rate climbed to 5 percent (American Nurses Association, 1996). The patient has the right to refuse treatment, and the nurse manager has an obligation to protect the patient's rights. It is incumbent on the employer to allow some flexibility in policy to protect the rights of both patients and employees.

PREGNANCY DISCRIMINATION

Another form of sexual discrimination is pregnancy discrimination. The Pregnancy Discrimination Act, passed in 1978, is an amendment to Title VII of the Civil Rights Act of 1964. This amendment states that female employees or applicants affected by pregnancy or related medical conditions will be treated in the same manner as other applicants or employees. The employee is entitled to up to 4 months of pregnancy leave once she is unable to continue her job duties as a result of pregnancy (U.S. Equal Employment Opportunity Commission, 1997c).

An employer may not refuse to hire a woman because of pregnancy as long as she can perform the major aspects of the job. Medical complications of pregnancy must be treated as any other medical condition, and the employee must be allowed to work as long as she is able to do her job. Jobs must be held open for pregnancy-related absences, the same as jobs are held open for employees on sick or disability leave (U.S. Equal Employment Opportunity Commission, 1997c). Although not specifically addressed by the ADA, most employers will make concessions for pregnant employees to ensure safety, such as not exposing the pregnant nurse employee to x-ray or rubella.

The Act prohibits discrimination against pregnant employees; however, it does not mandate that they receive preferential treatment. In *Alabama v. Flowers Hospital, Inc.* (1994), a pregnant nurse was fired for refusing to care for a patient with acquired immunodeficiency syndrome (AIDS). She sued under the Pregnancy Discrimination Act. A federal court found that the hospital did not discriminate against the nurse in that she was not treated differently from other employees, and that the nurse was in fact asking for preferential treatment.

Additionally, the Supreme Court ruled in *UAW v. Johnson Controls, Inc.* (1991) that polices that are written for fetal protection are in violation of Title VII. Therefore, employers can inform the applicant or employee of risks involved with the job, but must allow the pregnant applicant or employee to decide whether or not she accepts the job or assignment. It is incumbent upon the employer to ensure that the decision of the pregnant applicant or employee is an informed decision.

SEXUAL HARASSMENT

In 1980, the EEOC ruled that **sexual harassment** is a form of sex discrimination and a violation of Title VII. Box 13–1 further defines sexual harassment.

To meet the definition of sexual harassment, the conduct must be deemed **unwelcome conduct**. This means that the conduct was neither incited nor solicited and the conduct was felt to be undesirable and/or offensive. The victim does not have to be of the opposite sex. The victim also does not have to be the one harassed, but can be anyone affected by the offensive conduct (U. S. Equal Employment Opportunity Commission, 1997f).

There are two defined types of sexual harassment cases: quid pro quo and hostile working environment (Conners, 1996b). **Quid pro quo** (sometimes referred to as "something for something") sexual harassment occurs when a supervisor or other person in authoritative power over the employee demands sexual favor in exchange for not being fired, demoted, transferred, or the like (Conners, 1996b). The demand does not have to be verbal. It may be implied. Cases involving only a single incident of quid pro quo harassment have been upheld in the courts. (Conners, 1996b).

BOX 13–1

DEFINING SEXUAL HARASSMENT

The EEOC defines sexual harassment as:
Unwelcome sexual advances, requests for sexual favors, and other verbal or physical conduct of a sexual nature constitute sexual harassment when
- Submission to such conduct is made either explicitly or implicitly a term or condition of an individual's employment.
- Submission to or rejection of such conduct by an individual is used as a basis for employment decisions affecting an individual, or such conduct has the purpose or effect of unreasonably interfering with an individual's work performance or creating an intimidating, hostile, or offensive working environment.

Source: U.S. Equal Employment Opportunity Commission. (1997). *Facts about sexual harassment discrimination.* Washington, DC: Author.

A **hostile working environment** means that the workplace is intimidating or offensive, causing the employee to endure sexually inappropriate comments or conduct. The offender does not have to be a supervisor, but can be anyone within the employer's organization, including vendors, contract employees, volunteers, and consultant staff (Conners, 1996b). Inappropriate conduct may be verbal or physical. Examples of conduct that may be considered sexual harassment include:

- Offensive comments or insults of a sexual nature
- Jokes, stories, or gossip that has a sexual content
- Questions and /or comments about one's sexual life
- Photographs, cartoons, graphics, posters, or drawings of a sexual nature
- Sexually explicit computer screen savers in view of others
- E-mails of a sexual nature
- Obscene gestures, whistles, or touching the body (Conners, 1996b)

Constructive discharge is when the employee leaves employment because the discrimination is so intolerable that no reasonable person could be expected to work within the environment. The courts have treated constructive discharge as a termination by the employer, and it can be the basis of an EEOC or civil case (Arizona State Senate, 1997).

The employer has the obligation to investigate complaints of sexual harassment in a timely manner and take appropriate corrective action to ensure a harassment-free workplace and compliance with the law (Neubs, 1994). In *Farpella-Crosby v. Horizon Health Care* (1996), the court found that the employer failed to take prompt remedial action for 5 months after a nurse complained of abusive harassing behavior (Tammello, 1996).

The employee has the right to work in a harassment-free environment. Failure on the employer's part to take immediate and corrective action once a complaint of sexual harassment has been made increases employer liability. The law does not allow the employer to plead ignorance of the employees' environment. The law specifically addresses the employer's responsibility to take appropriate action when the employer knows or "should have known" that sexual harassment was taking place (Conners, 1996).

Many nurses are jointly responsible for nursing students within their employment organization. Title IX of the Education Amendment of 1972 prohibits sex discrimination in educational institutions that receive federal funds. Employers may also be liable for sexual harassment to a nursing student occurring within the employer's organization. College and university faculty members may hold similar liability when sexual harassment occurs within the college or university setting. It is important for administration to have polices in place for members of the faculty to follow when faced with sexual discrimination of students or staff. The explosive use of computers has opened up a new arena for "hostile environment" cases. The term **cyber liability** has surfaced in the literature. Exposure to sexually explicit computer images, messages, jokes, and the like can result in sexual harassment claims (Repa, 1998a). Retrieval of computer-deleted material also makes it easier to prove some of these cases. The Electronic Communications Privacy Act was enacted in 1986 before the prolific use of e-mail (Repa, 1998a). Most employees believe their e-mail communication is confidential, which is usually not the case. Employment lawsuits that were based on e-mail evidence have been won by employees (Heenam, Althen, & Roles, 1996).

AT WILL EMPLOYMENT

Most states have an **at will employment** law. Although there are some exceptions, the law basically states that an employer can terminate the employee's job for any reason at any time within the employment relationship. The employer's actions must be based on good faith under the at will law (Calfee, 1996). Examples would be insubordination, breach of policy and procedure, and failure to consistently perform the job as required by the employee's job description. The law also allows the employee the option of **resignation at will**. The at will law, however, does not protect the employer under Title VII. Wrongful termination suits are most commonly associated with at will termination (Fiesta, 1997). Examples of **wrongful termination** may be:

- Firing a nurse for voicing complaints about short staffing and patient safety issues
- Firing a nurse for "blowing the whistle" on the facility's illegal practices
- Firing a nurse for refusal to take part in illegal or unethical activities
- Firing a nurse in retaliation for filing a complaint with EEOC
- Firing a nurse after the nurse has filed a workers' compensation claim
- Firing a nurse for personal grudges

AGE DISCRIMINATION IN EMPLOYMENT ACT

Registered nurses in the U.S. workforce are definitely an aging population. In 1996 the average age of the registered nurse was 44.3 years. More than 62 percent of registered nurses are older than the age of 40. Additionally, the age of the nurse graduate has increased. In 1980, the nurse graduate's average age was 26.9 years. In 1991 it had increased to 33.5 years (American Nurses Association, 1994).

In 1967, the federal **Age Discrimination in Employment Act (ADEA)** was passed, which prohibits discrimination against persons 40 years of age or older. This law protects older workers against arbitrary termination based on age and applies to both employees and job applicants (U.S. Equal Employment Opportunity Commission, 1967). An important aspect of the law is that it protects older workers from being forced to retire, and it protects their pension rights when they leave. It also protects the worker from age discrimination in promotions, compensation, training, and assignments (U.S. Equal Employment Opportunity Commission, 1967).

ADEA applies only to workers age 40 and older and to institutions with 20 or more employees. Some states have age discrimina-

tion laws that provide employees with even greater protection than the ADEA (U.S. Equal Employment Opportunity Commission, 1967). The intent of the ADEA is for employers to evaluate and reevaluate employees on their ability and performance, not on their age. The employer that generalizes or stereotypes persons regarding age is in violation of the ADEA (U.S. Equal Employment Opportunity Commission, 1967).

Goodhouse v. Magnolia Hospital (1996) concerned the case of a 53-year-old nurse who was terminated after 23 years of employment during a reduction in force. She applied for another position that was available within the hospital but was not hired. She sued for age discrimination and was awarded $100,000. Additionally, the hospital was ordered to reinstate the nurse.

The court has also ruled that age-based harassment is a violation of employee rights. In *Madel v. FCI Marketing, Inc.* (1997), the employer was held liable for derogatory age-based comments. The word "old" was used in conjunction with lewd language, and sleeping quarters were referred to as the "geriatric wing" (Heenam, Althen, & Roles, 1997). The court stated its concerns with the "allegedly pervasive use of age-based epithets" (Heenam, Althen, & Roles, 1997). Employers may be held liable for a work environment that is hostile to seniors (Heenam, Althen, & Roles, 1997).

Many cases of age discrimination have been based on the employer's unintentional practice of age discrimination. If an employee believes that he or she has been the victim of age discrimination, he or she may have the right to file a complaint under state law, federal law, or both. According to a 1994 survey, the average award given in age discrimination cases was $302,914 (Blouin & Brent, 1996). This surpasses awards given in disability, race, or gender discrimination cases (Blouin & Brent, 1996).

REHABILITATION ACT OF 1973

The Rehabilitation Act of 1973 prohibits discrimination against handicapped applicants and employees by federal employers and recipients of federal financial aid. The Act's intent was to improve the opportunities available to persons with handicaps (U.S. Department of Health and Human Services, 1990). The Rehabilitation Act greatly facilitated the expansion of services for persons with disabilities. It proclaimed that no qualified individual shall be excluded from employment solely because of disability (U.S. Department of Health and Human Services, 1990). The Act mandated the removal of physical, attitudinal, and programmatic barriers to employment opportunities for persons with handicaps (U.S. Department of Health and Human Services, 1990). Box 13–2 provides examples of conditions that are considered a **handicap**.

The Act also established funding for evaluation, counseling, training, placement, and rehabilitation for those qualified individuals. The Act gave disabled persons a legal avenue to pursue discrimination charges. The Rehabilitation Act of 1973 served as a Bill of Rights for persons with disabilities. It was the first dynamic and progressive employment law that ensured that the rights of qualified persons with handicaps would be protected (U.S. Department of Health and Human Services, 1990).

AMERICANS WITH DISABILITIES ACT OF 1990

The **Americans with Disabilities Act of 1990 (ADA)** is a companion piece of legislation to the Rehabilitation Act of 1973. The ADA affects 6 million businesses and nonprofit agencies, 80,000 units of state and local government, and approximately 49 million people with disabilities (Civil Rights Division, Department of Justice, 1998). The ADA makes it illegal for employers with 15 or more employees to discriminate against persons with disabilities in hiring, firing, promotion, compensation, training, and benefits (U.S. Department of Health and Human Services, 1990). The ADA is enforced by the Equal Employment Opportunity Commission (EEOC) (Civil Rights Division, Department of Justice, 1998).

Complaints may be filed with the EEOC by employees who feel they have been the victim of employer discrimination. The EEOC will investigate the complaint, and, if the complaint is deemed to have merit and if efforts to obtain voluntary compliance have failed, the EEOC may refer the complaint to the Department of Justice (DOJ) (Civil Rights Division, Department of Justice, 1998). The ADA also gives the DOJ authority to regulate

BOX 13–2

EXAMPLES OF HANDICAPPING CONDITIONS

- AIDS
- Alcoholism
- Blindness or visual impairment
- Cancer
- Deafness or hearing impairment
- Diabetes
- Drug addiction
- Heart disease
- Mental or emotional illness

Source: U.S. Department of Health and Human Services. (1990).

Titles II and III of the ADA and to provide technical assistance and enforcement (Civil Rights Division, Department of Justice, 1998). The DOJ has the authority to file lawsuits in federal court to enforce the ADA. Under Title III, the DOJ may also obtain civil penalties of up to $50,000 for the first violation and $100,000 for subsequent violations (Civil Rights Division, Department of Justice, 1998). The DOJ has filed lawsuits for allegations of harassment, retaliation, involuntary reassignment, failure to promote, pregnancy discrimination, unlawful discharge, and religious discrimination (Civil Rights Division, Department of Justice, 1998).

The ADA is not meant to prohibit the employer from hiring the most qualified applicant, nor are there affirmative action obligations. It does, however, prohibit discrimination of qualified applicants or employees merely because of their disability (U.S. Department of Justice, 1990). Box 13–3 provides a broad definition of a **disability.**

The ADA defines **impairment** as a physiological disorder affecting one or more of a number of body systems or a mental or psychological disorder. The ADA definition of *impairment* does not include personality characteristics such as irresponsible behaviors, poor judgment and decision-making, and temper outbursts (U.S. Equal Employment Opportunity Commission, 1997a). Under ADA, the employer does not have to tolerate inappropriate behavior from the employee, even if the improper conduct results from the impairment. The employer

has the right to maintain a workplace free of violence, theft, and property destruction (U.S. Equal Employment Opportunity Commission, 1997a). The ADA allows employers to withhold employment from those individuals who pose a direct safety risk to themselves or others (U.S. Equal Employment Opportunity Commission, 1997a).

An employee with diabetes who takes insulin daily may be viewed by employers as not meeting the impairment definition established by the ADA (U.S. Equal Employment Opportunity Commission, 1997a). Diabetes is typically viewed as a disease that does not affect the employee's job. However, the diabetic employee is covered by the ADA. A disease or condition that requires the use of medications or auxiliary aids meets the definition of impairment, in that it substantially limits a major life activity (U.S. Equal Employment Opportunity Commission, 1997a).

An employee with a broken limb is not covered by the ADA, even if the employee is unable to perform essential job duties (U.S. Equal Employment Opportunity Commission, 1997a). The EEOC states that the ADA does not apply to an impairment that "does not substantially limit a major life activity if it is of limited duration and will have no long term effect" (U.S. Equal Employment Opportunity Commission, 1997a).

Pregnancy is not a physiological disorder and therefore is not covered by the ADA. The ADA considers extremes in height and weight as impairments. Body weight more than 100 percent over the norm is defined as

BOX 13–3

DEFINITION OF A DISABILITY

An individual with a disability is broadly defined as one who
- Has a physical or mental impairment that substantially limits one or more major life activities.
- Has a record of such an impairment.
- Is regarded as having such an impairment.

Source: U.S. Equal Employment Opportunity Commission. (1998). *Facts about the ADA.* Washington, DC: Author.

severe obesity and would most likely be covered under the ADA (U.S. Equal Employment Opportunity Commission, 1997a). Chronic conditions are typically covered under the ADA as well (U.S. Equal Employment Opportunity Commission, 1997a). These include conditions that substantially limit a major life activity, such as cancer, AIDS, heart disease, and chronic back pain. Hypertension may be considered an employment disability if it is an unresolved chronic condition with resultant medical restrictions (U.S. Equal Employment Opportunity Commission, 1997a).

In *Howard v. North Mississippi Medical Center* (1996), a home health aide claimed that her allergies and migraine headaches prevented her from making home visits and subsequently necessitated that she have a position in an office or clinic. The court found that the employer had made strong efforts to accommodate the employee but that her skills were not transferable to available positions and that migraines and allergies were not disabilities covered by the ADA.

A **major life activity** is defined by the ADA as the activities needed to care for oneself—standing, walking, seeing, speaking, hearing, learning, working, interacting with others, concentrating, and thinking (Corbett & Lane, 1995).

The ADA requires the employer to make reasonable accommodations for the qualified disabled applicant or employee. The following are some of the actions noted as a **reasonable accommodation** by the Equal Employment Opportunity Commission:

- Making existing facilities readily accessible
- Restructuring jobs, modifying schedules, and reassigning vacant positions
- Obtaining or modifying equipment and training materials and providing qualified readers or interpreters (U.S. Equal Employment Opportunity Commission, 1998)

Examples of assistive devices provided by employers include teletypewriters or telephone amplifiers for persons with hearing impairments, wooden blocks to elevate desks and tables for those persons in wheelchairs, and large-type computer terminals

and Braille printers to assist employees with visual impairments (U.S. Equal Employment Opportunity Commission, 1998).

The employer may not be required to make these accommodations if the employer can show that to do so would cause an **undue hardship**. Undue hardship is defined as "an action requiring significant difficulty or expense when considered in light of factors such as an employer's size, financial resources and the nature and structure of its operation" (U.S. Equal Employment Opportunity Commission, 1997a). The factors set out by the EEOC in establishing undue hardship are:

- Nature and cost of the accommodation
- Financial resources of the employer
- Nature of the business
- Accommodation costs already incurred (Corbett & Lane, 1995)

The employer is not held responsible if the employee has not informed the employer of the disability (U.S. Equal Employment Opportunity Commission, 1997a). The compliance with reasonable accommodation laws ensures that individuals with disabilities have the opportunity to perform jobs for which they qualify (U.S. Equal Employment Opportunity Commission, 1997a). The employer and nurse manager should structure the job descriptions to reflect the physical and mental skills necessary to perform the job. If a disabled nurse can perform the job, then the employer must not discriminate against the nurse. When job descriptions are unclear as to the physical and mental skills needed, it leaves the employer and nurse manager vulnerable to subjective decision-making and possible unintentional discrimination.

Questions regarding the nature or extent of the applicant's or employee's disability are prohibited under the ADA. They may be asked only about their ability to perform the job. Employers can make the job offer contingent on a medical examination, but only if medical examinations are required for all employees (U.S. Equal Employment Opportunity Commission, 1997a). The medical examination must have a job-specific focus and be congruent with the related employment needs. Employers must also be careful that they do not perceive disability when one does not exist (Heenam, Althen, & Roles, 1996). Lawsuits have been successfully won in cases where employees were denied employment because the employer perceived that the employee could not perform the job as a result of a disability (Heenam, Althen, & Roles, 1996).

There has been focus on the ADA in regard to psychiatric and substance abuse disabilities. The EEOC publishes a policy guide that may be helpful to employers called *The Americans with Disabilities Act and Psychiatric Disabilities.* The guide answers commonly asked questions about the ADA and mental impairment (Archives from The Jackson Lewis, 1997).

The employer may not ask an applicant questions related to mental disability before making an offer of employment. An exception exists, however, if an applicant asks for reasonable accommodations for the application process (U.S. Equal Employment Opportunity Commission, 1997a).

The ADA does not cover employees or applicants who engage in the use of illegal drugs. Additionally, disorders resulting from the current illegal use of drugs are not covered under the ADA. Illegal drugs includes the unlawful use of prescription-controlled medications (U.S. Equal Employment Opportunity Commission, 1997a). Employers have the right to screen all applicants for illegal drug use. Employees who use illegal drugs or abuse alcohol can be held to the same work performance criteria as all other employees according to the EEOC (U.S. Equal Employment Opportunity Commission, 1997a).

More than 12 percent of all ADA charges filed against employers with the EEOC involve alleged mental impairments (Archives from The Jackson Lewis, 1997). Box 13–4 provides examples of **mental impairments** potentially covered by the ADA.

Stress behaviors are not themselves covered by the ADA. However, stress may be related to a mental condition that is covered by the law (Archives from The Jackson Lewis, 1997). If an employee is taking medication for a mental impairment, he or she is covered by the ADA if there is evidence that the mental impairment left untreated (without the medication) would substantially limit a major life activity (Archives from The Jackson Lewis, 1997).

Psychiatric impairments may be more difficult for employers and supervisors to deal with in the workplace. Because of a general inability to recognize psychological impairment, employers must be educated and alerted to the needs and requests for accommodation for mentally impaired employees (Archives from The Jackson Lewis, 1997). Likewise, the employee must inform the employer of the disability and request accommodation when needed. Courts have termed this an interactive process, which may require a great deal of communication (Heenam, Althen, & Roles, 1996). Request for accommodation for mentally disabled employees many times may come in the form of

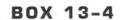

BOX 13-4

EXAMPLES OF MENTAL IMPAIRMENTS POTENTIALLY COVERED BY THE ADA

- Major depression
- Schizophrenia
- Anxiety disorders including panic disorder, obsessive-compulsive disorder, and posttraumatic disorder
- Bipolar disorder
- Personality disorders

Source: Heenam, Althen, & Roles, 1997.

a recommendation from a psychiatrist or psychologist to the supervisor (Archives from The Jackson Lewis, 1997).

Under the ADA, the employer must keep all medical information about applicants, employees, and former employees confidential. The ADA requires that medical information should be kept in separate confidential files apart from personnel files. Employee medical information may be shared with other employees such as supervisors, when deemed necessary for accommodation compliance (Conners, 1996a).

FAMILY AND MEDICAL LEAVE ACT

The **Family and Medical Leave Act of 1993 (FMLA)** (U.S. Department of Labor, 1993) is seen as the most compassionate law ever enacted to protect the employee's balance between job and family (Heenam et al., 1997).

The U.S. Department of Labor's Employment Standards Administration enforces FMLA. It allows employees to take up to 12 weeks of unpaid leave in a 12-month period for specified family and medical reasons. During this leave, the employee's job and benefits are protected. FMLA applies to all public employers and private employers with 50 or more employees. The employee must have worked for the employer for 12 months and worked at least 1250 hours over the past 12 months to be eligible for FMLA (Legal Shark, 1998).

Leave eligibility under FMLA includes:

- Birth and care of a newborn child of the employee
- Foster care placement or adoption of a child by the employee
- Care of an immediate family member—spouse, child, or parent—with a serious illness
- Serious illness of the employee (Legal Shark, 1998)

Upon return, the employee must receive his or her original job or equivalent job with equivalent pay. The latest enforcement report published by the Department of Labor states that most complaints stemmed from the employer's refusing to reinstate the employee to the same or equivalent job (Legal Shark, 1998). The complaints were successfully resolved with the employer's agreeing to comply with the law, usually after a telephone call in 90 percent of the cases (U.S. Department of Labor, 1997).

FAIR LABOR STANDARDS ACT

The **Fair Labor Standards Act of 1938 (FLSA)** was enacted to guarantee the employee's right to be paid for the work performed. The FLSA prohibits pay discrimination between male and female employees (U.S. Department of Labor, 1997).

The FLSA establishes the following:

- Forty-hour work week
- Federal minimum wage
- Requirements for overtime
- Restrictions on child labor (Repa, 1998b)

EQUAL PAY ACT

In 1963, the Equal Pay Act amended the FLSA. The Equal Pay Act prohibits discrimination of wages based on sex. It mandates that equal pay must be paid for equal work if the jobs performed are of "equal skill, effort and responsibility and are performed under similar working conditions" (Fair Labor Standards Act, Amended, 29 U.S.C. § 201, 1938). Pay differential must be based on seniority, merit, productivity, or job performance (Fair Labor Standards Act, 1938).

WHISTLEBLOWER LAWS

Most states have enacted **whistleblower laws** that prohibit the employer from discriminating or retaliating against an employee for reporting the employer's illegal acts. The law was enacted to encourage employees to report unsafe practices affecting the public. For example, nurses cannot be fired for reporting illegal practices by their employer, such as improper coding in insurance claims, false diagnoses to increase or ensure insurance money, improper or unethical treatment of elderly patients, misrepresentation of surgical assistants who are charted as physicians but are not licensed, falsifying medical records, and billing for services not rendered.

CONTRACT EMPLOYMENT AND INDEPENDENT CONTRACTORS

It is estimated that there are approximately 2.3 million workers employed in temporary help agencies in the United States. These workers are commonly referred to as **contingent workers** (Paskind, 1998). Many of these contingent workers are nurses hired to supplement core staffing. The EEOC has issued guidelines entitled *Guidance on Application of EEO Laws to Contingent Workers* (U.S. Equal Employment Opportunity Commission, 1997g) explaining when employers may be liable for discrimination against contingent workers (Paskind, 1998). Contingent workers are covered under the antidiscrimination statutes because they typically qualify as employees of the staffing firm, the company to whom they are assigned, or both (Paskind, 1998). The EEOC guidelines state:

- Staffing firms and their clients may not discriminate against these workers on the basis of race, color, religion, sex, national origin, age or disability.
- A staffing firm must take immediate and appropriate corrective action if it learns that its client has discriminated against one of the staffing firm's employees (U.S. Equal Employment Opportunity Commission, 1997g).

Employers may also hire independent contractors. What determines whether a worker is an employee or an independent contractor is a matter of law. **Employers** pay payroll taxes, Social Security/FICA, and unemployment taxes on employee salaries (Pelfrey & Theisen, 1995). Independent contractors are responsible for their own taxes. Recently the Internal Revenue Service (IRS) has looked more closely at the independent contractor–employer relationship in a belief that as much as $10 billion of lost tax revenue has occurred due to misclassification of the independent contractor (Pelfrey & Theisen, 1995).

Many of these contingent workers have employee contracts with an employer. A **contract** may be written, formal, or oral (Lindell, 1986) and has four requirements:

1. The job contracted for must be legal.
2. The parties agreeing to the contract must be legally competent and must be of legal age.
3. There must be a mutual agreement about the job to be performed.
4. There must be consideration or the promise of consideration (Lindell, 1986).

The IRS Code § 3401(d)(1) defines an **employer** as the "person having control of the payment of such wages." An **independent contractor** is defined by § 3508(b)(2) as "direct seller" or "a person hired to perform a task for another, who totally controls the means to be used in attaining the desired results, and is subject to control only in regards to the ends to be attained." (Pelfrey & Theisen, 1995). There are at least 20 factors that the IRS uses in determining whether the worker is an employee or independent contractor (Pelfrey & Theisen, 1995). These factors cover areas such as payment methods, reimbursement of expenses, location where the work is to be performed, the hours involved, reports, and the right to terminate (Pelfrey & Theisen, 1995).

There are critics of the 20-factor test who find it subjective and ineffective. The IRS is not restricted to using this test as the only means for determining worker status. Auditors will also look at the worker's behavior on the job, the finances of the worker, and the worker's relationship with the hiring facility in determining the worker's classification (Pelfrey & Theisen, 1995).

The nurse manager should be aware of the IRS guidelines and know whether employees under the nurse manager's supervision are at risk of reclassification by the IRS. The IRS considers misclassification of workers a serious offense. Reclassification of contract workers to employees can cost the employer back employment taxes as well as interest (Pelfrey & Theisen, 1995).

SUMMARY

Employment law encompasses many complicated laws that affect the nurse in the employment setting. Because of the constant change and evolving laws, it is imperative for nurses to stay abreast of current laws and court decisions affecting the employee-employer relationship. Nurse managers are responsible for hiring and supervising qualified and competent personnel. They must be fair and unbiased in hiring and terminating staff as well as in their supervisory duties. Discrimination based on race, national origin, age, religious preference, sex, pregnancy, or disability is against the law and applies to full-time employees as well as contract workers. Recent court decisions indicate that there is less tolerance for employer discrimination and unfair treatment of the employee than ever before. Nurses are often the largest group of employees in the health care organization and, therefore, may have the largest exposure to employment law violations. Nurses as leaders in their organizations have the ability and the responsibility to be the influencing factor in policy and procedure development in the area of employment law. Knowledge of these laws will help the individual nurse protect his or her rights as well as the rights of employees that the nurses may supervise.

POINTS TO REMEMBER

- Employment law is a specialized area of the law that is constantly changing and evolving. Nurses must have a basic knowledge of the employment laws to protect their rights and the rights of those they supervise.

- The Civil Rights Act of 1964 protects employees against employer discrimination based on race, color, national origin, sex, or religion.
- A victim of sexual harassment, a form of sexual discrimination, does not have to be of the opposite sex, nor does the victim have to be the one harassed, but can be anyone affected by the offensive conduct.
- Employees older than the age of 40 are protected against employer discrimination by the Age Discrimination in Employment Act.
- The Americans with Disabilities Act of 1990 protects the employees against employer discrimination based on the employee's disability. This includes not only hiring and termination, but also promotion, compensation, training, and benefits.
- The Family and Medical Leave Act allows employees to take up to 12 weeks of unpaid leave from work for specified family and medical reasons, without the fear of losing their jobs.
- Contract employees and independent contractors are covered under the antidiscrimination statutes because they qualify as employees of the firm that staffed them, the company to whom they are assigned, or both.

REFERENCES

The Age Discrimination in Employment Act of 1967, U.S.C.A. §§ 621–634 (1967).

Alabama v. Flowers Hospital, Inc., 33 F. 3d 1308 A-1 (1994).

American Nurses Association. (1994). *Nursing facts from today's registered nurse numbers and demographics.* Kansas City, MO: Author.

American Nurses Association. (1996, March). *Nation's nurses: National sample survey of registered nurses.* Unpublished American Nurses Association 1972 Inventory of Registered Nurses.

Archives from The Jackson Lewis: Prevention Strategies. (1997, Spring). *EEOC pronouncements on psychiatric disabilities and waivers of civil rights stir controversy among employers.*

Arizona State Senate. (1997). *Fact sheet for Senate Bill 1468* [On-line]. Available: http://www.azleg.state.azus/legtext/43/eg/lr/summary/s.1468.gr.htm.

Blouin, A. S., & Brent, N. J. (1994). Managing a culturally diverse staff: Legal considerations. *Journal of Nursing Administration*, 24(11), 13.

Blouin, A. S., & Brent, N. J. (1996). Downsizing and potential discrimination based on age. *Journal of Nursing Administration*, 26(11), 3.

Calfee, B. E. (1996, February). Labor laws working to protect you. *Nursing*, p. 34.

Chalmers v. Talon, No. 95-2594 (4th Cir. 1996).

Civil Rights Act, Title VII, U.S.C.A. (1964).

Civil Rights Division, Department of Justice. (1998). *Protecting the rights of all our nation's people*. Washington, DC: Author.

Conners, R. L. (1996, Winter). Law at work. 2(1). Online: http://www.law@work.com.

Conners, R. L. (1996, Spring). Law at work. *Sexual Harassment*, 2(2). Online: http://www.law@work. com.

Corbett, & Lane. (1995, April). *Employment Law Update*. Online: http://www.cklaw.com.

EEOC v. Townley Manufacturing, 859 F. 2d 610 (9th Cir. 1988).

Fair Labor Standards Act, Amended, 29 U.S.C. § 201 (1938).

Farpella-Crosby v. Horizon Health Care, 97 F. 3d 803 (Tex. 1996).

Fiesta, J. (1997, January). Labor law update: Part one. *Nursing Management*, p. 27.

Goodhouse v. Magnolia Hospital, 92 F. 3d 248 (5th Cir. 1996).

Heenam, Althen, & Roles. Newsletter. (1996a, August/September) Online: http://www.harlaw.com/newsletter.

Heenam, Althen, & Roles. Newsletter. (1996b, October/November). Online: http://www.harlaw.com/newsletter.

Heenam, Althen, & Roles. Newsletter. (1997, May/June). Online: http://www.harlaw.com/newsletter.

Howard v. North Mississippi Medical Center, 939 F. Supp. 505 (1996).

Kim v. The Southland Corp. Arlington HRC, Nos. 93-161-E and 93-195-E (1995).

Legal Shark. (1998). *The Family and Medical Leave Act*. Nolo Press. Online: http://www.legalshark.com/fmla/html.

Lindell, A. R. (1986, May/June). Legal and Ethical Issues: Clinical contractual agreements: Liability or blessing? *Journal of Professional Nursing*, p 138.

Little Forest Medical Center of Akron v. Ohio Civil Rights Commission, 631 N.E.2d 1068 (1993).

Long v. First Union Corp. of Virginia, E.D. VA, 68 FEP Cases 917, 1996.

Madel v. FCI Marketing, Inc., 116 F. 3d 1247 (8th Cir. 1997).

Murphy, S. S. (1995). *Legal handbook for Texas nurses* (p. 168). Austin, TX: University of Texas Press.

Neubs, H. P. (1994). Sexual harassment: A concern for nursing administrators. *Journal of Nursing Administration*, 24(5), 47.

New York Employment Law Forum (1998). *New York Employment Law*. [On-line]. Available: http://www.emplaw.com/lawtocz.html.

Odima v. Westin Tucson Hotel, No. 94-15839 (Ca. 9 1995).

Paskind, M. (1998, February). Beware: The dreaded GGG's have struck again. *Albuquerque Business Journal*. Online: http//www.abjournal.com.biz/pask/pask2-16.html.

Pelfrey, S., & Theisen, B. A. (1995, July/August). Independent contractor arrangements and IRS audits. *Journal of Nursing Administration*, 25(7/8) 63.

Repa, B. K. (1998a). *Computers and e-mail on the job: They're watching you*. Nolo Press. Online: http://www.nolo.com.

Repa, B. K. (1998b). *The Fair Labor Standards Act: Your right to get paid*. Nolo Press. Online: http://www.nolo.com.

Swart, J. C. (1996, July/August). Employment discrimination experiences of registered nurses. *Journal of Nursing Administration*, 26, 37.

Tammello, A. D. (1996, November). Liability for allowing hostile work environment. *The Regan Report on Nursing Law*, 37(6), p. 1.

UAW v. Johnson Controls, Inc., 55 Sup. Ct. 365 (1991).

U.S. Department of Health and Human Services. (1990). *Office of Civil Rights fact sheet*. Washington, DC: Author.

U.S. Department of Labor, Employment Standards Administration Wage and Hour Division. (1993). *The Family and Medical Leave Act of 1993* (Fact sheet No. 028). Washington, DC: Author.

U.S. Department of Labor. (1997, February 2). Labor Department Celebrates Family Medical Leave Act with Release of Print and Radio Public Service Announcements. [Press Release]. Washington, DC: Author.

U.S. Department of Labor, Bureau of Labor Statistics. (1998). *The employment situation news release: Employment situation summary*. Washington, DC: Author.

U.S. Department of Justice. (1990). *Americans with Disabilities Act*. [On-line]. Available: http://www.usdoj.gov/ert/ada/adahoml.htm anchor1151035.

U.S. Equal Employment Opportunity Commission. (1967). *Age Discrimination in Employment Act of 1967*. Washington, DC: Author.

U.S. Equal Employment Opportunity Commission. (1995). *Sexual harassment statistics: 1990-1995*. Washington, DC: Author.

U.S. Equal Employment Opportunity Commission. (1997a). *The ADA: Your responsibilities as an employer*. Washington, DC: Author.

U.S. Equal Employment Opportunity Commission. (1997b). *Facts about national origin discrimination*. Washington, DC: Author.

U.S. Equal Employment Opportunity Commission. (1997c). *Facts about pregnancy discrimination*. Washington, DC: Author.

U.S. Equal Employment Opportunity Commission. (1997d). *Facts about race/color discrimination*. Washington, DC: Author.

U.S. Equal Employment Opportunity Commission. (1997e). *Facts about religious discrimination*. Washington, DC: Author.

U.S. Equal Employment Opportunity Commission. (1997f). *Facts about sexual harassment discrimination*. Washington, DC: Author.

U.S. Equal Employment Opportunity Commission. (1997g). *U.S. Equal Employment Opportunity Commission issues guidance on application of EEO laws to contingent workers*. Washington, DC: Author.

U.S. Equal Employment Opportunity Commission. (1998). *Facts about the ADA*. Washington, DC: Author.

Valentin, I. (1997, August). Women's Educational Equity Act Title IX: A brief history. *Family Resource Center Digest*. Online: http://www.edc.org/womensequity/pubs/digest/digest-title9.html.

SUGGESTED READINGS

U.S. Department of Justice, Civil Rights Division. (1998, February). *Activities and programs*. Washington, DC: Author.

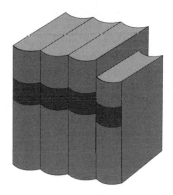

Chapter 14

MANAGED CARE
AND THE LAW

Susan Sportsman
Ana M. Valadez

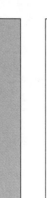

KEY WORDS

Apparent Agency
Appeals Process for
   Utilization Review
Capitation
Case Rate
Cost Containment
Credentialing
Diagnostic Related
   Groups (DRGs)
Direct Liability
Enterprise Liability
Gatekeeper
Generations of Managed
   Care
Health Maintenance
   Organization (HMO)
Health Mandates
Health Plan Employee
   Data and Information
   Setup (HEDIS)

Indirect Liability
Managed Care
Medical Necessity
Ostensible Agency
Oversight
Payer
Per Member, Per Month
   (pmpm)
Preferred Provider
   Organization (PPO)
Primary Care Provider
   (PCP)
Quality of Care Program
Regulatory Bodies
Respondeat Superior
Risk Sharing
Utilization Review
Vertical Integration
Virtual System

OBJECTIVES

Upon completion of this chapter, the reader will be able to:
- Discuss the impetus for and development of managed care.
- Evaluate the principles of liability that may occur as a result of managed care.
- Review state and federal health care mandates for managed care that result from actual or potential legislation.

INTRODUCTION— HISTORICAL CONTEXT

Since the early 1980s, the health care delivery system in the United States has been significantly altered by managed care. Its impact has clearly changed the roles and responsibilities of professional nurses, requiring them to integrate business principles into the clinical aspects of practice. As a result, the legal principles that govern nursing practice have been expanded. This chapter reviews the concept of managed care and its effect on health care and considers actions to ensure that cost-effective care is provided. In addition, this chapter emphasizes the legal implications of various strategies inherent in managed care.

IMPETUS FOR THE DEVELOPMENT OF MANAGED CARE

During the first half of the twentieth century, any patient who needed care paid the provider (physician, hospital, or clinic) directly after the service was rendered. In the 1950s, health care insurance became an increasingly popular employment benefit. The patient and/or employer purchased insurance from a company that was then obligated to reimburse the provider retrospectively for care through a fee-for-service mechanism. Because of the support of health care insurance, patients were financially responsible only for premiums and any deductibles that might have been required by their benefit plan. Access to insurance increased the number of citizens who could afford health care (particularly illness-related services), it is reducing the need for patients to be concerned about the specific charges they incurred.

Increased access to insurance was one of the factors that influenced the continuing escalation in health care costs in the 1970s and 1980s. However, increased access was not the only driving force. Other related influences had an effect on spiraling cost, including: (1) rising expectations of the consumer, provider, and supplier regarding health care; (2) emphasis on acute care rather than on illness prevention; (3) excess capac-

ity of hospitals and other providers; (4) inefficient management of health care resources; (5) high-priced technology; (6) escalating malpractice insurance rates and associated defensive medical practices; (7) antitrust regulations in the health care industry; and (8) the aging of the population.

HEALTH CARE COST INFLATION IN RELATION TO OUTCOMES

By the late 1980s, health care inflation had become a major economic problem for the United States. Inflation in health care far exceeded the gross national product (GNP) and threatened the economic competitiveness of this country. As a means of controlling costs in Medicare, **diagnostic related groups (DRGs)** were instituted in 1982. This reimbursement approach, which paid a designated amount for a specific diagnosis regardless of the charges by the providers, did little to slow the escalation of health care costs. Wyld (1996) noted that since the mid-1970s, health care inflation has mostly outpaced, often "out-raced," the overall inflation rate in the United States. As a result, health care administrators and providers were able to focus on building revenue rather than on controlling costs. As long as insurers would pay whatever the provider charged, caregivers could not be expected to voluntarily reduce their fees.

Spending a significant portion of the nation's GNP on health care might have been palatable had the outcomes of that care been excellent. However, despite significant advances in the technical aspects of care, the United States has not been the leader in many markers of good health for citizens. For example, in 1996, the life expectancies for men in the United States were below those in England, France, Switzerland, Canada, and Japan. The life expectancies of U.S. women, although higher than men, were below those of French, Swiss, Canadian, and Japanese women (Kalisch, 1996). In addition, the life expectancy of various minority groups in the United States is less than the overall average (U.S. Department of Health and Human Services, 1992).

There was also wide variation in the way

health care was delivered in different parts of the United States. This inconsistency may reflect a lack of use of scientific research in clinical decision-making. Dr. David Eddy of Duke University noted that 80 to 90 percent of clinical decisions are not based on controlled studies (Berkowitz, 1994). Wennberg (1994) found that use of surgical procedures varied greatly depending on the region of the country where they were performed. He also found that greater hospital bed capacity in a geographic area was associated with more dollars spent per person. Additionally, he discovered that higher levels of spending on outpatient services in a geographic area were not associated with a decrease in spending on inpatient care. Clearly, there was evidence that the costly health care in the United States may not have met the needs of those receiving services or produced the outcomes desired.

INITIATION OF MANAGED CARE

THE GOAL OF MANAGED CARE

As costs escalated, buyers of health care—including employers, various types of private insurance companies, and the federal government through Medicare and Medicaid programs—recognized they could not continue to pay for care as it was being delivered. They wanted value for the dollar spent and recognized that value in health care could be defined by the following equation:

$$\text{Value} = \text{Access} + \text{Quality}/\text{Cost}$$
$$(\text{Berkowitz, 1994})$$

In an effort to identify strategies to achieve this equation, the concept of managed care was born.

To the layman, managed care is synonymous with a **health maintenance organization (HMO)**. In reality, the term *managed care* covers a broad spectrum of arrangements for health care delivery and financing. A managed care plan can range from a closed-panel HMO with a staff and its own facilities to a traditional indemnity insurance policy that imposed utilization review protocols and requires policyholders to obtain prior authorization for selected services. Managed care plans may also include **preferred provider organizations (PPOs)**, point-of-service (POS) plans, and direct contracting arrangements between employers and providers. Regardless of the structure of the financing organization, each uses mechanisms for making health care more responsive to cost, consumer satisfaction, and health outcome (O'Neil, 1998). Increasingly common to all these organizational structures is that they have assumed some or all of the financial risks for providing care (American Nurses Association [ANA], 1998). Box 14–1 describes each of the payer organizations that are likely to use managed care strategies.

Managed care plans have been credited with controlling the medical cost of inflation in the late 1980s, as these plans have penetrated various geographic markets in the United States. For example, traditional fee-for-services plans had 52 percent of the health care market in 1992 but had fallen to just 15 percent by 1997, as managed care plans grew to 85 percent of the market (Blakely, 1998). The methods used to achieve the desired result have evolved over time.

GENERATIONS OF MANAGED CARE

The use of particular managed care strategies is more prevalent in some parts of the country than in others, often as a result of the length of time managed care has been in existence. The various stages that represent the evolution of managed care are described as the **generations of managed care**.

When managed care is first instituted in a geographic location, health care costs are considered only in the context of the utilization and price of the services offered. This approach is known as *first generation managed care*. The emphasis on utilization and price alone often results in an adversarial relationship between the payer and the provider. This, of course, spills over into the relation-

BOX 14-1

TYPES OF PAYER ORGANIZATIONS

- **Health Maintenance Organization (HMO)** — An entity that provides or arranges for the provision of coverage of health services needed by a plan member for fixed, prepaid premiums. HMOs are the most restrictive type of managed care plans, using gatekeepers, copayments, and utilization review stringently to control costs. HMOs are the second most common type of managed care health plans, comprising 30 percent of the total health insurance market (Blakely, 1998).
- **Preferred Provider Organization (PPO)** — The most common type of managed care plan, with 35 percent of the total market. These organizations offer patients significantly lower deductibles and coinsurance rates than they can get under conventional plans if the patients use physicians and hospitals that are a part of the PPO's network of providers. PPOs also allow enrollees to receive services from providers outside the network, but at a higher price than from those in the network (Blakely, 1998).
- **Point-of-Service (POS)** — Often known as HMO/PPO hybrids or open-ended HMOs. Enrollees may choose to receive services from providers who are not members of the plan's network as well as from those who are. When enrollees use network providers, a POS plan functions like an HMO. When they use other providers, those providers are paid on a fee-for-service basis and enrollees are responsible for deductibles and coinsurance payments. The POS is the third most common managed care plan, comprising 20 percent of the market (Blakely, 1998).
- **Utilization Review Organizations** — Some firms provide the utilization review function for other insurance companies. They may provide this service for the care of all the members of the plan or only for specific portions of the care, such as psychiatric or pharmaceutical services, where costs are typically difficult to control.

ship of each with the patient. Often both the payer and the provider communicate to the patient, directly or indirectly, that health care is not available because of the policies of the other. This may negatively influence the care delivered. As managed care evolves in a geographic area, *second generation managed care* becomes more prevalent. Under this philosophy, not only are utilization and price important, but access to care is also highlighted. As the market matures further, moving into *third generation managed care*, the quality of care (and the associated definition

of quality) also becomes important (Kalisch, 1996).

Third generation managed care is currently found in the areas of the country where managed care has been for some time. However, it is unclear whether the managed care market in these areas will continue to evolve into a fourth generation, where societal value and the health status of patients will be equally as important as quality, utilization, and price. Box 14–2 illustrates the concept of managed care generations via equations.

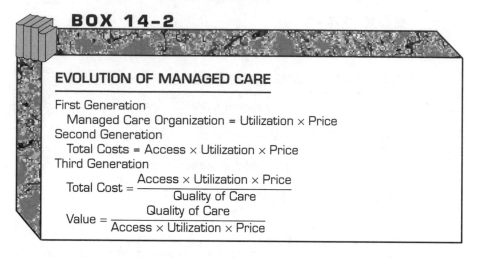

BOX 14-2

EVOLUTION OF MANAGED CARE

First Generation
Managed Care Organization = Utilization × Price
Second Generation
Total Costs = Access × Utilization × Price
Third Generation

$$\text{Total Cost} = \frac{\text{Access} \times \text{Utilization} \times \text{Price}}{\text{Quality of Care}}$$

$$\text{Value} = \frac{\text{Quality of Care}}{\text{Access} \times \text{Utilization} \times \text{Price}}$$

INTEGRATION OF PAYER AND PROVIDER

In recent years, there has been significant blurring of the lines between payer and provider organizations, generally through vertical integration or a virtual system of care. In **vertical integration**, a single entity owns or controls both the provider components and the insurance business. Organizations such as a staff-model HMO or a provider-owned delivery system provide a full spectrum of management, professional, and institutional services. In a **virtual system** of care, managed care companies contract for services with physician groups, hospital systems, home nursing agencies, and other health care providers (O'Neil, 1998). In either case, partnerships are formed to maximize the financial incentives of managed care. Box 14–3 provides definitions for such partnerships.

PURPOSE OF MANAGED CARE

The purpose of managed care is to ensure that the services provided to patients are necessary, efficiently provided, and appropriately priced. In general, managed care is designed to accomplish at least one of the following four objectives:

- Reduce the total cost of care, for example, by using case rate reimbursement strategies.
- Reduce the unit cost of care, for example, by requiring the use of a less expensive but equally effective medication to treat a medical condition.
- Maximize the effectiveness of care so that less will ultimately be needed.
- Reduce the need for intensive (and expensive) service by providing intervention before there is a need for intensive care and by providing increased alternative care options (B. Libby, personal communication, 1991).

FINANCING MECHANISMS IN MANAGED CARE

Cost containment, including cost sharing and price negotiation, although not the only purpose of managed care, is certainly its initial focus (Boland, 1993, p. 5). In traditional fee-for-service reimbursement mechanisms, the provider is paid a usual and customary fee. This is a standard fee in a specific geographic area based on the credentials of the provider. This approach provides little control when fees in a particular area are universally raised.

BOX 14-3

HEALTH CARE PARTNERSHIPS

- **Independent Practice Association (IPA)** — A physician organization composed of a loose network of primary and specialty physicians who maintain individual practices in terms of both autonomy and overhead. The IPA provides an entity that can contract with the physicians on an independent contractor, rather than an employer, basis. An IPA may accept full-risk physician capitation or discounted fee-for-service physician payments. This approach is especially suitable for solo practitioners and small groups because it has the potential for accessing sophisticated fiscal/managed care systems and provides a unified contracting option for payers.

- **Group Practice** — A medical group whose member physicians are employees of that group. Each physician is typically paid on an individual production basis. This approach has the advantage of a central administration, thereby reducing individual costs.

- **Medical Foundation** — A tax-exempt, nonprofit corporation that is either an affiliate or subsidiary of a hospital. The foundation owns and operates the facilities and equipment, employs all nonphysician personnel, and can contract directly with patients and third-party payers, billing in the name of the foundations. There is an associated physician entity that employs the individual physician and contracts with the foundation to provide physician services.

- **Physician-Hospital Organization (PHO)** — An entity jointly owned by a hospital and a physician group. The PHO contracts with hospitals and physicians for the delivery of health services to payers who have contracted with the PHO. The purpose of such an arrangement is to create an integrated delivery system of participating, independent providers. The PHO usually provides contract negotiation, marketing services to purchasers and third-party payers, management of risk through utilization review and quality control, financial incentives for controlling costs, and assistance in increasing operational efficiency of the hospital and physician practices to enable the parties to maximize revenues.

- **Management Services Organization (MSO)** — An organization that provides administrative support to a physician entity, either individual physicians or groups. The MSO is legally separate from any physician group, but owns the facilities, equipment, and supplies and employs all nonphysician personnel. The MSO contracts with the physician entity to provide supplies, personnel, and all necessary administrative services. The MSO is compensated by a fixed fee, budget, or percentage arrangement.

Source: Rogers, 1998.

DISCOUNTS FROM USUAL AND CUSTOMARY FEES

To assume more control over the process, payers may negotiate discounts from usual and customary fees. The payer contracts to pay the provider a discounted fee for particular services. In return, the payer may expect an increased number of referrals from that payer. A more stringent cost containment approach includes the payer's identification of the maximum allowable fee payable for a service regardless of the charge by the provider. The fee structure is published prior to entering the contract. Unfortunately, in the past, none of these containment approaches appreciably slowed the demand for health care services (Boland, 1993, p. 5).

THE CONCEPT OF RISK IN MANAGED CARE

As a further means of controlling costs, payers attempt to link patients' and providers' use of health care services directly to the associated cost. This relationship approach allows providers to share the financial risk with the payer for the care that is provided during a given length of time. Various types of prepaid reimbursement mechanisms, such as case rates and capitation, are examples of this approach. In general terms, the provider is given a budget for a particular case and must provide care under those financial parameters. If the care costs less than the budget, the provider will make a profit. If the care costs more than was budgeted, the provider will lose money. Under these circumstances, in order to be financially viable, providers must primarily care for patients who do not require long or expensive treatment beyond that which can be covered by the budget. For the same reason, it is not in the providers' best financial interest to care for high-risk patients. This reimbursement methodology requires the provider to accurately assess the aggregate costs of care for groups of patients assigned to them in order to successfully negotiate a risk-sharing contract.

CASE RATES

A **case rate** is a predetermined rate paid to a provider for a specified level of care. Case rates are usually determined according to the units of service offered, such as days of treatment or episodes of care. Diagnostic related groups (DRGs) are case rates that are paid according to the diagnosis rather than units of service. For example, a hospital may receive a certain amount from a payer such as Medicare for a designated surgical proce-

dure, regardless of the hospital's actual cost of caring for the patient.

CAPITATION

Capitation is a specified dollar amount established to cover the cost of health services delivered for a group of individuals for a specific time period. In most situations, a provider (usually known as a **primary care provider**, or **PCP**) will be assigned to a group of members in the health plan. The provider is then responsible for providing or arranging for any care these members may require. The reimbursement is prospective and paid as a **per member, per month (pmpm)** rate. Again, if the cost of the needed care for all the assigned members in a designated period is less than the negotiated contracted fee, the provider makes a profit. If the cost of the aggregate care is more than the contracted amount, the provider is still obligated to provide or arrange for the care, even if money will be lost, hence the notion of **risk sharing**.

MEDICAL NECESSITY

When providers are financially responsible for the care of a group of members wholly or in part, it is no longer in their best interest economically to provide the most intensive level of care for as long as possible. However, providers must be sure that their economic interest does not result in denying needed care. Therefore, there must be a mechanism to determine the **medical necessity** of the care provided. To accomplish this, PCPs serve as a gatekeeper for all care of members assigned to them, giving permission for care based on medical necessity. This gatekeeping responsibility is particularly necessary if the service is to be offered by a provider other than the PCP.

Capitation requires the provider to have more financial risk than any other reimbursement mechanism, even case rates or DRGs, because of the length of time for which the provider is responsible for the health care of the member. For this reason, it is particularly important to emphasize health promotion activities for members and to avoid a large number of high-risk patients in the member pool.

Capitation is a sophisticated approach to contracting for providers; however, it has had a documented effect of reducing the cost of care. According to Wyld (1996), patients under capitated health plans have 40 percent fewer inpatient admissions than those under traditional, fee-for-service reimbursement plans. In southern California, where the managed care market is extensive, inpatient utilization has dropped by as much as 50 percent since capitation became a predominant reimbursement mechanism (Wyld, 1996).

DELIVERY METHODS USED IN MANAGED CARE

Regardless of the type of organization involved or the specific reimbursement strategy used, managed care alters the decision-making of providers by interjecting a complex system of financial incentives, penalties, and administrative procedures into the provider-patient relationship. Effective managed care delivery systems control quality and use of services as well as clinical cost and operational expenses. Specific managed care interventions might include:

- Using providers proficient in managed care strategies
- Emphasizing case management to ensure continuity of care
- Decreasing the number of providers available to members to ensure control by the payer (use of core groups)
- Increasing the use of intermediate practitioners, such as nurse practitioners, to deliver primary care
- Regulating the average length of treatment by decreasing admissions to acute inpatient facilities and by reducing patient length of stays
- Evaluating medical (and nursing) practices and limiting reimbursement to those procedures and practices that show evidence of effectiveness
- Disseminating statistics on cost, quality, and outcomes to providers and consumers

- Soliciting competitive bids among providers
- Initiating practice management strategies, such as practice guidelines, clinical pathways, or care maps
- Implementing utilization management strategies, such as precertification and prospective, concurrent, or retrospective review

As a last resort, services may be rationed by denying access to health care to persons who cannot afford to pay or by limiting access to services or procedures regardless of eligibility or ability to pay. Although rationing does have significant legal and ethical implications, it does serve to reduce the cost of care.

Table 14–1 categorizes managed care strategies according to the specific objective to be accomplished and by the group, either payer or provider, that may implement the strategy.

MANAGED CARE LIABILITY

The legal implications of managed care evolved during the 1990s. Initially, the provider primarily held the legal risks; however, the **payer** (insurance companies, managed care companies, and/or employers) exerted more influence on the care authorized for patients. This influence affected legal risks associated with untoward outcomes, resulting in providers and patients becoming more and more resentful about the lack of accountability of payers. This influence has also stimulated the emergence of different theories of managed care liability that may be classified as direct liability, indirect liability, and the enterprise liability.

DIRECT LIABILITY

Direct liability holds the managed care organization responsible for the results of care unduly influenced by cost containment measures, such as improper denial of care or financial incentives to providers that result

TABLE 14–1. MANAGED CARE STRATEGIES

	Strategy	Used By
COST REDUCTION STRATEGIES	Case management	Payer, Provider
	Core groups of providers	Payer
	Decreased variations in care and diagnosis (practice guidelines)	Payer, Provider
	Discounts from usual and customary fees	Payer
	Employee cost sharing	Payer
	Limiting access via precertification	Payer
	Concurrent review	Payer, Provider
	Maximum allowable fees	Payer
	Reduction in access via a gatekeeper	Payer
	Retrospective review	Payer
	Second opinions	Payer
	Sharing risks via case rates (DRGs or per diem)	Payer
	Capitation (PCPs, carveouts)	Payer
	Using nonphysician providers	Payers
MAXIMIZING EFFECTIVENESS	Emphasizing and reimbursing for prevention	Payer, Provider
	Provider credentialing	Payer, Provider
	Provider privileging	Payer, Provider
	Outcomes management research	Payer, Provider
	Reducing variations in care via practice guidelines	Payer, Provider
REDUCTION IN INTENSIVE CARE	Developing alternative treatment that reflects the full continuum of care:	Provider
	Mobile crisis teams	
	Ambulatory care facilities	
	Telephone triage	
	Day hospitals	
	Subacute units	
	Home care	
	Rehabilitation units	Provider
	Evaluation of effectiveness of alternative treatment options	Payer, Provider
	Use of best practices and benchmarking	Payer, Provider
	Emphasis on primary care and prevention	Payer, Provider
	Facilitation of early diagnosis, treatment, and maintenance of the chronically ill in a noninstitutional setting	Payer, Provider

Source: Sportsman, S., & Hawley, L. (1998, January). *Case management in a managed care environment.* Web Based Course offered by University On Line /Health Executives Inc.

in a denial (Rogers, 1998). For example, as previously discussed, imposition of case rate, DRGs, or capitation methods of payment may encourage providers to ration services inappropriately, just as traditional fee-for-service reimbursement mechanisms may stimulate overuse of medical care. If cost containment policies stimulate cost-effective care by reducing wasteful spending, it is appropriate. If it discourages providers from prescribing necessary treatment, it is abusive.

Managed care organizations may also have direct liability if they fail to properly credential plan providers (Rogers, 1998). They must evaluate the credentials of providers in terms of education, training, experience, current fitness to practice, and past malpractice claims in the same way hospitals and other health care organizations have done for years. This evaluation must not only be done when the contract between the managed care organization and the provider is initiated, but also on a periodic basis thereafter.

The managed care organization may also be directly liable if there is a breach of contract, breach of warranty, bad faith, misrepresentation, or fraud (Rogers, 1998). Despite the slightly different legal definition of these concepts, in each the managed care organization is liable for failure to fulfill promises made to members in plan documents or in contracts with providers. Two legal cases illustrate this point.

In a 1997 landmark ruling by the California Supreme Court (*Engella v. The Permanente Medical Group*), the court found that the medical group had committed fraud in the administration of its arbitration program by unconscionable delays in resolution of disputed claims (Rogers, 1998). In another 1997 case, *McEvoy v. Group Health Cooperative of Eau Claire*, the Supreme Court of Wisconsin upheld the liability of the managed care organization for breach of contract. In this case, the medical director of the HMO initially authorized an out-of-network referral for inpatient treatment for a patient with anorexia nervosa. After 6 weeks of treatment, the director denied further care over the recommendation of both the psychiatrist and psychologist treating the patient, even though the patient had an additional 4 weeks for benefits remaining (Rogers, 1998).

INDIRECT LIABILITY

A managed care organization may be held indirectly liable because of its relationship with the provider of care. **Indirect liability** may be through the legal principle of *respondeat superior*, when the provider of care works directly for the managed care organization. It may also be through the principle of **ostensible agency**, or **apparent agency**. Under this principle, the managed care organization is liable for the negligence of plan providers who appear to the patient to be the agent of the managed care organization, even though they do not directly work for the company (Rogers, 1998).

ENTERPRISE LIABILITY

The most recent theory of liability to be used in managed care cases is that of **enterprise liability**. Enterprise liability grew out of product liability claims against manufacturers. The three principles in support for imposing strict liability against an enterprise include the need for (1) manufacturers to have more power than the consumers, (2) the risk to the manufacturer to be spread by insurance, and (3) the cost of safety to be a part of the cost of producing the product (Rogers, 1998). These principles seem to apply to managed care organizations as well as traditional manufacturing firms. Clearly, the payer is much more powerful than the individual consumer, in part because of the size of the organization and also because of the consumer's reluctance to challenge health care organizations. Managed care companies all carry liability insurance. This cost of insurance, as well as the cost of risk management activities, is included in the cost to the consumer.

CURRENT MANAGED CARE LEGISLATION

Managed care strategies have been shown to reduce the cost of health care. However, the public's perception of its negative impact on the quality of care has been significant. Drew Altman, president of the Kaiser Family Foundation, an independent nonprofit foundation that conducts research on health policy issues, notes that "Managed care is winning in the health care market place, but it is in danger of losing the battle for public opinion" (Blakely, 1998). In response to a Time/CNN poll, 75 percent of Americans think the health insurance system needs reform and 40 percent think it is in crisis (Ivins, 1998). As a result of the negative feelings toward managed care, there have also been increasing state and federal mandates to regulate the impact of managed care on quality of care.

STATE MANDATES

Because insurance is regulated at the state level, state legislatures were the first to respond to the public's concerns regarding managed care. From 1993 to 1998, state legislatures instituted various **health mandates** requiring insurance companies to implement consumer protection strategies. These mandates most commonly included a requirement to pay for a minimum hospital stay following childbirth and a guarantee for coverage for care provided by certain specialists and for emergency room care. According to the Blue Cross and Blue Shield Association, the national association of independent Blue Cross and Blue Shield companies, the number of state health mandates jumped nearly 20 percent to 1043 nationwide from 1993 to 1997 (Blakely, 1998). For example, during this time, Maryland passed 40 health care mandates, more than any other state, followed by Florida and Minnesota with 37 each, California with 33, and New York and Texas with 30 each. Idaho and Washington, DC, have the fewest health mandates; each has passed seven apiece (Blakely, 1998).

FEDERAL MANDATES

The President's Advisory Commission on Consumer Protection and Quality in the Health Care Industry was created in March 1997. The Commission developed a Consumer Bill of Rights and Responsibilities that addressed issues of information disclosure, choice of providers and plans, access to emergency services, participation in treat-

ment decisions, respect and nondiscrimination, confidentiality of health information, complaints and appeals, and consumer responsibilities.

The Commission also developed a report entitled *Quality First: Better Health Care for All Americans* in March 1998. The report documented quality problems in the areas of avoidable errors, underutilization of services, overuse of services, and variation in services. It included more than 50 recommendations to advance core aims for improvement as follows:

- Reducing underlying causes of illness, injury, and disability
- Expanding research on new treatments and evidence of effectiveness
- Ensuring the appropriate use of health care services
- Reducing health care errors
- Increasing patient participation in the care
- Addressing oversupply and undersupply of health care resources (ANA, 1998)

Stimulated by the work of the Commission and other concerns about managed care, in 1998 the 105th Congress considered bills that would institute federal health care mandates. According to Blakely (1998), Congress has introduced about 100 bills related to health care and more are being drafted. Box 14–4 outlines the major proposals currently under review, and Table 14–2 outlines some of the less comprehensive initiatives before Congress.

REDUCING LEGAL LIABILITY

Given the complexity of the health care delivery system and the blurring of lines between the payer and the provider, there is a real likelihood of legal liability for both payer and provider in today's environment. A network risk management approach is the safest course of action for reducing this liability. The following principles provide protection for both payers and providers:

- Institute a well-developed credentialing and privileging process.
- Develop a clear utilization review process.

(Text continued on page 251)

BOX 14-4

CURRENT COMPREHENSIVE MANAGED CARE LEGISLATIVE INITIATIVES

Patient Safety Act (H.R. 1165 and S. 2055), 1998

The Patient Safety Act was originally drafted by the American Nurses Association as a component of its "Every Patient Deserves a Nurse" campaign. The Patient Safety Act was introduced at the federal level in 1996 in the 104th Congress. The provisions of both the House and the Senate versions were drafted as conditions for participation in Medicare by health care institutions. It would require, at a minimum, health care institutions to make public specific information on the following staffing level, mix, and patient outcomes:

- The number of registered nurses (RNs) providing direct care.
- Numbers of unlicensed personnel used to provide direct patient care.
- Average number of patients per registered nurse providing direct patient care.
- Patient mortality rates.
- Incidence of adverse patient care incidents.
- Methods used for determining and adjusting staffing levels and patient care.
- Data regarding complaints filed with state agencies, HCFA, or accrediting agencies and related results

The Act also addressed the effect of mergers and acquisitions among health care institutions by requiring institutions to report to the Secretary of the Department of Health and Human Services regarding the impact on accessibility in:

- Primary, acute services and emergency services.
- Services for mothers and children.
- Services for the elderly.
- Services for the poor, uninsured, ethnic minority population, women, disabled persons, and lesbian and gay communities (ANA, 1998).

Patients' Bill of Rights Act (H.R. 3605 and S.B. 1891), 1998

This legislation writes into law the proposals of patients' rights developed by the President's Advisory Commission on Consumer Protection and Quality in the Health Care Industry. In addition to incorporating the recommendations of this committee into legislation, it also:

- Authorizes states to let patients sue employer-sponsored health plan.
- Requires a 48-hour minimum hospital stay for mastectomies and 24 hours for lymph node dissection.
- Provides whistleblower protection for providers.
- Provides antidiscrimination protection for health care providers on the basis of type of licensure.
- Allows a limited POS option by the HMO for employees who are offered only a closed-panel HMO; the employer would not be required to contribute to this option.
- Provides for adequacy of the provider network in terms of number, distribution, and variety of providers.

(Continued)

BOX 14-4

CURRENT COMPREHENSIVE MANAGED CARE LEGISLATIVE INITIATIVES (Continued)

- Requires a process for seriously ill individuals to select a specialist as a PCP and for accessing necessary specialty care without impediments.
- Allows women direct access to obstetrics/gynecology (OB/GYN) care and to designate an OB/GYN physician as a PCP.
- Provides access to pediatric specialists for children.
- Protects against disruptions in care, particularly with pregnancy, terminal illness, and institutionalization because of a change in plan or provider's network status.
- Provides access to emergency room care without prior authorization in a situation a prudent layperson would believe to be an emergency.
- Allows a process for certain plan members to participate in approved clinical trials, covering the routine patient costs associated with the trials.
- Provides for access to medications not on a plan's drug formulary when medically indicated.
- Prohibits discrimination of patients based on race, color, ethnicity, national origin, religion, sex, age, mental or physical disability, sexual orientation, genetic information, or source of payment.
- Provides specialized services related to prevention, detection, and treatment of the human immunodeficiency virus (HIV) and related illness, mental health services, and substance abuse services.

The legislation would also add whistleblower protections to Medicare law to protect health care providers who report or voice concerns about poor staffing from facing retribution. A violation of this provision would make the institution ineligible for Medicare participation (ANA, 1998).

Patient Access to Responsible Care Act (PARCA) (H.R. 1415 and S. 644)
This legislation outlines more than 300 new federal mandates on health insurance plans. Important among these are the following:

- Allowing patients to sue their managed care health plans and their employer who sponsors the plan for medical malpractice.
- Banning preauthorization requirements for emergency room care, or adoption of the prudent layperson threshold for defining a medical emergency.
- Guaranteeing access to a medical specialist when recommended by the treating physician, as well as a requirement that all health networks offer an option more flexible than an HMO.
- Limiting the ability of health plans to exclude doctors or certain other health care specialists.
- Creating independent grievance panels for patients and doctors to appeal adverse decisions by a managed care health plan (Blakely, 1998).

TABLE 14–2.
LESS COMPREHENSIVE LEGISLATION BEFORE CONGRESS

Bill Name and Number	Topic	Need	Summary of Provisions
H.R. 2174 S. 743	Equity in Prescription Insurance and Contraceptive Coverage Act of 1997	50% of indemnity plans and PPOs, 20% of POS networks, and 7% of HMOs cover no contraceptive methods other than sterilization.	• Require insurers and health plans that cover FDA-approved prescription drugs and devices to also cover FDA-approved prescription contraceptive drugs and devices. • Require plans to cover contraceptive services if they provide benefits for other outpatient services.
H.R. 306 S. 89	Genetic discrimination	Stresses the importance of protecting consumers from being denied coverage because of genetic information.	• Prohibit all insurers from denying or canceling insurance or varying the terms and conditions of coverage on the basis of genetic information in any circumstance. • Prohibit insurers from requesting or requiring an individual to disclose genetic information. • Prohibit insurers from disclosing genetic information without prior written consent.
H.R. 2854	Follow-up care for mothers and newborns	Addresses "drive through" deliveries and amends 1996 law that requires health plans to cover minimum hospital stays of 48 hours for vaginal deliveries and 96 hours for cesarean sections unless provider and mother agree that an earlier discharge is desirable.	• When an early discharge occurs, the insurer must provide follow-up care. The site (home or another outpatient setting) and the provider (registered nurse, nurse practitioner, nurse midwife, physician's assistant, or physician) must be selected by the mother and care provided within 24–72 hours after discharge.

(Continued)

TABLE 14–2. LESS COMPREHENSIVE LEGISLATION BEFORE CONGRESS *(Continued)*

Bill Name and Number	Topic	Need	Summary of Provisions
H.R. 815 S. 356	Access to Medical Service Act of 1997	Establishes a definition of a prudent layperson.	• Require health plans to cover emergency services if the patient presents a condition that a prudent layperson could reasonably expect would result in serious impairment of health. • Prohibit plans from requiring that patients obtain prior authorization before seeking emergency care. • Establish coverage standards for out-of-plans emergency care. • Allow plans to establish reasonable cost-sharing differentials when a patient chooses an emergency setting or an out-of-plan setting over an in-plan setting. • Provide a process for coordination of post-stabilization care, requiring timely communications between insurers and provider. • Require plans to educate their members on emergency care coverage and the appropriate use of emergency medical services, including use of 911.
H.R. 135 S. 142 H.R. 616 S. 249 H.R. 164 S. 609	Breast Cancer Patient Protection Act Women's Health and Cancer Rights Act Reconstructive Breast Surgery Benefits Act	Bills are in response to health plans encouraging or requiring short length of stay or outpatient treatment for mastectomy.	• Provide a minimum stay following mastectomies. • Require plans to pay for reconstructive surgery following a mastectomy.

(Continued)

TABLE 14-2. LESS COMPREHENSIVE LEGISLATION BEFORE CONGRESS *(Continued)*

Bill Name and Number	Topic	Need	Summary of Provisions
H.R. 1515 S. 729	Expansion of Portability and Health Insurance Coverage Act	Addresses the needs of small businesses to purchase health insurance for employees cost effectively.	• Allow small businesses to band together to purchase insurance through trade, church, or business organization. The new purchasing groups would be exempt from state health and consumer protection laws.
H.R. 3342	Patient Safety and Health Care Whistleblower Protection Act	Addresses the issue of provider protection when speaking out against unsafe practices.	• Prohibits retaliation or discrimination against a health care worker who, acting in good faith, advocates on behalf of patients with respect to care: 1. Outlines effective enforcement 2. Provides protection against false claims by disgruntled employees 3. Provides realistic burden of proof 4. Ensures confidentiality of patients and employees

Sources: American Nurses Association. (1998, June). *Successes and challenges in the federal legislative arena, 105th Congress 1997–98 Kansas City, MO: Author.* Blakely, S. (1998, July). The backlash against managed care. *Nation's Business*, pp. 16–24.

- Clearly define the process of delegation of oversight, if necessary.
- Ensure that medical necessity is clearly documented.
- Develop a quality of care program.
- Protect against gatekeeper liability (Rogers, 1998).

CREDENTIALING AND PRIVILEGING PROCESS

Organizations responsible, directly or indirectly, for the care of patients are required by **regulatory bodies** (Medicare, Joint Commis-sion on Accreditation of Healthcare Organizations [JCAHO], and Health Plan Employee Data and Information Setup [HEDIS]) to document that providers are competent to deliver necessary care and are of sound health to do so. To meet this responsibility, each payer and/or provider organization must validate the education, training, and experience of individual providers. These providers can then be approved to practice within the organization if their credentials meet the criteria established by the company. This process is known as **credentialing**.

The organization must also indicate what specialized tasks individual providers may perform based on their level of education and experience. For example, the family practice physician may be privileged by a hospital to deliver babies but not to perform more highly specialized gynecologic surgical techniques the obstetrics and gynecology specialist might be allowed to provide. Providers must be reprivileged regularly, based on established peer review processes to ensure that their knowledge and skills remain current. Organizations that do not maintain a well-documented credentialing and privileging process for clinicians are at high risk for legal action.

UTILIZATION REVIEW PROCESS

A **utilization review** process includes procedures by which designated health care professionals in each payer or provider group evaluates the appropriateness, quality, and medical necessity of services provided. To avoid liability, the services are well defined. The utilization review (UR) personnel are licensed in appropriate disciplines, and their training regarding the specific utilization process of the organization is documented. In addition, the UR personnel should comply with the requirements of the American Board of Quality Assurance and Utilization Review or other certification group. Physician reviewers review only in the medical area in which they are credentialed to practice (e.g., a psychiatrist must review psychiatric cases).

The utilization review process outlines the roles of the treating provider, the provider(s) responsible for prospective or concurrent review, and the organization's UR committee. In most UR processes, nonphysicians (nurse, social worker, or other appropriately qualified person) initially review the case. If they believe there is no evidence of medical necessity for the recommended treatment, they refer the case to the reviewing physician. If, after discussing the case with the treatment provider the physician continues to believe there is no medical necessity for the care in question, the denial is communicated to the provider of care. If the provider disagrees with the reviewing physician's decision, appeal policies are in place that require that the disputed care be further reviewed by the UR committee for the managed care organization.

The **appeals process for utilization review** is timely and reasonable to protect the rights of the patient. It includes appropriate specialists and provides a mechanism to inform the patient and the physician of their right to appeal at each stage of the process. When there is an appeal, the following questions are considered:

1. Did the UR committee contact the treating physician to obtain the medical records?
2. Did the UR committee consult with the treating provider prior to denial of a claim?
3. Did the UR committee arrange for an independent examination by a physician who performs objective tests if the reviewing party disagrees with the treating provider's recommendation? (Rogers, 1998)

Utilization review policies and procedures clearly state the appeals process. The contract between the managed care organization and the treating physician obligates the physician to appeal a denial decision if he or she believes the recommended treatment is medically necessary for the patient. Perhaps most importantly, the process provides for adequate communication to patient and physicians, distinguishing between coverage recommendations by the managed care organization and medical decisions by the treating physician (Rogers, 1998).

DELEGATION OF OVERSIGHT

When a utilization review process is applied in a manner that affects the treating physician's medical judgment or a credentialing program fails to ensure the use of qualified providers, each of the parties in the process has a potential exposure to liability due to **oversight.** A party cannot escape liability by delegating the performance of its duties, such as utilization review, to an independent contractor (Rogers, 1998).

Many managed care organizations delegate the utilization review or credentialing function to another organization or individual. This process of delegation is spelled out in the contract that designates the responsibility to credential all health care providers and continually monitor them for competence. The delegation also includes a statement indicating that the delegating organization has the ultimate discretion to determine medical necessity and to interpret plan documents, specifically the availability of benefits. The delegating organization maintains general and professional liability insurance with adequate limits of coverage for performance of the UR function. In addition, physicians performing UR functions are named as additional insureds under the policy (Rogers, 1998).

ESTABLISHMENT OF MEDICAL NECESSITY

The payer or provider establishes criteria for admission, continued stay, and discharge for the level of care provided, as a means of clarifying medical necessity. Without a clear definition of medical necessity, the physician who approves the level of care may be held liable for decisions that are made. For example, in *Van Vactor v. Blue Cross Association* (1997), the physician was held ultimately responsible for the outcome of the care because the medical necessity clause of the contract was vague (Roberts, 1998).

QUALITY OF CARE PROGRAMS

A quality assessment program consistent with quality standards required by JCAHO or the standards of the National Committee on Quality Assurance (NCQA) and/or the American Association of Health Plans (AAHP) is required of both the payer and the provider. In a **quality of care program**, outcomes of care are documented in addition to the results of monitoring of process indicators. Many payers as well as providers are beginning to publish "report cards of care," which provide the consumer with data to use when making decisions about the quality of care offered by providers or managed care companies. An example of such a report card includes the NCQA's **Health Plan**

Employee Data and Information Setup (HEDIS). HEDIS data focus on outcomes and document effectiveness of managed care organizations in caring for patients, accessibility and member satisfaction, financial and provider stability, cost of care treatment options, use of services, and provider clinical utilization and risk management activities.

GATEKEEPER LIABILITY

The provider is required to document the medical rationale for approving or denying a course of treatment. To do otherwise is to increase the **gatekeeper** liability. As previously discussed, admission, discharge, and continued stay criteria and clinical pathways or other management guidelines may be used to document that recommendations meet approved standards of care.

The danger of gatekeeper liability is particularly great with prospective payments. An understanding of the financial incentives in capitated contracts illustrates these risks. In such plans, PCPs assume much of the responsibility for the utilization review function, because they determine whether or not the service is covered under the capitation rate that has been negotiated. In addition, if certain goals are met by avoiding unnecessary tests and procedures, the PCP may receive financial incentive payments. As more citizens participate in managed care plans, there have been increasing concerns about incentive plans that tend to encourage reduced quality of care. For example, in *Hand v. Tavera* (1993), an emergency room physician recommended hospitalization for a patient, but the patient's PCP denied the request. The patient subsequently suffered a stroke. The court held the PCP liable even though the PCP had never met or treated the patient. The court further said that the physician-patient relationship in a prepaid plan begins when the PCP receives payment for the patient's care (Rogers, 1998). In contrast, treatment decisions in capitated plans are less likely to be attributed to adversely affecting patient care when there is a large number of providers and/or patients involved and when payments are calculated over a period of a year or more (Rogers, 1998).

SUMMARY

Managed care is not a short-term mechanism for addressing the ills of today's health care delivery system. O'Neil (1998) predicts that the market will continue to develop and use managed systems of care as the principal mechanisms for making health care more responsive to cost, consumer satisfaction, and health outcomes. Nurses and other health care providers must integrate the concepts inherent in the system into their practice, in ways that ensure cost-effective care and safe clinical practice.

POINTS TO REMEMBER

- The concept of managed care was developed in an effort to identify strategies to obtain the greatest value in health care for the dollar spent.
- Currently, there exists four generations of managed care in the United States.
- The initial focus of managed care is cost containment.
- The system of managed care alters the provider-patient relationship by interjecting economic considerations.
- Managed care organizations are exposed to direct, indirect, and enterprise liability.
- Managed care organizations monitor and reduce legal liability through the process of utilization review and credentialing of providers.

REFERENCES

American Nurses Association, Managed Care Working Group. (1998). *Managed care: Nursing's blueprint for action principles*. Kansas City, MO: Author.

Berkowitz, S. (1994, Summer). Putting the "effective" back into "cost effective." *Tarrant Co. Physician*, p. 20.

Blakely, S. (1998, July). The backlash against managed care. *Nation's Business*, pp. 16–24.

Boland, P. (1993). *Making managed health care work: A practical guide to strategies and solutions*. Gaithersburg, MD: Aspen Publishers.

Engella v. The Permanente Medical Group, Citation, 1997.

Hand v. Tavera, 864 S.W.2d 678 (Tex. –San Antonio 1993, n.w.h.).

Ivins, M. (1998, July 12). Tobacco first—now it's health insurance. *Fort Worth Star Telegram*, p. C-8.

Kalisch, P. (1996, October). *Seizing nursing and other clinical opportunities in the new managed care environment*. Seminar presented by Texas Tech University Health Sciences Center School of Nursing Continuing Nursing Education Program.

The McEvoy v. Group Health Comparative of Fau Claire, Citation, 1997.

O'Neil, E. (1998) Nursing in the next century. In E. O'Neil & J. Coffman (Eds.), *Strategic future of nursing: Changing roles, responsibilities and employment patterns of registered nurses* (pp. 211–221). San Francisco: The Center for the Health Professions at the University of California.

Patient's Bill of Rights Act (H.R. 3605 and S.B. 1891). 1998.

President's Advisory Commission on Consumer Protection and Quality in the Health Care Industry (1998, March). Quality First: Better Health Care for All Americans. Washington, DC: Author.

Rogers, E. (1998, February 26). *Shifting, shielding and spreading managed care liability through contract*. Presentation to the Greater Houston Society for Health Care Risk Management, Houston, TX.

Sportsman, S., & Hawley, L. (1998, January). *Case management in a managed care environment*. Web Based Course offered by University On Line/Health Executives Inc.

Wennberg, J. (1996). *The Dartmouth atlas of health care in the United States*. Hanover, NH: Dartmouth Medical School.

Wyld, D. (1996). The capitation revolution in health care: Implications for the field of nursing. *Nursing Administration Quarterly, 2*(12), 1–12.

U.S. Department of Health and Human Services, Public Health Department. (1992). *Healthy People 2000 summary report: National health promotion and disease prevention objectives*. Boston: Jones and Bartlett.

Van Vactor v. Blue Cross Association, 365 N.E. 2d 638 (Ill. Ct. App. 1997)

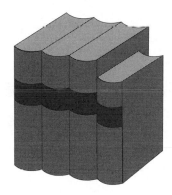

Chapter 15

ALTERNATE DISPUTE RESOLUTION IN NURSING

Mary E. O'Keefe

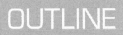

OUTLINE

Adhesion Contract	Med-Arb
Alternate Dispute	Mediation
Resolution (ADR)	Merits
Appraisement	Mini-Arbitration
Arbitration	Mini-Trial
Bifurcation of the Trial	Negotiation
Binding Arbitration	Neutral Expert
Burden of Proof	Nursing Supervisor
Capitation	Ombudsman
Collective Bargaining	Patient Care Analysis
Compromise	Test
Conciliation	Punitive Damages
Contractual Arbitration	Referee
Court-Annexed ADR	Reference
Enterprise Liability	Religious Tribunal
Ex Parte	Rent-a-Judge
Communications	*Respondeat Superior*
Fact-Finding	Risk Management
Good Faith	Satisfaction of Outcome
Impasse	Screening Panel
Interest of the Employer	Settlement
Test	Special Master
Judicial Arbitration	Summary Jury Trial
Limiting Statutes	Transaction Costs
Malice	Trial De Novo
Mandated	

Upon completion of this chapter, the reader will be able to:
- Define the various methods of alternate dispute resolution (ADR) used within the health care profession.
- Discuss court-annexed ADR procedures.
- Identify modern ADR approaches to dealing with malpractice claims within the health care profession.
- Demonstrate critical thinking in analysis of various scenarios in which ADR is used within the health care profession.
- Identify current issues and trends in the use of ADR within the health care profession.
- Discuss research and proposed research questions relative to nursing and ADR.

INTRODUCTION

The term **alternate dispute resolution (ADR)** encompasses a wide variety of methods used to settle health care disagreements quickly and cost effectively outside the courtroom, with minimal impact on the relationships between the opposing health care parties. ADR accelerates the resolution of health care disputes, facilitating either a compromise or settlement.

A **compromise** is a win/win method of amiably settling a health care dispute in which both parties give concessions. A compromise is designed to prevent or terminate litigation. A **settlement** results when the remaining conditions at issue are resolved, completing the compromise agreement, and the claim may be discharged (Alternate dispute resolution (f), 1981/1988; ADR: Employment Law (a) 1995).

The purpose of this chapter is to define ADR, discuss court-annexed ADR procedures, and identify ADR approaches to dealing with malpractice claims.

HISTORICAL PERSPECTIVE

Americans have preferred to settle their disputes without litigation since the days the first colonial settlements were established. Mediation, arbitration, and conciliation were used by the early Puritan, Quaker, and Dutch settlers to ensure conformity to community morals, using the legal system only as a last resort. In the nineteenth century, Mormons as well as Chinese and Jewish immigrants developed their own dispute resolution methods as protection from a broader society that they perceived as hostile (Alternate dispute resolution (a), 1981/1988).

In the 1970s, as attorneys were inaccessible to the poor and middle class, an informal, less expensive method of resolving disputes evolved known as alternate dispute resolution, or ADR. By the 1980s, ADR methods focused on providing confidentiality and limiting legal expenses (Alternate dispute resolution (a), 1981/1988; ADR: Employment law (b), 1995).

Historically, the American court system has used an adversarial system, headed by a neutral decision-maker, judge and/or jury, who makes a decision about the dispute *after* the opposing parties have presented their contested legal issues. ADR is nonadversarial; it uses a neutral person who helps the opposing or adversarial parties put together an agreement *while* the ADR process is ongoing.

There are two basic differences between the judicial/adversarial and ADR/nonadversarial processes. Within the adversarial system, one of the opposing parties must lose—the classic win/lose scenario—and disputes are resolved only when the neutral third party or judge applies the law. Within the nonadversarial system, a win/win situation is created, when the opposing parties create a solution to which both agree. The agreement is unique and not governed by any general principle of law, except to the extent to which the opposing parties agree it will be (Alternate dispute resolution (b), 1981/1988).

A review of the nursing and legal literature has revealed a scarcity of references on the use of ADR to settle disputes within nursing practice (see Appendix 15–A). Therefore, the definitions and principles that are applied in the use of ADR are borrowed from standard legal references, including: (1) *American Jurisprudence* and its supplements, and (2) *American Jurisprudence Trials* and its supplements. In most instances, the original reference cited in the legal source will not be cited again.

ALTERNATE DISPUTE RESOLUTION METHODS

The purpose of this section is to introduce nurses to the leading methods of ADR, which are:

- Collective bargaining
- Negotiation, including conciliation
- Mediation, including mediation-arbitration, or "med-arb"
- Arbitration
- Court-annexed methods of ADR, includ-

ing arbitration, mini-trial, summary jury trial, and fact-finding
- Alternative methods of ADR, including the use of a "rent-a-judge," religious tribunal, and ombudsman (Alternate dispute resolution (b), 1981/1988; ADR: Employment law (c), 1995).

ADR is generally a voluntary process. States have enacted statutes that require opposing parties to use ADR to resolve health care disputes. In some states:

- Compulsory arbitration or screening panels are required in malpractice actions.
- Compulsory arbitration is required in labor disputes and collective bargaining.
- Mediation is often required in divorce cases (Alternate dispute resolution (c), 1981/1988).

The provider must consider many factors before selecting the method of ADR that would be most effective in resolving a health care dispute. These factors may include:

- Nature of the relationship between the parties to the health care dispute
- Health care environment in which the dispute exists
- Health care issues involved
- Legal status of the case
- Costs of litigation
- Privacy issues
- Existence of an attorney-client relationship with one or both of the parties
- Probability of settlement of a dispute
- Effect of ADR on subsequent litigation (Alternate dispute resolution (d), 1981/1988).

Lawyers are hesitant to promote ADR to their clients. There are a variety of arguments against the use of ADR in resolving health care disputes. Over the last century an effort has been made to "professionalize" decision-makers within the system, for example, by using retired judges in ADR. Some legal professionals believe the use of physicians, nurses, and other health care providers as decision-makers reverses this process. Currently, in small claims courts, ADR may ultimately better serve the health care corporations whose consumers/patients have filed claims against them. Also, in health care facilities, there may be an overuse of ADR, with costs being borne by the public or groups other than the immediate user, such as dispute resolution centers (Alternate dispute resolution (e), 1981/1988). Nurses are usually introduced to ADR through the process of collective bargaining.

COLLECTIVE BARGAINING

The term **collective bargaining** means that, under the terms of the National Labor Relations Act (NLRA), employees have the right to form and join unions, designate representatives, and participate in negotiation and bargaining collectively (NLRA, 1994; Nusbaum, 1995). According to Catalano (1996 p. 272), collective bargaining is based on the principle that there is strength in numbers, with the goal "to equalize power between labor and management". The union is the primary unit of collective bargaining.

The passage of the NLRA in 1935 allowed for the legal recognition of collective bargaining. In 1944, the American Nurses Association (ANA), which to date does not serve as a bargaining agent, took the position that the State Nurses Association (SNA) could engage in collective bargaining on behalf of nurses (Tappen, 1995). In 1974, the amending of the Taft-Hartley Act allowed nurses in nonprofit hospitals to form collective bargaining units (Catalano, 1996, p. 272). Then, in 1991 a Supreme Court ruling allowed the National Labor Relations Board (NLRB) to define bargaining units for providers in all settings. A separate bargaining unit was identified for nurses (Catalano, 1996, p. 273).

The Service Employees International Union, representing approximately 400,000 nurses, is the major representative of nurses (Strickland & Fishman, 1994). The SNA represents approximately 140,000 registered nurses, in 840 collective bargaining units (Scott, 1993). But the NLRA does not consider nursing supervisors within the definition of employees, therefore, they are not protected under the act (NLRA, 1994, § 152(3) and § 164(a); Nusbaum, 1995, p. 1087).

**AREAS OF CONCERN
FOR COLLECTIVE BARGAINING UNITS**

- Economic issues such as salaries and benefits
- Shift differentials
- Overtime pay
- Personal days off
- Sick leave
- Maternity and paternity leave
- Uniform reimbursements
- Lunch and coffee breaks
- Health insurance
- Pension plans
- Severance pay
- Grievance procedures
- Maintenance and promotion of professional practice

Sources: Lippman, 1991; Tappen, 1995.

TEST: EMPLOYEE OR SUPERVISOR

Because nurses are often responsible for both directing and supervising personnel, along with providing patient care, their nursing practice is hard to categorize as exclusively supervisory or employment (Nusbaum, 1995, p. 1087). The NLRA provides a three-part test, of which each part must be met, to determine whether a nurse is an employee or a supervisor. First, a **nursing supervisor** must have the authority to perform any of the following activities, including hiring, transferring, suspending, laying off, recalling, promoting, discharging, assigning, rewarding, disciplining, adjusting grievances of, and/or directing the employee (NLRA, 1994, § 152(11); Nusbaum, 1995, p. 1090). Second, the judgment exercised by the nursing supervisor must be independent, not routine or clerical. For example, a nursing supervisor develops an individualized orientation for a new clinical nurse specialist. Finally, the power of a nursing supervisor is executed to the benefit and interest of the employer, not the patient. For example, the individualized orientation plan is designed to prepare a clinical nurse specialist who will expand the services of the health care provider/employer (NLRA, 1994, § 152(11); Nusbaum, 1995, p. 1090).

The NLRB adopted a test unique to the health care industry to determine whether nurses are supervisors, focusing on the *interest of the employer*. The NLRB test was known as a **patient care analysis test**. This test is used to determine whether the supervisory duties of the nurse were executed in the interest of the patient rather than the interest of the employer (Nusbaum, 1995, p. 1091).

The Supreme Court, in *National Labor Relations Board v. Health-Care & Retirement Corporation* (1994), held that the NLRB's *patient care analysis test* was contrary to the definition of a nursing supervisor under the NLRA, which focused on the *interest of the employer* (Nusbaum, 1995, p. 1092). The Supreme Court in *Health-Care* (1994) relied on two cases when interpreting whether or not the nurse's actions met the **interest of the employer test**. In citing the holding in *NLRB v. Yeshiva* (1980), the Supreme Court reasoned that patient care is the business of a health care provider/employer. Therefore, if the nurse attends to the patient or customer, then these nursing actions are conducted in the *interest of the employer.*

The Supreme Court also relied on *Packard Motor Car Co. v. NLRB* (1947) when determining elements of nursing actions conducted in the interest of the employer. The Court reasoned that the plain meaning of the phrase "in the *interest of the employer*" includes every nursing action of the employee acting within the terms of his or her job description.

THE EFFECT OF *NLRB v. HEALTH-CARE*

The immediate effect of the *NLRB v. Health-Care* (1994) ruling has been to adversely affect the organization and recognition of collective bargaining units within nursing, by: (1) disrupting the certification of collective bargaining units composed of nurses, (2) delaying certification of bargaining units, and (3) creating a backlog of NLRB-related cases. Based on the holding in *Health-Care* (1994), unfair labor practices in nursing have continued, as some employers have withdrawn recognition of collective bargaining units containing nurses, refusing to bargain with them as a collective group. Employers have also used the Supreme Court's ruling as a defense to other unfair labor practices or preemptive strikes against unions, such as wrongfully discharging or usurping their administrative authority (Nusbaum, 1995, pp. 1099–1100).

The full effects of the decision in *Health-Care* (1994) are still forthcoming. For example, the National Committee on Pay Equity feared the decision would have a "chilling effect" on unionization of nurses, preventing them from gaining protection against lower wages and further discrimination (Nusbaum, 1995, p. 1101).

Nurses may consider using their nursing organizations as a method to negotiate around the *NLRB v. Health-Care* (1994) holding. For example, nurses may conduct collective bargaining through their state nurses association, using these organizations to define the terms that distinguish an employee from a supervisor (Nusbaum, 1995, p. 1102).

Licensed practical nurses (LPNs) may also engage in collective bargaining. The United States Fourth Circuit (4th Circuit) has supported the NLRB ruling that unions can represent LPNs who are not supervisors. Beverly Enterprises, a nursing home, claimed its LPNs were supervisors under § 2(11) of the NLRA, as they were "in charge" for 8 hours each weeknight and for the entire weekend. Beverly Enterprises claimed that, although a registered nurse was on call at all times, the LPNs were the senior persons physically present at the nursing home (*Beverly Enterprises, West Virginia, Inc. v. National Labor Relations Bd.*, 1998; Strafford Publications, Inc., 1998(a)).

Beverly Enterprises also claimed the LPNs were performing supervisory functions when engaging in activities including:

- Instructing certified nurse assistants (CNAs) in their duties
- If abuse was suspected, removing the CNA from the building, even though they could not independently impose disciplinary measures
- Preparing written evaluations of the CNA's job performance, even though they could not recommend raises, promotions, or discharges (*Beverly Enterprises, West Virginia, Inc. v. National Labor Relations Bd.*, 1998; Strafford Publications, Inc., 1998(a))

The 4th Circuit held, with this set of facts, the " . . . LPN's did not exercise sufficient independent judgment to make them 'supervisors' . . . Each 'decision' was cabined to a few narrow, pre-selected choices . . . [or] no choice at all" (Strafford Publications, Inc., 1998(a), p. 218). The 4th Circuit also held:

- The LPNs could not independently have any effect on the employment status of anyone.
- The "direction" of the CNAs was in proportion to the LPN's higher level of training.
- The registered nurse on call during the night and on weekends was, in actuality, the supervisor (*Beverly Enterprises, West Virginia, Inc. v. National Labor Relations Bd.*, 1998; Strafford Publications, Inc., 1998(a)).

Nurses may use other methods of ADR to supplement, or as a substitute for, the collective bargaining process. In either employee or health care disputes, such nonadversarial methods as negotiation, mediation, and arbitration may be used.

NEGOTIATION

Once the collective bargaining unit is formed, the next step is to negotiate a contract with the employer. Management and employees form separate negotiating teams, with one person in each team designated as the spokesperson (Catalano, 1996, p. 276). Initially the teams meet separately to formulate negotiating positions and demands (Catalano, 1996, p. 276).

Negotiation, the most basic form of ADR, is usually the first relied on. Traditionally negotiation involves discussions on the terms of a proposed health care agreement and/or settlement of the terms and conditions of a health care transaction (ADR: Employment law (c), 1981/1988). Negotiation is also the process of conferring with colleagues to reach a settlement of some health care matter. When a neutral third party negotiates a health care issue, the disputants maintain control of the ADR process, deciding: (1) important health care facts and issues to be discussed, and (2) the best solution to the health care problem. Negotiation is an educational process, during which the disputants may be taught how to handle, settle, and prevent future health care disputes (Alternate dispute resolution (m), 1981/1988).

Conciliation, also known as facilitation, is an unstructured process of negotiation, which involves promoting communication between the parties to the health care dispute. Within the Age Discrimination in Employment Act, conciliation is defined as a voluntary process through which opposing parties attempt to reach a mutual understanding (Alternate dispute resolution (n), 1981/1988).

During conciliation, the facilitator is a neutral party, who (1) manages discussions between the opposing parties, (2) focuses the parties on identifying the health care problem, and (3) focuses the parties on resolving the disputed health care issues. Unlike a mediator, the facilitator does not offer settlement suggestions (Alternate dispute resolution (n), 1981/1988; Stulberg, 1984). When an impasse is reached in the contract negotiations between the collective bargaining unit and the employer, these stalemates may be resolved through mediation (Catalano, 1996, p. 277).

MEDIATION

Negotiation is usually the first form of ADR that is used in employee or other health care disputes. But, if negotiation fails and disputants wish to avoid trial, mediation is the next step. Mediation is the most popular form of ADR (ADR: Employment law (d), 1995). **Mediation** is a process by which opposing parties submit their health care dispute to an impartial third party, the mediator, who then attempts to help draw them together to agree on a mutual settlement (ADR: Employment law (c), 1995).

In mediation a decision is made to reach a voluntary settlement, enlisting a neutral third party. The neutral party assists the health care disputants in reaching a mutually acceptable agreement. Mediation is a more formal process than conciliation, with the mediator meeting first with both parties and then with each party separately until an agreement is reached. The mediator does not impose an agreement on the parties, that is, mediation is not binding. Mediators are usually invited to the mediation by the disputants. But courts or government agencies may select uninvited third-party mediators to health care disputes that are deadlocked and/or must be settled within a certain period of time (Alternate dispute resolution (o), 1981/1988). For example, the court may select an uninvited mediator to intervene in an employee-employer wage dispute to prevent the disruption of services to the critically ill patient.

Mediators may be: (1) judges or attorney's, although their code of professional responsibility offers them little guidance in functioning as a mediator; (2) laypersons; (3) factfinders; and/or (4) specialists in the area involved in the health care dispute (ADR: Employment law (c), 1995). Mediators in health care disputes primarily function to: (1) identify key issues, (2) explore a basis for an agreement, (3) explore consequences of not settling the health care dispute in a timely manner, and (4) encourage opposing parties to accommodate the interests of one another.

Mediators may not force the parties to produce evidence (Alternate dispute resolution (o), 1981/1988). Through mediation, the parties may see and hear the evidence of their adversary, weighing it against the strength of their case, which may, for example, facilitate the stronger party in obtaining an acceptable agreement, and the weaker party in avoiding the cost of litigation (ADR: Employment law (d), 1995).

The purpose of mediation is to resolve health care disputes as early as possible. Mediation works well with health care issues that cannot be resolved with all-or-nothing solutions, such as employment discrimination within the health care setting. Mediation is most effective in resolving health care disputes between parties who wish to maintain a long-term relationship but are unable to reach a decision on their own (Alternate dispute resolution (o), 1981/1988). For example, mediation is an effective mechanism to resolve disputes between administration and nursing management.

Parties may agree to mediate at the begin-

ning of their relationship, before litigation, or after a nursing malpractice lawsuit has been filed. Agreements to mediate may be prepared in writing as part of collective bargaining agreements, within an individual contract, or as a simple, specific agreement to mediate (ADR: Employment law (e), 1995).

The mediation process may be initiated by submitting a written request to the ADR organization and paying the filing fee to the organization. Mediation may be initiated to resolve health care employee disputes involving (1) wage payments, (2) interpretation of contract obligations, (3) benefits, and (4) issues surrounding employment termination.

Mediation can provide a mechanism by which both parties may "save face" while obtaining a "win/win" solution, or it can allow both sides to see the merits of their adversary's claims, providing possible support for needs that both may have. For example, parties to the mediation they agree insurance benefits may be paid to the patient when payments of claims were previously denied by the insurance company. (ADR: Employment law (e), 1995).

The method of selection of a mediator should be specified in the parties' original agreement to mediate. Some organizations appoint the mediator, for example, as does the American Arbitration Association. The

THE USE OF NURSES
IN ALTERNATE DISPUTE RESOLUTION

- Medical malpractice and personal injury cases
- Identifying standards and duties
- Interpreting the medical chart
- Determining the type and count of damages
- Determining causation of damages
- Identifying expert witnesses
- Identifying preexisting conditions
- Nurse Review Board actions
- Hospital nurse-doctor, nurse-nurse, and nurse-patient disputes
- Wrongful termination actions brought by nurses

Sources: Grant, 1995; LeFevre, 1997.

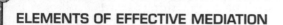

ELEMENTS OF EFFECTIVE MEDIATION

- Initiate communication.
- Initiate a working relationship.
- Focus on reality.
- Clarify interests, needs, and concerns.
- Explore creative options.
- Use external standards to measure the fairness of a compromise.
- Develop a durable agreement.

Source: Butler, 1998.

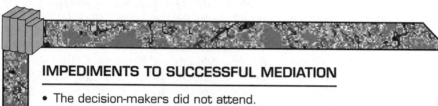

IMPEDIMENTS TO SUCCESSFUL MEDIATION

- The decision-makers did not attend.
- Parties are not separated from the issues.
- Extraneous issues are discussed.
- Inadequate information has been provided.
- The parties demonstrate inflexibility.
- The parties are negotiating too rapidly.
- Settlement was not the objective.

Source: Butler, 1998.

most essential qualification of the mediator is that he or she must be *impartial*. But opposing parties have been known to designate their legal counsel as comediators, if the neutral mediator becomes incapacitated during the mediation process (ADR: Employment law (f), 1995).

The mediator's authority includes: (1) in consultation with the parties, setting the date and time of the mediation session; (2) setting the location, which can be used as a strategic tool, for example, when one party has the mediation on their "home court"; (3) approximately 10 days prior to the first mediation session, requiring the submission to the mediator of a memorandum summarizing the disputed health care issues; (4) conducting joint and separate meetings with the opposing parties, recommending terms for

settlement; (5) participating in **ex parte communications**, which are communications with one party while the other is not present; and (6) with the consent of the parties who have previously agreed to pay expenses, obtain expert opinion(s) concerning complex health care issues (ADR: Employment law (g), 1995).

The guarantee of confidentiality is essential in health care mediation, as information learned by anyone participating in the mediation may not be discussed outside the mediation proceedings. The promise of confidentiality applies to the following: (1) health care records, reports, and all documents the mediator receives; (2) third parties, who may attend only after all parties and the mediator agree to their inclusion; (3) the mediator, who in most states cannot be

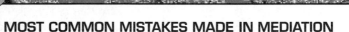

MOST COMMON MISTAKES MADE IN MEDIATION

During pre-mediation:
- Not identifying anyone who has authority to settle
- Changing the settlement offer

During the general caucus, discussing controversial issues such as:
- Veracity of one of the parties
- Severity of the injury
- Qualifications of opposing counsel
- Costs of litigation versus settlement

During private caucus, practicing:
- "Shooting the messenger"
- "Tit for tat" negotiations
- Refusing to listen to the mediator
- Trying to control opponent's next move

Source: Butler, 1998.

forced to testify in court or any related proceedings; (4) settlement discussions or settlement agreements; and (5) any offer to compromise or settle the health care dispute (ADR: Employment law (h), 1995).

The opposing parties' contract with the mediator should include at least the following terms: (1) specific hourly fees and to whom the fees are allocated; (2) a confidentiality provision; (3) procedural details, such as location, timing, and discovery; and, (4) the number and type of issues to be mediated (ADR: Employment law (i), 1995). Premediation activities should include execution and exchange of mediation agreements among the parties, document exchange, and payment or escrow of mediator fees (ADR: Employment law (i), 1995).

The mediation process generally progresses in the following sequence: (1) the introduction or explanation of the mediation process by the mediator; (2) the discussion of health care issues at dispute, presented by each party; (3) the exchange of emotions and feelings related to the issues, by each party; (4) caucusing with parties individually to discuss confidential information; (5) exploration of options or terms for resolution of the health care dispute; (6) settlement, by iden-tifying the terms of agreement; and finally, (7) agreement, by signing the instrument with the settlement terms (ADR: Employment law (i), 1995).

Health care mediation is designed to encompass both negotiation and advocacy. Although the mediator cannot impose an agreement on the parties, a persuasive mediator has a significant influence on the negotiations entered into during the mediation process. But counsel for both parties also act as advocates, convincing the mediator of the merits of their individual client's position.

In the initial phase of health care mediation, the mediator:

- Encourages active, good faith participation from both parties.
- Develops key facts of the health-care dispute.
- Identifies and defines the key health care issues (ADR: Employment law (j), 1995).

As the mediation evolves, the mediator moves the parties toward agreement by:

- Pressing opposing parties toward settling health care issues on which the parties are flexible.

- Obtaining reconsideration of health care issues on which the parties are deadlocked (ADR: Employment law (j), 1995).

An experienced mediator realizes that strong-arm tactics do not work, such as stating verbatim to one party the strongly held controversial positions of the opposing party. Such difficult positions must be presented to their adversary with a "honey coating" using a more palatable language (ADR: Employment law (j), 1995).

MEDIATION-ARBITRATION

Mediation-arbitration, or "med-arb," combines the benefits of mediation and arbitration. One neutral person acts as both mediator and arbitrator. **Med-arb** is a two-step process. First there is mediation, followed by formal arbitration, to decide any health care issues not resolved in mediation. As the parties know the mediator-arbitrator has more authority than the usual mediator and will resolve health care issues remaining after mediation, opposing parties are encouraged to be more open and honest in the mediation process. Med-arb results in a binding, final decision, including the terms of the mediation and the decision of the arbitration, both enforceable by the courts as a final arbitration award (Alternate dispute resolution (p), 1981/1988). Med-Arb may be successfully used to resolve employment issues that remain unsettled after collective bargaining has been completed. If mediation itself is unsuccessful in resolving the contract issues, the dispute may then be settled by an arbitrator (Catalano, 1996, p. 277).

ARBITRATION

Arbitration is the process through which a health care dispute is submitted to one or more impartial or neutral persons who make a final, binding decision on the outcome (ADR: Employment law (c), 1995; American Arbitration Association, 1993b). Arbitration may also be defined as a method of settling health care disputes through investigation and determination by one or more unofficial persons selected by the opposing parties instead of choosing a court proceeding (Alternate dispute resolution (p), 1981/1988; *Ferguson v. Ferguson*, 1937).

Binding arbitration legally holds all the parties to the arbitrator's final decision. Under the umbrella of binding arbitration, parties voluntarily agree to be bound by the decision of an impartial or neutral third person who is hired to function outside the court's system. The opposing parties to the health care dispute establish the rules, but the hearing is usually conducted within an informal setting (ADR: Employment law (s), 1995).

Health care arbitration may be conducted by a single arbitrator or a panel. The number of arbitrators may be specified at the time the contract for arbitration is entered into by the parties. An arbitrator may be a lawyer, a nonlawyer specialist in the area at issue, or a mixed group of experts in the field. The average arbitration takes 4 to 5 months, whereas litigation may take several years. The cost of arbitration compared with litigation is minimal, and in some cases may be free. There are two general forms of health care arbitration: (1) private or contractual, and (2) judicial arbitration (Alternate dispute resolution (f), 1981/1988).

Private contractual arbitration is the most common type of ADR. **Contractual arbitration** is characterized by the fact that the parties have negotiated a contract to settle their dispute via arbitration, and the court will enforce the arbitrator's decision. The power of the health care arbitrator stems from the appointment as an arbitrator. But the opposing parties to the arbitration can design the arbitration as the parties agree to, for example, limiting the number of health care issues to be arbitrated (Alternate dispute resolution (g), 1981/1988).

Arbitration may exclude the following rights and remedies of the disputing parties: (1) a right to trial by jury; (2) the benefit of jury instruction on the law by a judge; (3) the arbitrator's reasons for the decision, result, and/or reward; (4) a complete record of arbitration proceedings; and, (5) a judicial review of the decision, result, or reward. Under law, the agreement to arbitrate is not revocable at will, but may be enforced

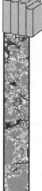

KEY QUESTIONS TO CONSIDER WHEN DECIDING WHETHER TO ARBITRATE A HEALTH CARE DISPUTE

- Is there an agreement to arbitrate?
- Which state law(s) control the arbitration?
- Is the disputed health care issue covered by the terms of the arbitration agreement?
- Has one of the parties waived or agreed to forego the right to arbitrate?
- Under what circumstances can this arbitrator's decision be changed or overturned?

Source: Schooler, 1998, pp. 22–30.

by either party to the health care dispute (Alternate dispute resolution (i), 1981/1988).

Arbitration may be distinguished from appraisement in health care, although some of the same general rules apply. **Appraisement** occurs when the parties need a neutral person to conduct some duty or act that will assist in resolving the health care dispute, such as helping the parties determine certain facts of the case. The agreement for appraisal extends to resolving only specific health care issues, such as actual cash value or amount of loss or health care damages. For example, a rehabilitation nurse may be used to appraise or determine the amount of actual and future medical damages due to a 20-year-old quadriplegic. This form of expert appraisement is called life care planning (see Chapter 23, Life Care Planning).

All other disputed issues are resolved in court. Neutral appraisers, such as the nurse who does life care planning, function in the following manner: (1) acting on their own skill and knowledge; (2) reaching individual versus group decisions; (3) meeting only to discuss individual differences in decisions; (4) without giving parties any formal notice or hearing evidence; (5) conducting ex parte or separate consultations and investigations, so long as parties are allowed to make statements or explain health care issues; and (6) if the agreement so specifies, making decisions regarding health care issues that are binding, such as, the amount of future

damages the 20-year-old quadriplegic will receive (Alternate dispute resolution (j), 1981/1988).

Arbitration may be distinguished from reference, although, again, some of the same general rules apply. **Reference** is conducted in a pending lawsuit to obtain facts at the order of the court. A **referee** is the person who conducts the reference or gathers the facts. For example, a psychiatric nurse practitioner may be ordered by the court to assess an inmate for fitness to retain custody of a child. The referee must report back to the appointing court, and the court may modify, correct, reject, or set aside the referee's report. However, if, for example, the dispute regarding the custody of the child is being heard before arbitrators, the arbitrators may ultimately have the final decision on the custody of the child (Alternate dispute resolution (k), 1981/1988).

Health care issues have been increasing in number on federal and state court dockets since the early 1990s. Arbitration has been firmly established as a grievance resolution method by the Supreme Court of the United States, making it the ADR method of choice, for example, in collective bargaining relationships (Alternate dispute resolution (s), 1981/1988).

In 1991, the Supreme Court held that an employee with a claim under the Age Discrimination Employment Act was obliged to submit the claim to binding arbitration under the terms of a contract signed by the employee with the employer (ADR: Employment law (t), 1995); *Gilmer v. Interstate/Johnson Lane Corp.*, 1991). Based on this holding, federal courts have enforced agreements to arbitrate, if the parties entered into the agreement knowingly and voluntarily. Courts traditionally have not upheld agreements to participate in ADR procedures if one of the parties: (1) has been forced to agree to pay for the cost of the ADR proceedings and/or (2) not file a complaint against the employer under the Equal Employment Opportunity Commission (ADR: Employment law (t), 1995).

Arbitration awards are difficult to overturn, but a dissatisfied party may do so if: (1) the award was obtained through fraud or corruption, (2) the award was based on arbitrator bias, and/or (3) the arbitration award was contrary to established principles of law. For example, under some state laws, if the plaintiff is 40 percent responsible for the damages, the defendant may not be required to compensate plaintiff for more than 60 percent of damages. The arbitration decision may also be overturned if the arbitrator: (1) demonstrates gross misconduct, such as refusing to hear key evidence that results in an unfair decision, such as attributing causation for damages to the wrong party, and/or (2) exceeds the powers expressed in the arbitration agreement. For example, the arbitrator exceeds his or her powers by bringing in health care issues outside the agreement established by the parties, such as causation when only damages are at issue (ADR: Employment law (u), 1995).

The arbitrator's award is also difficult to overturn, as the evidence required or **burden of proof** is hard to meet, for: (1) there may be no transcript of the arbitration proceeding, and/or (2) the arbitrator may not have provided a written report of the decision (ADR: Employment law (u), 1995).

The selection of the arbitrator is the step that should be the most carefully considered of any part of the arbitration process. Personal characteristics of the arbitrator(s) must include honesty, integrity, objectivity, and expertise in the health care matter at issue (ADR: Employment law (v), 1995).

Opposing parties may designate a single arbitrator, an arbitration panel, or an arbitration association at the initiation of their relationship or the arbitration proceeding. When the American Arbitration Association has been designated as the arbitration association, the number of arbitrators may be designated at the initiation of the proceedings. The American Arbitration Association will send the parties a list of 10 potential arbitrators: (1) allowing 10 days to make the selection, by striking three and listing the remaining in order of preference, the most highly preferred becoming the survivor; or (2) if the parties fail to select an arbitrator (ADR: Employment law (v), 1995).

If providers are involved in a complex health care case, then opposing parties must determine to what extent the arbitration process will mimic a trial. A prehearing may be advisable in large or complex health care cases, per request of either the parties or the arbitrator(s), discussing issues, including, but not limited to: (1) extent of and schedule for production of the health care documents; (2) number and length of depositions; (3) other discovery and motions; (4) location of the arbitration, for example, formal courtroom versus informal conference room atmosphere within the health care facility; (5) whether or not there will be a record or transcript of the arbitration, and who will pay for the transcript; (6) the health care issues to be arbitrated; (7) whether the decision will be given to the parties informally (verbally) or formally (in writing); and (8) the schedule for the entire arbitration process (ADR: Employment law (w), 1995).

Although the opposing parties may limit the award of damages or remedies, those remedies available in court will be equally available in arbitration. The arbitrator may award a variety of remedies to one or both parties to the dispute, including (1) an equitable remedy that may involve a court order that one party honor the health care contract, such as ordering an insurance company to pay for health care payment that had been refused; (2) payment of arbitration fees; (3) payment of other expenses of arbitration, such as attorney's fees for the winning party; and (4) payment of lost wages, back pay, and other damages (ADR: Employment law (x), 1995).

An arbitrator may decide to award **punitive damages**, or damages that are punishment to the errant party, designed to force compliance with the arbitrator's decision. Courts are more willing to enforce the award of punitive damages if the erring party acted with **malice,** or knowledge that their acts or inactions were likely to cause harm to the other party. The trend is to enforce the award of punitive damages if the award is within the arbitrator's powers or the opposing parties' arbitration agreement. The courts will also enforce the award of punitive damages if the parties agree to include such claims in the arbitration agreement, even if the state that governs the agreement excludes such claims (ADR: Employment law (y), 1995).

COURT-ANNEXED ADR

The purpose of this section is to discuss the types of **court-annexed ADR** (CA-ADR), or ADR that is ordered by the court, including: (1) arbitration, (2) mini-trial, (3) summary jury trial, and (4) fact-finding. CA-ADR is a frequently used ADR procedure, created in the early 1980s in the Northern District of Ohio, in Cleveland, in response to an overcrowded docket. Good faith or sincere, honest participation is required in CA-ADR (ADR: Employment law (o), 1995).

But, assuming the CA-ADR decision is nonbinding, opposing parties retain the absolute right to request a **trial de novo**, or new trial, if dissatisfied with the outcome. The CA-ADR procedure is nonbinding unless: (1) the parties agree in advance that the arbitrator's decision will be binding, and/or (2) the loser fails to file a request for a new trial (ADR: Employment law (o), 1995).

COURT-ANNEXED ARBITRATION

Judicial arbitration is also referred to as court-annexed arbitration, or CA-ARB, but not always considered a true CA-ADR method. It is **mandated**, or ordered by state or federal statute, and differs from contract arbitration in the following manner: (1) the decision of the arbitrator is binding and final only if the parties agree in advance that it will be; (2) if nonbinding, the parties have a right to a trial de novo; and (3) parties to a contractual arbitration generally dispute contract terms, whereas parties to a judicial arbitration may come to an agreement by chance. In a private arbitration the court is limited to enforcing the arbitration or the arbitrator's award of damages, discovery is limited, and the rules governing the health care evidence that may be admitted are more relaxed (Alternate dispute resolution (i), 1981/1988).

Numerous state and federal courts have adopted CA-ARB programs. Some courts automatically assign disputes to mandatory arbitration and a mandatory arbitration program if the amount in controversy does not exceed a certain limit. The court designates a hearing date within a specific time frame from the filing dates of the notice of arbitration as well as ordering the parties to engage in discovery and motion practice during that interim (ADR: Employment law (p), 1995).

The panel of arbitrators is usually composed of three local health care experts, including plaintiff's expert, defense expert, and, a neutral party who has expert knowledge of both plaintiff and defendant health care issues. The rules of evidence are modified in the following manner: (1) health care records are exchanged 20 days prior to the hearing, and those not subject to objection are admissible; (2) unless one party hires a stenographer at their own expense, no transcript is made; (3) testimony is taken under oath; and (4) the usual objections, as to hearsay and leading questions, may be posed (ADR: Employment law (p), 1995).

Procedurally, characteristics of the CA-ARB include the following parameters: (1) the average length of CA-ARB is a half day; (2) the expert panel caucuses immediately at the closure of the hearing to render a decision; (3) a copy of the decision is mailed to all participating counsel; (4) a disappointed litigant may file a Notice of Appeal to request a de novo jury trial within 30 days; (5) the arbitrator's award is inadmissible evidence; and (6) should one be made, a transcript of the arbitration is admissible at trial to impeach a witness (ADR: Employment law (p), 1995).

MINI-TRIAL

A **mini-trial** is a court-annexed mock or simulated trial, adversarial in nature, intended to move opposing parties who are stuck in their position, when negotiation and mediation have failed to settle the health care dispute. A mini-trial is used by the courts to supplement the negotiation process (ADR: Employment law (c), 1995).

The mini-trial is a structured settlement process that combines elements of negotiation, mediation and litigation (ADR: Employment law (n), 1995). The parties to the mini-trial choose an impartial third party or advisor who may be a former judge, eminent lawyer, law professor, or expert in the area of the disputed health care issues (Alternate dispute resolution (q), 1981/1988). The parties argue their case and question their opponents on relevant health care issues.

The neutral advisor has no authority and cannot rule on the admissibility of the health care evidence. However, the neutral advisor may: (1) moderate the opposing parties' discussions; (2) advise the parties on the strengths and weaknesses of their case; and/or (3) provide guidance and explanations on highly technical health care issues, if the advisor is an expert in the issues at dispute (Alternate dispute resolution (q), 1981/1988).

After the case is presented, and the opposing parties have seen and heard the strengths and weaknesses of both sides, the case is usually settled. If the parties reach an **impasse**, or cannot reach a decision, the neutral advisor may give a nonbinding, private opinion to the opposing parties, which is not admissible at trial (Alternate dispute resolution (q), 1981/1988).

Another variation of the mini-trial uses negotiators for the two sides, rather than a neutral advisor, when very complex health care issues are involved. If no agreement is reached, the mini-trial usually progresses to mediation, with the advisor becoming a mediator. However, the mini-trial is also often followed by a mini-arbitration. **Mini-arbitration** is a variation of the mini-trial, but the parties agree that the arbitrator's decision will be binding (Alternate dispute resolution (q), 1981/1988).

Parties in a mini-trial usually include plaintiff and defendant; legal counsel for both parties; and a neutral advisor, commonly a retired judge. The mini-trial may be held in a conference room or office, but is more commonly held in a hearing room. Discovery in health care issues is limited, as one of the goals of the mini-trial is to develop evidence to be presented at trial. For example, the number and length of depositions is usually limited (Alternate dispute resolution (q), 1981/1988).

The mini-trial is characterized by the following procedural characteristics: (1) counsel for opposing parties present their case in narrative form, including opening statement and summation, within a specific time limit; (2) counsel offers a summary of witnesses' testimony; (3) the neutral advisor helps each party's counsel resolve issues related to their presentations of testimony and/or commentaries prior to the actual mini-trial proceeding; (4) the mini-trial takes 1 day or less; (5) parties caucus, or meet, individually with the neutral advisor, sometimes without counsel, to discuss agreement terms; and (6) parties may meet individually with their counsel to write the final agreement (Alternate dispute resolution (q), 1981/1988).

SUMMARY JURY TRIAL

The **summary jury trial (SJT)** is a type of CA-ADR that is also a variation of the mini-trial, during which the health care case is presented before a jury. Characteristics of the SJT may include: (1) a trial, one-half to a full day in length; (2) a summarization of the case by the parties' counsel, before a 6-person jury; (3) a verdict, which is advisory and nonbinding; (4) a **bifurcation of the trial**, that is, after the verdict counsel may argue damage theories; (5) a postverdict conference with the jury, during which the judge permits counsel to talk with the jury regarding the reasons for their verdict; and, finally, (6) a settlement conference, held by the judge with the attorneys and opposing parties. If no settlement is reached, parties prepare for a full trial on the disputed health care issues (Alternate dispute resolution (r), 1981/1988).

COURT-ANNEXED SUMMARY JURY TRIAL

The summary jury trial is not widely accepted as a court-annexed ADR procedure. The reason may be that the U.S. Constitution guarantees opposing parties the right to a real jury trial, but does not give the court the power to impanel an "advisory" jury for a nonbinding ADR. The characteristics of the court-annexed summary jury trial is similar to that of the mini-trial, which include (1) a brief summary by counsel for the parties; (2) a jury, which is not told that their role is merely advisory; and (3) if stipulated by the parties, a nonbinding opinion, giving the parties an idea what opinion may be rendered in a real trial, which may include punitive damages (ADR: Employment law (q), 1995).

FACT-FINDING

Fact-finding is characterized by the following activities, conducted by a neutral expert or fact-finder: (1) a hearing regarding the health care issues at dispute; and (2) a written report, containing recommendations for settlement, which are nonbinding suggestions (Alternate dispute resolution (s), 1981/1988).

The **neutral expert**, or facilitator, is a health care expert who conducts ex parte communications, which are individual confidential communications with each of the parties. During these ex parte meetings, the neutral health care expert evaluates each party's health care claims. As in mediation, discussion between opposing parties is facilitated through the neutral expert. But contrary to the role of the mediator, the neutral expert gives an opinion or evaluation of the **merits,** or strength and validity, of the case. The neutral health care expert functions during the ADR procedure by discussing and then evaluating the settlement offers of both parties, reporting the evaluation of each

offer, or merely investigating the parties' settlement activities and writing a report to the court, serving no mediation function (ADR: Employment law (c), 1995; ADR: Employment law (r), 1995).

The court may appoint a neutral expert as a **special master**, a fact-finder who assists in resolving a dispute regarding health care issues when the opinions of the parties' experts differ sharply. For example, a neutral expert may be appointed if nursing experts differ sharply on the amount of and what caused damages to the patient (Alternate dispute resolution (s), 1981/1988).

Although the use of the court-appointed expert is not classically labeled ADR, it may serve to remove health care issues from the litigation process. For example, a court-appointed fact-finder may resolve issues related to life care planning for the teenage quadriplegic.

Parties to the health care dispute may assist the judge in selecting the neutral expert. The appointment of the expert is recommended in cases with highly technical health care issues. For example, a neutral health care expert may assist with the development of a settlement plan that provides for compensation for the long-term effects of exposure to a specific toxic chemical (Alternate dispute resolution (s), 1981/1988; ADR: Employment law (k), 1995).

Fact-finding may be a fairly formal ADR process occurring on one or a series of mutually scheduled sessions and conducted at a neutral location. The neutral expert or fact-finder may be required to follow a schedule. The type and number of health care issues are determined by opposing parties, including examination of health care records, experiments, and/or tests. Fact-finding involves independent questioning and investigation by the neutral health care expert, allowing the neutral expert to refuse to review certain health care evidence. The form of the neutral expert's final report may be requested by the parties, who may prefer informal, oral discussions rather than a formal written report (ADR: Employment law (l), 1995).

Once the final report is provided, the fact-finder may become the mediator. The functions of a fact-finder vary from that of a mediator in the following manner: (1) the fact-finder focuses on technical expertise, whereas the mediator focuses on conciliation skills; (2) fact-finding goes beyond the process of mediation, contributing facts necessary to formulate a decision in binding arbitration; (3) the fact-finder focuses on gathering information, not resolving the dispute; (4) the fact-finder may be given freedom to explore all relevant records of both parties, subject to rules of privacy and confidentiality; and, ultimately, (5) when the fact-finder has completed the tasks at hand, the report may facilitate new negotiations between the parties (ADR: Employment law (m), 1995).

COURT-ANNEXED FACT-FINDING

The fact-finder or neutral expert has become a more accepted method of ADR in federal courts. The neutral evaluator may be a volunteer. Regardless, the court usually requires the parties to meet with the neutral health care expert before significant discovery has been conducted (ADR: Employment law (c), 1995; ADR: Employment law (r), 1995). Court-annexed fact-finding may be used in cases involving federal health care workers, such as the investigation of a patient discrimination claim against a nurse working within the Veterans' Administration Health Care System.

The neutral expert, who is quite often a nurse and/or an attorney expert in the health care area, facilitates the fact-finding process by (1) requiring counsel for the parties to make a written presentation of the health care issues, or substance of the case; (2) by limiting the presentation staying within a 30- to 60-minute time period; (3) allowing counsel the option to also make oral presentations to supplement the written presentations; (4) making a nonbinding estimate of the liability and range of damages of the accused party; and (5) identifying areas and health care issues of agreement and disagreement and opposing parties' strengths and weaknesses. The neutral expert's evaluation of the health care dispute is strictly confidential, that is, not discoverable for, nor can be made part of, the court records of the case (ADR:

Employment law (c), 1995; ADR: Employment law (r), 1995.

ADR ALTERNATIVES

A variety of ADR procedures less commonly used also provide an alternative to settlement of health care disputes within the adversarial court system. These alternative ADR methods include the disputant's right to (1) rent-a-judge, (2) use a religious tribunal, or (3) solicit an ombudsman.

"RENT-A-JUDGE"

The practice of disputing parties deciding to **rent-a-judge** is also known as the practice of consensual reference or private judging. Advantages of this alternative method of ADR in resolving health care disputes include the ability to (1) select the neutral third party, obtaining a neutral expert in not only law but in the health care issue; (2) provide the opposing parties greater control over the schedule of the ADR procedure, including dates and times; (3) provide more flexibility in the type of ADR procedure used, such as making the expert's opinion binding versus nonbinding; (4) change procedural and/or evidentiary rules, for example, excluding some medical records and not others; (5) provide confidentiality, for example, avoiding publicity about the progress of a malpractice trial involving a well-known nurse practitioner; and (6) produce a rapid decision, usually within 20 days (Alternate dispute resolution (t), 1981/1988).

RELIGIOUS TRIBUNALS

The Jewish community originally developed alternate dispute resolution in response to what was perceived as the hostility of the European court to their religion. The practice of using religious tribunals continued in the United States. Currently, if the disputing parties are willing to accept the rabbinical authority as binding, the court system will not interfere with the parties' final settlement agreements (Alternate dispute resolution (u), 1981/1988.

A **religious tribunal** is one who has the authority to modify the terms of an arbitration agreement and rule on health care issues that had not been specifically submitted to arbitration. Courts have traditionally treated or viewed the religious tribunal form of ADR as common-law arbitration, ordering the agreement to be in writing in order to be enforceable through court, but refusing to order the tribunal to convene through court order, even if the parties have agreed to participate and be bound by such a proceeding (Alternate dispute resolution (u), 1981/1988).

OMBUDSMAN

The ombudsman functions to negotiate and resolve health care–related disputes between nurses and/or citizens and government health care or related agencies. For example, an ombudsman may intervene in a licensure revocation hearing on behalf of a registered nurse believed not to have been provided due process or the required procedural rights. The **ombudsman** is defined as a neutral person who is an officer of the legislature, who: (1) supervises the administration of the health care agency board; (2) intervenes in specific complaints between the public and administrative agencies, such as complaints between the nurse and the board of nursing; and/or (3) investigates, criticizes, and publicizes—but cannot reverse—the action of the agency or board (Alternate dispute resolution (v), 1981/1988).

A health care ombudsman functions by: (1) proposing solutions to specific complaints against the board or health care agency, but may not impose a decision; (2) investigating actions affecting nursing, requesting information, issuing subpoenas, and examining relevant nursing and health care records and documents; and (3) reporting the findings and/or recommendations directly to the nursing agency, the public, and/or the legislature. For example, an ombudsman may report to the legislature the state board of nursing for: (1) not providing for a mechanism to allow the

student nurse to enter a chemical dependency recovery program, and/or (2) not allowing that student nurse to become licensed within a reasonable period of time, after finishing the recovery and/or nursing program (Alternate dispute resolution (v), 1981/1988).

MODERN ADR METHODS OF DEALING WITH MALPRACTICE CLAIMS

The number of malpractice lawsuits has steadily increased over the years. The court system has been forced to deal with frivolous, unfounded malpractice lawsuits and unrealistic damage awards to plaintiffs. State legislatures have attempted to implement tort reform by enacting statutes that: (1) limit the amount of damages that may be recovered by plaintiffs, (2) require the submission of a malpractice claim to a pretrial screening panel of health care experts within the disputed area, and/or (3) send the health care dispute to arbitration (Physicians, Surgeons, etc. (a), 1981/1988).

STATUTES LIMITING AMOUNT OF RECOVERY

The cost of malpractice insurance is skyrocketing because of the amounts of damages being awarded to plaintiffs. State legislatures have, for example, adopted statutes designed to: (1) limit the amount of damages recoverable in a malpractice action or to be paid by an individual health care provider, that is, the individual or hospital; and (2) establish a patient compensation board similar to workers' compensation legislation, which screens damage awards. These **limiting statutes** apply proactively only, that is, limiting damage awards in future malpractice cases. But plaintiffs attack any limitation of their right to damages, claiming that limiting damages is a denial of their equal protection under the laws and a denial of their due process (Physicians, Surgeons, etc. (b), 1981/1988).

SCREENING PANELS

There are three primary types of ADR used to resolve disputes between patient and health care provider, including: (1) voluntary arbitration, (2) mandatory arbitration and mediation (all previously discussed), and (3) mandatory pretrial screening panels (Alternate dispute resolution (w), 1981/1988). Some states have enacted statutory provisions requiring the submission of a malpractice claim to a **screening panel** for the purpose of reviewing findings on the issues of liability and damages and encouraging settlement. The pretrial screening panel is typically composed of a judge, attorney, and a peer provider (Physicians, Surgeons, etc. (c), 1981/1988).

The malpractice claim review panel may be composed of as many as five voting members, for example, two health care providers, of which one must be a peer; one attorney, with experience in malpractice issues; and two lay persons. Courts generally do not view the use of pretrial panels as a denial of either party's due process. The possibility that the panel will favor and/or be greatly influenced by the health care provider is diminished by five members representing a variety of points of view, from within or as observers of the health care system. Research has demonstrated an insignificant statistical difference between the decision of a: (1) screening panel, when a malpractice case is presented to a panel of five voting members; and (2) jury, when a similar or the same case is presented at trial (Alternate dispute resolution (w), 1981/1988).

Pretrial screening panels have been attacked on the following constitutional basis, as a denial of (1) access to a court, (2) access to a jury, (3) equal protection under the law, and (4) due process under the law. Courts have both criticized and supported the malpractice screening panels, holding that state statutes creating pretrial panels (1) have allowed peers and other members of the screening panel to have the power to determine and freely apply the law in making the decision on the outcome of the malpractice issue; (2) have not required the screening panel to explain and/or justify its finding of

liability; and (3) cannot be applied retroactively (Physicians, Surgeons, etc. (c), 1981/1988).

Courts have generally upheld the use of the screening panels in malpractice and other health care disputes, as a jury will ultimately become the final arbitrator of the fact issues. The jury decides what weight to give the screening panel's recommendations, and consequently the individual parties' right to have access to the courts and a jury trial is not denied (Alternate dispute resolution (w), 1981/1988). For example, peer review panels are used by many state boards of nursing to screen out acts of malpractice by registered and/or licensed vocational nurses operating under the state's nurse practice act.

VOLUNTARY SUBMISSION TO AN IMPARTIAL SUBPANEL

The courts have allowed voluntary submission of malpractice claims to impartial subpanels for two purposes: (1) discouraging unfounded, frivolous malpractice claims against providers, and (2) making the testimony of health care experts available to legitimate malpractice claims. Because the impartial subpanel proceeding is voluntary, the participants may be able to revoke consent to participate prior to the subpanel's hearing, with reasonable notice of intention to withdraw and not participate. An impartial subpanel may be ideally used when the court believes that either party has a strong case but does not have the money to hire the experts necessary to either prove or defend the malpractice claim.

Procedurally, hearings before a health care subpanel generally involve the following components and considerations: (1) a hearing, in camera or in private; (2) possible testimony by the plaintiff and/or defendant provider; (3) cross-examination of either party by consent; (4) no rules of evidence, therefore, any relevant health care records or testimony may be relied on; and (5) no records or transcript. In summary, all proceedings, records, findings, and recommendations are confidential and may not be used or otherwise revealed without the consent of both parties (Physicians, Surgeons, etc. (d), 1981/1988).

The patient's medical malpractice claim may be dismissed if the patient fails to submit evidence to a review panel considering the health care dispute. In one such case, Lester Gleason II filed a complaint with the Indiana Department of Insurance, attributing complications related to his broken arm to acts of malpractice by his providers. Gleason and providers agreed to form a panel to review the claim, pursuant to the Indiana Medical Malpractice Act (*Gleason v. Bush*, 1997; Strafford Publications, Inc., 1998(b)).

Gleason failed to submit evidence to the review panel regarding his claim. Providers filed a motion to dismiss Gleason's malpractice suit when the 180-day deadline for the expert opinion by the review panel lapsed. Gleason claimed he had good reasons for failing to submit evidence supporting his claim, including statements: (1) he had no personal residence nor telephone services, having to get messages through friends; (2) he had changed mailing addresses three times in the preceding 9 months; and (3) he had no transportation. The Indiana Court of Appeals held that Gleason had not shown good cause for not timely providing evidence to the medical malpractice review panel (*Gleason v. Bush*, 1997; Strafford Publications, Inc., 1998(b)).

ARBITRATION OF MEDICAL MALPRACTICE CLAIMS

Arbitration has become the ADR procedure preferred to settle malpractice claims, as unlike decisions of expert screening panels, the decisions of arbitrators are final (Physicians, Surgeons, etc. (a), 1981/1988). Courts have long held that malpractice claims may be submitted to arbitration, thus it does not offend public policy. The major objectives of the health care provider in including an arbitration clause in a health care service agreement with the consumer or patient are to avoid or prevent a jury trial and to reduce liability and damages (Physicians, Surgeons, etc. (e), 1981/1988).

Arbitration clauses in health care agree-ments have been attacked for a variety of reasons. For example, an arbitration clause that required the entire arbitration process to be complete in 10 months was held to be unconstitutional because it violated the parties' right to due process (Alternate dispute resolution (x), 1981/1988).

The patient's personal representative is not always bound by the patient's agreement to arbitrate. In *Phillips v. Grace Hospital* (1998(c)), a patient by the name of Deborah Phillips was asked to sign an arbitration agreement on January 10, 1991, that would require arbitration of any claims against the hospital, employees, independent contractors, or any health care providers that arose out of "this hospital stay." Both Phillips and her providers understood the arbitration agreement related to her upcoming hysterectomy. Phillips visited the hospital on January 11 for preoperative tests (*Phillips v. Grace Hospital*, 1998; Strafford Publications, Inc., 1998(c), p. 227).

On January 14, 1991, Phillips returned for the hysterectomy and signed another arbitration agreement, identical to the agreement of January 10, 1991. The Michigan Medical Malpractice Act allows for the patient or his or her personal representative to revoke an agreement to arbitrate within 60 days after discharge by notifying the hospital in writing (*Phillips v. Grace Hospital*, 1998).

Phillips died after the hysterectomy, never having left the hospital. When Phillips' personal representative assumed control of her estate, she received copies of Phillips' medical records, with only the January 14, 1991, arbitration agreement. The personal representative filed suit against the hospital. The Michigan trial court allowed the personal representative to revoke the arbitration agreement entered into by the patient on January 14, 1991. But the representative did not learn of the arbitration agreement of January 11, 1991, until after she filed a lawsuit against the hospital (*Phillips v. Grace Hospital*, 1998).

The Michigan Court of Appeals held that the January 11 agreement to arbitrate was not enforceable as to the Phillips' personal representative. The Court of Appeals held that the 60-day revocation period began to run for Phillips' personal representative when the representative discovered or should have discovered that the arbitration agreement existed. The filing of the lawsuit by the personal representative served to revoke the agreement to arbitrate (*Phillips v. Grace Hospital*, 1998).

ISSUES AND TRENDS

The review of the nursing and legal literature indicates a number of issues and trends in the use of ADR measures in nursing practice and the resolution of health care disputes. Currently, the use of ADR within nursing practice is affected by trends related to: (1) enterprise liability for malpractice claims versus liability of the individual nurse, (2) the use of ADR plans by the enterprise or employer to settle health-care disputes, (3) the use of ADR to intervene in other health claims within the health care setting, and (4) malpractice countersuits by the provider.

ENTERPRISE VERSUS INDIVIDUAL NURSING LIABILITY

Under the theory of **enterprise liability**, responsibility and liability for a malpractice claim shifts from the individual provider to the employer, organization, or enterprise. The individual provider becomes immune from the malpractice action, with a role limited to providing background facts (Leone, 1994, p. 7).

Enterprise liability currently exists within the Veterans' Administration System and large staff-model health maintenance organizations (HMOs). Enterprise liability arises under two common areas: (1) negligent acts of the individual health care provider, such as physicians, nurses, and other health care employees; and (2) contested decisions of the provider's utilization review department (Leone, 1994, p. 8).

Use of the old fee-for-service basis of payment is decreasing, and individual health care professionals are being paid by staff-model HMOs via **capitation** payments, which are fixed monthly payments for each patient in the provider's practice covered by the HMO. This payment relationship places the focus of liability on the enterprise rather than the individual health care provider. The individual nurse is no longer an independent contractor, but receives a salary from the HMO. Plaintiffs may look to the "deeper pocket" and claim vicarious liability under the doctrine of *respondeat superior*, that is, the employer or superior is responsible for the act(s) of its employee-nurse health care provider.

Enterprise liability also arises for decisions made by the utilization review department (URD) in denying benefits to health care recipients. In *Wilson v. Blue Cross of California* (1990), although the provider determined that the patient needed 3 to 4 additional weeks of in-hospital care, the URD would not authorize more than 11 days of treatment. The patient was discharged and committed suicide. The primary provider then testified that the premature discharge of the patient was the cause of the suicide. The court held the hospital liable, noting the only reason the patient was discharged was because there was no insurance money to pay for the inpatient psychiatric care.

Potential enterprise liability exists for providers who are creating health care guidelines or protocols. If the patient/subscriber suffers injuries under the enterprise's guidelines or protocol, the enterprise may be held liable if the health care does not meet the community standard. Within the enterprise system of liability, ADR is well suited to, and is the method of choice in, resolving health care disputes.

ENTERPRISE ADR PLANS

As the trend in health care litigation is toward enterprise liability, health care organizations routinely incorporate ADR plans into their health care service agreements. The enterprise is the appropriate party to present the ADR plan to the patient, rather than the individual health care provider. The enterprise has an interest not only in resolving a malpractice claim while preserving the relationship with the patient, but must also preserve the relationship and the morale of the health care provider (Leone, 1994, p. 10). Leone (1994, p. 12) suggests that the enterprise's ADR procedure may be made more cost effective by using authoritative texts to establish the nursing standard and by using written expert reports, substituted for live testimony.

A number of national organizations have developed rules and procedures that are used by the enterprise to effectively implement ADR procedures. For example, the National Health Lawyers Association has developed specific rules and procedures for health care ADR. The American Arbitration Association has also adopted Health-Care Claim Settlement Procedures.

ADR INTERVENTIONS IN OTHER HEALTH CARE ISSUES

Bloom et al. (1995) identified other issues in the context of utilizing ADR in the health care setting. The following issues may arise during the drafting of an ADR agreement that is specific to the needs of the health care provider and the patient: (1) the type of ADR to utilize, (2) the ADR service to utilize, (3) the type of dispute "resolver" to obtain, and (4) whether or not to consult a decision tree in instances where the changing law effects one of the parties (Bloom et al., 1995, pp. 63–64). For example, parties may wish to use a decision tree in situations where the patient may be entitled to differing amounts and types of damages for malpractice within both state and federal court systems.

A number of issues that have arisen within the health care setting have been effectively addressed through ADR, including: (1) sexual harassment, (2) disruptive and impaired health care providers, (3) disputes between health care administration and individual providers, and (4) situations in which one or both of the parties desire privacy, for example, in issues of sexual exploitation (Bloom, Dempsey, Rothschild, Scanza & Hall, 1995, p. 67–70). ADR may also be used to address and interpret issues related to terms found in the employment contract of the individual health care provider. Neutral fact-finders

have been appointed to address issues related to utilization and quality assessment of health care data.

There are other situations in which ADR may not be appropriate to resolving health care issues, including, for example: (1) issues of public policy that need judicial guidance, such as right-to-die cases; (2) issues involving statutory or regulatory interpretation, such as patient dumping, fraud, and abuse; and (3) any issues that are sensitive and that the health care provider and/or patient wish to keep private (Bloom, Dempsey, Rothschild, Scanza & Hall, 1995).

According to Grant (1995, p. 53), ADR may also be used to intervene in both formal and informal suits. A formal dispute may include a grievance procedure or a wrongful dismissal lawsuit. An informal dispute may include, for example, a disagreement between staff members. Grant (1995, pp. 53–54) also notes that ADR procedures may be governed by internal and external sources in relation to the health care institution. An internal ADR organization may be used to intervene in health care disputes related to family complaints regarding services or conflicts between the multidisciplinary treatment team (MDTT) regarding patient care. External ADR organizations may be used to settle health care issues that arise related to a coroner's inquest, allegations of professional misconduct, and bioethical disputes.

MALPRACTICE COUNTER-SUITS BY PROVIDER

As medical malpractice claims have increased against health care providers, so have countersuits by providers against plaintiffs and/or their attorneys. Providers base these countersuits on claims that the plaintiff and/or the attorney filed a malpractice claim that: (1) was not a legitimate claim, (2) was brought in a malicious manner, and/or (3) was brought without proper investigation. The countersuits are usually filed in the form of actions for malicious prosecution, abuse of the legal process, and/or slander or defamation (Physicians, Surgeons, etc. (f), 1981/1988).

ETHICAL CONSIDERATIONS

The nursing and legal literature identifies specific ethical concerns related to the use of ADR within health care. These ethical issues relate to confidentiality and the principle of autonomy, for both the nurse and the patient, as well as other ethical principles involved in mediation.

CONFIDENTIALITY

The mediator who is a nurse and/or attorney must function under the rules requiring confidentiality, as specified in the state laws regulating ADR within the state the ADR is conducted. The mediator who is a health care professional must also function under the rules of confidentiality outlined in his or her respective professional codes. Whether the disputed health care issues relate to patient care or civil and criminal acts of coworkers involving patient care, the nurse attorney's duties related to confidentiality and questions of right to privacy will be governed by a unique combination of the professional standards under which the health care professional is licensed and the state and federal laws that control the actual ADR process (ADR: Employment law (h), 1995).

AUTONOMY

ADR processes provide autonomy for the participants. But issues related to autonomy also arise when the nurse participates in collective bargaining within the health care setting and when patients are forced to sign agreements to participate in ADR before receiving treatment from a provider or enterprise.

NURSING AUTONOMY

Court decisions distinguishing collective bargaining terms, such as nursing supervisor versus nursing employee, have: (1) reduced the nurse's freedom to bargain with manage-

ment, collectively and autonomously; and (2) determine the focus of nursing practice, that is, the "interest of the patient" versus the "interest of the employer."

Nursing organizations fear the *Health-Care* (1994) holding, which focuses nursing tasks on the interest of the employer rather than the interest of the patient, will impose a "gag rule" on nurse providers, placing nurses in the dilemma of either being a patient advocate or losing their job. Nurses will then find themselves within an ethical dilemma involving: (1) a duty of advocacy, or beneficence to the patient; and/or (2) a duty to the employer, or fidelity to the enterprise. This same ethical dilemma is recognized by the American Nurses Association, which fears the care of the patient will be compromised if nurses must focus their practice on the employer and not the patient (Nusbaum, 1995, p. 1102).

PATIENT AUTONOMY

Enterprise agreements, or health care provider agreements to participate in ADR, often do not provide for autonomy of the consumer or patient when formulating a decision to use ADR if a health care dispute arises with the provider. Arbitration clauses within the enterprise's health care agreements have been attacked on the grounds that such provisions are a contract of adhesion. An arbitration agreement that is an **adhesion contract** is defined as a standardized form agreement that: (1) does not allow the health care consumer to bargain on its terms; and (2) that must be agreed to on a "take it or leave it" basis, or the health care consumer does not receive the health care services (Physicians, Surgeons, etc. (l), 1981/1988; *Wheeler v. St. Joseph Hospital*, 1976). For example, an adhesion contract is created when an emergency room patient is forced to sign an agreement to arbitrate any future health care disputes before emergency services will be provided.

The enforceability of an adhesion contract involving health care arbitration depends on whether or not: (1) the terms providing for arbitration of the health care dispute are clear and conspicuous, in 10-point bold red type; (2) the terms are specifically pointed out to the patient and initialed; and (3) the health care provider explained the meaning of the terms of the arbitration agreement, its effect on the patient's rights during a health care dispute, and other dispute resolution options available to the patient (Physicians, Surgeons, etc. (l), 1981/1988; Alternate dispute resolution (x), 1981/1988).

OTHER ETHICAL PRINCIPLES INVOLVED IN HEALTH CARE DISPUTES

The actual agreement between parties to mediate, or use some other forms of ADR to resolve the health care dispute, will address issues related to a variety of ethical principles, including: (1) fidelity and veracity, requiring good faith or sincere participation in the ADR process, whether or not the agreement is in writing; (2) distributive justice, allocating to opposing parties the mediator's costs and expenses; (3) autonomy, providing for a method of independently selecting a mediator, location and timing of mediation, health care issues to be mediated, and guidelines for a mini-discovery process; and (4) privacy, spelling out a confidentiality provision (ADR: Employment law (i), 1995).

RECOMMENDATIONS FOR RESEARCH AND MALPRACTICE PREVENTION

No research was identified in a review of the nursing and legal literature regarding the effectiveness of ADR in the settlement of nursing-related issues. Therefore, research in related health care disciplines, such as medicine, was analyzed and the results applied to nursing practice.

The following research regarding health care–related ADR is recommended for replication and/or further investigation and follow-up to validate the findings and to determine the effectiveness of ADR as a malpractice prevention technique within

nursing practice. The purpose of this section is to discuss ADR research, which has been conducted regarding issues that effect: (1) the use of ADR, as a "pain reliever" in resolving health care disputes; (2) nursing, including beginning measurements of savings in cost and time when health care disputes are settled via ADR versus the litigation process; and (3) the law, analyzing the effectiveness of ADR strategies in resolving malpractice disputes.

RELIEVING THE PAIN OF HEALTH CARE DISPUTES

The St. Louis Health-Care Claims Committee of the American Arbitration Association (SLHC-AAA), working with the Alternative Resolution to the Court House (ARCH), examined the need for ADR in malpractice suits (Reeves, 1994). To determine how malpractice disputes developed, and how they might be better resolved, these two committees examined and described: (1) background perspectives and issues, or the disputes the plaintiff and provider bring to a malpractice action; (2) the psychological interaction between the patient and provider within the malpractice claim; (3) the costs of litigation; (4) less costly methods of ADR; (5) alternatives to litigation; and (6) a proposed pilot mediation program (Reeves, 1994, pp. 14–21).

BACKGROUND PERSPECTIVES

The malpractice claim is set within the background of the provider's and patient's perspective, or point of view, including their respective expectations. Reeves (1994, p. 14) noted that patients bring to their relationship with the provider the expectation that the provider will "make it better" and of "medical perfection." Whereas the provider brings the expectations that: (1) mistakes do happen, (2) poor results do occur, (3) the provider is the best decision-maker, and (4) patients should trust the provider (Reeves, 1994, p. 14). Further, the provider brings along the stress of managing a business, while meeting licensure requirements to stay current in the latest techniques in their area of expertise.

PSYCHOLOGICAL INTERACTIONS

The SLHC-AAA and ARCH also examined and described the psychological interactions between the patient and provider in a malpractice claim. According to Reeves (1994, p. 15), patients subjectively respond to their experiences within the health care system, whereas providers are taught to remain objective and dispassionate. Patients often describe the objectivity of the provider as lack of caring.

To complicate the problem, the provider may not communicate effectively and/or not provide enough information to the patient, such as informed consent. Reeves (1994, p. 15) notes that problem communication leads to distrust by the patient, reporting that the potential for provider liability increases as the level of distrust of that provider increases. Further, if the patient reports feelings of being abandoned, confusion, resentment, or suspicion of the provider, the patient may either expect a negative outcome or search for one. In summary, when the patient experiences anger and resentment, the intense hostility is usually expressed by a malpractice lawsuit (Reeves, 1994, p. 15).

COSTS OF LITIGATION

The most widely used method of resolving malpractice disputes is litigation, which has many disadvantages. The costs of litigation include not only a financial component, but also an emotional component. Reeves (1994, p. 15) examined and described four basic components of the costs of litigation. The first component, **transaction costs**, was described as: (1) out-of-pocket expenses; (2) the time and inconvenience of participating in the dispute; (3) resources consumed, such as neutral experts; and (4) lost opportunities.

The second component, **satisfaction of outcome**, or satisfaction with overall results, was determined by whether or not the parties' interests have been fulfilled and/or the dispute was fairly resolved (Reeves,

1994, p. 15). Both patient and provider described fairness in terms of being able to: (1) express their grievance against one another; (2) accept or reject the settlement agreement; and (3) participate in drafting the agreement (Reeves, 1994, p. 15).

The third element of describing the transaction costs was the long-term effect of the dispute on patient and provider. According to Reeves (1994, p. 15), costly long-term methods of dispute resolution, such as litigation, generate more hostility and tend to destroy relationships. Less costly methods of dispute resolution reduce hostility between the parties, while tending to preserve their relationship.

The last method of describing transaction cost lies in determining whether the settlement of the dispute tends to reduce the probability that the same dispute will arise in the future. Reeves (1994, p. 16) noted that the chance of recurrence of a malpractice suit is diminished if the parties participated in drafting the final settlement agreement and viewed the resolution as fair.

LESS COSTLY METHODS OF ADR

The goal of the pilot research project of the joint SLHC-AAA and ARCH committees was to identify the least costly methods of ADR for settling malpractice claims. The collaborating committees designed research whose overall purposes were to reduce: (1) transaction costs, specifically reducing fees incurred related to attorneys, experts, and discovery; (2) emotional costs, decreasing the time and energy taken away from family and business and the emotional drain of a trial; (3) the length of the dispute resolution process; (4) the dissatisfaction with the outcome of the litigation process, making the process and outcome a win/win situation for both parties; and (5) relationship costs, encouraging cooperation while preserving relationships (Reeves, 1994, p. 16).

ALTERNATIVES TO LITIGATION

The joint SLHC-AAA and ARCH committees placed selected ADR methods on a continuum in the following manner. At one end of the continuum, Reeves (1994, p. 16) described avoidance and unilateral power play as extreme, ineffective ADR methods, for the use of either results in total loss of control by both parties. Through avoidance, the patient believes there is a valid dispute, but does nothing about it. In a unilateral power play, one party settles the problem on his or her terms (Reeves, 1994, p. 16).

ADR, which leaves resolution of the malpractice issue to a neutral third party, such as with arbitration and litigation, was reported to have emotional costs, because decision-making power is given to another, and excessive financial and time costs. At the other end of the continuum, Reeves (1994, p. 17) presented the hypothesis that the greatest cost savings will result by implementing a system of dispute resolution based on early negotiation and mediation of health care disputes.

The joint SLHC-AAA and ARCH committees will explore the use of mediation as a result of the impact of the National Practitioner Data Bank of 1993 (NPDB) on settlement of malpractice claims (Reeves, 1994, p. 18). Under the terms of the NPDB, insurers who settle malpractice claims must report the payment to the Data Bank. The NPDB defines a malpractice act or claim as a written complaint or claim that demands payment based on actions or inactions of the provider in the delivery of health care Reeves, 1994, p. 18).

Other research questions arise regarding the relationship between the Data Bank and mediation. For example:

- If the malpractice claim is oral and settled in mediation, then must the payment on an oral agreement be reported to the Data Bank?
- If the claim is paid on the oral agreement, then what kind of record must be kept of the payment?
- If a written record of the payment claim is made, then must it be reported to the Data Bank? (Reeves, 1994, p. 18)

A PILOT MEDIATION PROGRAM

The SLHC-AAA and ARCH proposed a 1-year pilot mediation program that could be implemented to determine the effectiveness of ADR in preventing and/or reducing malpractice litigation. The pilot research program is composed of the following key players and functions:

- Hospital administration, who would coordinate the meetings and training of providers
- Hospital admission department, which would explain the mediation process to the patient and obtain permission for his or her participation
- Providers, who must sign a consent for participation
- Insurers, who must give permission for their patients to participate in the pilot program
- Risk managers, who must maintain copies of all consent forms and notify the American Arbitration Association if a lawsuit is filed
- American Arbitration Association, which must maintain a qualified panel of expert mediators and get the parties to the mediation table
- Medical claims committee, which must assist in the implementation of the program and training of providers, administration, and other key personnel (Reeves, 1994, pp. 18–19)

RESEARCH ON SAVINGS IN COST AND TIME

The Oakland, California, Kaiser Permanente Health Plan reported the following results in a study of the effects of their voluntary program of medical malpractice arbitration: (1) disputes were resolved in 33 months via litigation and in 19 months in arbitration; (2) the average trial lasted several weeks, the average arbitration lasted 2 to 4 days; (3) there were fewer excessive awards to plaintiffs; (4) the net average time spent defending health care claims was reduced by 22 percent; (5) net overall costs to the provider of defending the health care claim were reduced by 22 percent; (6) defense costs spent by health care providers in defending frivolous claims were reduced 59 percent; (7) frequency of filing claims against the provider decreased 63 percent; and (8) an increase in subscribers/patients and patient satisfaction (Leone, 1994, p.12).

Other research studies have also been conducted on the time and cost effectiveness of the use of ADR within the health care setting. The limited statistics gathered in a study by the American College of Obstetricians and Gynecologists of California indicated that the wide use of ADR had resulted in the resolution of malpractice claims more quickly and less costly than the national average (Leone, 1994).

Duke University Medical Center has incorporated an extensive and comprehensive ADR program into its health care provider agreement. This program uses the services of the American Arbitration Association in resolving any health care disputes that may arise (Leone, 1994).

RESEARCH ON EFFECTIVENESS IN RESOLVING MALPRACTICE DISPUTES

As noted previously, no research has been conducted regarding the effectiveness of ADR in settling health care issues within nursing practice. Therefore, analogies have been and will be drawn from the research conducted regarding the effectiveness of ADR in settling health care issues within medical practice.

The Medical Malpractice Program for the Private Adjudication Center is a nonprofit affiliate of Duke University School of Law. The Center, founded in 1987 through a grant, is designed to (1) teach, research, and provide ADR services to health care providers; (2) study the use of existing litigation procedures within the health care profession; (3) develop ADR methods for malpractice cases; and (4) advise opposing parties to a malpractice claim on ADR options (Metzloff, 1992, p. 429).

The Center identified the goals of ADR, within the context of a typical malpractice case, as including: (1) identifying and dismissing frivolous malpractice litigation, (2) providing a time and health care issue framework for voluntary settlement negotiations, and (3) providing a process to settle health care disputes that are not easily and voluntarily resolved (Metzloff, 1992, p. 431).

Potential benefits of malpractice ADR to the provider include: (1) the use of more qualified decision-makers, such as a panel of health care professionals experienced in resolving complex claims; (2) reduction in litigation costs, because the cost of litigating usually exceeds the amount paid in compensation to the plaintiff; (3) reduction in the trauma caused by the malpractice litigation, physically, emotionally, and financially; (4) improvement of the quality of expert witnesses, such as a court-appointed neutral health care expert; (5) facilitation of claims currently excluded, such as the modest low damages claim the average attorney will not try; and (6) its function as a screening tool, reviewing the merits of a potential malpractice case and weeding out frivolous health care claims (Metzloff, 1992, pp. 435–437).

The Center conducted research studies to describe the use and effectiveness of various ADR procedures in detecting, preventing, and/or intervening in malpractice suites. The Center reported the following research results for risk management, arbitration, mediation, screening panels, neutral evaluation, court-ordered arbitration, and summary jury trial.

RISK MANAGEMENT

Risk management is designed to monitor and improve the quality of nursing care through prevention of injuries, by monitoring health care equipment, and early, prompt identification of negligent injuries by health care providers. The Center found that most hospitals are not actively involved in the early detection and prevention of health care disputes before they are transformed into formal lawsuits (Metzloff, 1992, p. 438).

ARBITRATION

The impact of arbitration on the prevention of malpractice litigation is difficult to determine, because this ADR procedure does not currently have a critical role in nursing or medical malpractice cases. The research conducted does not show arbitration is pro-

provider, but actually plaintiffs prevailed slightly more often. There are several explanations why the use of arbitration is not more prevalent, including: (1) past hostility of the courts toward its use; (2) statutes providing protection to patients, which actually limit its use; (3) both plaintiff and defense attorneys' viewing the jury as the most appropriate dispute resolver; (4) the belief of some attorneys that arbitrators make more compromise decisions, for example, preventing their clients from receiving a larger award of money damages; and (5) the fear of insurers of health care providers that, if an expedited ADR process is developed, more malpractice claims would arise (Metzloff, 1992, pp. 438–440).

MEDIATION

Some states have passed legislation that allows trial judges to refer malpractice claims to ADR procedures. However, to date, there is no research that evaluates mediation (Metzhoff, 1992, p. 441).

SCREENING PANELS

Empirical studies have provided some indication that screening panels may eliminate cases with little merit or value. This may result because patients with low-merit malpractice cases are more willing to present their case to a health care screening panel for evaluation (Metzloff, 1992, p. 442).

NEUTRAL EVALUATION

Generally, the use of early neutral evaluation programs has been confined to health care lawsuits filed within federal court. There is no evidence as to the effectiveness of this ADR procedure in settling malpractice claims, because malpractice cases usually arise in state courts (Metzloff, 1992, p. 443).

COURT-ORDERED ARBITRATION

According to Metzloff (1992, p. 444), court-ordered arbitration programs have been subjected to intensive research. In general, research results reveal that patients are satisfied with the process of court-ordered arbitration, because this ADR process results in a more rapid resolution of malpractice claims.

SUMMARY JURY TRIAL

The effectiveness of the SJT is hard to assess because of its voluntary nature. This makes any study design regarding SJT inherently unsound, as random assignment of malpractice cases to control groups cannot be done, a step that is necessary in order to create a valid comparative study (Metzloff, 1992, p. 445).

RESEARCH THAT WILL PROMOTE MALPRACTICE PREVENTION

To facilitate the use of ADR and ensure that it is a valid method of malpractice prevention, the writing of Metzloff (1996) provided the basis for the following research questions, which can be applied to nursing:

- How can ADR be used within the nursing profession to prevent the filing of malpractice lawsuits?
- How can patients be encouraged to use ADR in nursing malpractice claims and/or lawsuits?
- How are nursing malpractice cases appropriate for the use of ADR?
- What qualifications are essential to provide credibility to the decisions of a member of an ADR panel hearing a health care dispute?
- Do ADR panels, as juries, award defendant health care providers definitive victories when the malpractice case has no merit?
- Are ADR panels as able as juries to value meritorious health care claims?
- Are ADR procedures more cost effective than traditional malpractice litigation?
- Does ADR involving malpractice claims more effectively use the testimony of health care experts?

SUMMARY

The various methods of alternative dispute resolution (ADR) used within the health care profession include negotiation, collective bargaining, mediation, and arbitration. There are also court-annexed ADR procedures, including the mini-trial and summary jury trial. Malpractice claims within the health care profession can be dealt with using the modern ADR approaches of screening panels and arbitration.

Current issues and trends in the use of ADR, such as (1) enterprise liability, (2) enterprise ADR plans, (3) ADR interventions in other health care issues, and (4) malpractice countersuits by providers, are affecting the use of ADR within the nursing profession.

There is no available literature relating to the effectiveness of ADR as it is applied to the nursing profession. Certain conclusions can be drawn from studies that have been conducted concerning the medical profession, but there are many actual and proposed research questions relative to nursing, ADR, and the health care profession that need to be addressed.

POINTS TO REMEMBER

- Americans have preferred to settle their disputes without litigation since the days the first colonial settlements were established.
- Historically, the American court system has utilized an adversarial system, headed by a neutral decision-maker, judge and/or jury, who make a decision about the dispute *after* the opposing parties have presented their contested legal issues.
- The leading methods of ADR are: (1) negotiation, including conciliation; (2) collective bargaining; (3) mediation, and (4) arbitration.
- State legislatures have attempted to implement tort reform by enacting statutes that limit the amount of damages that may be recovered by plaintiffs and/or require the submission of a malpractice claim to a pretrial screening panel of health care experts within the disputed area.
- There are three primary types of ADR used to resolve disputes between patient and health care provider, including: (1) voluntary arbitration, (2) mandatory arbitration, and mediation, and (3) mandatory pretrial screening panels.
- Currently, the use of ADR within nursing practice is affected by trends related to: (1) enterprise liability for malpractice claims versus liability of the individual nurse, (2) the use of ADR plans by the enterprise or employer to settle health care disputes, (3) the use of ADR to intervene in other health claims within the health care setting, and (4) malpractice countersuits by the provider.

REFERENCES

ADR: Employment law (a): In general. In *American Jurisprudence Trials* (2nd ed., Vol. 57, Chapter 255, Section 1). (1995). Rodchester, N.Y.: Lawyers Cooperative Publishing.

ADR: Employment law (b): Historical background. In *American Jurisprudence Trials* (2nd ed., Vol. 57, Chapter 255, Section 2). (1995). Rodchester, N.Y.: Lawyers Cooperative Publishing.

ADR: Employment law (c): Overview of types of ADR available. In *American Jurisprudence Trials* (2nd ed., Vol. 57, Chapter 255, Section 3). (1995). Rodchester, N.Y.: Lawyers Cooperative Publishing.

ADR: Employment law (d): Mediation: General. In *American Jurisprudence Trials* (2nd ed., Vol. 57, Chapter 255, Section 6). (1995). Rodchester, N.Y.: Lawyers Cooperative Publishing.

ADR: Employment law (e): Initiation of mediation. In *American Jurisprudence Trials* (2nd ed., Vol. 57, Chapter 255, Section 7). (1995). Rodchester, N.Y.: Lawyers Cooperative Publishing.

ADR: Employment law (f): Appointment of a mediator. In *American Jurisprudence Trials* (2nd ed., Vol. 57, Chapter 255, Section 8). (1995). Rodchester, N.Y.: Lawyers Cooperative Publishing.

ADR: Employment law (g): Scope of mediator's authority. In *American Jurisprudence Trials* (2nd ed., Vol. 57, Chapter 255, Section 9). (1995). Rodchester, N.Y.: Lawyers Cooperative Publishing.

ADR: Employment law (h): Privacy and confidentiality. In *American Jurisprudence Trials* (2nd ed., Vol. 57, Chapter 255, Section 10). (1995). Rodchester, N.Y.: Lawyers Cooperative Publishing.

ADR: Employment law (i): Practice and procedure checklist. In *American Jurisprudence Trials* (2nd ed., Vol. 57, Chapter 255, Section 11). (1995). Rodchester, N.Y.: Lawyers Cooperative Publishing.

ADR: Employment law (j): Mediation: Tactics. In *American Jurisprudence Trials* (2nd ed., Vol. 57, Chapter 255, Section 12). (1995). Rodchester, N.Y.: Lawyers Cooperative Publishing.

ADR: Employment law (k): Neutral evaluation or fact finding: In general. In *American Jurisprudence Trials* (2nd ed., Vol. 57, Chapter 255, Section 13). (1995). Rodchester, N.Y.: Lawyers Cooperative Publishing.

ADR: Employment law (l): Neutral evaluation or fact finding: Practice and procedure. In *American Jurisprudence Trials* (2nd ed., Vol. 57, Chapter 255, Section 15). (1995). Rodchester, N.Y.: Lawyers Cooperative Publishing.

ADR: Employment law (m): Neutral evaluation or fact finding: Relationship to negotiation and mediation. In *American Jurisprudence Trials* (2nd ed., Vol. 57, Chapter 255, Section 16). (1995). Rodchester, N.Y.: Lawyers Cooperative Publishing.

ADR: Employment law (n): Mini-trial: General. In *American Jurisprudence Trials* (2nd ed., Vol. 57, Chapter 255, Section 17). (1995). Rodchester, N.Y.: Lawyers Cooperative Publishing.

ADR: Employment law (o): Typical court annexed arbitration (CA-ARB). In *American Jurisprudence Trials* (2nd ed., Vol. 57, Chapter 255, Section 20). (1995). Rodchester, N.Y.: Lawyers Cooperative Publishing.

ADR: Employment law (p): Typical court annexed arbitration. In *American Jurisprudence Trials* (2nd ed., Vol. 57, Chapter 255, Section 21). (1995). Rodchester, N.Y.: Lawyers Cooperative Publishing.

ADR: Employment law (q): Court annexed ADR procedures: Summary jury trial. In *American Jurisprudence Trials* (2nd ed., Vol. 57, Chapter 255, Section 22). (1995). Rodchester, N.Y.: Lawyers Cooperative Publishing.

ADR: Employment law (r): Court annexed ADR procedures: Court annexed fact finding. In *American Jurisprudence Trials* (2nd ed., Vol. 57, Chapter 255, Section 23). (1995). Rodchester, N.Y.: Lawyers Cooperative Publishing.

ADR: Employment law (s): Binding arbitration, general. In *American Jurisprudence Trials* (2nd ed., Vol. 57, Chapter 255, Section 24). (1995). Rodchester, N.Y.: Lawyers Cooperative Publishing.

ADR: Employment law (t): Exclusivity of binding arbitration contracts. In *American Jurisprudence Trials* (2nd ed., Vol. 57, Chapter 255, Section 25). (1995). Rodchester, N.Y.: Lawyers Cooperative Publishing.

ADR: Employment law (u): Finality of awards. In *American Jurisprudence Trials* (2nd ed., Vol. 57, Chapter 255, Section 26). (1995). Rodchester, N.Y.: Lawyers Cooperative Publishing.

ADR: Employment law (v): Selection of arbitration. In *American Jurisprudence Trials* (2nd ed., Vol. 57, Chapter 255, Section 27). (1995). Rodchester, N.Y.: Lawyers Cooperative Publishing.

ADR: Employment law (w): Practice in complex cases. In *American Jurisprudence Trials* (2nd ed., Vol. 57, Chapter 255, Section 28). (1995). Rodchester, N.Y.: Lawyers Cooperative Publishing.

ADR: Employment law (x): Remedies. In *American Jurisprudence Trials* (2nd ed., Vol. 57, Chapter 255, Section 29). (1995). Rodchester, N.Y.: Lawyers Cooperative Publishing.

ADR: Employment law (y): Punitive damages. In *American Jurisprudence Trials Supplement* (2nd ed., Vol. 57, Chapter 255, Section 30). (1995). Rodchester, N.Y.: Lawyers Cooperative Publishing.

Alternate dispute resolution (a): General. In *American Jurisprudence* (2nd ed., Vol. 4, Section 1). (1981/1988). Rodchester, N.Y.: Lawyers Cooperative Publishing.

Alternate dispute resolution (b): Adversarial and non-adversarial dispute resolution. In *American Jurisprudence* (2nd ed., Vol. 4, Section 2). (1981/1988). Rodchester, N.Y.: Lawyers Cooperative Publishing.

Alternate dispute resolution (c): Mandatory and voluntary use of ADR procedures. In *American Jurisprudence* (2nd ed., Vol. 4, Section 3). (1981/1988). Rodchester, N.Y.: Lawyers Cooperative Publishing.

Alternate dispute resolution (d): Choice of alternative procedures. In *American Jurisprudence* (2nd ed., Vol. 4, Section 4). (1981/1988). Rodchester, N.Y.: Lawyers Cooperative Publishing.

Alternate dispute resolution (e): Objections to use of ADR methods. In *American Jurisprudence* (2nd ed., Vol. 4, Section 5). (1981/1988). Rodchester, N.Y.: Lawyers Cooperative Publishing.

Alternate dispute resolution (f): Introduction, generally. In *American Jurisprudence* (2nd ed., Vol. 4, Section 7). (1981/1988). Rodchester, N.Y.: Lawyers Cooperative Publishing.

Alternate dispute resolution (g): Arbitration, generally. In *American Jurisprudence* (2nd ed., Vol. 4, Section 8). (1981/1988). Rodchester, N.Y.: Lawyers Cooperative Publishing.

Alternate dispute resolution (h): Contractual (private) arbitration. In *American Jurisprudence* (2nd ed., Vol. 4, Section 9). (1981/1988). Rodchester, N.Y.: Lawyers Cooperative Publishing.

Alternate dispute resolution (i). Judicial arbitration. In *American Jurisprudence* (2nd ed., Vol. 4, Section 10). (1981/1988). Rodchester, N.Y.: Lawyers Cooperative Publishing.

Alternate dispute resolution (j): Nature of rights and remedies. In *American Jurisprudence* (2nd ed., Vol. 4, Section 11). (1981/1988). Rodchester, N.Y.: Lawyers Cooperative Publishing.

Alternate dispute resolution (k): Distinctions—appraisements. In *American Jurisprudence* (2nd ed., Vol. 4,

Section 12). (1981/1988). Rodchester, N.Y.: Lawyers Cooperative Publishing.

Alternate dispute resolution (l): Reference. In *American Jurisprudence* (2nd ed., Vol. 4, Section 13). (1981/1988). Rodchester, N.Y.: Lawyers Cooperative Publishing.

Alternate dispute resolution (m): Negotiation. In *American Jurisprudence* (2nd ed., Vol. 4, Section 14). (1981/1988). Rodchester, N.Y.: Lawyers Cooperative Publishing.

Alternate dispute resolution (n): Conciliation; facilitation. In *American Jurisprudence* (2nd ed., Vol. 4, Section 15). (1981/1988). Rodchester, N.Y.: Lawyers Cooperative Publishing.

Alternate dispute resolution (o): Mediation; role of mediators. In *American Jurisprudence* (2nd ed., Vol. 4, Section 16). (1981/1988). Rodchester, N.Y.: Lawyers Cooperative Publishing.

Alternate dispute resolution (p): Med-Arb. In *American Jurisprudence* (2nd ed., Vol. 4, Section 17). (1981/1988). Rodchester, N.Y.: Lawyers Cooperative Publishing.

Alternate dispute resolution (q): Mini-trial; mini-arbitration. In *American Jurisprudence* (2nd ed., Vol. 4, Section 18). (1981/1988). Rodchester, N.Y.: Lawyers Cooperative Publishing.

Alternate dispute resolution (r): Summary jury trial. In *American Jurisprudence* (2nd ed., Vol. 4, Section 19). (1981/1988). Rodchester, N.Y.: Lawyers Cooperative Publishing.

Alternate dispute resolution (s): Fact-finders; neutral experts. In *American Jurisprudence* (2nd ed., Vol. 4, Section 20). (1981/1988). Rodchester, N.Y.: Lawyers Cooperative Publishing.

Alternate dispute resolution (t): Rent-a-judge (consensual references). In *American Jurisprudence* (2nd ed., Vol. 4, Section 21). (1981/1988). Rodchester, N.Y.: Lawyers Cooperative Publishing.

Alternate dispute resolution (u): Religious tribunals. In *American Jurisprudence* (2nd ed., Vol. 4, Section 22). (1981/1988). Rodchester, N.Y.: Lawyers Cooperative Publishing.

Alternate dispute resolution (v): Ombudsman. In *American Jurisprudence* (2nd ed., Vol. 4, Section 23). (1981/1988). Rodchester, N.Y.: Lawyers Cooperative Publishing.

Alternate dispute resolution (w): Patient-doctor disputes, generally; screening panels. In *American Jurisprudence* (2nd ed., Vol. 4, Section 53). (1981/1988). Rodchester, N.Y.: Lawyers Cooperative Publishing.

Alternate dispute resolution (x): Voluntary and compulsory arbitration. In *American Jurisprudence* (2nd ed., Vol. 4, Section 54). (1981/1988). Rodchester, N.Y.: Lawyers Cooperative Publishing.

American Bar Association. (1996, August). American Bar Association resources for ADR. *American Bar Association Journal*, p. 62.

Bascalis, J. (1996, July). A better way to negotiate. *For the Defense*, pp. 12-14.

Benson v. Granowicz, 40 Mich. App. 167, 363 N.W.2d 238 (1984).

Beverly Enterprise, West Virginia, Inc. v. National Labor Relations Bd., No. 96-2778 (4th Cir. Feb. 13, 1998)

Bloom, A., Dempsey, M., Rothschild, I., Scanza, R., & Hall, J. (1995). Alternative dispute resolution in health-care. *Whittier Law Review, 16*, 61.

Bradstreet, A. (1996, July). Dealing with socialized gender-based behavior in negotiations. *For the Defense*, pp. 15-16.

Butler, R. (1998, February). *Mediation: Coming of age as a dispute resolution process.* Symposium conducted at the annual meeting of the Greater Houston Society of Health-Care and Risk Management, Houston, Texas.

Catalano, J.T. (1996). Contemporary Professional nursing. Philadelphia, PA: F.A. Davis.

Covey, J. (1989). *Seven habits of highly successful people.* New York: Simon & Schuster.

Ferguson v. Ferguson, 110 S.W.2d 1016 (Tex. Ct. App. Eastland, 1937).

Gilmer v. Interstate/Johnson Lane Corp., 500 U.S. 20, 114 L.Ed.2d 2, S.Ct. 1647 (1991).

Gleason v. Bush, 689 N.E. 2nd 480 (Ind. ct. App. 1997).

Goltz, P. (1996, August). Settling the score: Good negotiation skills pave the way for better settlements. *American Bar Association Journal*, p. 90.

Grant, A. (1995, August). Alternative dispute resolution. *Canadian Nurse, 91*(7), 53–54.

Kohane, D. (1996, July). Why you should mediate a dispute? *For the Defense*, pp. 22–23.

LeFevre, T. (1997, 1st Quarter). The use of nurses in alternate dispute resolution. *National Medical-Legal Journal*, 8(1), 4, 7.

Leone, A. (1994, September) Is ADR the Rx for malpractice? *Dispute Resolution Journal*, pp. 7–13.

Lippman, H. (1991). Legally speaking: Expect to hear about unions. *RN, 54*, 68–72.

Metzloff, T. (1992). Comment: Alternative dispute resolution strategies in medical malpractice. *Alaska Law Review, 9*, 429.

Metzloff, T. (1996) Comment: The unrealized potential of malpractice arbitration. *Wake Forest Law Review, 31*, 203.

National Labor Relations Act of 1988, 29 U.S.C.A. §§ 151–169 (West 1994).

National Labor Relations Board v. Health-Care & Retirement Corporation, 114 S.Ct. 1778 (1994).

NLRB v. Yeshiva, 444 U.S. 672 (1980).

Nusbaum, J. (1995). NLRB v. Health-Care & Retirement Corporation: Nurses as supervisors under the National Labor Relations Act. *Oregon Law Review, 74*, 1087.

Packard Motor Car Co. v. NLRB, 330 U.S. 485 (1947).

Phillips V. Grace Hospital, No. 195674 (Mich Ct. App. Mar. 20, 1998)

Physicians, surgeons, etc. (a): Modern approaches

to dealing with malpractice claims: Generally. In *American Jurisprudence* (2nd ed., Vol. 61, Section 372). (1981/1988). Rodchester, N.Y.: Lawyers Cooperative Publishing.

Physicians, surgeons, etc. (b): Modern approaches to dealing with malpractice claims: Statutes limiting amount of recovery. In *American Jurisprudence* (2nd ed., Vol. 61, Section 373). (1981-1988). Rodchester, N.Y.: Lawyers Cooperative Publishing.

Physicians, surgeons, etc. (c): Modern approaches to dealing with malpractice claims: Statutes requiring submission of malpractice claim to a pretrial panel. In *American Jurisprudence* (2nd ed., Vol. 61, Section 374). (1981/1988). Rodchester, N.Y.: Lawyers Cooperative Publishing.

Physicians, surgeons, etc. (d): Modern approaches to dealing with malpractice claims: Court rulings providing for voluntary submission of claim to an impartial subpanel. In *American Jurisprudence* (2nd ed., Vol. 61, Section 375). (1981/1988). Rodchester, N.Y.: Lawyers Cooperative Publishing.

Physicians, surgeons, etc. (e): Modern approaches to dealing with malpractice claims: Arbitration of medical malpractice claims. In *American Jurisprudence* (2nd ed., Vol. 61, Section 376). (1981/1988). Rodchester, N.Y.: Lawyers Cooperative Publishing.

Physicians, surgeons, etc. (f): Modern approaches to dealing with malpractice claims: Medical malpractice countersuits. In *American Jurisprudence* (2nd ed., Vol. 61, Section 377). (1981/1988). Rodchester, N.Y.: Lawyers Cooperative Publishing.

Reeves, J. (1994, September). ADR relieves pain of health care disputes. *Dispute Resolution Journal*, pp. 14-21.

Riskin, L. (1996, August). A quick course in mediation advocacy. *American Bar Association Journal*, pp. 56-57.

Schooler, L. (1998, March/April). Arbitration 1998: Developments in the law. *The Houston Lawyer*, pp. 22-30.

Scott, K. (1993). SNA representation means increased job satisfaction. *American Nurse*, 24, 2.

Stafford Publications, Inc. (1998(a), April 3). Labor Relations: Union can represent nursing home's licensed practical nurses who are not "supervisors." *Health Law Week*, 7(14), 217.

Stafford Publications, Inc. (1998(b), April 3). Malpractice. dismissal for failure to submit evidence to review panel was not above discretion. *Health Law Week*, 7(14), 218.

Stafford Publications, Inc. (1998(c), April 10). Arbitra-
tion: Arbitration forum is unfavorable as to patient's personal representative. *Health Law Week*, 7(15), 227.

Strickland, O., & Fishman, D. (1994). *Nursing issues in the 1990's*. Albany, NY: Delmar.

Stulberg. (1984). Negotiation concepts as advocacy skills: The ADR challenge. *Alabama Law Review*, 48, 719.

Tappen, R. (1995). Nursing leadership and management. Philadelphia: F. A. Davis.

Wheeler v. St. Joseph Hospital, 63 Cal. App. 3rd 345, 133 Cal. Rptr. 775, 84 A.L.R.3d 343 (4th Dist. 1976).

Wilson v. Blue Cross of California, 271 Cal. Rptr. 876, 222 Ca.3d 660 (Cal. App. 2 Dist. 1990). ed., Vol. 61, Section 373). (1981/1988). Rodchester, N.Y.: Lawyers Cooperative Publishing.

SUGGESTED READINGS

Canavati De Checa v. Diagnostic Center. Hospital, Inc., 852 S.W.2d 935 (Tex. 1993), rehearing of cause overruled (June 16, 1993) and remanded 995 F. 2d 74 (CA5 Tex.).

Federal Arbitration Act of 1925, 9 U.S.C.A. §§ 1 et seq. (West 1994).

Federal Mediation and Conciliation Act, 29 U.S.C.A. § 173 (a) (West 1994).

Ginsberg, W. (1996, July). The central role of the mediator. *For the Defense*, pp. 17-20.

Hoeffner, C. (1996, July). A guide to mediation. *For the Defense*, pp. 24-26.

Lucas v. United States, 807 F.2d 414 (CA5 Tex. 1986).

Mastrobuono v. Shearson Lehman Hutton, 131 L.Ed.2d 76, 115 S.Ct. 1212 (1995).

McKinstry v. Valley Obstetrics-Gynecology Clinic, P.C., 428 Mich. 167, 405 N.W.2d 88 (1987).

Moore v. Fragatos, 116 Mich. App. 179, 321 N.W.2d 781 (1982).

Pietrelli v. Peacock, 13 Cal. App. 4th 943, 16 Cal. Rptr. 2d 688, 93 CDOS 1301 (1st Dist. 1993).

Re Calongne, 447 So. 2d 1217 (5th Cir. 1984).

Reuben, R. (1996, August). Mandatory arbitration under fire. *American Bar Association Journal*, pp. 58-60.

Reuben, R. (1996, August). The lawyer turns peacemaker. *American Bar Association Journal*, pp. 54–62.

Wilson v. Kaiser Foundation Hospitals, 141 Cal. App. 3d 891, 190 Cal. Rptr. 649 (3rd Dist. 1983).

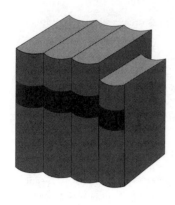

Chapter 16

THE LEGISLATIVE PROCESS

Susan Sportsman
Ana M. Valadez
Shirley Chater

A personal note of gratitude to James H. Willmann, JD, General Counsel, Texas Nurses Association, for his assistance with this manuscript.

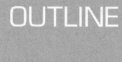

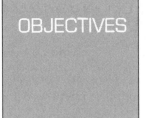

American Nurses
  Association Social
  Policy Statement
Board of Nurse
  Examiners (BNE)
Civil Law
Government Affairs
  Committee (GAC)
Grassroots Organization
Lobbying
N-STAT
Networking
Nurse Practice Act

Old Boy Network
Peer Review
Political Action
  Committee (PAC)
Political Networks
Politics
Professional Nursing
  Legislative Agenda
  Coalition (PNLAC)
Public Law
Public Policy
Safe Harbor Law
Whistleblower Laws

OBJECTIVES

Upon completion of this chapter, the reader will be able to:

- Develop a perspective on how the legislative process can help nursing promote quality care.
- Clarify the process of passing a bill.
- Enrich his or her cadre of skills to move nursing's issues and concerns forward to legislative agendas.
- Identify the opportunities nurses have to become involved in health-related legislative issues.

INTRODUCTION— HISTORICAL PERSPECTIVE

Since the days of Florence Nightingale, nursing has been involved in persuading influential government authorities to address concerns that affect patient/client care. However, because nursing has long ascribed to the notion that **politics** and quality care are incongruent partners, nurses have hesitated in becoming politically involved. The American Nurses Association (ANA), the professional organization for nurses, has served as an excellent role model for addressing legislative issues and has assisted nurses in reaching their political aspirations. Reviewing the legislative gains nursing has made since

the mid-1990s should provide an incentive for nurses to become involved in the political process.

THE LEGAL SYSTEM

Trandel-Korenchuk and Trandel-Korenchuk (1997) address the sources of law for U.S. citizens. They offer a perspective on law that includes principles and processes used to control behavior of humans so that orderly living can be enhanced and the need for force can be minimized. These authors readily admit that law is not an exact science because answers to legal problems can be ambiguous. Because the nursing profession covers a gamut of health care services, uncertainty about legal issues will always be there.

Civil law governs relationships with other private citizens, whereas **public law** governs relationships between citizens and the government. Public law is salient to the practicing nurse. Regulatory processes by which nurses are governed fall under public law; likewise, public law is what nurses seek to change when quality care issues are of concern.

The Constitution of the United States is the supreme law of the nation. It grants, as well as restricts, certain privileges to federal and state governments. The first 10 amendments of the Constitution place limits on federal power. In contrast, the Fourteenth Amendment places limitations on state governments. The Constitution also outlines due process and equal protection. In contrast, state constitutions organize state government and grant states power as well as limit it.

Legislative bodies, which initiate statutory law, are found in all of the three areas of government: federal, state, and local. However, regulation of nursing primarily comes from the state level. Thus, the state legislature becomes a key player with whom nurses must work and coalesce to effect changes in nursing practice.

REGULATORY PROCESSES FOR NURSING PRACTICE

The U.S. Constitution gives each state the authority to regulate health care providers. The day-to-day regulation of nursing practice in each state is by the **Board of Nurse Examiners (BNE)**. Therefore, those who serve on the BNE have tremendous power to effect nursing practice. Except for North Carolina, where members of the Board of Nursing are peer elected, states rely on the governor for appointments to the Board of Nursing (Gaffney, 1998). As a result, these boards usually include individuals who support the governor's philosophy and who have actively campaigned and provided resources (both monetary and time) that led

to the election of the governor. Through this political process, nurses can influence public policy regarding nursing practice through political action.

The BNE of each state develops rules and regulations to clarify the state's Nurse Practice Act and provide day-to-day regulation. Boards of nursing have delegated authority from a variety of law sources: (1) legislative, by public declaration of rules and regulations; (2) quasi-judicial, through hearings of contested matters; and (3) administrative, through licensure control (Guido, 1997). The ANA believes that state boards of nursing should be: (1) self governing; (2) approve or disapprove schools of nursing; (3) examine and provide licensure to bona fide nursing applicants; (4) issue, review, grant, and inactivate licenses; (5) provide regulation for specialty practice; and (6) discipline nurses who violate aspects of licensure law.

A **nurse practice act** is designed to protect the public, guide scope of practice issues, and define and set standards for nursing practice. The nurse practice act is by far the most important piece of legislation for nurses because of its overriding effect on all nursing practice. Nurse practice acts can fall into one of three categories: traditional, transitional, or administrative. The traditional approach limits states in defining or addressing advanced practice. The transitional category gives states some leeway in addressing advanced practice by the use of standing orders and physician supervision. The administrative category offers states a wider working perspective. It promotes a broader definition of nursing and allows incorporation of advanced practice, relying on the board's authority to define advanced practice regulation (Guido, 1997).

STATE MONITORING OF REGULATION

The public views nursing as a most trusted profession. Because of this trust and the expanding roles of professional nurses, accountability of the nurse for nursing interventions actions has increased. Consequently, malpractice acts naming nurses are now frequently seen, especially in traditional hospital settings. To diminish the possibility of being named in a lawsuit, nurses must remain fully informed regarding their scope of practice in the state in which they practice, particularly if and when multi-state licensure becomes a reality.

Sullivan and Mattera (1997) address how nurses may fall victim to state board investigations and even disciplinary action based on the perceived shortcomings in the nurse's practice. For instance, nurses may be charged with negligence because of substandard care, not doing their job, or being accused of patient neglect. Likewise, nurses may be found incompetent or not qualified to do a certain type of care (e. g., critical care unit [CCU] or critical nursing care). Nurses can also be viewed as abusive to patients/clients, and the abuse can be physical or verbal. Additionally, nurses can be accused of having a mental problem or a chemical or substance dependency that impairs practice. Fraud can also be a legal problem for nurses if they have lied about an arrest or academic record. The best way to ensure practice privileges is for the nurse to know and follow the nurse practice act of the state in which he or she practices, become familiar with the patient's bill of rights, and know the delegation rules as they apply when working with other health care personnels.

All nurses have the responsibility to report a peer if it appears the nurse practice act has been violated. Once the nurse has been reported to the state board of nursing, the board is obligated to investigate the allegation. All boards must adhere to due process in disciplinary hearings for the nurse who is alleged to have violated the nurse practice act. The severity of the nurse's action plus the concrete evidence to support the allegation dictate the board's recommended action. Boards can censure or reprimand nurses or place them on probation. The BNE may also revoke or suspend the nurse's license.

ISSUES AND TRENDS

The **American Nurses Association Social Policy Statement** (ANA, 1995) speaks to four features inherent in contemporary nursing practice:

- Assessing the person from a holistic view rather than focusing only on problems presented by the patient
- Integrating objective databases gleaned from the presenting patient's view
- Applying scientific rationale to diagnosis and treatment
- Exhibiting a caring bond that promotes health and healing

The Social Policy Statement also describes the nurses' scope of practice as being fluid, dynamic, and sensitive to changes related to various happenings, including the political environment and legal conditions. Although nursing care can be provided by both basic level and advanced practice nurses, all nurses are equally accountable for meeting standards of care. The nurse's accountability comes from the legal regulatory process of licensure and criminal and civil statutes. There are two kinds of self-regulation for nurses: self—having a knowledge base of the practice, and other—peer review of the nurse's practice. In both circumstances, knowledge of practice as well as legal and political issues is critical to this regulation.

In the recent past, nursing authors have described the hesitancy many nurses had about becoming involved in politics. However, times are rapidly changing. This change toward a more politically astute nurse can be attributed to several professional events. One such change is the strength of the **political action committee (PAC)** from the local to the national level. Skaggs (1997) addresses the crucial role PACs play in providing a mechanism for small contributors to have collective strength and influence. Another event, the First Nurses March on Washington, co-sponsored by the American Nurses Association (ANA, 1996), certainly proved to be a strengthening force for nurses to enter the political arena. The March brought workforce issues such as unlicensed assistive personnel and their impact on quality care to the consciousness of legislators. More recently, *The American Nurse* ("Five Nurses," 1998) reported on the five nurses running for House seats in November 1998. The fact that these nurses were actively seeking national offices can only serve as a motivator for other nurses to follow suit.

Robinson (1995) tells nurses that political involvement and influence require us to explore all types of political networks. **Networking** involves developing connections between people and opening channels to important information (Tappen, 1995). **Political networks** are valuable in two ways: they allow nurses to connect with the right influential people, and they promote the deliberate use of politics to accomplish a goal for the profession. Political networks offer nurses opportunities for advancing the profession, through three types of political networks. The first includes the **old boy network**, where older, more experienced nurses assist novice nurses in the political process. The second political network is designed to put expert nurses in contact with legislators. In this situation, for example, specialty nurses or advanced practice nurses might visit legislators to clarify a particular nursing issue. The third type of political network is a **grassroots organization** designed to quickly inundate legislators with information about a particular emerging health care issue. This type of political network includes the use of e-mail, faxes, telegrams, telephone calls, and letters to legislators that can influence the issue being addressed (Robinson, 1995). Bocchino and Sharp (1995) include political savvy as a nursing skill, with networking being the basis for political savvy. Networking is applicable to all nurses regardless of their area of practice albeit service or education. To what extent networking is used is really the choice of the individual nurse.

To be effective lobbyists, nurses have to first be registered voters who participate in the privilege of voting regularly. Nurses also need to know what, whom, how, and why to lobby. To address the "what" of **lobbying**, nurses need to be well versed on an issue and the policies affecting the issue. "Whom" to lobby is very important. Most nurses know federal legislators; however, few know state representatives and their key staff responsible for drafting proposals. It is important to communicate with the right legislator.

There are various resources, such as the League of Women Voters and the state nurses association that can assist the nurse in identifying whom to lobby. Being familiar with the legislative process and the status of the specific issue within the process helps the nurse with the "how" to lobby. The "why" of lobbying lies in wanting to shape health care policies for the betterment of patient care. One of the most influential ways for nurses to lobby is to coalesce with their professional organization on the local, state, and national levels. It is through this collective effort that gains for quality nursing practice have been achieved (Wray, Cohen, & Reinhard, 1998).

Aiken and Catalano (1994) offer the nurse the following 10 points on how to lobby effectively by: (1) developing a plan of action; (2) presenting the issue in a well-prepared manner; (3) answering a question truthfully, even if it means getting back to the legislator; (4) practicing patience, especially when waiting to see the legislator; (5) practicing courtesy; (6) being brief and concise when presenting a point of view; (7) being direct and to the point; (8) keeping it simple and clear; (9) keeping the group small to avoid a large distracting crowd; and (10) following the meeting with a thank you letter that clearly defines the issue and how the legislator can be of help.

Peer review is an example of an issue that has been promoted and encouraged on the national level by the ANA through their lobbying effort. ANA's lobbying team is the 78th most powerful lobbying group in Washington, exceeding several other lobbying groups such as the American Association of Medical Colleges and the American Academy of Family Physicians (Glazer, 1998). These lobbying efforts by ANA are possible because of ANA's Political Action Committee, which raises and contributes funds to politicians who support ANA's legislative agenda. The PAC continues to exceed $1 million in their fundraising efforts.

At the national level, there still must be input from nurses working on the state and local levels. **N-STAT** is a grassroots lobbying group of nurses who belong to the state nurses association. N-STAT is committed to write or call federal legislators representing their local areas when ANA notifies them of impending federal legislation. Last year N-STAT members contacted their legislators on average of four to six times during the legislative session. Such contacts provide an effective way to make a difference with legislation affecting nurses.

The Texas Nurses Association (TNA) has been very effective in accomplishing many legislative successes. Its success can be attributed to two forceful programs initiated by TNA, the **Government Affairs Committee (GAC)** and the **Professional Nursing Legislative Agenda Coalition (PNLAC)**. GAC begins its work long before the legislative session starts. It is at this time that the grassroots lobbying network is organized. If there is to be nurse-initiated legislation, bills are drafted, sponsors identified, and backup materials prepared. During the legislative session, GAC is responsible for lobbying contacts at legislative offices as well as organizing an RN Lobby Day at the Capitol.

PNLAC is a coalition of Texas nursing organizations whose main goal is to build consensus on legislative issues that affect all nurses. PNLAC is responsible for developing a legislative agenda for nursing and working actively to achieve the prescribed agenda. The synchronous work of these two political professional machines has afforded Texas nurses many legislative gains.

TNA has been proactive in addressing nursing issues that "blanket" all nurses. For example, they have responded to the PEW Commission challenge that states should address competency of regulated health care professionals. Legislation introduced by PNLAC and TNA in 1997 resulted in passage of S.B. 617, which authorizes the Texas Board of Nurse Examiners to pilot studies designed to include proactive peer review and targeted continuing nursing education. This legislation was built on TNA's Nursing Quality Assurance Act, which addressed peer review and mandatory reporting.

PASSAGE OF A BILL

IDEA FOR LEGISLATIVE CHANGE

The legislation dealing with the 1987 Nursing Quality Assurance Act originated from issues relating to the practice of medicine as well as the malpractice insurance crisis that Texas was experiencing. Prior to the 1987 legislative session, much publicity had been generated relating to malpractice insurance and lack of effective regulation of physicians who provided poor, inadequate care. Although the Chair of the Texas Senate Committee on Health and Human Resources was willing to introduce legislation to strengthen regulation for physicians and physician peer review committees, he did not believe the problem was unique to physicians. ("Nursing quality assurance bill," 1987; "Senate passes," 1987; "TNA enjoys," 1987; "TNA to sponsor quality," 1987; "TNA-supported quality," 1987). The Chair felt that it was not fair or appropriate to omit other professions such as nursing from this legislative effort. Hence, the TNA was asked to participate in drafting the nurse-related bill and to work closely with the office of the Chair of the Senate Health and Human Resources.

DEVELOPMENT OF PROPOSAL

Working closely with the GAC, TNA's Board of Directors identified major components of the bill and asked the GAC to draft a bill that would address two main areas: (1) mandatory reporting to the Board of Nurse Examiners of registered nurses who engaged in unsafe practice, and (2) peer review for professional nurses. The work of TNA resulted in the introduction of the Professional Nursing Quality Assurance Act of 1987.

During this step, the GAC worked closely with lobbyists and solicited their input. Likewise, the TNA staff worked with lobbyists to develop draft language for legislation.

PROPOSAL DISCUSSED WITH PROFESSIONAL ORGANIZATIONS

Because of the size of the state and number of media markets, a public relations campaign to the public was not practical. However, the legislation was publicized among professional nursing groups and input was sought and included.

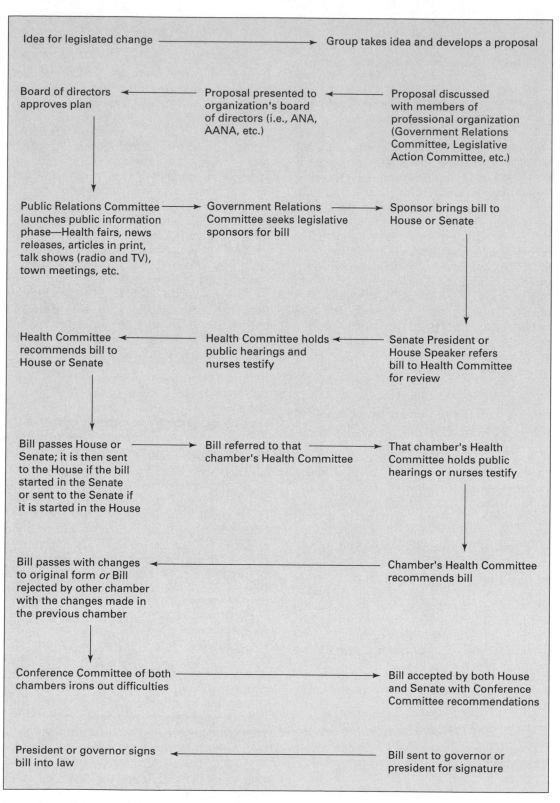

FIG. 16–1. Path of a bill from conceptualization to law. (From Aiken, T. D., & Catalano, J. T. (1994). *Legal, ethical and political issues in nursing.* Philadelphia: F.A. Davis.)

LEGISLATIVE SPONSORS

The legislative sponsors of the bill in the Senate and House of Representatives were selected based on their interest in the bill and their influence in passing bills in the Texas legislature. Having the Chair of the Committee on Health and Human Services as one of the Senate sponsors greatly increased the chance for passage of the bill, because it was this committee that originally proposed such a bill. The House sponsor of the bill was selected because she was a registered nurse and had been active on the TNA's GAC prior to running for a legislative position.

HOUSE AND SENATE COMMITTEE HEARINGS, NURSING TESTIMONY, BILL PASSAGE

The 1987 TNA official legislative publication, *NurseWatch*, reports on the numerous events that reflect the tedious work involved in making a bill a reality. Retooling of the bill and testimony by several nurses in support of the bill are documented ("TNA-supported quality," 1987). *NurseWatch* helped nurses throughout the state to monitor the progress of the bill as it advanced through the legislative process. A communications network used at that time, Nurse Telephone Trees, was quite effective in reaching nurses so that letters could be sent to legislators asking them to support the bill ("Nursing quality assurance bill," 1987; "Senate passes," 1987; "TNA enjoys," 1987). The bill finally passed and became law in May 1987.

Figure 16–1 illustrates the steps taken to bring a bill from its inception into law. The description of events that led to the 1987 Nursing Quality Assurance Act for Texas nurses closely correlate with the steps in this figure.

SUBSEQUENT AMENDMENTS TO THE BILL

In 1993, the peer review law was strengthened to address due process. The 1995 amendments expanded peer review to licensed vocational nurses. In 1997, an amendment was added to give the registered nurse the right to request peer review if he or she is requested to engage in conduct that violates duty to a patient. The amendment also provides a **safe harbor law** to protect the nurse while peer review is pending. In June 1998, the Texas Supreme Court upheld the validity of the provisions in the Nurse Practice Act that prohibits retaliation against persons who report unsafe care. These **whistleblower laws** were enacted as a part of the 1987 Professional Nursing Quality Assurance Act.

PUBLIC POLICY: INFLUENCING FACTORS

Policy that is developed by governmental bodies, such as legislation passed by Congress, is **public policy**. Nursing can pride itself on the influence nurses have had on public policy through their support of candidates who share nursing's view on health care and by electing nurses to political offices in the 1990s (Mason & Leavitt, 1998). Although no one can deny the milestones nursing has accomplished in shaping many aspects of health care for Americans, the need to demystify politics and policy making for nurses is still there. Why is this so? Perhaps the answer is that policy needs to be correlated with the nurses' practice arena so that personal and professional experiences can be seen as political. Therefore, aspects of bedside nursing need to be directly related to policy and politics (Mason & Leavitt, 1998). Chater (1998) views public policy in the context of a wheel (Fig. 16–2). She views public policy as the hub of the wheel with several spokes, representing values, timing, politics, cost and economics, and knowledge base, that influence the hub (public policy). All five spokes are interrelated and affect each other in varying degrees. This analogy is clearly visible with the legislative passage of the Texas Professional Nursing Quality Assurance Act of 1987. The values of politicians, as well as of the nurses, melded together into a passion for peer review to

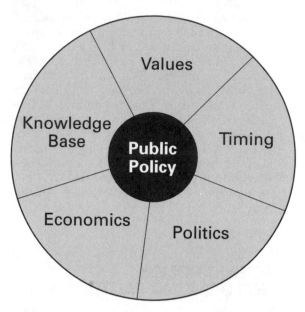

FIG. 16–2. Public policy as a wheel. (From S. Chater, 1998.)

ensure quality care. Likewise, the economics of increasing litigation concerning safe care mirrored and shaped the politics of that era. A sound knowledge base about quality care and how to monitor its aspects helped nursing to succeed in passage of the bill. Finally, the timing—having a sense of when, where, and how to introduce public policy—was also evident. The fact that physicians were already exploring assurance of quality care led to successful nurse-physician collaboration that resulted in the nurse bill.

SUMMARY

All nurses should have an understanding of a broad overview of the law and the significance of public law to the nursing profession. Knowledge of the legislative process, including the related issues of networking and lobbying, is essential for nurses to be effective in influencing the development and passage of laws that affect public policy as it relates to health care. The

tracking of one state's success with a professional nurse quality assurance act demonstrates the detail and time needed to affect the legislative process. Political activism for nurses is not only needed but essential for quality care. Viewing public policy as the hub of a wheel surrounded by influencing spokes provides a guiding map to follow when addressing public policy.

POINTS TO REMEMBER

- The legislative process has long been used by nurses to influence quality patient care.
- All nurses, irrespective of their practice area, need to know how the legislative process works on the federal, state, and local levels.
- All nurses need to understand the role and function of the Board of Nurse Examiners in the state in which they practice.
- All nurses should know how the political environment affects nursing practice and how political involvement by the profession is essential.

- Steps necessary for passage of a bill are essential knowledge for nurses.
- The influence of public policy by nursing is noteworthy and continues to grow.

REFERENCES

Aiken, T. D., & Catalano, J. T. (1994). *Legal, ethical and political issues in nursing*. Philadelphia: F.A. Davis.

American Nurses Association. (1995). *Nursing's social policy statement*. Washington, DC: American Nurses Publishing.

American Nurses Association. (1996). *First nurses march on Washington* [On-line]. Available: http:\\www.nursing world.org\press rel\1996\march.htm

Bocchino, C. A., & Sharp, N. J. (1995). Chapter, Health Care Policy Issues: Nursing Politics and Power. In K. W. Vestal (Ed.), *Nursing management: Concepts and issues*. Philadelphia: J.B. Lippincott.

Chater, S. S. (1998, March). *The Voice of Nursing in Public Policy*. Paper presented to Texas Nurses Association Convention.

Five nurses running for house seats. (1998, September/October). *The American Nurse*, 3(5) 9.

Gaffney, T. (1998). State Government. In D. J. Mason & J. K. Leavitt (Eds.), *Policy and politics in nursing and health care*. Philadelphia: W.B. Saunders.

Glazer, G. (1998). The time is now—How? *Online Journal of Issues in Nursing*, 1–3. [On-line]. Available: http://www.nursingworld.org/ojintpclg/leg_5.htm

Guido, G. W. (1997). *Legal issues in nursing* (2nd ed.). Stanford, CT: Appleton & Lange.

Mason, D. J., & Leavitt, J. K. (1998). *Policy and politics in nursing and health care*. Philadelphia: W.B. Saunders.

Nursing quality assurance bill advances. (1987, May). *NurseWatch*, 3(5) 1–2.

Robinson, C. (1995). Networking Strategies. In K. W. Vestal (Ed.), *Nursing management: Concepts and issues*. Philadelphia: J.B. Lippincott.

Senate passes nursing quality assurance bill without dissent. (1987, April). *NurseWatch*, 3(4) 1–2.

Skaggs, B. (1997). Political Care Action in Nursing. In J. A. Zerwekh & J. C. Clayborn (Eds.), *Nursing today: Transition and trends* (2nd ed.). Philadelphia: W.B. Saunders.

Sullivan, G. H., & Mattera, M. D. (1997). *RNs legally speaking*. Montvale, NJ: Medical Economics.

Tappen, R. M. (1995). *Nursing leadership and management: Concepts and practice* (3rd ed.). Philadelphia: F.A. Davis.

TNA enjoys busy but successful session. (1987, June). *NurseWatch*, 3(8) 1.

TNA to sponsor quality assurance bill for RNs. (1987, January). *NurseWatch*, 1(1) 1–2.

TNA-supported quality assurance bill for RNs nears introduction. (1987, February). *NurseWatch*, 1(2) 1.

Trandel-Korenchuk, D. M., & Trandel-Korenchuk, K.M. (1997). *Nursing & the law* (5th ed.). Gaithersburg, MD: Aspen Publication.

Wray, R., Cohen, S., & Reinhard, S. (1998). Lobbying Policymakers: Individual and Collective Strategies. In D. J. Mason & J. K. Leavitt (Eds.), *Policy and politics in nursing and health care*. Philadelphia: W.B. Saunders.

SUGGESTED READINGS

Marquis, B. L., & Huston, C. J. (1992). *Leadership roles and management functions in nursing: Theory and application*. New York: J. B. Lippincott.

Nickitas, D. C. (1997). *Quick reference to nursing leadership*. Boston: Delmar Publishers.

Texas Nurses Association. (1998a). *Legislative government affairs: Beating the odds* [On-line]. Available: http://www.texasnurscs.org/legis.htm

Texas Nurses Association. (1998b). *Legislative government affairs: What is PNLAC?* [On-line]. Available: http://www.texasnurses.org/legis.htm

Willmann, J. H. (1998). *Annotated guide to the Texas Nursing Practice Act* (3rd ed.). Austin, TX: Texas Nurses Association.

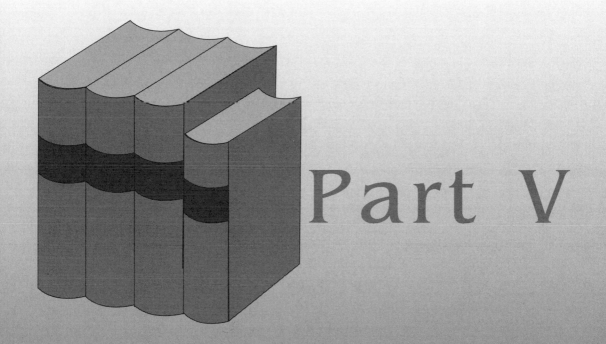

Part V

NURSING LAW
AND
SPECIALIZATION

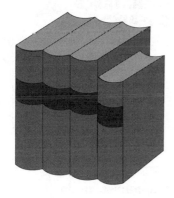

Chapter 17

ADVANCED PRACTICE NURSING

Victoria Berry
Taralynn R. Mackay

KEY WORDS

Advanced Practice Nurse (APN)
Agency for Health Care Policy and Research (AHCPR)
Certified Registered Nurse Anesthetists
Clinical Guidelines
Clinical Nurse Midwife (CNM)
Clinical Nurse Specialist (CNS)
Critical Pathways
Institutional Practice Guidelines

Joint Commission on Accreditation of Healthcare Organizations (JCAHO)
Licensure
Midlevel Providers
Mutual Recognition Model
Nurse Practitioner
Physician's Assistant
Registration
Standards

OBJECTIVES

Upon completion of this chapter, the reader will be able to:
- Analyze the laws which control advanced practice nursing.
- Discuss the standards and clinical practice guidelines which regulate advanced practice nursing.
- Identify the clinical areas in which advanced practice nurses specialize.

INTRODUCTION— HISTORICAL PERSPECTIVE

Before physicians became organized in the late 1800s and developed medical practice acts and legislation for the delivery of health care, there were nurse practitioners and midwives. With the advent of nurse practice acts, nurses were restricted to nursing functions and their independent functions were abolished. Throughout the 1900s, the role of the nurse was expanded to reflect the nurse's clinical expertise, educational preparation, and training. The expanded role allowed nurses to perform some acts, such as cardiopulmonary resuscitation (CPR), withdrawing blood, and starting intravenous lines, that had been considered the practice of medicine (Safriet, 1992).

In the 1960s, there was an increased demand for health care providers as a result of Medicare and Medicaid changes that increased the number of individuals entitled to governmental aid (Safriet, 1992). There were not enough physicians to fill the demands being made for health care, especially in medically underserved populations. The result was the establishment of midlevel providers. **Midlevel providers** consist of advanced practice nurses and physician's assistants.

Dr. Eugene Stead, the director of the first program for physician's assistants, looked for a health care provider who could provide quality medical care, especially in medically underserved areas (Younger, Conner, Cartwright, Kole, Forsyth, 1997). The concept of a health care provider who was a physician extender/assistant was initially proposed as an advanced medical education program for clinical nurses (Younger et al., 1997). However, because this new midlevel practitioner was based on the "medical" theory model rather than the "nursing" theory model, the National League of Nursing opposed the program for nurses (Younger et al., 1997). So Dr. Stead selected ex-military corpsmen who had received medical training during their military service as the pool for this new type of health care provider, which became known as physician's assistants (Younger et al., 1997).

A **physician's assistant** functions as an assistant to a supervising physician. Although supervised by a physician, the constant physical presence of the physician is not required, because physician's assistants can perform their functions under protocols or standing orders. Although the supervision requirements in most states differ for physician's assistants and for advanced practice nurses, physician's assistants function under the same or similar prescribing laws as advanced practice nurses.

In 1965, an advanced program based on nursing theory was started at the University of Colorado by Loretta Ford, RN, EdD, and Henry Silver, MD (Loeb, 1992). The program

was initiated to instruct nurses in new clinical roles that would increase their responsibilities and would enable nurses to function in nontraditional nursing settings (Loeb, 1992). In 1971 Idaho was the first state to enact laws recognizing advanced practice nursing as encompassing diagnosis and treatment as part of its practice scope (Safriet, 1992). By 1980, there were advanced practice certification programs in all 50 states (Loeb, 1992). The role of the advanced practice nurse continues to increase because state legislatures are recognizing the capabilities, the usefulness, and the cost-effectiveness of the advanced practice nurse.

DEFINITIONS

ADVANCED PRACTICE NURSE

An **advanced practice nurse** (APN) is a registered nurse who has received advanced training. The majority of APNs receive their advanced training in master's programs, although some receive training in certificate programs that require an additional 2 years of clinical training beyond the master's degree. APNs care for children and adults in practically all health care settings. Currently, 25 states allow some types of APNs to practice independently (Pearson, 1998). The testimony quoted in Box 17–1 gives the rationale for APNs to independently care for families. Even if an APN is practicing independently, the APN should still be in a collaborative relationship with a physician, because of the need to refer patients.

However, advanced practice nursing is not without complications. There is controversy surrounding the APNs' competition or their perceived competition with physicians for patients. In response to the controversy, there have been several studies performed on the efficiency and cost effectiveness of APNs. The findings show that APNs are becoming recognized more frequently for their ability to save consumers money, while providing quality care to patients. A 1992 study revealed that APNs were 20 percent

BOX 17-1

TESTIMONY OF A FAMILY NURSE PRACTITIONER

". . . Nurses are well-positioned to fill many of the current gaps in accessibility and availability of primary and preventive health care services. Advanced practice nurses are trained to provide from 80 to 90 percent of the necessary primary care services of the nation. Primary care services include: preventive care and screening, physical examinations, health histories, basic diagnostic testing, diagnosis and treatment of common physical and mental conditions, prescribing and managing medication therapy, care of minor injuries, education and counseling on health and nutrition issues, minor surgery or assisting at surgery, prenatal care and delivery of normal pregnancies, well-baby care, continuing care and management of chronic conditions, and referral to and coordination with specialty caregivers."

Source: Folkerts, 1994.

BOX 17-2

CONTROVERSY INVOLVING SOME ADVANCED PRACTICE NURSES

Physician: "One issue that looms large in the debate is the nurses' desire for greater status and recognition within what has been a highly hierarchical system of medical care delivery. . . . The main question is, perhaps, whether medicine can be practiced at graduated levels of competence and education, starting at less than a professional degree and residency, without a hierarchy. Should a practitioner who does not possess a complete medical education be allowed to decide when she or he requires assistance?" (Rudy, 1995a)

Nurse's response: "Advanced practice nurses who do wish to become independent practitioners are not interested in independently practicing medicine: they are interested in practicing *nursing*, just as they have been trained to do. Quality health care by a primary care provider does not always require medical acts, but when it does, NPs have historically either performed those medical acts for which they have been properly trained or referred the patient to a physician who can. It does not require a 'complete medical education' but rather sound judgment to know when consultation is necessary, and our value of patient outcomes prevents NPs from attempting what is beyond our capabilities." (Ruppert, 1995)

Physician's response: "At first blush, it is difficult to disagree with much of what she says. She writes that NPs do not wish to be independently practicing medicine. However, they do wish to be independently practicing nursing. To too many of her colleagues, that means making 'nursing diagnoses' (as opposed to 'medical diagnoses'?), prescribing treatments, etc. Fine, one is tempted to suppose. However, I am not beguiled by the velvet touch. What is the difference between nursing and medical diagnoses? . . . The nurse's independence would evolve within the relationship between him or her and the physician who is responsible." (Rudy, 1995b)

BOX 17-3

FURTHER CONTROVERSY INVOLVING SOME ADVANCED PRACTICE NURSES

American Medical Association, Board of Trustees Report:
"Nurses are not qualified by their education and training to practice as independent practitioners to meet the broad spectrum of needs of patients. . . . Nurses' education does not prepare them to serve as the first point of contact for all the patient's medical and health care needs." (American Medical Association, 1993)

American Association of Colleges of Nursing, response to the AMA's Board of Trustees Report:
"Physicians do not have a monopoly on health care knowledge, nor are they the only qualified independent providers of health care. It does not take 11 years of medical training to competently immunize a child, treat an ear infection or sore throat, give a physical exam, or even manage diabetes or high blood pressure. APNs not only are providing this level of care, but can be prepared at almost one-fifth the cost of expensive and prolonged medical education." (American Association of Colleges of Nursing, 1994)

less expensive than physicians in treating two conditions (otitis media and sore throat) and that the APNs were at least as effective as the physicians in treating the patients (Salkever, Skinner, Steinwachs, & Katz, 1992). However, it was pointed out by a physician that the APNs saw two-thirds the number of patients that the physicians saw and, thus, were able to provide more time to the patients (Rudy, 1995a). The physician also noted that the nurses ordered "twice as many laboratory studies as did physicians on cases of otitis media, while physicians ordered nearly twice as many follow-up visits on cases of sore throats . . . [and] the cost of care was comparable in the two groups" (Rudy, 1995a). However, another study done in 1994 showed that when a geriatric nurse practitioner was involved in the care of nursing home patients along with a physician, the average cost was 42 percent lower than when care was provided by a physician alone (Burl et al., 1994). Boxes 17–2 and 17–3 discuss some of the controversies surrounding APNs.

Currently, APNs specialize in the four fields described in the following sections. Throughout this chapter a nurse who is involved with advanced practice will be referred to in general terms as an APN.

NURSE PRACTITIONER

According to the American Academy of Nurse Practitioners, **nurse practitioners** (NPs) are "advanced practice nurses who provide primary health care and specialized health services to individuals, families, groups, and communities" (American Academy of Nurse Practitioners, 1993). NPs practice in the areas of family care, women's health, neonatal care, pediatrics, adult health, and acute care (Guido, 1995). The practice of a NP focuses on health promotion, health maintenance, including treatment of acute and chronic diseases, and disease prevention (American Academy of Nurse Practitioners, 1993). There were approximately 53,753 NPs in the United States as of 1992 (Department of Health and Human Services, 1992).

CLINICAL NURSE SPECIALIST

The field of the **clinical nurse specialist** (CNS) originated as a graduate program in psychiatric nursing, but it has expanded to many other areas. The focus of CNS practice is not diagnosing the patient nor treating the patient with medications, but rather treating the patient through education, consultation, and therapy. The CNS must earn a graduate degree that represents educational preparation and advanced clinical practice related to the specialty. Because of the manner of practice, a CNS usually works in a hospital or a clinic, which can decrease the CNS's autonomy (Guido, 1995).

CERTIFIED NURSE MIDWIFE

Clinical nurse midwives (CNMs) have practiced for years in many countries. They have been in the United States since the 1920s (American Nurses Association). Their function is to provide care of the pregnant woman before, during, and after the birth of the infant. They also administer care to the newborn infant. CNMs are also involved in family planning and gynecology (American Nurses Association). Since 1982, CNMs have been in a collaborative practice with the American College of Obstetricians and Gynecologists (American Nurses Association).

CERTIFIED REGISTERED NURSE ANESTHETIST

A **certified registered nurse anesthetists** (CRNA) evaluates the patient's overall physical health in anticipation of the administration of anesthesia and provides anesthesia to patients, which includes the selection and administration of drugs, intravenous fluids, and ventilator techniques. CRNAs administer more than 65 percent of the anesthesia given each year and do so in more than 85 percent of rural hospitals (American Association of Nurse Anesthetists, 1998). Some states require that the CRNA work under the supervision of a physician, not specifically an anesthesiologist. Other states allow CRNAs to work independently or in collaboration with physicians.

STATUTORY LAW REGULATING NURSING PRACTICE

Individual states are responsible for licensing and regulating nursing professionals within the state's boundaries (Box 17–4). The early nursing laws from the 1900s were registration or certification acts (Safriet, 1992). Only those individuals who registered with the state and proved that they were trained to perform the duties were allowed to be called registered nurses (Safriet, 1992). By the 1930s, states were requiring a license to practice nursing (Box 17–5).

Each state has a nurse practice act that was established by the legislature and is enforced by the executive branch of the government through the state's regulatory agencies. Some states regulate APNs through the state nursing board, some states regulate APNs through the state medical board, and other states use a combination of nursing and medical boards to regulate APNs. In order to administer the state's statutory law regarding APNs, the designated regulatory board issues rules and regulations that govern specific acts performed by the APNs. Regulatory agencies are also responsible for establishing licensure application requirements, the requirements for maintaining the license, and disciplinary actions. Therefore, in order to practice safely, the APN should be familiar with the regulatory board's rules and regulations regarding practice as well as the state's licensing and practice act.

State legislatures have addressed the boundaries of prescriptive authority for APNs in various ways. A 1998 survey of the states' laws revealed that 17 states allowed APNs to prescribe medications autonomously, 31 states allowed APNs to prescribe medications with physician involvement or physician delegation, and 2 states did not allow APNs to prescribe medications (Pearson, 1998).

BOX 17-4

COMPARISON BETWEEN LAWS AND REGULATIONS

Texas Nursing Practice Act:
"'Professional Nursing' shall be defined as the performance for compensation of any nursing act (a) in the observation, assessment, intervention, evaluation, rehabilitation, care and counsel, and health teachings of persons who are ill, injured or infirm or experiencing changes in normal health processes; (b) in the maintenance of health or prevention of illness; (c) in the administration of medications or treatments as ordered by a licensed physician, including a podiatric physician licensed by the Texas State Board of Podiatric Medical Examiners, or dentist; (d) in the supervision or teaching of nursing; (e) in the administration, supervision, and evaluation of nursing practices, policies, and procedures; (f) in the requesting, receiving, signing for, and distributing of prescription drug samples to patients at sites at which a registered nurse is authorized to sign prescription drug orders. . ." (Texas Nursing Practice Act, 1998)

Board of Nurse Examiners for the State of Texas, Rules and Regulations:
"The responsibility of the Texas Board of Nurse Examiners (Board) is to regulate the practice of professional nursing within the State of Texas. The purpose of defining standards of practice is to identify roles and responsibilities of the registered professional nurse (RN) in any health care setting. The standards for professional nursing practice shall establish a minimum acceptable level of professional nursing practice. The RN shall:
1. know and conform to the Texas Nurse Practice Act and the board's rules and regulations as well as all Federal, State, or local laws, rules or regulations affecting the RN's current area of nursing practice;
2. provide, without discrimination, nursing services regardless of the age, disability, economic status, gender, national origin, race, religion, or health problems of the client served; . . ."
This section is composed of 20 standards of professional nursing practice that further expand on the definition of professional nursing as set out in the Texas Nursing Practice Act (Board of Nurse Examiners for the State of Texas, 1999).

BOX 17-5

DIFFERENCES BETWEEN REGISTRATION AND LICENSURE

Registration is the process by which an individual completes documents and submits the documents to the state. The state accepts the individual's representation that the individual is trained and competent. Thus, the individual has stated that he or she has qualifications that allow the individual to be maintained on a state registry.

Licensure means that the state has established the requirements and education that are the basis for licensure. The state also requires verification of the individual's competence. The documentation required is usually more complex and the licensure process is more time-intensive than registration. If an individual is licensed, the state is representing that the individual has met educational or training requirements that have been established for a license.

COMMON LAW REGULATING NURSING PRACTICE

Courts, both federal and state, play a role in developing the laws under which APNs practice. Whereas the legislature and the regulatory agencies are responsible for statutory law, courts create case law or common law based on the judges' decisions in various lawsuits. The courts also interpret the regulations and statutes under which APNs practice.

Two significant court cases helped the movement toward establishing APNs as an independent profession (Guido, 1995). In 1983, the Missouri Supreme Court held that when the nursing practice act was enacted, the legislature intended for APNs to be able to practice within their knowledge and capabilities because of the broad language used to define professional nursing (*Sermchief v. Gonzales*, 1983). The Court further stated:

Professional nursing ... is in a period of rapid and progressive change ... [and a] nurse may be permitted to assume responsibilities heretofore not considered to be within the field of professional nursing so long as those responsibilities are consistent with her or his specialized education, judgment and skill based on knowledge and application of principles derived from the biological, physical, social and nursing sciences (*Sermchief v. Gonzales*, 1983).

The Texas Court of Appeals, in 1985, held that the state nursing board, under its regulatory power, could define the education required of nurses and the scope of practice of nurses under the board's jurisdiction (*Bellegie v. Board of Nurse Examiners*, 1985).

STANDARDS

Standards are considered to be the minimum requirements for nursing activities. However, they are not absolute, because they depend on subjective determinations about what are the minimum acceptable behaviors. *Standards of care, clinical guidelines*, and *standards of professional performance* are terms that are often confused and used interchangeably. Standards of care involve standards of nursing process, whereas standards of professional performance involve standards relating to the professional behavior of nurses. Clinical guidelines are patient-focused recommended courses of action (which are discussed later). Various organizations have established standards. APNs should look to their specialty organizations, as well as the organizations described in this chapter, for standards that have been adopted for their specialty.

The **Joint Commission on Accreditation of Healthcare Organizations (JCAHO)** is an independent nonprofit entity that establishes standards for the delivery of health care and conducts surveys to evaluate health care establishments. Although JCAHO uses the term *standard of care*, its standards are actually more similar to clinical guidelines because they are patient focused.

In 1996, JCAHO redesigned its standards so that they are patient centered, performance focused, and organized around functions common to all health care organizations (JCAHO). JCAHO believes that nursing standards are the backbone of nursing and establish the parameters for nursing activities (JCAHO). Furthermore, JCAHO requires the development of nursing standards as well as a process for evaluating those standards (JCAHO).

The American Nurses Association (ANA) explains the need for standards of practice by stating that "a profession must seek control of its practice in order to guarantee the quality of its service to the public" (American Nurses Association). The various divisions on nursing practice within the ANA have formulated standards, and there is an overall, broad collection called the Standards of Clinical Nursing Practice (American Nurses Association). The ANA also has position statements available that set out its opinion regarding various issues. For example, there is a booklet specifically for APNs that addresses the standards and scope of practice applicable to APNs. The ANA divides the standards of nursing practice into two subgroups: Standards of Care and Standards of Professional Performance.

The ANA Standards of Care involve nursing process and activities directly surrounding patient care. The nursing activities are:

- Assessment
- Diagnosis
- Outcome identification
- Planning
- Implementation
- Evaluation (American Nurses Association)

The ANA Standards of Professional Performance involve professional nursing behavior. These activities describe competent behavior in a professional nurse. All nurses are expected to engage in these activities as appropriate based on their education and position:

- Quality of care
- Performance appraisal
- Education
- Collegiality
- Ethics
- Collaboration
- Research
- Resource utilization (American Nurses Association)

Finally, the legal definition of standard of care is what a reasonable and prudent nurse would do in the same or similar situation. Some courts apply this standard to a reasonable and prudent nurse in the same or similar situation in the same locality rather than in a similar locality. For example, a nurse who practices in a rural health clinic should be judged by what a nurse in a rural health clinic would have done in the same or similar situation. The rural health nurse should not be judged by what a nurse in a major city hospital would do in the same or similar situation. Other courts are attempting to apply a national standard, but this is an evolving area of the law.

CLINICAL PRACTICE GUIDELINES

Clinical guidelines are the clinical steps for patient management. Guidelines are recommended practices for meeting standards of care. They are detailed, patient-focused, and based on diagnosis, procedures, or clinical conditions. Clinical guidelines are being pushed in view of managed care because guidelines are seen as a way to control the costs of health care. They are also seen as a way to provide continuity and quality of care.

AGENCY FOR HEALTH CARE POLICY AND RESEARCH

The **Agency for Health Care Policy and Research (AHCPR)** was established in 1989 under the Omnibus Budget Reconciliation Act of 1989 and became part of the Department of Health and Human Services. The mission of AHCPR is to compile and provide research information to health care providers and professionals and to consumers and to develop clinical practice guidelines. AHCPR has several clinical practice guidelines available, but there will not be any further guidelines in the current format because the AHCPR is redesigning its approach to the guidelines. Box 17–6 lists the nineteen clinical guidelines available from the agency's website.

DEVELOPMENT OF CLINICAL PRACTICE GUIDELINES

The APN may develop clinical guidelines as an operational tool to assist in clinical decisions. These clinical guidelines provide a range of acceptable practices and options that can be adapted to specific patient needs. Standards provide the APN with process; the clinical guidelines provide research-based information. Standards are rigid, whereas clinical guidelines may be flexible to meet patient needs. Clinical guidelines do not take the place of standards, but rather provide a research-based option for decisions. APNs should ensure that the clinical guidelines adapted for their practice are up to date and based on valid review and opinion. Once clinical guidelines are in place and utilized in practice, the APN should be cognizant of the need to document any deviation from the

BOX 17-6

NINETEEN CLINICAL GUIDELINES FROM THE AHCPR

1. Acute Pain Management (February 1992)
2. Urinary Incontinence in Adults (March 1992)
3. Prevention of Pressure Ulcers (May 1992)
4. Cataract in Adults (February 1993)
5. Depression in Primary Care (April 1993)
6. Sickle Cell Disease in Infants (April 1993)
7. Early HIV Infection (January 1994)
8. Benign Prostatic Hyperplasia (February 1994)
9. Management of Cancer Pain (March 1994)
10. Unstable Angina (March 1994)
11. Heart Failure (June 1994)
12. Otitis Media with Effusion in Children (July 1994)
13. Quality Determinants of Mammography (October 1994)
14. Acute Low Back Problems in Adults (December 1994)
15. Treatment of Pressure Ulcers (December 1994)
16. Post-Stroke Rehabilitation (May 1995)
17. Cardiac Rehabilitation (October 1995)
18. Smoking Cessation (April 1996)
19. Early Identification of Alzheimer's Disease and Related Dementias (November 1996)

Available from the Agency for Health Care Policy and Research (AHCPR) website at http://www.ahrq.gov

use of the guideline and the clinical rationale for such deviation.

INSTITUTIONAL PRACTICE GUIDELINES

There has been a growing interest in the use of **institutional practice guidelines** as a means to reduce organizational cost. As a result, many institutional definitions of quality of care include edicts of practice guidelines. One of the nation's largest preferred provider organizations announced that more than 250 of their acute care hospitals have contributed to some 700 clinical pathways in an "cooperative program to address quality, clinical outcomes and cost of care issues" (Multiplan, Inc., 1997).

Managed care companies have used practice guidelines as indicators of quality. Although there is discussion and debate as to the validity of the outcomes, many practitioners are held to certain practice guidelines within their organizations. Organizational guidelines typically focus on resource allocation and utilization and outline the minimum acceptable standard of care. They may limit patient care and options of treatment. APNs may find themselves in the company of physicians in their obligation to adhere to organization guidelines that may be ethically questionable.

CRITICAL PATHWAYS

A critical pathway is defined as "a structured, multidisciplinary patient care plan in which diagnostic and therapeutic interventions performed by physicians, nurses and other staff for a particular diagnosis or procedure are sequenced on a timeline" (Ireson, 1997). **Critical pathways** were developed in 1985 by Bower and Zander (Carpenito, 1996). Critical pathways are simply timelines that dictate when a patient activity should be accomplished. Critical pathways have typically been used in the inpatient setting to reduce costs and length of stays. Although some studies would seem to indicate that critical pathways do control costs while providing quality of care, this is debatable.

The APN should be wary of clinical pathways that appear to replace standards and nursing diagnosis. Not every patient will not follow the same critical pathway for a particular illness. Pathways may be utilized as tools or reminders, but not as a plan of care. The APN is still responsible for using sound judgment and providing individualized care.

LEGAL IMPLICATIONS

Malpractice law requires establishment of certain elements, and duty to the patient is one of those elements. Both clinical practice guidelines and standards are used to establish a minimum duty in courts. There is an argument that guidelines and standards should not be used in court as a determination for what the nurse's duty was in a particular situation because they are professional tools only to aid the professional and the patient. However, when a court reviews a nurse's actions or omissions, the court has to look to some established duty for guidance in order to determine what is the usual intervention in the practice of nursing for a situation like or similar to the one before the court.

SPECIALTY NURSING PRACTICES

It is difficult to determine the exact number of APNs in the United States because of variations in licensing laws. One body of research suggests that in March 1996, of the approximately 71,000 registered nurses with formal preparation as nurse practi-

tioners, 31 percent were family nurse practitioners, 18 percent were adult nurse practitioners, 18 percent were pediatric nurse practitioners, and 33 percent were other types of nurse practitioners (Bureau of Health Professions, Health Resources and Services Administration, Division of Nursing, 1996).

Some states require that nurse practitioners have a certification through the state board of nurse examiners. Other certifying bodies are the American Nurses Credentialing Center (ANCC), the National Certification Board of Pediatric Nurse Practitioners and Nurses (NCB), the National Certification Corporation of the Obstetric, Gynecological and Neonatal Nursing Specialties (NCC), the American Academy of Nurse Practitioners (AANP), and the National Association for Nurse Practitioners in Reproductive Health (NANPRH). Box 17–7 indicates the breakdown of the employment location for Nurse Practitioners who work in an ambulatory care settings. Box 17–8 lists the various certifications that APNs may hold.

Numerous state and national organizations representing nurse practitioners have developed with the growth of the field. Both certified nurse midwives and nurse anesthetists have national organizations; however, many other specialty nurse practitioner associations have developed. Some of these associations are listed in Appendix 17–A.

ISSUES AND TRENDS

NURSING

A 1994 document from the PEW Health Professions Commission stated that because of the shortages of primary care physicians, the number of APN graduates must double by the year 2000 in order to meet the demand for health care. The document further attacks the restrictions some states have on APNs' autonomy and prescribing privileges (PEW Health Professions Commission, 1994).

There has been some speculation that midlevel providers, such as APNs, will soon replace family practitioners as the initial caregiver and medical evaluator in managed

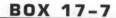

BOX 17-7

EMPLOYMENT LOCATION FOR NURSE PRACTITIONERS WHO WORK IN AMBULATORY CARE SETTINGS

- 36% in physician's practice sites
- 16% in public health or school sites
- 14% in community health centers
- 10% in hospital outpatient settings
- 4% in health maintenance organizations (HMOs)
- 24% in rural areas

Source: Bureau of Health Professions, Health Resources and Services Administration, Division of Nursing, 1996.
Based on 36,800 nurse practitioners in ambulatory care settings.

BOX 17-8

TYPES OF ADVANCED PRACTICE NURSE CERTIFICATIONS

CNS – Clinical Nurse Specialist
NNP – Neonatal Nurse Practitioner
PNP – Pediatric Nurse Practitioner
FNP – Family Nurse Practitioner
ACNP – Acute Care Nurse Practitioner
ANP/ARNP – Adult Nurse Practitioner
GNP – Gerontological Nurse Practitioner
CNM – Certified Nurse Midwife
OGNP – OB/GYN Nurse Practitioner
CRNA – Certified Registered Nurse Anesthetist

care organizations. Whatever occurs, in order for APNs to advance their practice, they will have to obtain the ability to function independently, to be reimbursed equitably for their services, and to practice without location restrictions (Guido, 1995). Another way to help promote APN practice is to have only the nursing boards regulate APNs, instead of the medical boards (Guido, 1995).

LAW

There is ongoing discussion regarding nursing practice across state lines. The **mutual** **recognition model** of nurse licensure is being evaluated by various APN associations and certifying bodies (Sharp, 1998). The proposal would allow nurses to practice in other states, either actual physical practice or electronic practice, without having a license in the other states (Sharp, 1998). The proposal would function similarly to the way driver's licenses are recognized across state lines. Thus, the nurse would have a license in the nurse's home state, but if the nurse chooses to practice in another state, the nurse would be subject to the other state's laws (Sharp, 1998).

Another issue for APNs is third-party

reimbursement. APNs are seeking to be reimbursed in full for the treatment they render. Currently, Medicare usually reimburses APNs for a percentage of the care they render compared to 100 percent of the care rendered by a physician for the same treatment (there are some exceptions where APNs may be reimbursed 100 percent). Most insurance companies follow Medicare's lead on reimbursement, so APNs are usually not receiving full payment for the care and treatment given to patients. Federal and state legislative sessions involve efforts toward total reimbursement for advanced practice nursing.

There are also campaigns in various states to obtain full prescribing authority for APNs, which would include the authority to prescribe controlled substances (Pearson, 1998). More than half the states currently allow some prescription of controlled substances. In the other states that do not allow APNs to prescribe controlled substances, APNs argue that limiting their prescriptive authority is limiting the care they are able to provide to the public.

Finally, there is a concern that APNs need to be recognized by all state legislatures and that all APNs need to be governed by the states' board of nurses. The argument is that until the legislatures statutorily acknowledge APNs, their status remains substandard, and that only nurses have the knowledge and experience to govern nurses.

ETHICAL ISSUES AND CONSIDERATIONS

Ethical issues in the nursing profession are not new. Nurses have traditionally listed staffing patterns, allocation of resources, and informed consent as important ethical issues. However, because of increased autonomy and independent judgment responsibilities, APNs may face even more complex ethical dilemmas than nurses in more traditional roles.

Situations in which patients have not provided advance directives may put APNs in an ethical dilemma in the area of artificial nutrition, hydration, and the prolonging of life. Disagreements about what constitutes "extraordinary means" may also arise. What decision does the APN make when the physician is not available and an urgent action beyond the APN's scope of practice is needed to care for the patient? What does the APN do when his or her values and beliefs regarding the welfare of the patient conflict with those of the physician?

The APN may face conflict with right to die issues and do not resuscitate (DNR) orders. As an independent practitioner, the APN may also face dilemmas in the areas of the right to treatment, informed consent, and unnecessary treatment. End-of-life decisions, cost containment issues that affect patient welfare, issues in human immunodeficiency virus/acquired immunodeficiency syndrome (HIV/AIDS) care, and providing futile care may confront the APN. Issues of advocacy and professional boundaries and responsibilities also will continue to be ethical dilemmas for many APNs.

Ethical issues that traditionally were faced by physicians may increasingly be faced by APNs. For example, managed care mandates that have traditionally focused on the physician may now include APNs. Moral dilemmas concerning organ harvesting and transplants, euthanasia, abortion, reproductive and genetic medicine, and pain management will become more commonplace for APNs. As heath care technology increases and the APN's role continues to evolve, it is imperative that each nurse know the laws regulating those issues of ethical concern. It is equally important that there is a formal or informal avenue for professional discussion and resolution when the APN is faced with ethical dilemmas that affect clinical judgment and decision.

RECOMMENDATIONS FOR RESEARCH

MALPRACTICE PREVENTION

The number one action to prevent malpractice or other problems is for the APN to become familiar with the laws, statutes, rules, regulations, standards, and practice guidelines that govern APN practice.

APNs should know the boundaries of their practice and should ensure that they do not extend their practice beyond those boundaries. Likewise, APNs should refer patients when the care required exceeds their capabilities or practice restrictions.

Because of the changing environment in which APNs find themselves, it is prudent for APNs to stay current. APNs should subscribe to a professional APN journal in order to monitor the changes in advanced nursing practice. Another method is to monitor the various websites on the Internet that involve advanced practice and other pertinent nursing issues.

Furthermore, because the status of APNs is changing and the potential is unknown, it would be beneficial for the APN to become active in a state or national organization that promotes APN practice and that seeks to change or implement legislation to aid APNs. Many nurses steer away from political activities, but they really can make a difference in the manner in which their profession is treated.

SUMMARY

Advanced practice nurses (APNs) are registered nurses who have received advanced education and training. Most APNs have master's degrees, but a smaller number have received an additional 2 years of clinical training along with the master's degree. APNs care for all age groups in various health care facilities, clinics, and private homes. APNs generally treat the patient from a holistic approach, rather than a disease-oriented approach.

APNs have become more and more a part of health care delivery since their inception in the 1960s and 1970s. As a result of the changes in health care, the increasing longevity of the population, and the decreasing number of general health providers, APNs are being looked to as the solution to the health delivery problems.

This trend is not occurring without controversy. APNs are seen as a threat to physi-

cians in that many physicians perceive APNs as receiving less education but nonetheless taking the place of medical doctors in the treatment of patients. However, the nature of health care today shows that there is a need for APNs, and there are studies that support the competency of APNs.

POINTS TO REMEMBER

- APNs are governed by regulatory agencies.
- Advanced nursing practice is regulated by statutes, which are enacted by the legislature, and by regulations, which are put in place by regulatory agencies.
- Court cases also affect APN practice along with standards of clinical guidelines.
- Advanced nursing practice is divided into four categories of practice: nurse practitioners, clinical nurse specialists, certified nurse midwives, and certified registered nurse anesthetists.

REFERENCES

Agency for Health Care Research and Quality. (1999) Nursing Clinical Guidelines from the AHCPR. [Online]. Available: http://www.ahrq.gov

American Academy of Nurse Practitioners. (1993). *Position statements.* Austin, Texas: Author.

American Association of Colleges of Nursing. (1994, May). *Media backgrounder: Expanded roles for advanced practice nurses.* Washington, DC: Author.

American Association of Nurse Anesthetists. (1998). *Information—Questions and Answers About a Career in Nurse Anesthesia.* Park Ridge, IL: Author.

American Medical Association. (1993, December). *Board of Trustees Report: Talking points (Addendum) to economic and quality of care issues with implications on scope of practice—physicians and nurses.* Chicago, IL: Author.

Bellegie v. Board of Nurse Examiners, 685 S.W.2d 431 (Tex. Ct. App.–Austin, 1985).

Board of Nurse Examiners for the State of Texas, Rules and Regulations Relating to Professional Nurse Education, Licensure and Practice, 22 Texas Administrative Code § 217.11 (1999).

Bureau of Health Professions, Health Resources and Services Administration, Division of Nursing. (1992,

March). *National sample survey of registered nurses.* Rockville, MD: Author.

Burl, J. B., et al. (1994, December). Demonstration of the cost-effectiveness of a nurse practitioner/physician team in long-term care facilities. *HMO Practice, 8,*157–161.

Carpenito, L. J. (1996, January–March). Editorial: Critical pathways: A wolf in sheep's clothing. *Nursing Forum, 31*(1), 3.

Department of Health and Human Services, Department of Nursing. (1992, March). *The registered nurse population: Findings from the national sample survey of registered nurses.* Washington, DC: Author.

Folkerts, D. J. (1994, March 8). *ARNP: Testimony before the Senate Finance Committee on Health Care Reform.* Kent, WA: Nurse Practitioner Support Service.

Guido, G. W. (1995, February). Advanced nursing practice: Legal concerns. *AACN Clinical Issues, 6*(1) pp. 99–104.

Ireson, C. L. (1997, June). Critical pathways: Effectiveness in achieving patient outcomes. *Journal of Nursing Administration, 27*(6), 1.

Loeb, S. (1992). *Nurse's handbook of law & ethics.* Philadelphia: Springhouse Corporation.

Multiplan, Inc. (1997, December 1). *Press release: Library of critical pathways enrolls 250 hospitals in debut release.* New York: Author.

Pearson, L. J. (1998, January). Annual update of how each state stands on legislative issues affecting advanced nursing practice. *The Nurse Practitioner, 23*(14) pp. 14–16.

Pew Health Professions Commission. (1994, April). *Nurse practitioners: Doubling the graduates by the year 2000.* San Francisco: University of California, Center for the Health Professions.

Rudy, D. R. (1995a, January). Advanced practice nurses: Should they be independent? *Archives of Family Medicine, 4,*14-16.

Rudy, D. R. (1995b, August). MD: Letter to the editor: In reply. *Archives of Family Medicine, 4,* 674.

Ruppert, N. (1995, August). RN: Letter to the editor. *Archives of Family Medicine, 4,* 674.

Safriet, B. J. (1992, Summer). Health care dollars and regulatory sense: The role of advanced practice nursing. *Yale Journal on Regulations, 9,* 417.

Salkever, D. S., Skinner, E. A., Steinwachs, D. M., & Katz, H. (1992). Episode-based efficiency comparisons for physicians and nurse practitioners. *Medical Care, 20,*143–153.

Sermchief v. Gonzales, 660 S.W.2d 683 (Mo. Banc, 1983).

Sharp, N. (1998). The drama of a paradigm shift: Looking at APRN licensure after the rear 2000. *The Nurse Practitioner, 23,* 142-143.

Texas Nursing Practice Act, Vernon's Annotated Civil Statutes, Article 4517 § 5 (Supplement, 1998).

Younger, P, Conner, C, Cartwright, K, Kole, S, Forsyth, J. (1997). *Physician assistant legal handbook.* Gaithersburg, MD: Aspen Publishers.

APPENDIX 17-A

SPECIALTY NURSE PRACTITIONER ORGANIZATIONS

American Academy of Nurse Practitioners (AANP)
Capitol Station, LBJ Bldg.
PO Box 12846
Austin, TX 78711

American College of Nurse Practitioners (ACNP)
503 Capitol Court, NE, #300
Washington, DC 20002

National Association of Nurse Practitioners in Reproductive Health (NANPRH)
1090 Vermont Ave., NW, #800
Washington, DC 20005

Uniformed Nurse Practitioner Association (UNPA)
Health Care Resources
1153 Bergen Parkway, M181
Evergreen, CO 80439

National Conference of Gerontological Nurse Practitioners (NCGNP)
PO Box 270101
Ft. Collins, CO 80527

National Association of Pediatric Nurse Associates and Practitioners (NAPNAP)
1101 Kings Highway North, #206
Cherry Hill, NJ 08034

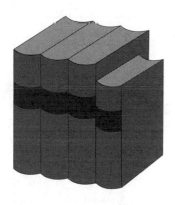

Chapter 18

HOME HEALTH NURSING

Anthony K. Cutrona

Supervision of Unlicensed Personnel by the
Registered Nurse
Usual Delegated Nursing Tasks
IMPLEMENTATION OF OASIS
**RECOMMENDATION FOR RESEARCH AND
MALPRACTICE PREVENTION**
MALPRACTICE ISSUES
AVOIDING MALPRACTICE
SUMMARY
POINTS TO REMEMBER
REFERENCES

KEY WORDS

Abandonment
Balanced Budget Act
 of 1997
Certified Agencies
Diagnostic Related
 Groups (DRGs)
Discharge Planner
Endpoint
Homebound
Home Health
 Agency (HHA)
Home Health Nursing
Home Health Providers

Hospital-Based Agencies
Interim Payment
 System (IPS)
Interpretive Guidelines
Medicare Conditions of
 Payment
Operation Restore Trust
Outcome Assessment
 System Information
 Set (OASIS)
Per Beneficiary Limit
Proprietary Agencies
Skilled Nursing Service

OBJECTIVES

Upon completion of this chapter, the reader will be
able to:
- Describe the primary elements of providing home
  health nursing care.
- Describe basic patient eligibility requirements under
  the Medicare home health benefit.
- Describe documentation requirements under the
  Medicare home health benefit.
- Identify and assess issues of legal risk in home
  health nursing.

HOME HEALTH CARE INDUSTRY

Home health care is a diverse and dynamic part of the U.S. health care industry. More than 20,000 providers deliver home care services to approximately 7 million individuals who have acute illnesses, long-term health conditions, chronic disabilities, or terminal illnesses (HCFA Health Standards and Quality Bureau, 1996a).

The first home care agencies were established in the 1880s. The number of agencies has grown from 1100 in 1963 to more than 20,000 as of December 1996. Of those providers, 10,027 are Medicare-certified home health agencies (**certified agencies**), 2154 are Medicare-certified hospices, and 8034 are home organizations that do not participate in the Medicare program (Table 18–1) (National Association of Home Care, 1996). **Home health providers** include visiting nurse associations, health departments, community-based nursing services, hospital-based agencies, nursing registries, hospices, independent professional practices, and proprietary agencies. **Hospital-based agencies**, those that are owned by and located in close geographic proximity to a hospital, constitute approximately 25 percent of all certified agencies. However, free-standing or **proprietary agencies** now constitute almost half of all certified home health agencies (Table 18–2) (National Association of Home Care, 1996).

HOME HEALTH NURSING

Home health nursing can be defined as the provision of nursing care to acute, chronically ill, and well clients of all ages in their homes while integrating community nursing principles that focus on health promotion and on environmental, psychosocial, economic, cultural, and personal health factors affecting an individual's and family's health status (American Nurses Association, 1992).

Home care providers employ more than 145,000 registered nurses and 40,000 licensed vocational/practical nurses (Table 18–3) (U.S. Department of Labor Statistics, 1994). The practice of home care nursing will continue to grow, not only in the number of nursing professionals choosing to provide health care in the home setting, but also in the rapidly increasing types of treatments that are now available outside an institutional setting.

MEDICARE HOME HEALTH BENEFIT

The growth of home care services was fueled by the enactment of Medicare in 1965.

TABLE 18–1. HOME CARE AGENCIES: MEDICARE-CERTIFIED AND OTHERS, 1989–1996

| Year | Total | MEDICARE-CERTIFIED AGENCIES | | |
		Home Health	Hospices	Other
1989	11,097	5,676	597	4,824
1990	11,765	5,695	774	5,296
1991	12,433	5,780	898	5,755
1992	12,497	6,004	1,039	5,454
1993	13,959	6,497	1,223	6,239
1994	15,027	7,521	1,459	6,047
1995	18,874	9,120	1,857	7,897
1996*	20,215	10,027	2,154	8,034

*1996 data as of December 31, 1996.
Sources: NAHC inventory of home care agencies for total agencies and HCFA Health Standards and Quality Bureau and Bureau of Policy Development for Medicare-certified agencies.

TABLE 18–2. NUMBER OF MEDICARE-CERTIFIED HOME CARE AGENCIES, BY AUSPICE, FOR SELECTED YEARS, 1967–1996

	Freestanding Agencies						Facility-Based Agencies			
Year	VNA	Comb	Pub	Prop	PNP	Oth	Hosp	Rehab	SNF	Total
1967	549	93	939	0	0	39	133	0	0	1,753
1975	525	46	1,228	47	0	109	273	9	5	2,242
1980	515	63	1,260	186	484	40	359	8	9	2,924
1985	514	59	1,205	1,943	832	4	1,277	20	129	5,983
1990	474	47	985	1,884	710	0	1,486	8	101	5,695
1991	476	41	941	1,970	701	0	1,537	9	105	5,780
1992	530	52	1,083	1,962	637	28	1,623	3	86	6,004
1993	594	46	1,196	2,146	558	41	1,809	1	106	6,497
1994	586	45	1,146	2,892	597	48	2,081	3	123	7,521
1995	575	40	1,182	3,951	667	65	2,470	4	166	9,120
1996	576	34	1,177	4,658	695	58	2,634	4	191	10,027

Sources: HCFA, Center for Information Systems, Health Standards and Quality Bureau.

VNA: Visiting Nurse Associations are freestanding, voluntary, nonprofit organizations governed by a board of directors and usually financed by tax-deductible contributions as well as by earnings.

Comb: Combination agencies are combined government and voluntary agencies. These agencies are sometimes included with counts for VNAs.

Pub: Public agencies are government agencies operated by a state, county, city, or other unit of local government having a major responsibility for preventing disease and for community health education.

Prop: Proprietary agencies are freestanding, for-profit home care agencies.

PNP: Private not-for-profit agencies are freestanding and privately developed, governed and owned nonprofit home care agencies. These agencies were not counted separately prior to 1980.

Oth: Other freestanding agencies that do not fit one of the categories for freestanding agencies listed above.

Hosp: Hospital-based agencies are operating units or departments of a hospital. Agencies that have working arrangements with a hospital, or perhaps are even owned by a hospital but operated as separate entities, are classified as freestanding agencies under one of the categories listed above.

Rehab: Refers to agencies based in rehabilitation facilities.

SNF: Refers to agencies based in skilled nursing facilities.

TABLE 18–3. NUMBERS OF HOME HEALTH CARE WORKERS, 1994 (BLS) AND MEDICARE-CERTIFIED AGENCY FTEs, 1996 (HCFA)

Type of Employee	Number of Employees[1]	Number of FTEs[2]
Registered Nurse	112,217	144,390
Licensed Practical Nurse	39,774	32,733
Physical Therapists	9,378	13,651
Home Care Aides	242,291	136,495
Occupational Therapist	3,626	3,569
SP	2,758	2,096
Social Worker	7,508	7,489
Other	137,848	64,536
Totals	555,400	404,959

Sources: [1]U.S. Department of Labor. Bureau of Labor Statistics, National Industry-Occupation Employment Matrix, data for 1994. Excludes hospital-based and public agencies.

[2]Unpublished data on full-time equivalents (FTEs) in Medicare-certified home health agencies as of December 1996 from the HCFA Center for Information Systems, Health Standards and Quality Bureau.

Medicare provided home care services, primarily skilled nursing care and therapy, to the nation's elderly population (Dolan, 1990). In 1983, implementation of a new hospital reimbursement system related to the assessment of a patient's medical diagnosis, called **diagnostic related groups (DRGs)**, brought major changes in patient treatments. Because hospitals were paid a predetermined amount based on the DRG, hospitals were forced to find ways to shorten time periods for inpatient care. As a result, patients began being discharged from hospitals to home at earlier stages of recovery with medical conditions requiring more acute and intensive nursing care. This further fueled the growth of health care being provided in the home setting (Richardson, 1994).

In 1997, the Congressional Budget Office estimated that Medicare home health expenditures would increase by 14.2 percent that year. In response to the Congressional Budget Office report, Congress passed major reforms of the Medicare home health benefit. Under the **Balanced Budget Act of 1997**, Congress implemented the **interim payment system (IPS)**. Under IPS, a per beneficiary limit averaging approximately $3500 per patient became law (Balanced Budget Act of 1997, 1997). The **per beneficiary limit** capped the amount home health agencies would be reimbursed annually for the home health services provided, regardless of the medical needs of the patient. As a result of IPS, home health agencies were forced to reduce the amount of home health services, while still providing the patient with the reasonable and necessary treatments (Institute for Heath Care Research and Policy, 1998).

IPS was designed to further limit the future growth of Medicare home health expenditures and resulted in the closure of many home health agencies. Despite the dramatic changes in the Medicare home health benefit, patients prefer medical treatment provided in the home. Since home care is less costly than institutional care, home health will continue to be a vital and essential part of the U.S. health care community (U.S. Department of Labor Statistics, 1994).

ISSUES AND TRENDS

HOME HEALTH SERVICES PROVIDED UNDER THE MEDICARE HOME HEALTH BENEFIT

Home care professional and personal care services covered by Medicare include skilled nursing, physical therapy, occupational therapy, speech-language pathology, medical social services, and services by home health aides. Medical supplies, durable medical equipment, and some intravenous drug therapy services are also included (HCFA Health Standards and Quality Bureau, 1996a, § 204.4). To be eligible to receive Medicare reimbursement for home health services rendered to eligible beneficiaries, the home health agency must comply with the requirements set forth in the **Medicare Conditions of Payment**, the State Operations Manual (SOM), and various other state and federal statutes (HCFA Health Standards and Quality Bureau, 1996b, § 2180; U.S.C. § 1861 (o)). The agency must pass an initial compliance survey, which is usually conducted by each individual state's health department (Public Health 42 C.F.R. § 409.49; U.S.C. § 1861 (m)).

Medicare patients are most often referred to home health services from their individual physicians or through posthospitalization discharges. In those referrals directly from the physician's office, the doctor, the patient, and the patient's family should discuss the home health options. In a hospital setting, a hospital-employed **discharge planner** is usually included in the consultations regarding home care services (Gingerich & Ondeck, 1994). Although the physician or discharge planner may recommend a home health agency, the patient still has the right to choose which Medicare-certified home health agency is to deliver the home health services. A failure to honor the patient's right to choose could result in legal liability (Gingerich & Ondeck, 1994).

Once a home health agency is chosen, the patient's primary physician may issue a written or verbal order to the home health agency to provide an assessment of the patient's medical condition. Under the Conditions of Payment, if a physician refers a patient under a plan of care that cannot be completed until after an evaluation visit, the registered nurse consults with the physician to obtain approval for additions or modifications to the original plan of care (Public Health 42 C.F.R. § 484.18(a)). In practice, the development of the plan of care is the duty of the registered nurse who performs the initial evaluation visit. The doctor should review and approve the plan of care; lack of interaction between the nurse and physician gives rise to a variety of legal problems. Because the patient is legally under the care and treatment of the physician, the physician retains ultimate responsibility and liability for the patient. However, home health agencies find that many physicians are apathetic or ignorant of their role in the provision of home health care services. This perception was validated by an audit conducted by the Office of Inspector General, in which physicians were found to have "failed to properly supervise the implementation and monitoring of the patient's plan of care" (Office of Inspector General, 1997).

Physicians rely on the recommendations and instructions provided to them by the home health care providers, especially the nursing personnel. The physician's abrogation of professional responsibility for supervising the patient's care places home health nurses at a high risk of incurring liability. It is critical that the home health agency personnel communicate with the physician regarding the patient's medical condition and any changes in it (Public Health 42 C.F.R. § 484.18(b)).

COVERAGE REQUIREMENTS UNDER THE MEDICARE HOME HEALTH PATIENT BENEFIT

To qualify for home health services, a Medicare beneficiary must meet each of the following requirements:

- Be homebound
- Need reasonable and necessary intermittent skilled services (skilled nursing, phys-

ical therapy, speech-language pathology, or continuing occupational therapy)
- Be provided services under a plan of care developed and approved by a physician (Public Health 42 C.F.R. § 409.42)

There are serious consequences for providing home health services to those patients who do not meet these coverage requirements. Billing Medicare for home health services that do not meet Medicare regulations can constitute false claims and subject the home health agency and its personnel to civil and criminal allegations of fraud and abuse (Money and Finance 31 U.S.C. § 3729(a)(1)). It is critical that the home health nurse have full knowledge of all Medicare clinical guidelines governing home health services, especially homebound status, medical necessity, and the plan of care, as discussed in the following sections.

HOMEBOUND STATUS

Whether a patient is considered **homebound** is one of the most scrutinized elements of the Medicare home health benefit. Under a nationwide government antifraud initiative entitled **Operation Restore Trust**, 39 percent of the home health beneficiaries claims that were reviewed were denied payment for not meeting Medicare guidelines (Office of Inspector General, 1997). Of those denials, 70 percent of the denials were made because the beneficiaries were not homebound, at least according to the intermediary responsible for making coverage decisions. In addition, approximately 96 percent of the Medicare reimbursement monies, which home health agencies were required to refund to Medicare, were a result of coverage denials based on homebound status guidelines (Office of Inspector General, 1997).

Under Medicare, in order for a patient to be eligible to receive covered home health services, the law requires that a physician certify that the patient is confined to his or her home. An individual does not have to be bedridden to be considered as confined to the home. However, the condition of these patients should be such that there exists a normal inability to leave home, and consequently, leaving home would require a considerable and taxing effort (HCFA Health Standards and Quality Bureau, 1996a, § 204.1). If the patient does in fact leave the home, the patient may nevertheless be considered homebound if the absences from the home are infrequent and for periods of relatively short duration or are attributable to the need to receive medical treatment. Where the patient is leaving the home to receive medical treatment, there is no limit to the number and length of time the patient is away from home. However, there is still the requirement that it takes a considerable and taxing effort to leave the home (HCFA Health Standards and Quality Bureau, 1996a, § 204.1).

Homebound status requires there be a normal inability to leave home. That inability can be due to physical or psychiatric limitations. If the patient is confined to the home because of the patient's psychiatric condition, it must be shown by either a refusal to leave home or that the condition makes it unsafe for the patient to leave home. If the patient is confined to the home because of physical limitations, it must take a considerable and taxing effort to leave the home, which generally requires the use of supportive devices, special transportation, or the assistance of others to leave home (HCFA Health Standards and Quality Bureau, 1996a, § 204.1).

Homebound status must not only be determined on the initial assessment, but must be an ongoing evaluation. If the patient's condition improves and he or she is no longer homebound, the patient must be discharged from home health service (HCFA Health Standards and Quality Bureau, 1996a, § 204.1).

NEED FOR SKILLED SERVICES

Although the Medicare home health benefit also covers physical therapy, speech-language pathology, and continuing occupational therapy, this section focuses on the legal requirements for coverage when the patient needs skilled nursing services. A **skilled nursing service** must be provided by a registered nurse, or by a licensed practical/vocational nurse under the supervision of a registered nurse (HCFA Health Standards and Quality Bureau, 1996a, § 205.1(A)(1)). To determine whether a service requires the skills of a nurse, inherent complexity of the service, the condition of the patient, and accepted standards of medical and nursing practice must be considered. Depending on the case, medical complexity is sufficient to qualify for skilled nursing service (HCFA Health Standards and Quality Bureau, 1996a, § 205.1(A)(1)).

Observation and Assessment

An important element of the provision of skilled nursing services includes the observation and assessment of the patient's condition by a licensed nurse. Observation and assessment are reasonable and necessary skilled services when: (1) the likelihood of change in a patient's condition requires skilled nursing personnel to identify and evaluate the patient's need for possible modification of treatment; or, (2) initiation of additional medical procedures, until such time as the patient's treatment regimen is essentially stabilized (HCFA Health Standards and Quality Bureau, 1996a, § 205.1(B)(1)).

Further, such indications as abnormal or fluctuating vital signs, weight changes, edema, symptoms of drug toxicity, abnormal or fluctuating laboratory values, and respiratory changes on auscultation may justify skilled observation and assessment. When these indications increase the likelihood that skilled observation and assessment by a nurse will result in a change to the treatment of the patient, the services would be covered. Observation and assessment by a nurse are not reasonable and necessary to the treatment of the illness or injury when these indications are part of a chronic condition and there is no modification in treatment modalities (HCFA Health Standards and Quality Bureau, 1996a, § 205.1(B)(1)).

Management and Evaluation of a Patient Plan of Care

Skilled nursing visits for management and evaluation of the patient's care plan are reasonable and necessary when underlying conditions or complications require that only a registered nurse can ensure that essential nonskilled care is achieving the desired outcomes. The complexity of the unskilled services that are a necessary part of the medical treatment must require the involvement of licensed nurses. If nursing visits are not required in observing and assessing the efficacy of the nonskilled services being provided, skilled nursing care would not be considered reasonable and necessary to treat the illness or injury (HCFA Health Standards and Quality Bureau, § 205.1(B)(2)).

Endpoint

When skilled nursing services are being provided on a daily basis (5, 6, or 7 days per week) and the visits are expected to last more than a short period of time (defined as more than 3 weeks), there must be a finite and predictable endpoint to the daily skilled nursing visits. This endpoint must be documented in the medical record and may be stated in days, weeks, months, or a specific date for ending daily nursing visits. Upon admission, the stated **endpoint** may be the physician's and the nurse's best guess of when the skilled nursing services will be reduced to less than daily. This endpoint should be adjusted if it becomes apparent that the original endpoint is not realistic. Once justified, an adjustment of the endpoint should be made immediately, in either the nurse's notes or the medical record. As always, documentation should be provided to validate the adjustment of the endpoint (HCFA Health Standards and Quality Bureau, 1996a, § 205.1(C)(3)).

If it becomes clear that there is not a finite and predictable endpoint to daily skilled nursing visits, then the patient no longer qualifies for Medicare home health coverage. The Medicare home health benefit was not established to provide daily skilled nursing services, but to provide intermittent skilled nursing services. The only exception to this rule is for a patient who requires and qualifies for skilled nursing services to perform daily insulin injections (HCFA Health Standards and Quality Bureau, 1996a, § 205.1(C)(3)).

PLAN OF CARE DEVELOPED AND APPROVED BY A PHYSICIAN

Medicare covers home health services only if a physician initially establishes a plan of care, certifies the need for care, reviews the plan, and recertifies the need for care at least every 62 days. A standardized method of data collection, HCFA Form 485, Home Health Certification and Plan of Care, has been developed by the Health Care Financing Administration (HCFA) to assist the physician, the home health agency, and the Medicare intermediary, the entity responsible for making coverage determinations and issuing the actual reimbursement checks to the home health agency (HCFA Health Standards and Quality Bureau, 1996a, § 204.2).

HCFA Form 485: Home Health Certification and Plan of Care

The HCFA Form 485 (Fig. 18–1) is the physician's plan of care for the patient. It lists the physician's orders for treatment for skilled services, medications, and the patient's functional limitations and permitted activities. This form is designed to meet federal regulatory requirements for both the physician's home health plan of care and home health certification and recertification requirements. The form is completed by the physician and the home health agency. It must be signed and dated by the physician before the claim is submitted for reimbursement. The ability of a home health nurse to prepare an accurate plan of care, one that provides a clear and individualized assessment of the patient's medical condition, is the most important tool in providing home health services in compliance with Medicare regulations. Accordingly, a comprehensive knowledge and polished documentation skills in completing a HCFA Form 485 is critical in reducing the risk of nursing malpractice in the home health setting (HCFA, Health Standards and Quality Bureau, 1996a, § 234).

HCFA Form 486: Medical Update and Patient Information

HCFA 486 Form, Medical Update and Patient Information (Fig. 18–2), contains descriptions of changes in the patient's status and treatment since the HCFA Form 485 was initially completed. It also provides information on the patient's status and needs on admission and at recertification (HCFA Health Standards and Quality Bureau, 1996a, § 234).

HCFA Form 487: Addendum

The HCFA Form 487, Addendum, is available to allow space for additional documentation of data elements contained in the HCFA Forms 485 and 486 (HCFA Health Standards and Quality Bureau, 1996a, § 234).

DOCUMENTATION REQUIREMENTS UNDER THE MEDICARE HOME HEALTH BENEFIT

The key to receiving proper reimbursement for the home health services provided to patients is proper documentation. When patients do not receive the benefits to which they are entitled or agencies are denied reimbursement for the delivered services, inadequate documentation is often to blame. Medicare auditors have focused on inadequate documentation, and this has resulted in a dramatic decrease in erroneous claims. A 1998 Medicare audit of all types of health care providers showed that undocumented and inadequately documented claims accounted for nearly 13 percent of all erroneous claims, down from nearly 30 percent in 1997 (Office of Inspector General, 1998).

Adequate documentation is required to achieve the necessary communication be-

tween the provider and the intermediary regarding the patient's home health care needs. In addition to the HCFA Forms 485, 486, and 487, Medicare requires very specific and precise information in order to make coverage decisions.

MEDICARE CONDITIONS OF PARTICIPATION

The **Medicare Conditions of Participation** (COP) are the federal regulations that govern the provision of Medicare home health services. HCFA delegates the responsibility for determining a home health agency's compliance with the COP to each individual state's health department. Those state surveyor agencies conduct the initial survey of the **home health agency (HHA)**, which determines whether the HHA meets Medicare certification requirements (HCFA Health Standards and Quality Bureau, 1996b). The state surveyor agencies also conduct annual surveys and complaint surveys to ensure that the HHA remains in compliance with the federal COP and any state regulation that governs home health services. In making the determination as to whether an individual condition of participation is met, the surveyor uses the State Operations Manual, which includes the Interpretive Guidelines for Surveyors (HCFA Health Standards and Quality Bureau, 1996b, § 2198). The **Interpretive Guidelines** serve to interpret and clarify the COP for HHAs. They merely define or explain the relevant statute and regulations and do not impose any requirements that are not otherwise set forth in statute or regulation (HCFA Health Standards and Quality Bureau, 1996b, Appendix B). If the surveyor determines that the HHA is not in compliance with any condition of participation, the HHA may be subjected to termination of its Medicare certification, and depending on the alleged deficiency, the individual nurse may be subject to sanctions.

Although a nurse who specializes in home health should be familiar with all conditions of participation, this section focuses on those specifically dealing with the provision of clinical services and the documentation of

HCFA FORM 485: PLAN OF TREATMENT

Department of Health and Human Services
Health Care Financing Administration

Forms Approved
OMB No. 0938-0357

HOME HEALTH CERTIFICATION AND PLAN OF CARE

1. Patient's HI Claim No. 2. Start of Care Date	3. Certification Period From: To:
4. Medical Record No.	5. Provider No.
6. Patient's Name and Address	7. Provider's Name, Address and Telephone Number

8. Date of Birth	9. Sex ☐ M ☐ F	10. Medications: Dose/Frequency/Route (N)ew (C)hanged
11. ICD-9-CM	Principle Diagnosis	Date	
12. ICD-9-CM	Surgical Procedure	Date	
13. ICD-9-CM	Other Pertinent Diagnosis	Date	

14. DME and Supplies	15. Safety Measures:
16. Nutritional Reg	17. Allergies

18. A. Functional Limitations

1 ☐ Amputation
2 ☐ Bowel Bladder (incontinence)
3 ☐ Contracture
4 ☐ Hearing
5 ☐ Paralysis
6 ☐ Endurance
7 ☐ Ambulation
8 ☐ Speech
9 ☐ Legally Blind
A ☐ Dyspnea With Minimal Exertion
B ☐ Other (Specify)

18. B. Activities Permitted

1 ☐ Complete Bedrest
2 ☐ Bedrest BAP
3 ☐ Up As Tolerated
4 ☐ Transfer Bed Chair
5 ☐ Exercises Prescribed
6 ☐ Panial Weight Bearing
7 ☐ Independent At Home
8 ☐ Crutches
9 ☐ Cane
A ☐ Wheelchair
B ☐ Walker
C ☐ No Restrictions
D ☐ Other (Specify)

continues

19. Mental Status   1 ☐ Oriented   3 ☐ Forgetfulness   5 ☐ Disenchanted   7 ☐ Agitated

2 ☐ Comatose   4 ☐ Depressed   6 ☐ Lethargic   8 ☐ Other

20. Prognosis   1 ☐ Poor   2 ☐ Guarded   3 ☐ Fair   4 ☐ Good   5 ☐ Exellent

21. Orders for Discipline and Treatment (Specify Amount/Frequency/Duration)

22. Goals/Rehabilitation Potential/ Discharge Plans

23. Nurse's Signature and Date of Verbal SOC Where Applicable:	24. Physician's Name and Address
25. Date HHA Recieved Signed POT	26. I certify/recertify that the patient is confined to his/her house and needs intermittent skilled nursing care, physical therapy and/or speech therapy or continues to need occupational therapy. The patient is under my care, and I have authorized the services on this plan of care and will periodically review my plan.
27. Attending Physician's Signature and Date Signed	28. Anyone who misrepresents, falsifies, or conceals essential information required for payment of Federal funds may be subject to fine, imprisonment, or civil penalty under applicable Federal laws.

FIG. 18-1. HCFA Form 485: Plan of Treatment.

HCFA FORM 486: MEDICAL UPDATE AND PATIENT INFORMATION

Department of Health and Human Services Health Care Financing Administrations	Forms Approved OMB No. 0938-0357

HOME HEALTH CERTIFICATION AND PLAN OF CARE

1. Patient's HI Claim No.	2. Start of Care Date	3. Certification Period From: To:

4. Medical Record No.	5. Provider No.

6. Patient's Name and Address	7. Provider's Name

8. Medicare Covered: ☐ Y ☐ N	9. Date Physician Last Saw Patient:

10. Date Last Contacted Physician:

11. Is the Patient Receiving Care in an 1861(j)(1) Skilled Nursing Facility or Equivalent?
☐ Y ☐ N ☐ Do Not Know

12. ☐ Certification ☐ Recertification ☐ Modified

13. Dates of Last Inpatient Stay: Admission Discharge	14. Type of Facility

15. Updated Information: New Orders/Treatments/Clinical Facts/Summary from Each Discipline

16. Functional Limitations (Expand Forms 485 and Level of ADL) Reason Homebound/ Prior Functional Status

17. Supplementary Plan of Care of File from Physician Other than Referring Physician: ☐ Y ☐ N
(If Yes, Please Specify Giving Goals/Rehab, Potential/Discharge Plan)

18. Unusual Home/Social Environment

19. Indicate Any Time When the Home Health Agency Made a Visit and Patient was Not Home and Reason Why if Ascertainable	20. Specify Any Known Medical and/or Non-Medical Reasons the Patient Regularly Leaves Home and Frequency of Occurrence

21. Nurse or Therapist Completing or Revising Form	Date (Mo.,Day,Yr.)

FIG. 18-2. HCFA Form 486: Medical Update and Patient Information.

those services. The home health nurse must provide clinical services in strict compliance with the following conditions of participation, including the acceptance of patients, plan of care, and medical supervision. Patients are accepted for treatment on the basis of a reasonable expectation that the patient's medical, nursing, and social needs can be met adequately by the agency in the patient's place of residence. Care follows a written plan of care established and periodically reviewed by a doctor of medicine, osteopathy, or podiatric medicine (Public Health 42 C.F.R. § 484.18).

Plan of Care

The plan of care developed in consultation with the agency staff covers all pertinent diagnoses, including mental status, types of services and equipment required, frequency of visits, prognosis, rehabilitation potential, functional limitations, activities permitted, nutritional requirements, medications, safety measures to protect against injury, instructions for timely discharge or referral, and other appropriate items (Public Health 42 C.F.R. § 484.18(a)).

Periodic Review of Plan of Care

The total plan of care is reviewed by the attending physician and HHA personnel as often as the severity of the patient's condition requires, but at least once every 62 days (Public Health 42 C.F.R. § 484.18 (b)).

Conformance with Physician's Orders

Drugs and treatments are administered by agency staff only as ordered by the physician. The nurse or therapist immediately records and signs oral orders and obtains the physician's countersignature (Public Health 42 C.F.R. § 484.18 (b)).

Duties of the Registered Nurse

The registered nurse makes the initial evaluation visit, regularly reevaluates the patient's nursing needs, initiates the plan of care and necessary revisions, furnishes those services requiring substantial and specialized nursing skills, initiates appropriate preventive and rehabilitative nursing procedures, prepares clinical and progress notes, coordinates services, informs the physician and other personnel of changes in the patient's condition and needs, counsels the patient and family in meeting nursing and related needs, participates in inservice programs, and supervises and teaches other nursing personnel (Public Health 42 C.F.R. § 484.30 (2)).

Assignment and Duties of the Home Health Aide

Duties of a home health aide include the performance of simple procedures as an extension of therapy services, personal care ambulation and exercise, household services essential to health care at home, assistance with medications that are ordinarily self-administered, reporting changes in the patient's conditions and needs, and completion of appropriate records (Public Health 42 C.F.R. § 484.36 (c)).

Clinical Records

A clinical record containing pertinent past and current findings in accordance with accepted professional standards is maintained for every patient receiving home health services. In addition to the plan of care, the record contains appropriate identifying information: (1) name of physician; drug (2) dietary, treatment, and activity orders; (3) signed and dated clinical and progress notes; (4) copies of summary reports sent to the attending physician; and (5) discharge summary (Public Health 42 C.F.R. § 484.48).

A finding that the HHA has failed to comply with any of the cited documentation-related conditions of participation may subject the individual nurse responsible for the compliance deficiency to legal liability. Further, depending on the nature and severity of the deficiencies, the HHA may be subject to allegations of fraudulent or abusive practices.

SELECTED LEGAL ISSUES

PREVENTING PATIENT ABANDONMENT IN HOME HEALTH CARE

The Balanced Budget Act of 1997 has brought the issue of patient abandonment to the forefront for all home health providers. It imposed dramatic reductions in reimbursement for home health services and resulted in a major reduction in the quantity of home health services provided. The reduction and termination of services resulted in home health agencies' and the individual home health nurses' incurring greater risk of legal liability for patient abandonment. It is essential for home health nurses to understand what constitutes abandonment and to take steps to reduce the risk of such a claim.

In December 1997, HCFA sent a written alert to selected state agencies responsible for overseeing home health agency compliance, requesting that they document complaints of patient abandonment. The letter further instructed the state surveyors to contact any home health agency against which a complaint was filed to inform the provider's administrator that denial or discontinuation of services that are not consistent with the Medicare COP may place the home health agency at risk for termination of its Medicare provider agreement (Min DePearle, 1977).

In determining whether a termination of services is warranted, even though nursing needs remain, the home health nurse must evaluate the individual situation. For example, when the patient or his or her primary caregiver is noncompliant with the treatment or medicine regimen, or when the home or family environment is unsafe for the home health agency's clinical personnel, the nurse should consider discharging the patient. However, the most common patient discharge situation may be as a result of shorter treatment periods necessitated by the reduction in reimbursement for home health services.

Home health providers must remember that one of the most important elements of home health care, from both a legal and ethical perspective, is to ensure that patients understand the rights provided to them under the law. Under federal law, a patient is entitled to be (1) informed of the care or treatment to be provided by the home health agency and any changes to such care or treatment, (2) informed of the patient's liability, if any, for payment of services rendered, and (3) given reasonable notice (except in emergency situations) prior to discharge by the home health agency (Public Health 42 C.F.R. § 484.10). A violation of these rights can result in a claim of patient abandonment when it arises by the failure of a home health agency to follow proper protocol in the discharge of a patient.

Abandonment is defined as the unilateral termination of the health care provider-patient relationship, without proper reasonable notice and when there is still the necessity of continuing medical attention (*Lee v. Dewbre*, 1962). To be liable for patient abandonment, it must be proved that (1) the health care treatment was unreasonably terminated; (2) the termination of health care treatment was contrary to the patient's will or without the patient's knowledge; (3) the health care provider failed to arrange for care by another appropriate skilled health care provider; (4) the health care provider should have reasonably foreseen that harm to the patient would arise from the termination of the care; and (5) the patient suffered actual harm or loss as a result of the discontinuance of care (*Katesetos v. Nolan*, 1976). A patient who is improperly discharged may file a lawsuit against the home health agency and the individual nurse for damages resulting from the wrongful discharge. If a lawsuit is filed, a referral to the state board governing nursing practice is very likely. A comprehensive understanding of discharge standards and the implementation of policy and procedures addressing patient abandonment is critical to prevent liability claims.

The home health agency and the treating nurse may avoid a claim for patient abandonment by providing the patient with reasonable notice of discharge before termination of services. A determination of what is reasonable notice depends on the specific situation of each individual patient. Those agency personnel who treat that individual patient should conduct a case conference to determine what constitutes reasonable notice for that patient. When determining a reasonable notice period, participants in the case conference must account for all relevant factors, such as the physical and mental condition of the patient and the accessibility of alternative care sources. Once a reasonable notice period is determined, the patient must be notified in writing, with the written notices being delivered to the patient's home, if consistent with the agency's policies and procedures. Because there is no federal regulation that mandates a minimum notice period for patient discharges, it is imperative that all nursing personnel consult their relevant state regulations that govern patient rights or discharges. As claims for patient abandonment increase, home health nurses must be knowledgeable about the issue and take positive steps to avoid such liability.

DELEGATION OF SELECTED NURSING TASKS BY REGISTERED NURSES TO UNLICENSED PERSONNEL

HOME HEALTH AIDE SERVICES

An important sector of home health services and one that is a source of potential liability for nurses is that of home health aide services. A nurse's failure to properly delegate and supervise the home health aide can result in the nurse's being held liable for negligence caused by the aide.

In order to qualify for Medicare home health aide services, the patient must meet the coverage requirements previously described (homebound, under physician's care, and in need of skilled services). In addition, the services provided by the home health aide must be intermittent, meet the definition of home health aide services, and be reasonable and necessary to the treatment of the patient's illness or injury (HCFA Health Standards and Quality Bureau, § 206.2).

Medicare coverage for home health aide services requires that hands-on personal care be provided to the patient or that services are

needed to maintain the patient's health or to facilitate treatment of the patient's illness or injury. The physician's order should indicate the frequency of the home health aide services required by the patient. These services may include:

- Personal care, including bathing, dressing, grooming, hair care, nail and oral hygiene, changing the bed linens of an incontinent patient, shaving, deodorant application, skin care with lotions and/or powder, foot care, and ear care; feeding; assistance with elimination (including enemas, unless skills of a licensed nurse are required because of the patient's condition); routine catheter care and routine colostomy care; assistance with ambulation; changing positions in bed; and assistance with transfers.
- Simple dressing changes that do not require the skills of a licensed nurse.
- Assistance with medications that are ordinarily self-administered and do not require the skills of a licensed nurse to be provided safely and effectively.
- Routine care of prosthetic and orthotic devices (HCFA Health Standards and Quality Bureau, 1996a, § 206.2 (a), (b), (c) and (e)).

GENERAL CRITERIA FOR DELEGATION

Depending on individual state laws, registered nurses (RNs) can delegate nursing tasks to nonlicensed personnel, within certain restrictions. Because the registered professional nurse is responsible for the nature and quality of all nursing care that a patient receives under her or his direction, a failure to properly supervise those to whom nursing tasks are delegated can result in a possible loss of his or her nursing license. The full utilization of the services of a RN may require a delegation of selected nursing tasks to unlicensed assistive personnel (UAP). Although UAPs may be used to complement the nursing services, such personnel may not be used as a substitute for the RN (22 Texas Administrative Code, 1999, § 218.1). If a UAP commits an act that would subject him or her to possible liability as a result of an improper delegation of nursing task or failure by the RN to properly supervise the UAP, the RN will also be subjected to liability. Accordingly, the RN must practice in compliance with basic requirements to avoid liability for improperly delegating nursing tasks and/or failure to properly supervise.

The RN must make an assessment of the client's nursing care needs. The RN should, when the client's condition allows, consult with the client to identify the client's nursing needs prior to delegating nursing tasks. The actual delegated nursing task must be one that a reasonable and prudent RN would find is within the scope of sound nursing judgment to delegate and must be one that, in the opinion of the delegating RN, can be properly and safely performed by the UAP involved without jeopardizing the client's welfare. The delegated nursing tasks must be based on the needs of the client and the knowledge and skills of the individual selected to perform such tasks. The nursing task *must not* require the UAP to exercise nursing judgment or intervention except in emergency situations. The UAP to whom the nursing task is delegated must be adequately identified. The RN must either instruct the UAP in the delegated task or verify the UAP's competency to perform the nursing task. The RN must adequately supervise the performance of the delegated nursing task in accordance with the supervision requirements set out in the following section. It is critical that the registered nurse realize that he or she retains full accountability and responsibility for the delegated nursing task (22 Texas Administrative Code, 1999, § 218.3).

SUPERVISION OF UNLICENSED PERSONNEL BY THE REGISTERED NURSE

The registered professional nurse shall provide supervision of all nursing tasks delegated to unlicensed persons. The degree of supervision required shall be determined by the RN after an evaluation of appropriate factors involved, including, but not limited to, the stability of the condition of the client; the training and capability of the unlicensed person to whom the nursing task is delegated; the nature of the nursing task being delegated; and the proximity and availability of the RN to the unlicensed person when the nursing task will be performed (22 Texas Administrative Code, 1999, § 218.4(1)).

When the RN delegates nursing tasks to unlicensed persons, the RN or another equally qualified RN shall be available in person or by telecommunications and shall make decisions about appropriate levels of supervision based on the health care setting and patient's condition. In the home health setting, the RN is required to assess, plan, intervene, and evaluate the client's unstable and unpredictable condition and need for skilled nursing services. The RN shall be responsible for the nursing care rendered and shall make supervisory visits at least every 2 weeks. The RN shall assess the relationship between the UAP and the client to determine whether health care goals are being met (22 Texas Administrative Code, 1999, § 218.4(1)(B)).

When the patient has stable and predictable health care needs, the RN shall make supervisory visits when, in consultation with the individual client and, when appropriate, with family and significant others, the RN determines it is necessary to ensure that safe and effective services are provided. The ability or desire of the client to participate in the supervision of the care provided by the UAP should be considered when establishing the frequency of supervisory visits (22 Texas Administrative Code, 1999, § 218.4(1)(C)).

USUAL DELEGATED NURSING TASKS

The following tasks are within the scope of sound professional nursing practice to be delegated, regardless of the setting, provided the delegation is in compliance with the general criteria and supervision requirements previously described:

- The collecting, reporting, and documentation of data, including, but not limited to, vital signs, height, weight, intake and output, Clinitest and hematest results, changes from baseline data established by the RN, environmental conditions, client or family comments relating to the client's care, and behaviors related to the plan of care

- Ambulation, positioning, and turning
- Personal hygiene and elimination
- Feeding, cutting up food
- Socialization activities
- Activities of daily living, limited to bathing, dressing, grooming, routine hair and skin care, meal preparation, feeding, exercising, toileting, transfer and ambulation, and assistance with self-administered medications
- Reinforcement of health teaching planned and/or provided by the RN (22 Texas Administrative Code, 1999, § 218.9).

IMPLEMENTATION OF OASIS

In January 1999, HCFA published new Conditions of Participation to require that home health agencies begin to collect the **Outcome Assessment System Information Set (OASIS)** and to report OASIS to their state survey agency. OASIS data items encompass sociodemographic, environmental, support system, health status, and functional status attributes of nonmaternity, adult patients. In addition to measuring patient outcomes, OASIS data have three important uses in the areas of patient assessment and care planning, individual agency case mix reports that contain aggregate statistics on various patient characteristics, and internal home health agency performance improvement.

Specifically, the condition of participation addressing OASIS requires that each patient must receive, and an HHA must provide, a patient-specific comprehensive assessment, which must accurately reflect the patient's current health status. The assessment should include information that may be used to demonstrate the patient's progress toward desired outcomes. It must identify the patient's continuing need for home care and demonstrate that the provision of home health services will meet the patient's medical, nursing, rehabilitative, social, and discharge needs. For Medicare patients, the HHA must verify the patient's eligibility for the Medicare home health benefit, including homebound status both at the time of initial assessment visit and again at the time of completion of the comprehensive assessment. The comprehensive assessment must incorporate the current version of the OASIS (Public Health 42 C.F.R. § 484.55).

Further, the OASIS condition of participation requires that the HHA conduct an initial assessment visit to be performed by a registered nurse only. The initial visit must establish eligibility homebound status and must be held either within 48 hours of the referral or within 48 hours of the patient's return home or on the physician-ordered start of care date. In addition, the HHA must complete a comprehensive assessment, which must be completed in a timely manner, consistent with the patient's immediate needs, but no later than 5 calendar days from the start of care. The RN must complete the comprehensive assessment and determine eligibility for the Medicare benefit, including homebound status (Public Health 42 C.F.R. § 484.55 (a), (b)).

RECOMMENDATION FOR RESEARCH AND MALPRACTICE PREVENTION

MALPRACTICE ISSUES

In addition to the issues specific to home health care nursing discussed earlier, nurses have to remain aware of the areas of risk inherent in all types of practice. The following issues have been identified as areas of potential nursing malpractice and unprofessional conduct under state nurse practice laws, and they can subject a nurse to serious consequences: (1) a failure to act in an appropriate manner in any patient situation; (2) a failure to report changes in the patient's condition to the physician; (3) a failure to provide appropriate nursing care based on the patient assessment; (4) a failure to follow physician orders; (5) a failure to properly delegate nursing tasks to; or, (6) properly supervise, unlicensed personnel; and patient abandonment.

AVOIDING MALPRACTICE

Nurses may reduce the risks of malpractice and avoid legal problems by ensuring they are educated in the individual state nursing practice law, the state and federal regulations governing home health care, and the specific policies and procedures of the home health agency where employed. In addition, there are affirmative measures that nurses may take to help reduce the risk and help avoid malpractice claims. For example, when the nurse is unclear on the appropriate nursing intervention, guidance and authorization from the home health administration or supervising nurse or the patient's physician should be sought. Because of the extensive documentation requirements under the Medicare home health benefit, the ability to properly prepare clear and detailed nursing notes is critical in avoiding malpractice claims and allegations of fraud or abuse. Nurses must strictly comply with all mandatory reporting requirements of the state or individual home health agency. Liability claims may arise against the best of nurses; therefore, malpractice insurance, with sufficient coverage amounts, is highly recommended.

SUMMARY

Nursing professionals practicing in the home health care arena must be aware and knowledgeable of those issues with an inherent risk of nursing malpractice. Nurses must have an understanding of the myriad of federal and state laws that govern home health agencies. In addition, they should be knowledgeable of the standards governing home health nursing practice and incorporate them into their daily practice. It is essential that home health nurses be aware of the coverage requirements under the Medicare home health benefit, including homebound status, medical necessity, and patient assessment and documentation requirements under the Conditions of Participation, specifically OASIS. Further, home health nurses must be aware of how to avoid liability regarding patient abandonment and the delegation of nursing tasks and supervision of unlicensed personnel.

Despite the reduction in home health agencies resulting from the implementation of the interim payment system, the increasing geriatric population, along with the general preference patients have for receiving medical care in their homes, will ensure that the demand for home health care will be strong. Those nurses who realize and appreciate what a privilege it is to be invited into the patient's home, will enjoy rewarding nursing careers in home health care.

POINTS TO REMEMBER

- More than 20,000 providers deliver home health care services to approximately 7 million individuals who have acute illnesses, long-term health conditions, chronic disabilities, or terminal illnesses.
- Home care providers employ more than 145,000 registered nurses and 40,000 licensed vocational/practical nurses.
- The growth of home care services was fueled by the enactment of Medicare in 1965.
- Home care professional and personal care services covered by Medicare include skilled nursing, physical therapy, occupational therapy, speech-language pathology, medical social services, and services of home health aides.
- Establishing whether or not the patient is homebound is one of the most scrutinized elements of the Medicare home health benefit.
- Medicare covers home health services only if a physician initially establishes a plan of care, certifies the need for care, reviews the plan, and recertifies the need for care at least every 62 days.
- The key to receiving proper reimbursement for home health services is proper documentation.
- The Balanced Budget Act of 1997 imposed dramatic reductions in reimbursement for home health services and resulted in a major reduction in the quantity of home health services provided.
- A nurse's failure to properly delegate and supervise the home health aide can result in the nurse's being held liable for negligence caused by the aide.
- When the RN delegates nursing tasks to

unlicensed persons, the RN or another equally qualified RN shall be available in person or by telecommunications and shall make decisions about appropriate levels of supervision based on the health care setting and patient's condition.

REFERENCES

American Nurses Association. (1992). *A statement of the scope of home health nursing practice.* Washington, DC: American Nurses Publishing.

Balanced Budget Act of 1997, p. 105–33 (1997).

Dolan, M. (1990). *Community and home health care plans.* Springhouse, PA: Springhouse.

Examining Boards 22 Texas Administrative Code § 218.1, .3, .4(1), .4(1)(C), .4(2)(B), .9, (1999).

Gingerich, B., & Ondeck, D. (1994). *Discharge planning for home health care: A multi-disciplinary approach.* Gaithersburg, MD: Aspen Publishers.

HCFA Health Standards and Quality Bureau. (1996a, December 31). *Home health agency manual* [HCFA Pub. 11, §§ 204.1, .2, .4; § 205.1A1, .1B1, .1B2, .1C3; § 206.2(a),(b),(c) and (e); § 234]. Washington, D.C.: Author.

HCFA Health Standards and Quality Bureau. (1996b, December 31). *State Operations Manual* [HCFA Pub. 7, §§ 2180, 2198, and Appendix B]. Washington D.C.: Author.

Institute for Health Care Research and Policy. (1998, March). *The Balanced Budget Act of 1997: Effect on Medicare's home health benefit and beneficiaries who need long-term care.* Washington, DC: Georgetown University for the Commonwealth Fund.

Katesetos v. Nolan, 368 A. 2d 172 (Conn. 1976).

Lee v. Dewbre, 362 S.W.2d 900 (Tex. Civ. App. 7th 1962).

Min DePearle, N. (1997, December). *HCFA Letter*, pp.1–2 .

Money and Finance 31 U.S.C. § 3729(a)(1) (1994).

National Association of Home Care. (1996, December). *Inventory of home health agencies.* Washington D.C.: Author.

Office of Inspector General. (1997). *Financial audit report of the health care financing administration.* Washington, DC: Author.

Office of Inspector General. (1998). *Financial audit report of the health care financing administration.* Baltimore, MD: Author.

Public Health 42 C.F.R. §§ 484.55(a) and (b); 409.42, .49; 484.10, .18(b), .30(a), .36(c), .48 (1990-1991).

Richardson, H. (1994). Long term care. In A. R. Kovner (Ed.), *Jonas health-care delivery in the United States* (pp. 194–231). New York: Springer.

Social Security Act of 1861 U.S.C. § 1861 (m) and (o) (1995).

U.S. Department of Labor Statistics. (1994). *The National Center of Health Statistics: 1994 health interview surveys.* Washington, D.C.: Author.

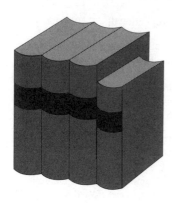

Chapter 19

LONG-TERM CARE NURSING

Anthony K. Cutrona

KEY WORDS

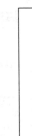

Abuse	Long-term Acute Care Hospital
Activities of Daily Living (ADLs)	Long-term Care
Advance Directives	Long-term Care Facilities
Assisted-living Facility	Minimum Data Set (MDS)
Bill of Resident's Rights	Nursing Facilities
Capacity	Older Persons
Competency	Omnibus Budget Reconciliation Act of 1987 (OBRA)
Directive to Physician	
Do Not Resuscitate (DNR) Order	Personal Care Facility
Durable Power of Attorney	Resident Assessment Instrument (RAI)
Gerontological Nursing	Restraint
Incompetency	Skilled Nursing Facilities (SNFs)
Instrumental Activities of Daily Living (IADLs)	Terminal Condition
Life-Sustaining Procedure	
Living Will	

OBJECTIVES

Upon completion of this chapter, the reader will be able to:
- Describe the primary elements of providing long-term nursing care to the elderly.
- Identify the various types of long-term care settings.
- Identify and assess issues of legal risk in long-term care nursing.

LONG-TERM CARE NURSING

Although long-term care includes patients of all ages, the coming explosion in America's elderly population will offer many challenges to our health care system. Professional nurses will be leaders in meeting the challenges inherent in providing medical services to the diverse population of patients needing long-term care. These challenges include ensuring the availability and accessibility of community-based and institutional care, so that those with chronic medical needs are provided with appropriate health care services.

Long-term care provides physical, psychological, spiritual, social, and economic services to help people attain, maintain, or regain their optimum level of functioning. It encompasses a range of services, provided throughout the life span to people who have lost their capacity to function independently because of a chronic illness or condition (National Center for Health Statistics, 1997). Long-term care is commonly thought of as caring for older adults in nursing homes. However, of those 65 years and older, only 4 percent lived in nursing homes in 1996. However, the percentage of those older adults living in nursing homes increased dramatically with age, ranging from 1 percent for persons 65 to 74 years to 4 percent for persons 75 to 84 years and 20 percent for persons 85 years and older (U.S. Bureau of the Census, 1998).

Of the 12.6 million Americans in need of long-term care, 81 percent reside in the community. Of those, about one-third are non–older adults and children (U.S. Bureau of the Census, 1997). Patients needing long-term care may include persons with mental retardation or chronic mental illness, disabled adults and children, those with chronic illnesses, persons with acquired immunodeficiency syndrome (AIDS), as well as the elderly. As discussed later, these patients may be treated in a variety of settings besides nursing homes. Generally, the nature and severity of their medical condition requires constant care and treatment, usually extending for the duration of their lives.

DEMOGRAPHICS

INCREASE IN OLDER PERSON POPULATION

Although it encompasses a wide variety of settings and types of patients, the focus of long-term care nursing practice is on the care of **older persons**, generally defined as those individuals aged 65 and older. The older person population is the fastest growing demographic group in the United States. According to statistics compiled by the Administration on Aging, a federal government agency, the older person population numbered 34.4 million in 1998. They represented 12.7 percent of the U.S. population, approximately one in every eight Americans. The number of older Americans has increased 9.1 percent since 1990, compared with an increase of 7 percent for the under-65 population. Since 1900, the percentage of Americans older than 65 years has more than tripled (4.1 percent in 1900 to 12.7 percent in 1998), and the number has increased 11-fold, from 3.1 million to 34.1 million. The older population itself is getting older. In 1998, the 65 to 74 age group was eight times larger than in 1900, but the 75 to 84 age group was 16 times larger. More important to long-term care issues, the population of those aged 85 years and older (3.9 million) was 33 times larger (National Center for Health Statistics, 1997; U.S. Bureau of the Census, 1996/1997).

The older population will continue to grow significantly (Fig. 19–1). The older population will burgeon between the years 2010 and 2030 when the "baby boom" generation reaches age 65. By 2030, there will be approximately 70 million older persons, more than twice their number in 1997. People aged 65 and older are projected to represent 13 percent of population in the year 2000 but will increase to 20 percent by 2030 (National Center for Health Statistics, 1997; U.S. Bureau of the Census, 1996/1997).

HEALTH AND HEALTH CARE

In 1997, 27 percent of older persons assessed their heath as fair or poor, compared with 9.4

Global Aging

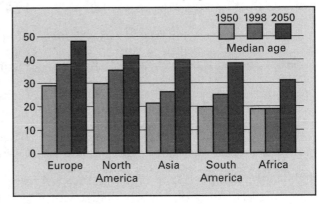

FIG. 19-1. Global aging. Source: United Nations Population Division.

percent for all persons. Limitations on activities because of chronic conditions increase with age. In 1996, 36.3 percent of older persons reported they were limited by chronic conditions. In contrast, only 13.9 percent of the total population were limited in their activities. In 1994 and 1995, more than half of the older population reported having at least one disability, with one-third reporting a severe disability. The percentages with disabilities increase sharply with age. More than 4.4 million (14 percent) had difficulty in carrying out **activities of daily living (ADLs)**, and 6.5 million (21 percent) reported difficulties with **instrumental activities of daily living (IADLs)**. ADLs include bathing, dressing, eating, and getting around the house. IADLs include preparing meals, shopping, managing money, using the telephone, doing housework, and taking medication (U.S. Bureau of the Census, 1997).

Most older persons have at least one chronic condition and many have multiple conditions. In 1994, the most frequently occurring conditions for older persons were arthritis, hypertension, heart disease, hearing impairments, cataracts, orthopedic impairments, sinusitis, and diabetes (U.S. Bureau of the Census, 1997).

As the older person population grows, the need for long-term care facilities and the nurses to staff them will experience dramatic growth. The ability to properly identify the special medical needs of elderly patients will be required of all nurses practicing in this area.

LONG-TERM CARE FACILITIES

Long-term care facilities include nursing facilities, skilled nursing facilities, long-term acute care hospitals, and assisted-living or personal care facilities. Each facility varies in the type and level of nursing care provided; however, because the overwhelming majority of their patients are elderly, they share common areas of nursing practice.

NURSING FACILITIES

Nursing facilities, commonly known as nursing homes, have standards defined by federal law. A nursing facility must care for its residents in such a manner and in such an environment as will promote maintenance or enhancement of the quality of life of each resident (Requirements for Nursing Facilities, 1990 § 1396r(b)(1)(A)). A nursing facility must provide services and activities or maintain the highest practicable physical, mental, and psychosocial well-being of each resident (Requirements for Nursing Facilities, 1990).

Federal statute also mandates various and specific types of care that a nursing facility must provide to its patients. A nursing facility must provide (or arrange for the provision of) nursing and related services and specialized rehabilitative services; medically related social services; pharmaceutical services; dietary services; an ongoing program, directed by a qualified professional, or activities designed to meet the interests and the physical, mental, and psychosocial well-being of each resident; routine dental services; and treatment and services required by mentally ill and mentally retarded residents. The services provided or arranged by the facility must meet professional standards of quality (Requirements for Nursing Facilities, 1990).

Further, federal law mandates that a certain level of professional doctor and nursing services be provided by the nursing home. It must "provide twenty-four (24) hour licensed nursing services, which are sufficient to meet the nursing needs of its residents, and must use the services of a registered professional nurse for at least eight (8) consecutive hours, seven (7) days a week. The nursing facility must require that the health care of each resident be provided under the supervision of a physician (or other licensed persons who may be allowed under state law), provide for having a physician available to furnish necessary medical care in case of an emergency and maintain clinical records on all residents" (Requirements for Nursing Facilities, 1990).

SKILLED NURSING FACILITIES

Skilled nursing facilities (SNFs) provide skilled nursing services to individuals who require extended inpatient care and are classified as hospital-based, free-standing, or swing-bed providers by Medicare for payment purposes (Post-hospital SNF Care, Coverage of Services, 1990). As a condition of Medicare participation, all SNFs are required to have a transfer agreement with a hospital in effect.

LONG-TERM ACUTE CARE HOSPITALS

Long-term acute care hospitals are hospitals that are primarily engaged in providing medical services to patients whose average length of stay exceeds 25 consecutive days (Long-term Care Hospitals, 1990).

ASSISTED-LIVING OR PERSONAL CARE FACILITIES

An **assisted-living facility**, also called a **personal care facility,** is not governed by federal law. Individual state laws provide guidance on the extent of health services these type facilities must provide. For example, under Texas law, a personal care facility must provide food and shelter and personal care services, including assistance with meals, dressing, movement, bathing, or other personal needs or maintenance (Assisted Living Facility Licensing Act, 1999).

Medicare may pay for personal care services, such as assistance with bathing, dressing, grooming, movement, eating, or toileting, under the home health benefit only if the facility has not contracted with the resident to provide those services directly (HCFA Health Standards and Quality Bureau, 1996). This type of facility is the fastest-growing segment of long-term care, so future federal regulatory control is likely.

ISSUES AND TRENDS

GERONTOLOGICAL NURSING

Gerontological nursing includes the delivery of direct care, management and development of nonprofessional caregivers, and the evaluation of care and services for the older client. All professional nurses caring for geriatric clients must have the basic knowledge and skills to develop the care plan by using the nursing process; establish a therapeutic relationship with the client and family; recognize age-related changes; collect data to determine health status and functional ability; function as a member of the interdisciplinary team; participate with clients, families, and other health care providers in making ethical decisions; act as an advocate for the aging client and family members; teach clients and families about measures that promote independence, maintain and restore health, and promote comfort; act as a source of referrals to other professionals or agencies, as appropriate; apply existing knowledge in geriatrics to nursing practice and interventions; protect the client's rights and autonomy; participate in continuing education, state and national professional organizations, and certification; and apply the standards of gerontological nursing practice to improve the clients' quality of care and quality of life (Acello, 1998).

The American Nurses Association (ANA), a national organization of nurse professionals, sets practice standards for nursing. The ANA *Scope and Standards of Gerontological Nursing Practice* provides a tool for which to measure accountability. Measurement criteria are listed for each standard so that nurses may assess their own performance and managers can assess staff members' performance (ANA, 1976a).

The *Standards of Clinical Gerontological Nursing Care* (ANA, 1976a) and *Standards of Professional Gerontological Nursing Performance* (ANA, 1976b) address health promotion, maintenance, disease prevention, and self-care standards. These current standards address the full scope of gerontological nursing practice in two parts, as follows:

STANDARDS OF CLINICAL GERONTOLOGICAL NURSING

The following standards of clinical gerontological nursing care describe the basic tools necessary to properly treat older patients.

Assessment by collecting client health data
Diagnosis by conducting an analysis of the assessment data
Outcome Identification individualized to the client
Planning by developing a care plan that prescribes interventions necessary to attain expected outcomes

Implementing of the interventions listed in the care plan
Evaluating of the client's progress toward attainment of expected outcomes (ANA, 1976a)

STANDARDS OF PROFESSIONAL GERONTOLOGICAL NURSING PERFORMANCE

The following standards of professional performance describe competent levels of care, performance appraisal, education, collegiality, ethics, collaboration, research, and resource utilization. Gerontological nurses are expected to engage in appropriate activities for their level of education, position, and practice setting. Gerontological nurses should seek activities such as membership in professional organizations, special certification, further academic education, or advanced practice education. The standards are described as follows:

Quality of Care by conducting an evaluation of the effectiveness of the quality of nursing care
Performance Appraisal by using applicable standards, statutes, and regulations to evaluate the individual nursing performance
Education by maintaining knowledge of current nursing practices
Collegiality by contributing to the professional growth of others by sharing information (clinical, research, etc.)
Ethics by behaving ethically when making decisions and performing actions that affect clients (ANA, 1976b)

MEDICARE RESIDENT ASSESSMENT REQUIREMENTS FOR LONG-TERM CARE FACILITIES

On December 23, 1997, the Health Care Financing Administration (HCFA) issued a final rule establishing a resident assessment instrument for use by long-term care facilities participating in the Medicare and Medicaid programs when conducting a periodic assessment of a resident's functional capacity. The **resident assessment instrument (RAI)** consists of a minimum data set of elements, common definitions, and coding categories needed to perform a comprehensive assessment of a long-term care facility resident. A state may choose to use the federally established resident assessment instrument or an alternative instrument that is designed by the state and approved by HCFA. These regulations establish guidelines for use of the data set and designation of the assessment instrument.

The RAI is intended to produce a comprehensive, accurate, standardized, reproducible assessment of each long-term care facility resident's functional capacity. The final rule is now codified as part of the Medicare Conditions of Participation Governing Long-Term Care Facilities (Conditions of Participation and Long-term Care Requirements, 1990). A combination of those sections that detail the new long-term facility resident assessment requirements is set out as follows:

1. *Resident assessment instrument.* A facility must make a comprehensive assessment of a resident's needs, using the resident assessment instrument (RAI) specified by the State. The **minimum data set (MDS)** required of each RAI must include at least the following:

    (i) *Identification and demographic information*, which includes information to identify the resident and facility, the resident's residential history, education, the reason for the assessment, guardianship status and information regarding advance directives, and information regarding mental health history.

    (ii) *Customary routine*, which includes the resident's lifestyle prior to admission to the facility.

    (iii) *Cognitive patterns*, which include memory, decision-making, consciousness, behavioral measures of delirium, and stability of condition.

    (iv) *Communication*, which includes scales for measuring hearing and communication skills, information on how the resident expresses himself or herself, and stability of communicative ability.

    (v) *Vision patterns*, which includes a scale for measuring vision and vision problems.

    (vi) *Mood and behavior patterns*, which includes scales for measuring behavioral indicators and symptoms and stability of condition.

    (vii) *Psychosocial well-being*, which includes the resident's interpersonal relationships and adjustment factors.

    (viii) *Physical functioning and structural problems*, which includes scales for measuring activities of daily living, mobility, potential for improvement, and stability of functioning.

    (ix) *Continence*, which includes assessment scales for bowel and bladder incontinence, continence patterns, interventions, and stability of continence patterns.

    (x) Disease diagnosis and health conditions, which includes active medical diagnoses, physical problems, pain assessment, and stability of condition.

    (xi) *Dental and nutritional status*, which includes information on height and weight, nutritional problems and accommodations, oral care, and problems and measure of nutritional intake.

    (xii) *Skin condition*, which includes current and historical assessment of skin problems, treatments, and information regarding foot care.

    (xiii) *Activity pursuit*, which gathers information on the resident's activity preferences and the amount of time spent participating in activities.

    (xiv) *Medication*, which contains information on the types and numbers of medications the resident receives.

    (xv) *Special treatments and procedures*, which includes measurements of therapies, assessment of rehabilitation/restorative care, special programs and interventions, and information on hospital visits and physician involvement.

(xvi) *Discharge potential*, which assesses the possibility of discharging the resident and discharge status.

(xvii) *Documentation of summary information*, regarding the additional assessment performed through the resident assessment protocols.

(xviii) *Documentation of participation in assessment*.

The assessment process must include direct observation and communication with the resident, as well as communication with licensed and nonlicensed direct care staff members on all shifts.

A long-term care facility must conduct a comprehensive assessment of a resident as follows:

(i) Within fourteen (14) calendar days after admission, excluding readmissions in which there is no significant change in the resident's physical or mental condition;

(ii) Within fourteen (14) calendar days after the facility determines, or should have determined, that there has been a significant change in the resident's physical or mental condition; or

(iii) Not less often than once every twelve (12) months (Resident Assessment, 1998).

ETHICAL CONSIDERATIONS AND CONFLICTS

PATIENT RIGHTS IN LONG-TERM CARE FACILITIES

There are approximately 17,000 Medicare/ Medicaid dually certified nursing homes in the United States, with more than 1.5 million residents (National Center for Health Statistics, 1997). In 1987, in an effort to improve the care of residents of long-term care facilities, the U.S. Congress passed the first federal resident rights provisions as part of the **Omnibus Budget Reconciliation Act of 1987 (OBRA)**. The provisions set out below outline the minimum standards of health, safety, patient autonomy, notice requirements, and fiduciary duties of facilities. All states are also required to have a **Bill of Resident's Rights** that are at least as protective as the federal statutes.

The Residents' Rights are as follows:

1. *Freedom of Choice:* A resident shall have the right to choose a personal attending physician; to be informed in advance about care and treatment; to be informed in advance about any changes in care and treatment which could affect resident well-being; and to participate in changes in care and treatment or planning care and treatment (Resident Assessment, 1990, § 483.10(d); Requirements for Nursing Facilities, 1990, § 1395i-3c(1)(A)(I),(v), § 1396r(c)(1)(A),(v)).

2. *Freedom from Abuse and Restraints:* Residents should expect to be free from physical or mental abuse, corporal punishment, involuntary seclusion, and any physical or chemical restraints imposed for purposes of discipline or convenience and not necessary to treat a medical symptom (Resident Assessment, 1990, §483.13; Requirements for Nursing Facilities, 1990, § 1395i-3(c)(1)(A)(i),(ii), § 1396r(c)(1)(A)(ii)).

3. *Privacy:* A resident should have a right to privacy regarding accommodations, medical treatment, written and telephonic communications, visits, and meetings of family and resident groups (Resident Assessment, 1990 § 483.10(e) (1); Requirements for Nursing Facilities, 1990, § 1395i-3 (c)(l)(A)(iii), § 1396r(c) (1)(A)(iii)).

4. *Confidentiality:* A resident has a right to confidentiality regarding medical and personal records (Resident Assessment, 1990, § 483.10(e)(2); Requirements for Nursing Facilities, 1990, § 1395i-3(c)(1) (A)(iv),(c)(3)(E), § 1396r(c)(1) (A)(iv),(c) (3)(E), § 3027(a)(12)).

5. *Grievances:* The resident shall have the right to voice complaints about care without fear of discrimination or reprisal for voicing concerns. The resident shall have the right to prompt action by the facility to resolve grievances, including

those about the behavior of other residents (Resident Assessment, 1990, § 483.10(f); Requirements for Nursing Facilities, 1990, § 1395i-3(c)(1)(A)(vi), § 1396r(c)(1)(A)(vi)).

6. *Accommodation of Needs:* The resident shall receive services with reasonable accommodation of individual needs and preferences, except where granting such accommodation would endanger the health and safety of others (Resident Assessment, 1990, § 483.15, § 483.20, § 483.25; Requirements for Nursing Facilities, 1990, § 1395i-3(c)(1)(A)(v)(1), § 1396r(c)(1)(A)(v)(1)).

7. *The Right to Participation in Resident and Family Groups:* The residential facility must promote and protect the right of residents to organize and participate in resident groups in the facility and the right of the resident's family to meet in the facility with the families of other residents in the facility; the resident has the right to participate in social, religious, and community activities that do not interfere with the rights of other residents (Resident Assessment, 1990, § 483.15(c), (d); Requirements for Nursing Facilities, 1990, § 1395i-3(c)(1)(A) (vii),(viii),(c)(3), § 1396r(c)(1)(A) (vii), (viii),(c)(3)).

8. *Access and Visitation Rights:* A nursing facility must permit immediate access to a resident by any representative of the Secretary, by any representative of the state, by an ombudsman or an advocate for the mentally or developmentally disabled, or by the resident's individual physician; permit immediate access to a resident, subject to the resident's right to deny or withdraw consent at any time, by immediate family or other relatives of the resident; permit immediate access to a resident, subject to reasonable restrictions and the resident's right to deny or withdraw consent at any time, by immediate family or other relatives of the resident; permit reasonable access to a resident by any entity or individual that provides health, social, legal, or other services to the resident, subject to the resident's right to deny or withdraw consent at any time; permit representatives of the state ombudsman, with

the permission of the resident—or the resident's legal representative and consistent with state law, to examine a resident's clinical record (Resident Assessment, 1990, § 483.10a; Requirements for Nursing Facilities, 1990, § 1395i-3(c)(3)(A)-(E), § 1396r(c)(3)(A)(E), 1990).

9. *Equal Access to Quality Care:* A nursing home must establish and maintain identical policies and practices regarding transfer, discharge, and the provision of services required under the state plan for all individuals regardless of the source of payment (Resident Assessment, 1990, § 483.12(c); Requirements for Nursing Facilities, 1990, § 1395i-3(c)(4)(A), § 1396r(c)(4)(A)).

10. *Rights of Incompetent Resident:* In the case of a resident adjudged incompetent under the laws of a state, the rights of the resident under this title shall devolve upon, and to the extent judged necessary by a court of competent jurisdiction, be exercised by, the person appointed under state law to act on the resident's behalf (Resident Assessment, 1990, § 483.10(a)(3); Requirements for Nursing Facilities, 1990, § 1395i-3(c)(1)(C), § 1396r(c)(1)(C)).

11. *Admissions Policy:* A nursing facility must, in respect to admission policy, not require individuals applying to reside or residing in the facility to waive their rights to benefits under the Medicare or Medicaid program; not require oral or written assurance that such individuals are not eligible for, or will not apply for, benefits under Medicare and Medicaid; prominently display in the facility written information, and provide oral and written information, about how to apply for and use such benefits and how to receive refunds for previous payments covered by such benefits; not require a third-party guarantee of payment to the facility as a condition of admission to, or expedited admission to, or continued stay in, the facility; and in the case of a Medicaid recipient, not charge, solicit, accept, or receive, in addition to any amount otherwise required to be paid under the state plan, any gift, money, donation, or other consideration as a

precondition of admitting, or expediting the admission of, the individual to the facility or as a requirement for the individual's continued stay in the facility (Resident Assessment, 1990, § 483.12(d); Requirements for Nursing Facilities, 1990, § 1395i-3(c)(5)(A)(i)(I)-(III),(A)(ii), § 1396r(c)(5)(A)(i)(I)-(III),(A)(ii),(A)(iii)).

12. *Transfer and Discharge Rights:* A resident has the right to remain in a facility and must not be transferred or discharged unless the transfer or discharge is necessary to meet the resident's welfare and the resident's welfare cannot be met in the facility; the transfer or discharge is appropriate because the resident's health has improved enough that the resident no longer requires the services provided by the facility; the health and safety of individuals in the facility are otherwise endangered; the resident has failed, after reasonable notice, to pay an allowable charge imposed by the facility for an item or service which the resident requested and for which the resident may be charged above the basic rate; the facility ceases to operate (Resident Assessment, 1990, § 483.12(a)(2); Requirements for Nursing Facilities, 1990, § 1395i-3(c)(2), § 1396r(c)(2)).

13. *Right to Preparation and Orientation:* A facility must provide sufficient preparation and orientation to a facility to ensure sage and orderly transfer or discharge (Resident Assessment, 1990, § 483.12(a)(7); Requirements for Nursing Facilities, 1990, § 1395i-3(c)(2)(C), § 1396r(c)(2)(C)).

14. *Right to Notice of Bed-Hold Period:* Before a resident is transferred for hospitalization or therapeutic leave, a facility must provide written information to the resident and a family member or legal representative concerning the period during which the resident will be permitted to return and resume residence in the facility under the state plan, and the policies of the facility regarding such bed-hold period. At the time of transfer of a resident to a hospital or for therapeutic leave, a nursing facility must provide written notice to the resident and a family member or legal representative of the bed-hold period (Resident Assessment, 1990, § 483.12(b)(1),(2); Requirements for Nursing Facilities, 1990, § 1396r(c)(2(D)(i),(ii)).

15. *Right to Priority Readmission:* A nursing facility must establish and follow a written policy under which a resident who is eligible for medical assistance for nursing facility services under a state plan, who is transferred from the facility for hospitalization or therapeutic leave, and whose hospitalization or therapeutic leave exceeds a period paid for under the state plan for the holding of a bed in the facility for a resident, will be permitted to be readmitted to the facility immediately upon the first availability of a bed in a semi-private room in the facility if, at the time of readmission, the resident requires the services provided by the facility (Resident Assessment, 1990, § 483.12(b)(3); Requirements for Nursing Facilities, 1990, § 1396r(c)(2)(D)(iii)).

16. *Relocation:* A resident is entitled to receive notice before the room or roommate of the resident is changed in the facility (Resident Assessment, 1990, § 483.15(e)(2); Requirements for Nursing Facilities, 1990, § 1395i-3(c)(1)(A)(v)(II), § 1396r(c)(1)(A)(v)(II)).

17. *Payment Obligations—Right to be Informed:* A nursing facility must inform each resident who is entitled to medical assistance at the time of admission to the facility or, if later, at the time the resident becomes eligible for such assistance of the items and services that are included in nursing facility services under the state plan and for which the resident may not be charged and of those other items and services that the facility offers and for which the resident may be charged and the amount of the charges for such items and services, and of changes in the items and services or in charges imposed for items and services included in the state plan; and inform each other resident, in writing before or at the time of admission and periodically during the resident's stay, of services available in the facility and of related charges for such services, including any charges for services not covered under Title 18 or by the facility's basic per diem charge (Resident Assessment, 1990, §

483.10(b)(5); Requirements for Nursing Facilities, 1990, § 1395i-3(c)(1)(B)(iii), § 1396r(c)(1)(B)(iii)).

18. *Right to Inspect Survey Results:* Upon reasonable request, the facility must provide the results of the most recent survey of the facility conducted by the Secretary or a state with respect to the facility and any plan of correction in effect with respect to the facility. The facility must also protect and promote this right to examine survey results (Resident Assessment, 1990, § 483.10(g); Requirements for Nursing Facilities, 1990, § 1395i-3(c)(1)(A)(x), § 1396r(c)(1)(A)(x)).

19. *Personal Funds:* A facility may not require residents to deposit their personal funds with the facility. Once a facility has accepted written authorization from the resident for the safekeeping of a resident account, the facility must hold, safeguard, and account for such personal funds under a system established and maintained in accordance with the following:

- The facility must deposit any resident's funds in excess of $50 in an interest bearing account (or accounts separate from any of the facility's operating accounts and credits all interest earned to the account). With respect to other funds, the facility must maintain such funds in a non-interest-bearing account or petty cash funds.
- The facility must assure a full and complete separate accounting of each resident's personal funds, maintain a written record of all financial transactions involving a resident's personal funds, and afford the resident or their legal representative reasonable access to such record.
- The facility must notify each resident receiving Medicaid when the amount in the resident's account reaches $200 less than the applicable resource limit, and that if the amount in the account (in addition with the resident's other resources) reaches above the allowable resource limit, the resident may lose income eligibility for Medicaid or SSI.
- Upon the death of the resident with an account, the facility must promptly convey the resident's personal funds and an accounting to the estate (Resident Assessment, 1990, § 483.10(c); Requirements for Nursing Facilities, 1990, § 1395i-3(c)(6), § 1396r(c)(6)).

20. *Right to be Informed about Rights:* A nursing facility must inform each resident, orally and in writing at the time of admission to the facility, of the resident's legal rights during the stay at the facility; make available to each resident, upon reasonable request, a written statement of such rights, which shall include a description of the requirements for protection of personal funds and a statement that a resident may file a complaint with a state survey and certification agency respecting resident abuse and neglect and misappropriation of resident property in the facility. Written statements of rights must be updated when changes are made in rights provided by state or federal law (Resident Assessment, 1990, § 483.10(b)(1); Requirements for Nursing Facilities, 1990, § 1395i-3(c)(1)(B)(i),(ii), § 1396r(c)(1)(B)(i),(ii)).

A failure to provide appropriate clinical care can result in not only a medical malpractice, but also a claim that the patient's rights have been violated. For example, in Florida a son was awarded $719,064.02 in compensatory damages and $2 million in punitive damages after his father died as a result of severe bedsores obtained at the nursing home facility. The Appeals Court upheld the damage award under a statute providing for a civil action based on a violation of rights of a nursing home resident. The Court held that the damages were not limited by the Wrongful Death Act when such a violation resulted in a patient's death. Furthermore, a claim for the resident's pain and suffering prior to death was valid (*Beverly Enterprises–Florida, Inc. v. Spilman*, 1995).

Accordingly, nurses practicing in the long-term care area must have a full understanding of the Residents' Rights. Each individual state may implement more expansive patient rights than the federal residents' rights just described. Each long-term facility and its nursing staff must know their state's residents' rights and ensure that strict compliance is inherent in providing care to those patients.

COMPETENCY

Determining whether a patient is competent to make his or her own health decisions is one of the most difficult areas of gerontological nursing practice. The legal implications of assuming that a patient is competent, without fully assessing the ability of the patient to understand the consequences of accepting or refusing specific medical treatments, can subject the nurse to legal liability. Under the Residents' Rights, the elderly person, unless adjudicated legally incompetent by a court, is presumed competent to make his or her own decisions. If the patient's competency is questionable, the nurses must consult with the physician, facility administrator, and family members, if any. Competence and capacity must be determined before considering the patient's health care decisions, and if not satisfactorily determined, the courts may become involved. This is an area of nursing where, too often, nurses may be called on to make legal decisions outside their expertise. An understanding of the differences in competency, capacity, and incompetency will assist the long-term nurse in navigating this difficult issue.

Competency may be defined as follows: of legal age, without mental disability or incapacity, legally fit and qualified to give testimony or execute legal documents. In the law, with regard to health care decisions, there is no definitive test for competency (Aiken, 1994).

Incompetency may be defined as an inability to understand information needed to reason and deliberate, an inability to make decisions in one's best interests. A patient who is unconscious and completely unable to communicate because of some gross impairment is incompetent. However, for most patients, competency may fluctuate, making a decision difficult to execute.

Capacity may be defined as possession of a set of values and goals, the ability to communicate and understand information, and the ability to reason and deliberate about one's choices (Eliopoulos, 1994).

ADVANCE DIRECTIVES

Advance directives allow individuals to choose in advance of physical or mental incapacity what health care treatments or life-sustaining measures are to be received or withdrawn and who may assist in making those decisions. Under federal law, health care providers are required to provide its patients with information on advance directives (Reqirements for Nursing Facilities, 1990, § 1395cc). Even though these documents have life or death consequences, few patients or providers are comfortable discussing the legal ramifications of such declarations. It is ironic that clinical personnel are responsible for providing such critical legal advice and seldom have they been provided with sufficient legal guidance.

There are several types of documents that are categorized as advance directives. Three of those most closely related to health care issues are the do not resuscitate (DNR) order, the durable power of attorney for health care, and the directive to physician, commonly known as the living will.

DO NOT RESUSCITATE ORDERS

A **do not resuscitate (DNR) order** is a legal document that provides instructions to health care providers related to the patient's right to refuse specific life-saving treatments. Under the Residents' Rights, the patient has the right to refuse treatment, regardless of his or her health condition. However, the patient must have the capacity to refuse treatment.

All long-term facilities should have DNR policies developed in consultation with medical and nursing staffs and other appropriate facility staff. The policies should address conflict resolution and shared decision-making between the health care staff and the patient's family. In order for the DNR order to be effective, the patient must be competent when the DNR order is made. Supporting documentation should include client's current condition, prognosis, summary of decision-making, and the parties involved in the decision. It should also include designation of a future date for review of the DNR order (Joint Commission on Accreditation of Healthcare Organizations [JCAHO], 1998).

DNR orders address the refusal of life-saving treatment; a related area is the issue of withdrawing existing medical treatment. The withdrawal of life-prolonging care presents a major ethical dilemma. However, the withdrawal of nutrition and/or hydration, which may be an exception to the patient's right to withhold or withdraw treatment, has been addressed by the American Medical Association (AMA) and the American Nurses Association (ANA). The AMA, in its *Statement on Withholding or Withdrawing Life Prolonging Medical Treatment*, indicated that the insertion of a feeding tube or intravenous feeding is medical treatment. Accordingly, it is the AMA's position that nutrition and hydration may be refused.

In contrast, the American Nurses Association Committee on Ethics stated that the provision of food and fluid is nursing care. Accordingly, the withholding or withdrawing nutrition and hydration is generally not morally permissible, except if a patient is harmed more by being fed than by refusing.

This conflict between the positions of the ANA and the AMA is a source of potential liability for the long-term care nurse. Because the nurse's duties may include application of a nasally inserted feeding tube or starting an intravenous infusion through which nutrition and hydration could be provided, the withdrawal of this nursing care may raise ethical and legal issues. Consultation with the facility administrative staff and other legal counsel would be advised in such a situation.

DURABLE POWER OF ATTORNEY FOR HEALTH CARE

Durable power of attorney for health care is a legal document that allows a patient to designate an agent to make health care decisions for the patient. Because there is not a standardized form promulgated under federal law, several states have enacted state laws addressing this issue. The elements of a durable power of attorney for health care discussed in this section are based on the revised statutes promulgated in Texas (Ad-

vance Directives Act, 1999). Nurses practicing in long-term care should always be familiar with the relevant laws of their state.

The power authorized by the statute takes effect only when the patient's attending physician certifies in writing that the patient lacks the capacity to make health care decisions. However, the patient *need not be competent* to revoke the power. A durable power of attorney for health care can be revoked by *any* notification by the patient to the agent or a care provider, or by any act "evidencing a specific intent to revoke the power" (Advance Directives Act, 1999).

The health care agent must make health care decisions according to knowledge of the patient's wishes or using best judgment of what is in the patient's best interest. The patient may further limit the agent's authority and should do so in writing. In some states, the power of attorney may authorize the agent to withdraw or withhold life-sustaining procedures, as in a directive to physician (Advance Directives Act, 1999).

Generally, witnessing requirements prohibit any employee of the treating health care facility from being a witness to the execution of any type of advance directive. However, under the new Texas law, of the two witnesses required, one may now be an employee of a treating health care facility, making it easier for a hospitalized patient to execute the advanced directive (Advance Directives Act, 1999). The witnessing requirements for advance directives may vary according to state law, but must always be strictly adhered to.

DIRECTIVES TO PHYSICIANS

Most people are familiar with the term **living will**, legally known as a **directive to physician**. Almost all states have passed legislation allowing any adult to sign a directive instructing his or her physician to withhold or withdraw life-sustaining procedures in the event of a terminal condition.

As with the durable power of attorney for health care, individual state laws govern the termination or refusal of life-sustaining procedures. Further, state laws provide guidance for care providers as to their evaluation and acceptance of and duties under the directives and should include guidance for the patient's family in making the decision, in conjunction with a physician, to withhold or withdraw life-sustaining procedures (Advance Directives Act, 1999).

In general, directives to physicians state that life-sustaining procedures shall be withheld or withdrawn in the event of a terminal condition. A **life-sustaining procedure** is a medical procedure, treatment, or intervention that utilizes mechanical or other artificial means to sustain, restore, or supplant a vital function and, when applied to a person in a terminal condition, serves only to prolong the process of dying. In Texas, a **terminal condition** is statutorily defined as an incurable or irreversible condition caused by injury, disease, or illness that would produce death without the application of life-sustaining procedures according to reasonable medical judgment and in which the application of life-sustaining procedures serves only to postpone the moment of death. A terminal condition must be certified in writing by the examining physician (Advance Directives Act, 1999). Some states may require the certification of more than one physician.

A directive must be made a part of the patient's medical record. The attending physician must comply with the directive unless the physician believes that the directive does not reflect the present desire of the patient. When a qualified adult has designated a health care agent to make treatment decisions, that agent and the attending physician may make the decision to withhold or withdraw life-sustaining procedures from the patient (Advance Directives Act, 1999).

Generally, health care providers are not criminally or civilly liable for failing to carry out the directive of a patient. If an agent, guardian, or family member complies with the statutory rules, he or she should not be held liable. Liability should only arise if the agent, guardian, or family member acts in total disregard of the patient's known wishes or fails to take reasonable steps necessary to ascertain the patient's wishes concerning life-sustaining procedures (Advance Directives Act, 1999). However, a failure to honor a patient's clear instructions concerning treatment may violate the rights of the patient.

To avoid liability, long-term care facilities must implement policies and procedures addressing the termination or withholding of life-sustaining procedures and ensure that all facility staff understand and comply with such policies.

PHYSICAL RESTRAINTS

Restraint may be defined as the use of a chemical substance, mechanical device, and/or physical restriction by one or more persons that limits the activity of another. In accordance with an individual treatment plan, safe and proper nursing care may include the use of protective devices and restraints. However, these measures are indicated only under limited and specific situations where (1) the patient's treatment plan indicates it is necessary as an integral part of the plan to protect the safety of the patient or others and not for the convenience of the staff or facility; (2) there is an authorizing physician's order based on personal observation and assessment of the patient, consistent with state regulations and institutional policy; and (3) a good faith effort to use the least restrictive measures has been attempted prior to applying the more severe and restrictive restraint (Resident Assessment, 1990, § 405.1121).

PATIENT ABUSE AND NEGLECT

Abuse or neglect of a resident of a long-term care facility is illegal under federal and state laws. Any employee who has cause to believe that the physical or mental health of a resident of a health care facility has been adversely affected by abuse or neglect must report it to the appropriate state agencies. Most states have mandatory reporting laws that require the reporting of elder abuse or neglect to the proper law enforcement authorities and provide penalties for a failure to report.

Patient abuse or neglect may give rise not only to a civil suit for violation of civil rights and breach of contract and negligence, but also to possible criminal prosecution. Despite the efforts of enforcement officials, the elderly in nursing homes are subject to patient abuse, and tremendous problems remain in the care and safety of the elderly. Proper and professional nursing care is essential to prevent abuse and neglect and provide long-term patients with the care they deserve.

RECOMMENDATIONS FOR RESEARCH AND MALPRACTICE PREVENTION

MALPRACTICE ISSUES

In addition to the issues specific to long-term care nursing previously discussed, nurses have to remain aware of the areas of risk inherent in all types of practice. The following issues have been identified as areas of potential nursing malpractice and unprofessional conduct under state nursing practice laws, conduct that can subject a nurse to serious consequences: (1) a failure to act in an appropriate manner in any patient situation; (2) a failure to report changes in the patient's condition to the physician; (3) a failure to provide appropriate nursing care based on the patient or resident assessment; and (4) a failure to follow physician orders.

As a result of reductions and changes in the reimbursement methods for long-term care facilities, there are financial constraints that may raise malpractice issues. The following are areas of concern that may arise because of those changes: (1) a failure to adequately monitor a patient as a result of possible staff reductions; (2) a failure to properly delegate nursing tasks to unlicensed personnel, such as certified nursing assistants; and (3) a failure to properly supervise unlicensed personnel, such as certified nursing assistants.

AVOIDING MALPRACTICE

Nurses may reduce the risks of malpractice and avoid legal problems by ensuring that they are fully educated in the following areas: (1) the individual state nurse practice law; (2) the state and federal regulations governing long-term care; (3) the specific policies and procedures of the long-term facility where employed; and (4) the standard governing long-term and gerontological nursing practice.

In addition, there are affirmative measures that nurses may take to help reduce the risk and help avoid malpractice claims. For example, when the nurse is unclear on the appropriate nursing intervention, guidance and authorization from the facility administration or management should be sought. The development of good documentation skills is critical in avoiding malpractice claims. Nurses must strictly comply with all mandatory reporting requirements of the state or the individual facility. Because liability claims may arise against the best of nurses, malpractice insurance, with sufficient coverage amounts, is highly recommended.

SUMMARY

Those nursing professionals practicing in the long-term care arena must be aware and knowledgeable of those issues with an inherent risk of nursing malpractice. Nurses must have an understanding of the myriad of federal and state laws that govern long-term care facilities. In addition they should be knowledgeable of the standards governing gerontological nursing practice and incorporate them into their daily practice. It is essential that long-term care nurses be aware of issues such as patient rights, patient competency, advance directives, and patient abuse and neglect in order to avoid the associated legal risks.

The growth of the older person population along with the continuing increase in life span will ensure that the demand for those nursing professionals well versed in long-term care will be strong. The elderly, along with our children, are our most vulnerable and valuable citizens. Those nurses who choose to provide professional and compassionate nursing care will ensure that our elders' twilight years are quality years. They will also enjoy rewarding nursing careers in long-term care.

POINTS TO REMEMBER

- Long-term care nursing provides physical, psychological, spiritual, social, and economic support and services.
- Of the 12.6 million Americans in need of long-term care, 81 percent reside in the community; of those, approximately one-third are non–older adults and children.
- Most older persons have at least one chronic condition and many have multiple conditions.
- Long-term care facilities include nursing facilities, skilled nursing facilities, long-term acute care facilities, and assisted living or personal care facilities.
- Federal statutory law mandates various and specific types of care that a nursing facility must provide to its patients.
- The resident assessment instrument (RAI) is intended to produce a comprehensive, accurate, standardized, reproducible assessment of each long-term care facility resident's functional capacity.
- There are approximately 17,000 Medicare/Medicaid dually certified nursing homes in the United States, with more than 1.5 million residents.
- The conflict between the ANA's and the AMA's position on withholding or withdrawing life-prolonging medical treatment is a source of potential liability for the long-term care nurse.

REFERENCES

Acello, B. (1998). *The geriatric survival handbook*. Englewood, CO: Skidmore-Roth Publishing.

Advance Directives Act, Health and Safety Code, Vernon's Texas Codes Annotated, Chapter 166 *et seq.* (1999).

Aiken, T. D. (1994). *Legal, ethical, and political issues in nursing*. Philadelphia: F.A. Davis.

American Nurses Association. (1976a). *Standards of clinical gerontological nursing*. Kansas City, MO: Author.

American Nurses Association. (1976b). *Standards of professional gerontological nursing performance*. Kansas City, MO: Author.

Assisted Living Facility Licensing Act, Health and Safety Code, Vernon's Texas Codes Annotated, Chapter 247 *et seq.* (1999).

Beverly Enterprises-Florida, Inc. v. Spilman, 661 So. 2d 867 (Fla. 1995).

Conditions of Participation and Long-term Care Requirements, 42 C.F.R. § 488.3 (1993).

Convalescent and Nursing Homes and Related Institutions, Health and Safety Code, Vernon's Texas Codes Annotated, Chapter 242 *et seq.* (1997).

Eliopoulos, C. (1994). *Gerontological nursing* (3rd ed.). Philadelphia: J.B. Lippincott.

HCFA Health Standards and Quality Bureau. (1996, December 31). *Home health agency manual* [HCFA Pub. 11, § 200.2]. Washington, D.C.: Author.

HCFA Health Standards and Quality Bureau. (1996, December 31). *Medicare home health agency manual*. [HCFA Pub. 11, § 202.2].

Joint Commission on Accreditation of Healthcare Organizations. (1998). *Manual for accreditation*. Oakbrook Terrace, IL: Author.

Long-term Care Hospitals, 42 C.F.R. § 412.23 (e)(1) (1990).

National Center for Health Statistics. (1997, January 23). *An overview of nursing homes and their current residents: Data from the 1995 National Nursing Home Survey*. Hyattsville, MD: Genevieve W. Strahan.

Omnibus Budget Reconciliation Act of 1987, Public Law 100–203.

Post-hospital SNF Care, Coverage of Services, 42 C.F.R. § 409.20–36 (1990).

Requirements for Nursing Facilities, 42 U.S.C § 1395i *et seq.*; 1396r *et seq.*, 3027(a) (1990).

Resident Assessment, 42 C.F.R. § 483 *et seq.* (1998).

U.S. Bureau of the Census. (1996, February). Population projections of the United States by age, sex, race and Hispanic origin: 1995–2050. *Current Population Reports*, pp. 25–1130.

U.S. Bureau of the Census. (1997, August). Americans with Disabilities, 1994–95. *Current Population Reports*, pp. 70–615.

U.S. Bureau of the Census. (1998). Household and family characteristics: March 1998. *Current Population Reports*, pp. 20–515.

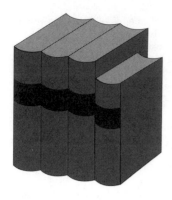

Chapter 20

PSYCHIATRIC NURSING

Cynthia J. Weiss-Kaffie

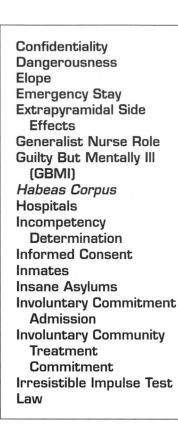

Confidentiality
Dangerousness
Elope
Emergency Stay
Extrapyramidal Side
   Effects
Generalist Nurse Role
Guilty But Mentally Ill
   (GBMI)
Habeas Corpus
Hospitals
Incompetency
   Determination
Informed Consent
Inmates
Insane Asylums
Involuntary Commitment
   Admission
Involuntary Community
   Treatment
   Commitment
Irresistible Impulse Test
Law

Long-Term Stay
Major Tranquilizers
Miracle Drugs
M'Naghten Rule
Neuroleptics
Not Guilty by Reason of
   Insanity (NGRI)
Nurse Practitioner (NP)
Order of Protective
   Custody
Outpatient Commitment
Parens Patriae
Patients
Petition
Police Power
Preventive Commitment
Privacy Rights
Psychiatry
Public Hospitals
Residents
Short-term Stay
Testimonial Privilege
Voluntary Admission

OBJECTIVES

Upon completion of this chapter, the reader will be able to:

- Describe the care of mentally ill persons from a historical perspective.
- Explain how state powers allow hospitalization of mentally ill persons.
- Compare and contrast voluntary hospitalization, involuntary commitment hospitalization, and discharge processes.
- Examine how the judicial incompetency procedure affects mentally ill persons' rights, treatment, and decision-making.
- Apply landmark legal cases to admission, treatment, and personal and civil rights of mentally ill persons.
- Describe forensic psychiatric concepts.
- Differentiate roles of professional registered nurses in psychiatric settings.
- Relate present-day case law regarding nurses' behavior in caring for mentally ill persons.

INTRODUCTION

This chapter acquaints nurses employed in inpatient and community mental health care settings with legal concepts that form the basis of psychiatric professional nursing practice. Many of these concepts also relate to nurses employed in medical/surgical treatment centers, home care, and community health agencies when mentally ill persons are physically ill or injured.

A historical perspective from the early care era through institutional and de-institutional eras is provided. Historical background assists nurses in understanding that present-day legal principles evolved as a result of needs of mentally ill individuals and needs of citizens.

An overview of two legal principles enabling states to hospitalize mentally ill persons against their will is then presented. Landmark legal cases that govern how clients are admitted, treated, and discharged are included. Client rights, forensic concepts, and nurse roles expected of generalist and advanced practice registered professional nurses in the care of mentally ill clients are addressed. Present-day case law regarding nurse concerns in caring for mentally ill persons are also included.

HISTORICAL PERSPECTIVE

EARLY CARE ERA

During early and colonial years in the United States, mentally ill persons were many times cared for by their families. Generally, these mentally-ill relatives were kept in attics or in areas away from other family members and often spent much of their time alone. Those persons who exhibited extremely bizarre and dangerous behavior were jailed along with common criminals and were called **inmates**. Certainly, they received no treatment measures and there were no laws to govern their confinement.

In the middle 1800s, large **insane asylums** were constructed well away from popu-

lated areas. Persons whose behavior was frightening or deranged were placed in large asylums. Confinement in these large warehouse-like asylums was easily accomplished. Admission decisions were made by families and asylum administrators, again, without legal protection, medical examination, or due process. Conditions were better than jails, yet far from wholesome, and again, little or no scientific treatment approaches were used.

During the middle to late 1800s, crusaders such as Dorothea Lynde Dix brought attention to persons confined because of their strange and dangerous behaviors. She and other activists called attention to conditions in the asylums, and as a result, the public realized that a need existed for legal, rational approaches for admission of mentally ill persons to institutions (Saphire, 1976).

Statutes requiring trial by jury for those unwilling to enter hospitals willingly came about from activist efforts on behalf of mentally ill persons. When asylums became **hospitals**, terminology referring to persons restricted to these institutions slowly began to change and they were referred to as **patients**. Scientific treatment for mentally ill patients remained a futuristic concept.

INSTITUTIONAL ERA

Large **public hospitals** for care of mentally ill persons continued to be located away from urban areas. Distance from family homes to hospitals made visits by relatives and friends nearly impossible. Thus, patients, or **residents** as terminology changed, lived not as members of families or communities, but were "warehoused" in self-contained hospital communities. Many persons lived out their entire lives as patient-residents in public institutions.

New drugs for the treatment of mentally ill individuals were introduced in the early 1950s. These drugs, called **neuroleptics**, or **major tranquilizers**, marked the beginning of scientific psychopharmacological treatment. Drugs such as Thorazine, Mellaril, and Stelazine profoundly affected and reduced patients' bizarre and dangerous behaviors.

Mentally ill patient-residents who, before taking the new major tranquilizing drugs, were unable to attend to therapeutic approaches or deal with unlocked units where they could come and go within limits, were suddenly able to behave in ways that allowed fewer liberty restrictions and new therapy approaches. Although these drugs were hailed as **miracle drugs**, the treatment team was unaware that long-term use of these drugs would cause irreversible **extrapyramidal side effects,** bizarre and life-threatening neurological behaviors and symptoms. These symptoms and syndromes made it extremely difficult for mentally ill persons to be accepted by society outside the hospital setting.

DE-INSTITUTIONAL ERA

Major tranquilizing drugs provided the means to reduce unruly and dangerous behavior often exhibited by the mentally ill. In addition, large amounts of financial support were required to maintain the large 1000-plus bed mental hospitals. As patient behaviors were modified, patient rights surfaced as an issue. Thus, these three factors ushered in the de-institutional era.

The federal government passed **community mental health legislation** beginning in the 1960s, which released large numbers of mentally ill institutionalized persons to communities where, theoretically, they could lead more normal lives near families and friends while remaining in treatment during the day or night at local community mental health care facilities. Inpatient numbers of publicly housed mentally ill persons, now referred to as **clients**, were reduced from approximately 1000 or more to 400 or so in the state facilities.

Intent of the federal community mental health legislation was altruistic. However, problems arose when funds needed to finance the community mental health movement were less than adequate to administer quality community programs.

Most states reexamined their mental health care statutes in the mid-1970s. Laws addressing admission and discharge criteria were revised to support the federal community mental health legislation. Admission standards and due process rights with mandated case review intervals were defined. Patient/client rights moved clearly to the forefront, and new treatment requirements were initiated by new or revised state statutes. Although each state devises and passes its own mental health care statutes, most state laws throughout the United States are similar in content. Nurses, therefore, must be responsible and accountable to know the requirements of the mental health laws in the state where they practice.

LAW: INDIVIDUAL RIGHTS VERSUS SOCIETY RIGHTS

Law and psychiatry interact to form a delicate and tenuous relationship. Both law and psychiatry deal with human behavior. **Law** addresses both individual behavior outcomes and rights as well as the safety of society. **Psychiatry** addresses the meaning of individual behavior and life satisfaction. The law enables society to function as smoothly as possible, but cannot consider individual quality of life issues. Psychiatry focuses on individual behavior as well as quality of life issues. Thus, even though both law and psychiatry focus on human behavior, neither one can totally meet the needs of society and individuals.

POLICE POWER AND *PARENS PATRIAE* LEGAL DOCTRINES

States possess legal powers required to hospitalize persons believed to be mentally ill. Two doctrines give states these rights.

The **police power** doctrine enables states to protect its citizens from dangerous acts of mentally ill persons, whereas the *parens patriae* doctrine allows states to hospitalize citizens who are unable to care for themselves, as in the case of mentally ill individuals. Most liberty restrictions of mentally ill persons by states for protection of society occur under the state's police power. Police power is used most often to hospitalize the mentally ill, which allows states to give up the business of providing care to the mentally ill because of budgetary restrictions. Use of police power rather than *parens patriae* to admit mentally ill persons to facilities also accentuates issues of liberty, individual rights, and treatment.

ADMISSION PROCEDURES

Mentally ill persons may be admitted to treatment facilities either voluntarily or involuntarily. Whether an admission is voluntary or involuntary determines some treatment decisions and governs how elopement and discharge procedures are handled.

VOLUNTARY ADMISSION

Voluntary admission allows persons to admit that they are in need of treatment. Family members, friends, physicians, and police officers, for example, may suggest to an individual that he or she is ill and in need of treatment. Additionally, the person himself or herself may decide treatment is needed and voluntarily or willingly enter a hospital by simply filling out the facility admission forms. Examination of the person and treatment, if needed, are then initiated.

INVOLUNTARY COMMITMENT ADMISSION

When persons are unaware that their behavior indicates they have a mental illness and refuse to enter a treatment facility voluntarily, an involuntary commitment admission procedure may be initiated. Friends, family, physicians, or police officers may initiate the involuntary commitment admission procedure through use of a petition. The **petition** outlines why the person is in need of treatment by submitting behavioral evidence that the person is mentally ill.

Involuntary commitment admission procedures are usually based on a state's police power, which is the authority possessed by the state to protect society from dangerous acts of mentally ill persons. In rare circumstances, the state may initiate an involuntary commitment admission procedure under the state's *parens patriae* power, which allows the state authority to provide care for mentally ill individuals who cannot care for themselves.

Under the state's police power authority, grounds for an **involuntary commitment admission** are based on dangerousness. Evidence is presented regarding the level of danger the person presents to himself or herself and/or to others. Other criteria that may be used to support an involuntary commitment procedure include behaviors that indicate the person is mentally ill or is unable to meet his or her own needs.

Determination of **dangerousness** involves several aspects and may be quite difficult to establish. First, the nature of harm or conduct is taken into account—is the harm likely to be in the form of bodily harm, harm to property, or is it more likely to be psychological in nature? Second, the magnitude of the behavior is considered—is the danger likely to result in murder, suicide, assault, or verbal abuse? Third, the probability or likelihood that the behavior will occur is weighed—how likely is it that the behavior will take place? Fourth, imminence or how quickly the threat is likely to take place is investigated—is the behavior likely to happen in the immediate future or in a few weeks or months? Fifth, frequency or how often the threat will take place is studied—is it likely the behavior will be an isolated incident or happen time and time again?

Three avenues may be used to accomplish an involuntary commitment admission procedure. Evidence regarding an individual's level of dangerousness may be presented to the court or an administrative panel or may take place via medical certification. A psychiatric examination of the person is done. Decisions made by an administrative panel or medical certification are used rarely, generally only in emergencies, and both approaches are subject to judicial review. Judicial review is necessary because the 14th Amendment to the U.S. Constitution provides citizens protection against loss of liberty and ensures due process rights.

Involuntary commitment admissions, in most states, involve three lengths of stay depending on the severity of the individual's mental illness and how well the client responds to therapy. Generally, the three lengths of commitment stay consist of an emergency stay, a short-term stay, and a long-term stay.

An **emergency stay** is usually 24 hours in length. A 24-hour stay, sometimes referred to as a 24-hour emergency detention, provides time for a psychiatric evaluation, observation, and treatment decisions. A **short-term stay**, in some states called an **order of protective custody**, most often allows hospitalization for a month or so. A short-term stay is selected for sicker persons when a longer period for examination, observation, and treatment is needed. A **long-term stay**, usually 90 days in length, often called a 90-day stay or detention, is used for persons who are severely ill and difficult to treat. If commitment is needed for longer than 90 days, mandated case reviews at specified time intervals must be held or the person will be discharged.

INVOLUNTARY COMMUNITY COMMITMENT

A fairly new form of commitment is beginning to show some promise for the purpose of treating the mentally ill. Community commitment to treatment allows clients to remain in their homes as outpatients, yet requires and guarantees that they receive proper treatment.

Involuntary community treatment commitment is used for persons who have serious and persistent mental illness and a history of dangerousness to self or others. These clients must meet certain guidelines, some of which include an interest in and previous failure when living in the community, capacity to understand the stipulations placed on them in the community, and ability to follow the prescribed treatment plan.

There are three ways mentally ill persons can be committed to treatment and remain in the community. The first is outpatient commitment; the second, preventive commitment; and the third, conditional release from the hospital.

Outpatient commitment requires the client to follow a court-ordered course of outpatient treatment. **Preventive commitment** may be used for persons who do not yet meet usual inpatient commitment criteria. A predicted deterioration standard may be used as criteria for persons to qualify for preventive commitment in that they are in need of treatment to prevent a relapse that is likely to happen. **Conditional release** from the hospital requires continued supervision after discharge regarding specific conditions outlined prior to release of the client, such as medication clinic visits, outpatient group therapy sessions, or time spent in prescribed aftercare programs. Conditional release can be used to test whether or not the client can effectively and responsibly deal with living in the community.

Of the three alternative involuntary community commitment approaches, the preventive commitment process requires the closest scrutiny. Involuntarily committing persons in the community in the event that "they might relapse" allows a great many personal injustices. Anyone may relapse, just as anyone may commit a serious crime against another human being or property. Without clear application criteria, any person could justifiably be involuntarily committed to treatment in the community or arrested by police on the outside chance that their behavior might deteriorate or they might commit a serious crime. Personal liberty and freedom may be in jeopardy in this approach to treatment.

These new commitment approaches are interesting concepts. Each approach needs to be studied in relation to outcomes. Cost containment and managed care require that health teams explore alternative, more economical ways of treating mental illness because many health benefit plans do not include mental illness benefits. Further, the number of persons who are underinsured or have no insurance benefits at all increases at an astounding pace.

INCOMPETENCY DETERMINATION

In some states, involuntary commitment to treatment automatically carries an **incompetency determination**, which essentially means that the individual is incapable of making personal decisions. In these states, persons who are involuntarily committed to treatment for a mental illness are stripped of their civil rights that are guaranteed by the Constitution. These rights include the right to vote, serve on a jury, enter into a contract, marry or divorce, execute a will, drive, obtain and maintain a professional license, and sue or be sued.

Most states, however, do not impose an incompetency determination on persons who are involuntarily committed to treatment for a mental illness. Thus, in these states, a judicial procedure beyond the involuntary commitment procedure must be initiated in those cases where the client is deemed unable to make appropriate decisions on his or her own behalf. Incompetency hearings examine evidence regarding the client's ability to make sound decisions. In cases in which clients are found incompetent, a guardian is appointed by the court to make treatment and course of living decisions for the client in question. Nurses must be responsible and accountable to know how the state in which they practice handles the incompetency determination.

TREATMENT AND CLIENT RIGHTS

Law has and continues to have an impact on all aspects of caring for and treating mentally ill persons. Client rights, liberty and due process, treatment and treatment setting, in addition to admission and discharge procedures, are subject to landmark legal case law verdicts.

LIBERTY AND DUE PROCESS RIGHTS

In a 1975 Supreme Court case out of the District Court for the Northern District of Florida, a former patient who had been involuntarily committed under civil commitment procedures to a state mental hospital brought action against the hospital superintendent and others alleging that the defendants had intentionally and maliciously deprived him of his constitutional right to liberty for 15 years without benefit of treatment. The Court held that a state cannot constitutionally confine a nondangerous individual who is capable of safely living free in the community with assistance from family and friends. Thus, an individual cannot be detained without cause (*O'Connor v. Donaldson*, 1975).

The Supreme Court reviewed a 1975 Texas case regarding procedural proof required when involuntarily committing patients to mental hospitals for indefinite periods. The Supreme Court found that the preponderance of the evidence standard was too lenient, but that the standard of beyond a reasonable doubt was too high. The Court determined that the middle standard, clear and convincing evidence, was appropriate for these cases. Thus, the standard for taking away one's liberty by commitment to a mental hospital should be higher than those used in civil cases and lower than in criminal cases (*Addington v. Texas*, 1979).

Commitment of minor children by their parents or guardians to mental hospitals was addressed by the Supreme Court in the class action Georgia case of *Parham v. J.R. et al.* (1979). The minor children alleged they had been deprived of their liberty rights via Georgia state commitment law. The Supreme Court held that although the law was reasonable and consistent with constitutional guarantees, the risk of possible error in decision-making by parents and/or guardians is so great that a panel of neutral fact-finders should conduct an inquiry to determine whether statutory requirements are met.

The Supreme Court of the State of New York heard the case of *Pilgrim Psychiatric Center v. Christian F.* (1994) regarding admission status. The hospital sought to have a patient's voluntary admission status changed to involuntary in order to administer electroconvulsive therapy treatments to the patient. The Court held that a patient's admission status could be changed only on recommendation of a hospital psychiatrist in addition to certification of two examining physicians pursuant to the state Mental Hygiene Law. The Court held that the hospital cannot initiate a change in admission status on its own volition.

TREATMENT RIGHTS

A petition for *habeas corpus* by a patient involuntarily committed to a mental hospital after being acquitted of an offense by reason of insanity, complaining he had received no treatment, was denied by the U.S. District Court for the District of Columbia. On appeal to the U. S. Court of Appeals District of Columbia Circuit, the Court held that a person who is involuntarily committed to a mental hospital after being acquitted of an offense by reason of insanity has a right to individualized accepted psychiatric treatment, confinement in a humane psychological and physical environment, and qualified staff in sufficient numbers. The purpose of commitment to a psychiatric hospital under these circumstances, therefore, is treatment, not punishment (*Rouse v. Cameron*, 1966).

The District Court for the Eastern District of Pennsylvania denied a plea by a mother of a mentally retarded individual involuntarily committed to a state institution for constitutional rights to safe conditions of confinement, freedom from bodily restraint, and training or habilation. The case eventually found its way to the U.S. Supreme Court, and the Court held that the respondent had a constitutionally protected liberty interest under the due process clause of the Fourteenth Amendment to reasonably safe conditions of confinement, freedom from unreasonable bodily restraints, and minimally adequate training (*Youngberg v. Romeo,* 1982).

The most widely publicized case addressing the right to treatment is the 1971 Alabama class action case of *Wyatt v. Stickney*. A class action suit was brought by guardians of patients involuntarily confined at a state mental hospital and by some employees assigned to the hospital. The District Court having jurisdiction over the case found that programs of treatment in use at the state mental hospital in question were scientifically and medically inadequate and deprived patients of their constitutional rights. The Court, however, reserved ruling to provide state officials 6 months to promulgate and implement proper standards of treatment (*Wyatt v. Stickney*, 1971).

LEAST RESTRICTIVE TREATMENT SETTING RIGHTS

Dixon v. Weinberger (1975) was a class action case brought by patients confined in a federal mental institution based on the Hospitalization of the Mentally Ill Act of the District of Columbia. The plaintiffs declared they had a right to treatment that includes placement in facilities outside the institution when such placement is determined to be consistent with the rehabilitative purposes of the Act. The District Court of the District of Columbia held that plaintiffs have a right to the treatment sought, when the institution has determined that such treatment is appropriate. The Court further held that primary responsibility for exploring and providing alternative facilities at the commitment level is on the District of Columbia. However, in the case of patients still in need of psychiatric care despite readiness for placement in alternative facilities, the Court held that the duty to provide such treatment by placement outside the institution is a joint responsibility of the District of Columbia and the federal government.

REFUSAL OF TREATMENT RIGHTS

Once treatment and treatment setting rights were established, right to refuse treatment issues were brought to the courts. Involuntary treatment is in conflict with freedom of thought and the right to control one's life and behavior, so long as they do not interfere with the rights of society. Most often these cases addressed whether or not psychotropic medications could be forced against client wishes. The issue of psychotropic medications concerns the potential of untreatable medication side effects such as tardive dyskinesia.

John Rennie and others brought a class action case against Ann Klein and other state human services officials and psychiatric hospital administrators, addressing their right to injunctive relief against forcible administration of drugs. The United States District Court, District of New Jersey, in *Rennie v. Klein* (1979), held that, indeed, patients did have the right to refuse drug treatment. Specifically, the Court determined (1) both voluntary and involuntary patients have due process and privacy rights provided by the Federal Constitution, which include a qualified right to refuse treatment and due process rights before drugs could be forcibly administered; (2) voluntarily admitted patients have an absolute right to refuse treatment; (3) consent must be obtained from patients, which includes information on drugs and patient rights; (4) a patient advocacy program must analyze cases when treating physicians certify that patients are incapable of providing their own consent; and (5) informal review by an independent psychiatrist must be done prior to forcing treatment on involuntarily committed patients.

Another class action suit was argued in 1980. *Rogers v. Okin* (1980) originated in Massachusetts and later became *Mills v. Rogers* (1980). *Mills* was heard by the Supreme Court. *Rogers*, again, addressed the issue of forcible medication administration. The U.S. Court of Appeals, First Circuit, brought the concept of emergency into play, holding that a definition of emergency that would justify administration of drugs over the patient's objection should include situations in which immediate administration of drugs is reasonably believed to be necessary to prevent further deterioration in the patient's mental health. Additionally, the Court determined that absent emergency, judicial finding of incapacity of the patient to make treatment decisions must be made before the state may rely on its *parens patriae* powers to forcibly medicate, but added that the state is not required to seek guardian approval for decisions to treat incompetent patients with psychotropic drugs.

In a Wisconsin case, *Virgil D. v. Rock County* (1994), the State Supreme Court found that the appellant-petitioner could rightfully refuse psychotropic medication administration even though he did recognize he had a mental illness. He was, however, able to testify that there were no advantages to taking psychotropic drugs, and that many disadvantages did exist where these drugs were concerned.

Thus, the treatment team must determine that three criteria be met to force medication without client consent. The client must exhibit behavior that is dangerous to self or others; the medication ordered by the physician must have a reasonable chance of providing help to the client; and clients who refuse medication must be judged incompetent to evaluate the benefits of the treatment in question.

PERSONAL RIGHTS

Personal rights of mentally ill persons basically have two foundations. Federal and state statutes and treatment facility policies provide rights mentally ill persons may expect to be awarded on their behalf.

COMMUNICATION

Mentally ill persons have the right to communicate with persons outside the confinement facility. Exercise of this **communication right** may occur through in-house visits from family and friends. Additionally, clients may place and receive calls and send and receive unopened mail. In-house visits and telephone and mail privileges are governed by the treatment facility policies. Communication rights may be restricted if the treatment team members can make the case that these rights would be harmful to the patient or hinder the client's treatment and recovery.

PERSONAL EFFECTS

Mentally ill persons admitted to treatment facilities have the right to bring personal effects with them based on facility policy. Items of considerable monetary value are usually placed in the facility safe or vault or sent home with family members.

Personal property capable of harming oneself or others is removed and maintained by the facility until the person is discharged. Items commonly removed from clients include knives, glass containers, metal nail files, medication, razor blades, and any other item believed to be a danger. Suicidal clients also are likely to have belts and shoelaces removed as well.

EDUCATION

Minor children have the right to education. Treatment facilities most often contract with local school districts for this service. According to the contract, teachers are provided by the district, and the facility provides resources needed for education. Children attend to their studies each day as part of their treatment plans.

INFORMED CONSENT

Unless found to be incompetent, mentally ill persons of majority age have the right to exercise informed consent regarding treatment decisions. Consent for treatment of minor children must be obtained from a parent or court-appointed guardian. For mentally ill persons hospitalized in states that assume incompetency when involuntarily admitted for treatment, and for those who are determined to be incompetent via additional judiciary proceedings, court-appointed guardians exercise informed consent on their behalf.

The right to **informed consent** mandates that adequate information be provided on a level appropriate for the client's understanding in his or her primary language. Intended results and common side effects of the treatment must be communicated to the client or guardian, in addition to any alternative treatments and likely outcomes if the treatment is refused. Physicians communicate this information to clients or guardians, and nurses act as witnesses and are responsible to answer or seek answers to questions clients and family members may ask after they have received the treatment information. Nurses are also responsible to contact the physician when clients or guardians express doubt or lack of understanding about the treatment or the consent. Signed consent forms are maintained as part of the client's medical record.

For safe professional care, nurses must know the legal age of majority in the state in which they are employed. They must also know the law in the state regarding incompetency judgments.

INDEPENDENT PSYCHIATRIST EXAMINATION

Emergency admission statutes often require that clients may request a psychiatric examination by a physician of his or her choice. Generally, the client will be discharged immediately if the independent physician finds that the client is not mentally ill.

PRIVACY AND CONFIDENTIALITY

Privacy rights are also acknowledged for persons who are mentally ill. Clients may keep personal information completely secret that does not affect their mental illness.

Confidentiality rights are the same for mentally ill clients as they are for medical-surgical patients. **Confidentiality** mandates that no information regarding the client or his or her treatment be communicated to anyone who is not involved in the care of the client. The right to release information belongs to the client. Treatment facility policy governs confidentiality. Clients must sign release forms outlining the specific information and the source to whom the information is released. These forms become a part of the medical record.

TESTIMONIAL PRIVILEGE

Testimonial privilege is closely related to privacy and confidentiality rights, but applies to court-related proceedings. **Testimonial privilege** is afforded communication between spouses, attorney and client, physician and patient, and clergy and parishioner. As in confidentiality, the person who speaks maintains the right to release the information; the listener is obliged to remain silent.

In the case of physician and patient, testimonial privilege allows the patient the confidence required to disclose detailed information about the chief complaint. Without a degree of detail, appropriate treatment could not be initiated.

Most states do not extend testimonial privilege to health care providers beyond the physician. Some states, however, extend the privilege to psychotherapists. This extension came about through the ruling in *Tarasoff v. Regents of the University of California et al.* (1974). In *Tarasoff*, a student confided to his university-based therapist that he intended to kill his former girlfriend, identified by name, when she returned to school from vacation. The therapist maintained the client's confidence. When the young woman returned for classes, the former boyfriend followed through with his intention and killed her. The parents brought suit against the university, and the Court held that therapists have a duty to warn by engaging in affirmative action when specific information detailing intended harm is shared in the course of the therapy relationship.

An advanced practice psychiatric–mental health **clinical nurse specialist (CNS)** or **nurse practitioner (NP)** who provides psychotherapy may be included in the testimonial privilege regarding professional communication between the parties in a therapist-client relationship. These nurses are responsible to contact the professional nursing board in the state in which they are licensed regarding testimonial privilege. If there are no provisions in the state nursing practice act, the CNS or NP should exercise the privilege unless ordered by the court to testify regarding client information.

HABEAS CORPUS

Clients admitted for treatment of a mental illness against their will may execute a writ of *habeas corpus* (written request) for speedy release on the grounds that they are sane and able to be released. Originally *habeas corpus* was provided for prisoners; however, the scope has been extended to cover all constitutional issues. When a person believed by authorities to be mentally ill is hospitalized involuntarily and exercises the right to *habeas corpus*, the treatment team

who wish to detain the client must successfully defend their intent in a court hearing or the person will be released.

CIVIL RIGHTS

Civil rights are personal, natural rights guaranteed and protected by the Constitution and enjoyed by all citizens. These rights include the right to vote, marry and divorce, enter into a contract, execute a will, obtain and maintain a professional license, and sue and be sued.

All mentally ill persons who admit themselves voluntarily for treatment maintain their civil rights. Persons who are involuntarily admitted for treatment also maintain their civil rights in most states, although some states have laws that automatically restrict an involuntarily committed person's civil rights. Additional judicial proceedings must be initiated to restrict the civil rights of involuntarily committed clients in states where civil rights are maintained. To remove civil rights, evidence must be shown that, because of the mental illness, the client is unable to make personal decisions, and legal guardians are appointed to act on the client's behalf. Nurses are obligated to investigate the mental health admission statute in the state in which they are employed so they do not unlawfully restrict civil rights of hospitalized clients.

Specifically, in states where civil rights are maintained, involuntarily committed clients may enter into a contract if the person understands the circumstances and consequences of the agreement. Involuntarily committed clients also may execute a legal will if he or she knows, in general terms, the nature and extent of the assets and knows who the friends and/or family are and what these relationships mean.

FORENSIC PSYCHIATRY

Forensic psychiatry deals with persons who commit crimes and are judged **not guilty by reason of insanity (NGRI)**. Because of public outcry against the NGRI ruling, which, in actuality, is not a commonly used criminal defense, the ruling **guilty but mentally ill (GBMI)** is gaining in popularity. These persons are believed to have committed the crime, in a large part as a result of their mental illness. This ruling is based on the humanitarian value that people should not be held responsible for crimes they did not realize they were committing or if they could not stop themselves from following through with the criminal behavior.

Three standards have been applied over the years to determine whether a person was insane at the time of the crime: the M'Naghten Rule, the irresistible impulse test, and the American Law Institute (ALI) standard. Currently, most states use the ALI standard.

Under the **M'Naghten Rule**, the court attempts to determine whether, at the time of the crime, the person had sufficient mental capacity to know and understand what he or she was doing and whether he or she knew and understood that it was wrong and a violation of the rights of another. Essentially, was the person able to understand the nature and quality of the act and to distinguish between right and wrong at the time of the offense (*M'Naghten's Case*, 1843).

The **irresistible impulse test** is broader in scope than the M'Naghten Rule. Under this test, a person may avoid criminal responsibility even if he or she is able to distinguish between right and wrong and is fully aware of the nature and quality of the act. But the person must establish that he or she was unable to refrain from acting (*Commonwealth of Pennsylvania v. Walzack, 1976*).

The **American Law Institute (ALI) standard** (American Law Institute, 1985) is used most frequently today. The ALI test requires that the person was unable to appreciate the wrongfulness of an act or to conform his or her behavior to the requirements of the law. This standard, however, excludes the sociopath.

DISPOSITION OF PERSONS JUDGED NGRI/GBMI

Persons who are found not guilty by reason of insanity (NGRI) or guilty but mentally ill

(GBMI) by the courts are sent to special forensic psychiatric hospitals or prisons to be treated in hopes they will regain their sanity. Prisoners in general population prisons who begin to exhibit mentally ill behaviors also may be transferred to forensic treatment centers. Another group of persons who may be sent to special forensic treatment locations are those who are found incompetent to stand trial. A person who is incompetent to stand trial is unable to understand the charges and cannot assist the attorney with his or her defense strategy.

Nurses come in contact with these prisoners as members of the treatment team. In forensic treatment centers, both security and treatment are prime concerns. Nurses who wish to work in these settings need to engage in a fair amount of self-awareness to discover their true attitudes regarding care of criminals. They also need an orientation to the security responsibility performed by the guards. Many times, the security focus and the treatment focus seem to be diametrically opposed. This conflict of providers makes it difficult for both groups to deal with, and the patient is often caught in the middle of philosophical differences. The nurse must investigate forensic laws in the state where he or she is employed to prepare for caring for inmates.

DISMISSAL PROCEDURES

Discharge approaches depend on the admission status of the client. Those admitted voluntarily face a simpler discharge process than those involuntarily committed or classified as forensic patients.

DISCHARGING THE VOLUNTARILY ADMITTED CLIENT

Any person who was and remains a voluntary client may be discharged on his or her own initiative via a request letter. This discharge is analogous to the **against medical advice (AMA)** discharge occasionally initiated by medical-surgical patients in general care hospitals and treatment facilities.

These patients decide on their own that they are ready to leave and write a letter to the administrator or treatment team indicating they wish to leave. After initiating the letter request, they are asked to remain in the facility for a specified time (generally 4 or so hours) as identified in the treatment facility policy. This short time period allows time for the psychiatrist to visit the client, write discharge orders, or initiate a court hearing to retain the client if his or her behavior is such that involuntary commitment is needed. Generally, the client is allowed to leave the facility.

Some clients make the decision to "**elope**" or run away from the treatment facility. In the case of the voluntarily admitted client, no attempt on the part of the treatment team is made to return him or her to the facility. These persons are free to go where they want, unless the treatment team deems it necessary to initiate an involuntary commitment based on the degree of mental illness exhibited by the client.

Lastly, the treatment team may discharge the client when the mental illness has been brought under control. Discharge orders are written with scheduled follow-up appointments and treatment.

DISCHARGING THE INVOLUNTARILY COMMITTED CLIENT

In most states, after the length of time specified in the commitment has elapsed, the treatment team may discharge the involuntarily committed client. Again, discharge orders are written and a follow-up plan of care is initiated. Some states, however, require through their mental health statutes that the court be informed when the treatment team determines that the client is ready for discharge. Another hearing may be held by the court before the discharge may be ordered.

Involuntarily committed clients also make the decision to elope from the treatment facility. If these clients do not return on their own, and family or friends fail to return them, police are notified and they are forcibly returned for treatment.

DISCHARGING THE FORENSIC PRISONER

State law determines how this population leaves the forensic setting. If the prisoner was transferred from the general prison population for mental health care and treatment and the illness is controlled, he or she is returned to the same or another general prison to complete the terms of the sentence.

If, however, the prisoner was found by the trial court to be NGRI and the mental illness behaviors have improved, he or she may be sent to the prison where the incarceration would have taken place had the NGRI verdict not been handed down. In other instances, the person may be discharged, most often with the court's approval. Conservatism persists, however, in the courts in cases in which persons have been found to be NGRI. State law determines how or where additional prison time or treatment will be initiated.

In states where the GBMI judgment is used, these persons are transferred to another prison setting to complete their sentences. When mentally ill prisoners escape, exhaustive attempts are made to return them to confinement.

NURSE ROLES

Nurses who choose to work with mentally ill clients and/or forensic prisoners must be familiar with the state nursing practice act, in the case of registered nurses, and the titling act, in the case of licensed vocational/practical nurses. Both nursing practice acts and titling acts govern the practice of registered and licensed nurses. Professional nursing practice is also guided by the American Nurses Association (ANA) Statement on Psychiatric-Mental Health Clinical Nursing Practice and the Standards of Psychiatric-Mental Health Clinical Nursing Practice (ANA, 1994). Nurses must also be familiar with the state mental health statute in the state in which they practice. In addition to these statutes, agency policies and procedures identify specifically how nurses will function within the treatment agency.

Nurses occupy two main category roles when caring for mentally ill clients. One is that of the **generalist nurse role**, which is filled by nurses educated in diploma, associate degree, and baccalaureate degree schools of nursing. These nurses are direct care providers and client advocates, and sometimes they may act as coleaders for group interventions.

The other role is that of the **advanced practice nurse** (APN), occupied by nurses who have completed graduate educational programs. These nurses have earned designations of psychiatric mental health clinical nurse specialist or nurse practitioner. Registered nurses who are advanced practitioners must be familiar not only with the state nursing practice statute and mental health statute, but must also know the parameters contained in the advanced practice section of the state nursing practice act in the state in which they are employed.

Advanced practice nurses also provide direct client care and act as client advocates along with generalist nurses. Additionally, they may act as psychotherapists, providing either individual one-on-one therapy or group therapy for approximately 10 or so clients at a time. Some advanced practice nurses, depending on their educational preparation and statute provisions, have prescriptive privileges, which means they may initiate psychopharmacology treatments as indicated by client diagnosis and behavior.

When advanced practice nurses provide psychotherapy, they may be covered by testimonial privilege regarding information they learn as a result of the therapist-client relationship. The advanced practice section of the state nursing practice act may provide guidance regarding testimonial confidentiality. Whether or not guidance is found in the statute, advanced practice nurses would be wise to practice as if they have the privilege until they are notified otherwise.

However, testimonial privilege does not apply to specific information regarding planned harm to a named individual or individuals divulged by the client to the therapist. In *Tarasoff v. Regents of the Univer-* *sity of California et al.* (1974), a client told his university-based therapist he intended to kill his former girlfriend when she returned to classes at the university after vacation. The therapist, holding to the rules of client confidentiality, withheld this information. The young man did, in fact, kill the girl when she returned to the campus. The parents sued, and the Court held that the therapist under these specific circumstances, when the intended victim or victims are named, was required to take affirmative action to prevent a dangerous outcome. Thus, it seems to follow that under the same circumstances, the nurse therapist could be held to the same standard.

Both generalist and advanced practice nurses occupy the role of citizen in the community and state in which they reside. The role of citizen also carries responsibilities. Nurses as citizens need to keep themselves aware of mental illness issues and causes in their local area. Nurses are valuable members of mental health associations, self-help groups in the community, and state alliances that advocate for mentally ill persons. In the role of alliance member, they may be called on to testify in the Congress regarding important mental illness legislation.

CASE LAW

Various sets of circumstances come into play in the care and treatment of psychiatric clients. Nurses need to keep themselves attuned to case law outcomes in the specialization area of psychiatry and mental health.

PSYCHIATRIC PATIENT RAPED AT HOSPITAL: FAILURE TO ADHERE TO OBSERVATION PROTOCOLS

In *Genao v. State* (1998), a psychiatric patient was raped at the hospital. Ms. Genao was admitted to New York's South Beach Psychiatric Center after speaking about suicide, inability to sleep, bouts of crying, and complaints of hearing voices. She was subsequently given an injection of Haldol and was placed under observation in what was known as the "quiet room." By the time the Haldol was administered, lithium, Ativan, and Cogentin also had been administered. At 6:45 P.M., a staff member heard "whimpering" coming from a room and investigated. As a result of the investigation, it was noted that the patient had been raped by a fellow patient on the unit. The patient brought suit against the state of New York for the injuries sustained in the rape.

The Court of Claims held that the hospital was not liable under the theory of medical malpractice, but that the hospital had negligently supervised the patient. The patient was awarded $200,000 for past pain and suffering and $50,000 for future pain and suffering. Nurse Braithwaite made the last three entries on the patient record at 5:30, 6:00, and 6:30 P.M., but testified she did not rely on visual observation. Testimony also revealed that the nurse could not recall the victim's specific whereabouts on the unit for any of the three early evening entries. Evidence revealed that the victim had not attended the evening meal.

The Court found that the defendant, acting by and through its staff, was negligent in its supervision of the patient and that the defendant failed to use reasonable care to protect the patient from "a not unforeseeable occurrence," and did not adhere to its own 30-minute observation standard.

PSYCHIATRIC PATIENT IMPROPERLY "PUNISHED" BY SECLUSION AND RESTRAINT

Nurses who restrain patients must be very careful to follow the facility policies and procedures outlining use of medical and physical restraint and seclusion or such containment can be construed as punishment. Mr. Alt was involuntarily admitted to John Umstead Hospital, a state psychiatric hospital in November 1989 after claiming to have overdosed on Tylenol (*Alt v. John Umstead Hospital*, 1997). The patient did not respect staff members unless they had doctoral degrees and had poor relationships with those who held the high degree, often

calling them derogatory names. After a stay on the unit, a physician and social worker met with the patient about a job and residence placement in the community. The physician wrote a discharge order effective that day with a note stating, "Patient does not appear to be an acute danger to himself or others and did not voice suicidal or homicidal thoughts." Later in the day the physician amended the note to allow the patient to be picked up in the morning. At the 5:30 evening meal, the patient threw his dinner tray against the wall, all the while shouting obscenities. Nurse DeBerry ordered the patient into seclusion and leather restraints and called the physician for an order to seclude and restrain for up to 8 hours. At 11:40 P.M., the physician visited the patient in seclusion and restraints, and the patient remained under strict confinement the rest of the night. The patient brought suit against the hospital and filed a complaint with the Industrial Commission. The Deputy Commissioner denied the claim, and the patient appealed to the Full Commission. The Full Commission reversed the decision and ordered damages. The hospital appealed.

The Court of Appeals of North Carolina affirmed the judgment of the Full Commission, holding that evidence was sufficient to support findings that the actions of the employees were not in keeping with the applicable standards of psychiatric practice. The findings held that the patient's behavior did not constitute imminent danger to others and did not warrant the degree of restraint applied.

PSYCHIATRIC PATIENT "DISAPPEARS"—DEATH PRESUMED: NURSES SUED

Dr. Ahn was voluntarily admitted to Carrier Clinic for severe depression on March 22, 1998, after complaining that he "worried a lot, felt hopeless and useless, and felt he was a bad doctor." The admitting physician made the diagnosis of major affective disorder, depressed, noting specifically high anxiety level with agitation, guilt and pessimistic ruminations, and suicidal ideations. The physician, however, did not restrict the patient to the unit for observation, rather the patient was placed on an open unit with various ground privileges. This decision was later called into question. Nurse Baxter was replaced by Nurse Manuell at shift change, and Nurse Schilp came on as supervisor. The patient was last seen on the unit at 5:00 P.M., and a subsequent search by hospital personnel and town police with search dogs and helicopters did not locate the patient.

Five years after the patient's disappearance, the wife filed a petition to have her husband declared legally dead. The widow then brought suit against the clinic, two nurses, and others. The trial court found that the defendants had been negligent in the care of the patient, but that negligence had not caused his death. Judgment was entered for the defendants, and the plaintiff appealed.

The Superior Court, Appellate Division, reversed the judgment of the lower court, and further review was ordered. The Supreme Court held that a retrial on issues of negligence and causation would be necessary (*Ahn v. Kim*, 1996). This case illustrates that nurses should be keenly aware that once a health care professional is admitted as a patient, he or she must be treated exactly as any other patient.

NURSE HAS PROBABLE CAUSE TO DETAIN AND MEDICATE PATIENT

On April 15, 1991, when Robert Heater came home from work, he told his mother that he "needed help." The family called Southwood Psychiatric Center, and the intake counselor determined that Robert met the criteria for a 72-hour hold in that he was agitated and threatening people. At approximately 10:30 P.M., the patient became combative, threatening to "kill them all." The nurse on duty read the patient a Detainment Advisement and at about 2:00 A.M. injected the patient with Ativan. This injection was repeated because the patient, who was in restraints, continued to struggle and was highly combative. Subsequently, the patient brought suit against the nurse and the psychiatric center. The Superior Court, San

Diego County, determined that the defendants were immune from liability and granted the defendants' motion to dismiss. The patient appealed.

The California Court of Appeals affirmed the judgment of the trial court, ruling that the nurse had probable cause to detain the patient, and further, she acted within the applicable standard of care in medicating the patient. The Court of Appeals did order a probable cause hearing regarding the involuntary detention (*Heater v. Southwood Psychiatric Center*, 1996).

NURSE ATTACKED: SUIT AGAINST PROVIDERS

In *Charleston v. Larson* (1998), a patient receiving general duty nursing care threatened Nurse Charleston that he "would break her neck" and, in fact, attacked and beat her without provocation. Nurse Charleston filed a complaint against both Dr. Larson, a licensed physician practicing psychiatry at CPC Streamwood Hospital, and the patient, alleging claims based on negligence and intentional tort. Nurse Charleston filed an affidavit by a psychiatrist who stated that at the time of the patient's admission he was a high-risk patient with a history of alcohol, drugs, and sexual abuse and engaged in self-mutilation. Hospital records did not indicate that an initial complete workup was performed by Dr. Larson, and there was no indication that the hospital staff was informed of the patient's "dangerous condition." Dr. Larson filed a motion to dismiss the complaint, which was granted by the Circuit Court, Cook County, Illinois. The nurse appealed.

The Appellate Court of Illinois affirmed the lower court's decision that the defendant psychiatrist did not have a duty to protect the nurse from the attack by the patient. Illinois law, in general, does not impose a duty to protect another from a criminal attack by a third person unless the attack is reasonably foreseeable and the parties stand in a "special relationship." The Court was not willing to characterize the relationship that Dr. Larson had with the patient as the type of special relationship that would trigger a duty to warn.

In the case of *Turner v. Jordan* (1997), Nurse Turner at Hubbard Hospital was attacked and severely beaten by Tarry Williams, a psychiatric inpatient admitted by Dr. H. Jordan. The patient was diagnosed as bipolar and manic and had been a psychiatric patient at Hubbard on five separate occasions. On three of those occasions, he had been found to be a danger to himself or others and had been committed to the Middle Tennessee Mental Health Institute. On one of the Hubbard hospitalizations, the patient attempted to attack Dr. Jordan, and the hospital staff intervened. After the treatment team discussed the Williams case, Dr. Jordan wrote: "This patient presents no behavior or clinical evidence suggesting that he is suicidal. He is aggressive, grandiose, intimidating, combative and dangerous. We will discharge him soon by allowing him to sign out against medical advice." That evening the patient attacked Nurse Turner, inflicting severe head injuries. She then sued Dr. Jordan for medical negligence, alleging that he violated his duty to use reasonable care in the treatment of his patient. The jury returned a verdict in favor of Nurse Turner allocating 100 percent of fault to Dr. Jordan and no fault to the patient. Dr. Jordan appealed. The Davidson Circuit Court did not approve of the trial judge's instructions to the jury that resulted in the allocation of fault and reversed the judgment and granted a new trial. Nurse Turner appealed.

The Supreme Court of Tennessee held that a psychiatrist owes a nurse a duty of care to protect her from violent patients. The standard of care requires that, if a patient is found to be dangerous, the patient must be prevented from acting on that, staff must be informed of the patient's danger, and the patient must be medicated if necessary to prevent his acting in a manner that endangers himself or others, restrained to prevent aggressive behavior, or transferred to a treatment setting equipped to handle such behavior. Dr. Jordan had testified that he did not recall the patient or any information about the danger the patient presented, even though he, himself, had been a victim of an attempted attack by the same patient.

Unfortunately, the Supreme Court was compelled to uphold the Davidson Circuit Court reversal of the trial court's ruling in favor of the nurse regarding the allocation of fault that the Court determined to be prejudicial to Dr. Jordan. This case illustrates how convenient it is for a physician to say, "I don't remember this patient." Who would expect that the physician would be unable to remember treating a patient who attacked him?

STUDENT NURSES BLOW WHISTLE: NURSE TERMINATED FOR ABUSING PATIENTS

Over the years, suits have been brought against health care providers who allegedly abuse both mentally ill and mentally retarded patients. In this New York case (*Marrello v. Carter*, 1996), two student nurses alleged that they witnessed Nurse Marrello abusing two patients, a mentally retarded patient and a 93-year-old patient suffering from Alzheimer's disease, on more than one occasion. Based on the student nurses' alleged complaint, the hospital adopted a Hearing Officer's findings of fact and conclusions of law and terminated Nurse Marrello's employment. The County Commissioner of Hospitals found that the nurse was guilty of misconduct meriting her termination. The nurse brought a proceeding to review the determination by the County Commissioner.

The Supreme Court of New York, Appellate Division, Third Department, dismissed the nurse's petition, finding that the judgment that the nurse was guilty of misconduct meriting termination was supported by substantial evidence. The testimony by the two student nurses who witnessed alleged abuse of the two patients was "direct and unshakable" and far more credible than the nurse's conflicting testimony.

One cannot help but admire the student nurses for blowing the whistle on the nurse in question. All too often, colleagues are intimidated by abusive behavior and are reluctant to report nurses or other health care providers who abuse patients. It is hoped that this finding will inspire nurses to report caregiver abuse of patients.

COMBATIVE PATIENT INJURES NURSE: PHYSICIAN'S DUTY TO WARN

On June 8, 1992, James Elgart, a patient treated for delirium tremens in the medical-surgical unit of South Nassau Communities Hospital, attacked and injured Nurse Adams. The patient had exhibited violent behavior twice before during the 3 days preceding the June 8th incident; each time the treating physician, Dr. Seiden, was notified. After the June 8th attack, Nurse Adams brought suit against the patient and Dr. Seiden, alleging the defendant doctor was negligent in admitting the patient to the medical-surgical floor instead of the psychiatric unit, failing to transfer the patient after learning of his violent behaviors, and failing to warn the nurse that the patient could become violent. The Supreme Court of New York, Nassau County, granted Dr. Seiden's motion for summary judgment. Nurse Adams appealed.

The Court noted that the law is well settled that "a defendant generally has no duty to control the conduct of third persons so as to prevent them from harming others, even where as a practical matter a defendant can exercise such control." One of the deciding factors in this case was that often patients undergoing treatment for and as a result of drug and alcohol will, in severe cases, manifest bizarre behavior. The Court further found that the injured nurse was not at a particular risk because the patient had not "specifically threatened her."

There are several issues that the Court failed to address. Among them were whether the physician was negligent in failing to transfer the patient to a psychiatric unit. The defendant physician could be seen as not only putting Nurse Adams at risk, but also subjecting all others involved in the care and treatment of the patient to an unnecessary and unwarranted risk. There was some evidence that Nurse Adams was, in fact, aware of the patient's likelihood to be vicious, because of the diagnosis. It seems

that physicians, nurses, and all other health care providers have a duty to warn other caregivers of a patient's tendency to exhibit vicious or dangerous behavior that might cause death or serious injury (*Adams v. Elgart*, 1972).

SUMMARY

An understanding of the historical treatment of the mentally ill can help those practicing psychiatric nursing to gain perspective on the present-day care of mentally ill persons. It is important for these nurses to have a general understanding of the principles involved in committing mentally ill persons to treatment, including state police power and *parens patriae* doctrines, as well as the laws governing voluntary and involuntary admission procedures, forensic care, and discharge procedures. Most mentally ill patients retain the same rights as medical-surgical patients, and nurses involved in their care must be aware of their clients' rights regarding treatment, treatment setting, refusal of treatment, and personal and civil rights. Knowledge of state and federal laws governing the rights of the mentally ill patient is necessary for nurse generalists as well as advanced practice nurses. As citizens, nurses should also keep abreast of mental illness issues in their local area. Recent judgments in court cases concerning mental illness care and treatment are helpful in highlighting the many issues inherent in the field of psychiatric nursing.

POINTS TO REMEMBER

- Historical perspectives have a direct bearing on laws governing present-day care of mentally ill persons.
- Nurses are held responsible for knowing content of state nursing practice or titling acts that dictate the practice of professional and vocational nurses.
- Advanced practice nurses are responsible to know the parameters of the state nurs-

ing practice act section that provides guidance for advanced practitioners.
- State statutes define how mentally ill patients are admitted and discharged from psychiatric treatment facilities.
- Landmark legal cases have determined treatment, treatment setting, and civil rights issues for psychiatric patients.
- Working with forensic prisoners requires self-awareness and an understanding of nurse caregiver and security roles.
- Three rules or standards govern whether criminals can mount an insanity defense.
- Nurses in psychiatric treatment facilities include those practicing at the generalist and advanced practice levels.
- Nurses have responsibilities in their roles of community and state citizens to advocate for the mentally ill.
- Nurses are responsible for understanding case law rulings in regard to caring for mentally ill clients.

REFERENCES

Adams v. Elgart, 623 N.Y.S. 2d 637 (N.Y. 1972).
Addington v. Texas, 99 S. Ct. 1804 (1979).
Ahn v. Kim, 678 A. 2d 1073 (N.J. 1996).
Alt v. John Umstead Hospital, 479 S.E.2d 800 (N.C. 1997).

American Law Institute. (1985, June). Model penal code: Complete statutory text. Chicago, IL: American Bar Association.
American Nurses Association. (1994). *Statement on psychiatric-mental health clinical nursing practice and standards of psychiatric-mental health clinical nursing practice.* Washington, DC: Author.
Charleston v. Larson, 696 N.E.2d 793 (IL 1998).
Commonwealth of Pennsylvania v. Walzack, 468 PA. 360 A.2d 914, 919 (1976).
Dixon v. Weinberger, 405 F. Supp. 974 (1975).
Genao v. State, 679 N.Y.S. 2d 539 (N.Y. 1998).
Heater v. Southwood Psychiatric Center 49 Cal. Rptr. 880 (1996).
Marrello v. Carter, 640 N.Y.S. 2d 679 (1996).
Mills v. Rogers, 457 S. Ct. 291 (1982).
M'Naghten's Case, 8 Eng. Rep. 718 (1843).
O'Connor v. Donaldson, 95 S. Ct. 2486 (1975).
Parham v. J.R., 99 S.Ct. 2493 (1979).
Pilgrim Psychiatric Center v. Christian F., 610 N.Y.S. 2d 962 (A.D. 2 Dept. 1994).
Rennie v. Klein, 476 F. Supp. 1294 (1979).
Rogers v. Okin, 634 F. 2d 650 (1980).
Rouse v. Cameron, 373 F. 2d 451 (1966).
Saphire, R. B. (1976). The civilly committed public mental patient and the right to aftercare. *Florida State University Law Review, 4,* 229–242.
Tarasoff v. Regents of the University of California et al., 529 P. 2d 553 (1974).
Turner v. Jordan, 957 S.W.2d 815 (1997).
Virgil D. v. Rock County, 524 N.W.2d 894 (WI 1994).
Wyatt v. Stickney, 325 F. Supp. 781 (1971).
Youngberg v. Romeo, 102 S. Ct. 2452 (1982).

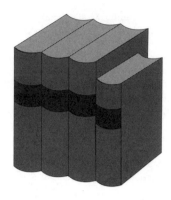

Chapter 21

EMERGENCY NURSING

Cheryl Pozzi
Nancy E. Purtell

THE SUSPECTED CRIMINAL PATIENT
LIVING WILLS
ORGAN DONATION
WORKPLACE VIOLENCE
GOOD SAMARITAN
ADVANCED PRACTICE NURSES
COMMON PITFALLS IN EMERGENCY
          DEPARTMENT NURSING PRACTICE
ETHICAL CONSIDERATIONS
RESEARCH SUGGESTIONS
SUMMARY
POINTS TO REMEMBER
REFERENCES
SUGGESTED READINGS

KEY WORDS

Abuse
Advance Directive
Against Medical
  Advice (AMA)
Battery
Consent
Consolidated Omnibus
  Budget Reconciliation
  Act (COBRA)
Critical Incident Stress
  Management (CISM)
Diagnosis
Emergency
Emergency Medical
  Treatment and
  Labor Act
Emergency Nursing
Employee Assistance
  Program (EAP)
ENA Code of Ethics
Exclusionary Rule
Expressed Consent
False Imprisonment

Federal Emergency
  Medical Services
  System Act of
  1973 (FEMA)
Hill-Burton Act
Horizontal Violence
Implied Consent
Incompetent
Informed Consent
In Loco Parentis
Living Will
Natural Death Act
Nursing Diagnosis
Omnibus Budget
  Reconciliation Act
  of 1987 (OBRA)
Prudent Layperson
Rape
Screening Examination
Triage
Uniform Anatomical
  Gift Act
Workplace Violence

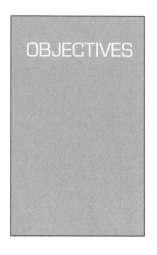
Upon completion of this chapter, the reader will be able to:
- Discuss the nursing and legal history of emergency nursing.
- Analyze general legal principles that regulate emergency nursing practice.
- Identify general legal duties of the emergency nurse.
- Identify duties of the emergency nurse to the incompetent patient.
- Analyze functions of the advanced practice emergency nurse.
- Identify emergency health care situations that require mandatory reporting.

INTRODUCTION

The emergency department (ED, used interchangeably with ER) is one of the most diverse and challenging practice areas for nurses, because it presents a high risk for exposure to malpractice. The ED is the practice area within the health care system where issues regarding triage, accurate communication, thorough documentation, detailed treatments, decisions regarding life-sustaining treatment, offers of organ donation, and suspected criminal activity all may be channeled through the nurse. Compounding these issues are the numbers of patients and the short time period for case management. Today's nurses are faced with a greater number of patients waiting for treatment, ultimately leading to frustrations and anger on the part of both patient and nurse. Reality forces physicians to select patients with more severe injuries, while those with lesser injuries or illnesses are forced to wait, sometimes very long hours. The potential for many legal issues is present in the emergency room. For example, missed or untimely diagnoses and assessments by nurses and/or physicians can lead to a high risk for medical malpractice.

HISTORY OF EMERGENCY NURSING

Historically speaking, Florence Nightingale was an emergency nurse. Providing emergency care for the ill and injured in the battlefields during war was found to be such a worthy activity that it evolved into a full-time profession. Consequently, morbidity and emotional well-being in the ED have been progressively improved following the advent of Nightingale's efforts (Johnstone, 1994, p. 13).

Emergency nursing has become an area of advanced nursing practice only since the early 1970s. The definition of **emergency nursing** encompasses the care of individuals of all ages, with perceived or actual physical or emotional alterations of health, which are undiagnosed or require further interventions (Newberry, 1992). The scope of emergency nursing practice involves assessment, diagnosis, treatment, and evaluation of perceived, actual or potential, sudden or urgent, physical or psychosocial problems that are primarily episodic or acute and occur in a variety of settings (Emergency Nurses Association [ENA], 1990).

Emergency nursing can occur in hospital emergency department, pre-hospital and military settings, clinics, health maintenance organizations, and ambulatory services; business, educational, industrial, and correctional institutions; and other health care environments. Emergency care is delivered where the consumer works, plays, and goes to school (ENA, 1989b).

Emergency nursing is a specialty type of nursing that continues to change as the needs of the consumer and principles of health care evolve.

LEGAL HISTORY

The emergency room is considered a practice area with high legal risk (Hemelt & Mackert, 1982). Emergency care by its very nature involves issues that call for solutions based in disciplines of law and health care (Hemelt & Mackert, 1982). Some legal issues may pertain directly to physicians, the hospital organization, or to the nurses. It is important for nurses to be aware of laws pertaining to nursing and other providers or institutions in order to define the scope of practice. Nurses have been named in lawsuits; for example, when physicians have ordered inappropriate interventions, and the nurse followed through without questioning or advocating hospital policy, procedure, and/or appropriate laws (Pozgar, 1990).

Historically, issues have arisen relative to the duty to provide care as employees of a hospital and/or a physician. These issues have frequently involved the nurse. For example, assessments must be made regarding the patient's ability to independently pay for health care versus payments by an insurance coverage. Patients, while being ill, have been wrongfully refused health care because hospital beds were full, transferred to another hospital, instructed to go home and call their private physician, and/or instructed to drive themselves to a different hospital (Pozgar, 1990). Fortunately, because of requirements of the Joint Commission on Accreditation of Healthcare Organizations (JCAHO), state laws, state licensing regulations, health department regulations, and

"antidumping" legislation passed by Congress, hospitals may no longer turn away emergency room patients, but must provide at least minimal care before transfer.

The New York State Emergency Medical Services Act of 1983 provided that every general hospital must admit any person who is in need of immediate health care. Any licensed health care practitioner who refuses to treat a person arriving at a general hospital for emergency medical treatment is guilty of a misdemeanor, subject to up to 1 year in prison and/or a fine not to exceed $1000 (Pozgar, 1990). Emergency medical technicians, ambulance personnel, and paramedics have a duty to report any facility refusing health care.

The **Hill-Burton Act** required each state to submit a plan that would provide adequate hospital and other facilities for all persons residing within its boundaries. The 1970 amendments to the Act placed a special emphasis on emergency services, with some states explicitly requiring hospitals to provide some degree of emergency care (Pozgar, 1990). In addition, the Act provides that any hospital receiving funds under this program must make available a reasonable number of free services to persons unable to pay. In 1972, regulations by the Department of Health and Human Services established the numerical guidelines defining a "reasonable volume of services."

An antidumping provision approved by Congress as part of the **Omnibus Budget Reconciliation Act of 1987** (OBRA) forbids hospitals from turning away emergency room patients or dumping them on another institution for inability to pay for services. Failure to follow these antidumping provisions results in a $25,000 penalty, per occurrence (Pozgar, 1990).

The **Emergency Medical Treatment and Labor Act** (also referred to as COBRA) contains an antidumping provision, which states that a hospital must provide a medical screening examination to any patient coming into the emergency department. If an emergency medical condition is present, the hospital must provide treatment to stabilize the patient's medical condition. However, the patient may request a transfer in writing; and if a physician certifies that the benefits of the transfer in an unstable condition outweigh the risks, then the patient may be transferred (Furrow et al., 1995).

The Supreme Court of South Dakota, in *Fjerstad v. Knutson* (1978), held the hospital liable for the failure of the on-call physician to respond to an emergency (Pozgar, 1990). In *Thomas v. Corso* (1972), the court sustained a verdict against a hospital and physician who did not respond at once to an emergency, failing to arrive in time to provide treatment. In this case, the patient had been struck by a car, and the hospital nurse notified the on-call doctor. As the patient's condition had worsened and the nurse had failed to notify the physician, the nurse was also held liable. Under the doctrine of *respondent superior*, the nurse's negligence was the basis for holding the hospital liable as well (Pozgar, 1990). A similar set of facts received the same verdict in *Citizens Hospital Association v. Schoulin* (1972), as the nurse also failed to inform the doctor of the deteriorating condition of the patient in the emergency room (Pozgar, 1990).

Hospitals have a duty to render care in a timely fashion, as held in *Marks v. Mandel* (1985). The issue in that case related to the response time of the on-call physician, who failed to meet the standard and respond within 30 minutes of being notified (Pozgar, 1990). In the case of *Wilmington General Hospital v. Manlove*, the nurse advised the parents of an infant that the hospital could not provide treatment because the child was already under the care of a pediatric physician. Liability in negligence resulted when the nurse advised the parents to make an appointment with the physician at the pediatric clinic, without determining the acuity of the child's condition (Pozgar, 1990).

GENERAL LEGAL PRINCIPLES

Medicolegal authorities agree that only physicians should diagnose an emergency (Pegalis & Wachsman, 1982). **Diagnosis** usually refers to the conclusion reached on the condition of a patient, as determined by an adequate examination, history, and pertinent laboratory work (Pegalis & Wachsman, 1982). An **emergency** is a threat to life and/or a threat of disability or serious aggravation of an existing disablement (Pegalis & Wachsman, 1982). A **nursing diagnosis** is the conclusion of the nurse's assessments and findings, by labeling the patient's responses. The term **triage** is derived from the French word *trier*, which means to sort out (Pegalis & Wachsman, 1982). ED nurses perform the function of the initial patient screening, but the ultimate responsibility for the triage decisions remains with the senior resident (Wickens, 1978). The nurse is the first set of eyes and ears for the treatment team in the hospital setting. The judgment and assessment abilities of the nurse, combined with training and experience, must result in conclusions beneficial for the patient and the smooth flow of the ED. Although everyone who presents to the ED feels the emergency is serious, the level of severity varies. Under antidumping law, everyone who presents to the ED must be evaluated and appropriately stabilized. However, first sorting through those requesting care can be a tense, unstable, and legally risky experience.

MEDICAL RECORDS

At one time, emergency medical records were minimal, because of the nature of the admission. Today federal, state, and JCAHO regulations mandate specific standards regarding the contents, storage, and maintenance of medical records. The admission personnel are responsible for initiating the medical record, which should contain at a minimum the following information: (1) how the patient was found; (2) what type of injury was present on admission; (3) what care was provided at the accident scene; and (4) level of consciousness, including vital signs. The written record is also transferred with the patient to any facility to which the patient is transferred. Under the standards of the American Hospital Association (AHA), the medical records must be factual, complete, statements identified as such and contain signed consents when appropriate.

JCAHO's standards for medical records include the following requirements: (1) patient identification; (2) time and means of arrival; (3) pertinent history of the illness or injury and physical findings, including the patient's vital signs; (4) emergency care given to the patient prior to arrival; (5) diagnostic and therapeutic orders; (6) clinical observation, including results of treatment; (7) reports of procedures, tests, and results; (8) diagnostic impressions; (9) conclusions at the termination of evaluation and treatment, including final disposition, the patient's condition on discharge or transfer, and any instructions given to the patient or family, or both, for follow-up care; and (10) documentation of any patient who leaves against medical advice (AMA) (Hemelt & Mackert, 1982).

Nurses can be held liable, as a servant of the hospital, for not meeting identified standards for emergency care. Usually, after a proper history is first taken, the nurse's assessment is the basis for the initiation of treatment and care. For example, liability may arise in situations in which the nurse is ordered to discharge a patient with "take home" or follow-up instructions.

In the case of *Baldwin v. Knight* (1978), the patient was struck in the calf of his leg with a piece of wire while mowing the lawn. The nurse noted "patient has a puncture type wound, received while mowing grass, from a broken bottle." The emergency room physician assumed the patient cut his leg on a broken glass when cutting the lawn and sutured the wound without first doing an x-ray examination. A piece of wire was later found imbedded in the leg, and the patient successfully sued under the legal theory of negligence.

The AHA suggests the following additional policies and procedures for emergency patient care as legal safeguards:

- The standard of care provided in the emergency department must be maintained at a level equal to that provided elsewhere in the hospital and community.
- All personnel within the ED must meet licensure requirements, be reasonably competent, and have the ability to communicate with patients, but also know the extent and limitations of professional duties.
- The patient must be given explicit directions on follow-up care on discharge, which are clearly understood and confirmed in writing (Pegalis & Wachsman, 1982, p. 158).

JCAHO requires that hospitals develop appropriate procedures and nursing service coverage for the ED (Pegalis & Wachsman, 1982, p. 164). There must be written policies and procedures specifying the scope and conduct of patient care to be rendered, which must be approved by hospital administration and medical staff. Standards help define issues concerning nurses "floating" from another department into the ED during busy or understaffed periods. The hospital has a duty to provide an appropriate number of staff to fulfill the needs of the department; however, underqualified staff in the ED can be hazardous. If additional staff is pulled from a unit to be placed in the ED, float personnel should be from similarly related areas, such as from the intensive care unit (ICU) or a trauma care unit. These providers can also be assigned to simple tasks appropriate to their level of experience.

The American College of Surgeons also set forth standards for "early care" of the injured patient (Pegalis & Wachsman, 1982, p. 166). These standards help set the guidelines for the Emergency Medical Services (EMS) and early emergency room care of the patient. The **Federal Emergency Medical Services System Act of 1973 (FEMA)** has developed provisions and guidelines for coordinating health care services during emergency and disaster situations (Pegalis & Wachsman, 1982, p. 177). It should be noted that additional procedures nurses perform within the emergency room setting that extend the standard scope of practice must be based on established policy, procedure, and appropriate training. Nurses in the ED develop advanced skills to assist in the rapid delivery of care. These extended skills must be preceded by appropriate training and demonstration of competency before they are incorporated into ED nursing practice.

MANAGED CARE IN THE EMERGENCY DEPARTMENT

Nurses cannot refuse to evaluate a patient, because that refusal would violate the antidumping provisions of the **Consolidated Omnibus Budget Reconciliation Act (COBRA)**, which would ultimately subject the hospital to a fine and loss of Medicare revenue (Herr, 1998). However, the exact definition of screening has not been spelled out by federal regulations. The recommendation is to offer a **screening examination**, which at a minimum standard must include vital signs and chief complaint. An ethical and legal dilemma occurs when the patient withdraws a request to be transferred because of inability to pay, refuses care, and/or seeks discharge. Documentation is then critical, along with a modified AMA form to reflect refusal of care (Herr, 1998).

Some states have passed legislation that makes managed care accept the prudent layperson definition of emergency. This means the managed care plan must pay for any ED visit prompted by signs or symptoms that a so-called **prudent layperson**—a person in the community who possesses an average level of understanding and medical knowledge—would think is an emergency (Herr, 1998).

LEGAL DUTIES

DUTY TO OBEY PHYSICIAN ORDERS

Nurses have the duty to follow physicians' orders (Pozgar, 1990, p. 91). Nurses face many ethical dilemmas because of a need to determine the best interest of and advocate for the patient, while following (1) hospital policy and procedure, (2) physicians' orders, (3) nursing practice standards, (4) state and federal laws, and (5) standards for personal safety. In *Toth v. Community Hospital at Glen Cove*, nurses were held negligent when failing to follow the physician's orders for delivery of oxygen to a set of twins. The physician had ordered oxygen to be administered at the rate of 6 liters per minute for the first 12 hours and then 4 liters per minute

thereafter. The nurses were held negligent when they delivered 6 liters per minute continuously over several weeks, creating blindness in one twin and severe damage to one eye in the other twin.

DUTY TO REPORT NEGLIGENT PHYSICIANS

Nurses have the duty to report physician negligence (Pozgar, 1990, p. 92). In *Goff v. Doctors General Hospital* (1958), a nurse determined that a postpartum patient was in critical condition subsequent to the physician's negligently suturing after delivery. The nurse contacted the physician, who was not in the hospital. The nurse knew that the patient was in grave condition and would die with no emergency intervention. The nurse failed to notify a supervisor of the patient's deteriorating condition. The patient died and the nurse was found negligent, for evidence was sufficient to find that the nurses who attended the patient were aware of the excessive bleeding. The nurses were found negligent, and their negligence was held to be a contributing cause of the patient's death.

DUTY TO QUESTION PATIENT DISCHARGE

If there is reason to believe a patient discharge may be injurious to the health of the patient, the nurse has the duty to question the discharge (Pozgar, 1990, p. 92). In *Koeniguer v. Erkrich* (1988) the jury found that the nurses had a duty to attempt to delay the patient's discharge if conditions warranted continued hospitalization, and that delay in treatment, resulting from premature discharge, contributed to the patient's death.

DUTY TO REPORT PATIENT CHANGES

Nurses have the responsibility to report changes in the patient's condition that may adversely affect the patient's well-being (Pozgar, 1990, p. 92). In *Darling v. Charleston Community Memorial Hospital* (1965), the patient had his broken leg set in a cast. He began complaining of pain almost immediately. Later, his toes became swollen and dark, then cold and insensitive. Nurses checked his leg only a few times a day and failed to report its worsening condition. After 3 days, the cast was removed to reveal a necrotic leg, which had to be amputated (Ford, 1987, p. 116). (For similar cases involving nurses who failed to report significant changes or who failed to adequately monitor the patient's condition, see *Cline v. Lund* (1993) and *Sanchez v. Bay General Hospital* (1981), respectively.)

The emergency room receives an ever-evolving number of patients who need constant monitoring, because of a high level of acuity and undiagnosed conditions. Constant attention, monitoring and communication with the physician are critical to avoid unnecessary delays in treatment or misinterpretation of a patient's signs and symptoms. It is imperative to follow nursing practice guidelines within hospital ED policy and procedure. Reporting changes involves more than just the physiological assessment of whether symptoms warrant immediate attention, for emergencies usually also involve a psychiatric component.

THE INCOMPETENT PATIENT

The **incompetent** patient is one who for various reasons is unable to speak for himself or herself, unable to comprehend, and/or is legally termed unable to make a decision because of medical condition or age. Examples of incompetent patients include minors, unconscious patients, the mentally ill, those diagnosed with organic illnesses creating delirium or dementia, and the mentally retarded. The issues that arise regarding these patients generally involve consent for treatment, use of restraints, and involuntary commitment. For example, issues may arise involving the minor patient who is injured beyond the ability to comprehend informed consent, yet requiring a decision about immediate life-saving treatments, whose parent's religious beliefs preclude the appropriate treatment (Pozgar, 1990, p. 127).

Restraints

Restraining and/or detaining a patient inappropriately is **false imprisonment** (Ford, 1987, p. 87). Federal law dictates the parameters for the use of restraints, through implementation of the Mental Health Code Law. Each individual state determines how the law is applied within the state. If a patient is a danger to self, others, or the health care staff, restraints can be applied. If restraints are applied to a patient considered competent and not a danger to self or society, false imprisonment charges could be filed. Once restraints are applied, the patient should be closely monitored for changes in medical condition, possibility of restraints becoming loose, or maintenance of adequate circulation (Ford, 1987, p. 1430). Positional asphyxia has unfortunately occurred in cases where patients have been restrained unmonitored and the position unchanged.

Hospital policy and procedure should reflect the uniqueness of the state law on restraints. These policies and procedures must specify the length of time the patient may be restrained. Most states require the written order of a physician before restraining the patient. Emergency situations are the exception. Restraints are not to be used as a means of punishment, for the convenience of the provider, or as a substitute for treatment programs. Restraints are not to be used without treatment and/or the rehabilitation necessary to integrate the person into society (Ford, 1987, p. 142; *O'Connor v. Donaldson*, 1975). In *Big Town Nursing Home v. Newman* (1970), Mr. Newman attempted to escape from the nursing home where his son had placed him. The nursing home attempted to restrain Mr. Newman. Mr. Newman finally escaped and sued, under the legal theory of false imprisonment. The courts held in favor of Mr. Newman, for the court had not declared him incompetent.

Prisoners can be lawfully restrained on the orders of law enforcement authorities. However, in most cases, law enforcement personnel remain with prisoners throughout treatment and hospitalization. In addition, patients with a communicable disease may be considered a threat to society if a request is made to leave the hospital AMA. The hospital may choose to involuntarily detain this patient until a restraining order is obtained and/or law enforcement personnel are able to assist with the detention (Ford, 1987, p. 88).

A hospital also has the duty to protect a suicidal patient from self-harm (Furrow, 1995, pp. 152, 600). This duty exists whether the patient is voluntarily or involuntarily committed. In *Abille v. United States* (1980), the physician had not ordered suicide precautions for the patient. The patient had been admitted and diagnosed as suicidal, which normally results in a patient not being able to leave the health care facility without an escort. The nursing staff allowed him to leave the ward, and he subsequently jumped from a window, committing suicide. The Alaska court held that the failure to protect the patient from self-harm was a breach of the standard of care.

Consent for Treatment

Consent is the voluntary agreement by a person who is in possession and exercise of sufficient mental capacity to make an intelligent choice between proposed alternatives (Pozgar, 1990, p. 116). Consent of this nature is considered **informed consent**. The principle of informed consent was articulated by Justice Cardozo, in language quoted in *Schloendorf v. Society of New York Hospital* (1914): "Every human being of adult years and sound mind has a right to determine what shall be done with his own body" (cited in Furrow, 1995, p. 266; Pozgar, 1990). Consent may be expressed or implied. "**Expressed consent** can take the form of a verbal agreement or can take place through a signed form. **Implied consent** has been authorized" (Furrow, 1995, p. 116). Consent must be obtained from the patient and if that is impossible, then by a person representing the patient. Treating a patient without consent is an intentional touching without consent, or a **battery**. A parent or legal guardian must provide consent for a minor. In the case of a life-and-death decision, another family member may give consent for

treatment. In extreme cases, the physician may proceed to treat the patient in a life-and-death situation without obtaining consent from an authorized patient representative.

Generally, in order to provide informed consent, individuals must be given adequate information to make an intelligent decision about the choices available for their treatment (Ford, 1987, p. 64; Pozgar, 1990, p. 117). The patient also has the right to refuse treatment, even if the health care is advisable (Ford, 1987, p. 74). The patient must have a personal understanding of the physician's explanation of the risks of treatment and possible consequences. The needs of the patient relative to informed consent depend on age, maturity, mental status, language barriers, and ethical and religious considerations.

The rights and requests of a competent patient may not be disregarded even if the outcome of the refusal may be detrimental to health. In *Erickson v. Digard* (1962), the patient refused a blood transfusion and the court held that his requests must be honored (Pozgar, 1990, p. 122).

Temporary guardianship can be granted in cases in which the patient is critical, a treatment decision must be made immediately, and attempts are made to contact family members or persons of authority to provide consent. In the case of *In re Estate Dorone* (1987), a 22-year-old male patient was brought to the hospital by helicopter following an automobile accident. Providers determined that the patient would die without immediate cranial surgery, which would require a blood transfusion, a procedure contrary to the patient's religious beliefs. The Court of Common Pleas appointed the hospital administrator as temporary guardian, allowing this executive to authorize the consent for emergency treatment (Pozgar, 1990, p. 124).

Minors

When providing informed consent for minors, the nurse must consider either the individual state's statutorily defined age of emancipation and/or marital status. While attempting to acquire consent from the legal parent(s) or the person acting **in loco parentis** (the person who is providing consent for the child in the absence of the parent), treatment should not be delayed or withheld to the detriment of the child.

Ethical dilemmas arise when the minor is involved in a situation he or she has requested to be kept in confidence from the parents. Issues regarding the protection of the patient's privacy and confidentiality must be addressed; however under some state laws, consent may need to be obtained from the parents. For example, if a girl presents with abdominal pain and needs surgery for a miscarriage, the parent's consent may need to be obtained, whether or not it ultimately breaches the minor patient's right to confidentiality.

In the case of *Carter v. Cangello* (1980), a 17-year-old girl had run away from home and was living in the home of a woman who provided a place to stay in exchange for household chores. The parents knew of the daughter's living arrangements but had been contributing to their daughter's schooling and medical care. The court held in favor of the girl's right to consent to her own surgery, and further held that the physician was free from any liability to the parents for treating the minor daughter without parental consent (Pozgar, 1990, p. 124).

LEGAL REPORTING OBLIGATIONS

CHILD ABUSE

Most states have statutorily imposed a specific mandatory obligation on nurses to report physically abused or neglected children. The most difficult related issue is the adequate and fair determination of what constitutes abuse, the determination of whether the injury was intentional or whether there is a possibility of an accident having occurred. The welfare of the child must be considered at all times. In the past, reporting of such concerns was done reluctantly (Pozgar, 1990, p. 139). Parents could sue providers on the grounds of defamation or invasion of privacy if the charges were not proven true. Fortunately, society has learned

to place a greater interest on the safety and welfare of the child versus the privacy and character claims of a parent.

In 1874, child abuse gained attention when a church worker by the name of Etta Wheeler found a 9-year-old girl, Mary Ellen, chained to her bed. As New York had no laws to protect children, the American Society for the Prevention of Cruelty to Animals agreed to intervene. One year later, the case reached the courts, and New York adopted its first child protection law.

Today, all states and the District of Columbia have enacted laws to protect abused children. Most states also protect the persons reporting the incidents, by providing immunity from prosecution. The first statutory law mandating reporting of child abuse resulted from a 1963 report by the Children's Bureau of the Department of Health, Education, and Welfare. Subsequently, most states created legislation protecting children from child abuse by 1970. In 1973, the Early Childhood Project Education Commission published a model law to provide uniformity in the diverse interpretations of laws against child abuse. In 1973, Congress also passed the Child Abuse Prevention and Treatment Act. This act required states to meet uniform standards in order to be eligible for federal assistance in setting up programs to identify, prevent, and treat problems of child abuse. There are two common features of state implementation of this legislation: (1) the empowering of social welfare and/or law enforcement bureaus to receive and investigate reports of actual or suspected abuse, and (2) the granting of legal immunity from liability for defamation or invasion of privacy to any person reporting an incident of actual or suspected abuse (Ford, 1987, p. 136).

Emergency nurses are frequently the first to suspect or discover abuse or neglect. The nurse has a duty to comply with the laws requiring the mandatory reporting of suspicions of abuse or neglect to the appropriate authorities. The nurse may need to photograph injuries, but only with consent of the patient being photographed (Ford, 1987, p. 137), depending on state law and hospital policy. Thorough objective documentation is imperative, while keeping personal reactions separate from the facts recorded. **Abuse** is generally defined as serious physical injury caused by another, which has not occurred by accidental means (Pozgar, 1990, p. 140). Some state mandatory reporting laws require the following information: (1) name and address of the child, (2) the person responsible for the child's care, (3) the child's age, (4) the nature and extent of the child's injuries, and (5) any other information that might be helpful in establishing the cause of the injuries, such as photographs of the injured child and the identity of the perpetrator (Pozgar, 1990, p. 140).

In *Awkerman v. Tri-County Orthopedic Group* (1985), a minor child and his mother brought an action for damages against physicians for failing to diagnose disease and filing erroneous abuse reports. The court held that the child abuse reporting statute provided immunity to the persons who filed the child abuse reports in good faith, even if the reports were filed because of the negligent diagnosis of the child's frequent bone fractures, eventually diagnosed as osteogenesis imperfecta (Pozgar, 1990, p. 140). But the court also held that immunity from liability did not extend to damages for malpractice that may have resulted from the failure to diagnose the child's disease, as long as the elements of negligence were present.

DOMESTIC VIOLENCE

The state of California enacted a bill mandating that incidences of persons with wounds or injuries inflicted as a result of domestic violence must be reported to law enforcement officials by health care workers (McLain, 1998). A research team studied police records to determine whether the law had created an increase in reporting of domestic violence (McLain, 1998, citing California Penal Code 11160, 1994). The authors concluded:

The mandatory law requiring medical professionals to report physical domestic violence to law enforcement officials has been ineffective in increasing medical personnel referral to the Los Angeles County Sheriff Department (LACSD) during the two years after the law [was enacted] (Sachs, Peek, Baraff, & Hasselblad, 1998).

Possible explanations for this outcome include (1) the provider's ignorance of the law; (2) noncompliance with reporting laws, e.g., following a victim's wish that a report not be made; (3) knowledge that the incident was already reported to the police by the victim before arriving at the medical facility; and/or (4) the victim's misrepresentation of the cause of the injuries, because of awareness of the law and not wishing the incident to be reported (Herr, 1998). Other states may have similar laws, requiring at least the reporting of violence, if there is a concern for the safety of minor children within the home environment. In such situations, the nurse is faced with the ethical dilemma of respecting the patient's wishes of nonreporting/confidentiality versus following the mandatory provisions of reporting law.

RAPE

Rape is a criminal act that is reportable. It previously encompassed three general elements: (1) carnal knowledge of a woman, (2) lack of consent to this carnal knowledge, and (3) use of force to accomplish this act (Kravis et al., 1987). Professionals have recognized that this definition of rape is inadequate. The elements of rape were interpreted too narrowly, for carnal knowledge was construed as penetration of the vagina by the man's penis, lack of consent was construed as forcible resistance, and the use of force was considered to be physical violence and/or use of a weapon (Carrow, 1980). The definition of rape no longer includes the element of penetration. The definition has been expanded to include the following acts of abuse: (1) aggravated assault, (2) attempted rape, (3) indecent assault, (4) involuntary sexual intercourse, (5) sexual abuse, and (6) statutory rape (Kravis et al., 1987).

Programs for sexual assault nurse examiner (SANE) have been successfully operating throughout portions of the United States since 1976 (Hohenhaus, 1998). These specially trained nurses understand the issues and laws governing sexual assault and conduct specific forensic examinations and documentation designed for this emergency.

North Carolina introduced Senate Bill 320, which became law on August 6, 1998, allowing nurses to perform sexual assault examinations and to be paid directly by third-party payers (Hohenhaus, 1998). The bill mandates that SANEs be trained in North Carolina in approved programs, to ensure supervision and control of the quality of the education provided to the nurse examiners (Hohenhaus, 1998). The benefits of such programs allow victims to bypass long waits in the ED, be evaluated and treated by professionals who understand the specifics of the emergency, and have thorough documentation by nurse experts, who can later testify in court to the evidence collected. Some of the SANE programs have been established as an adjunct to the ED, whereas others are free standing.

COMMUNICABLE DISEASES

A provider's duty to maintain confidentiality may conflict with a duty to disclose information to third parties, such as warning of a risk of violence, a contagious disease, or some other health risk (Furrow, 1995, p. 151). Reportable conditions include disease in newborns and communicable diseases.

Courts have cited the Restatement (Second) Torts, § 324A, which provides in part that one who provides services to another may be liable to a third person for harm resulting from his failure to exercise reasonable care, "if the harm is suffered because of reliance of the other person upon the undertaking" . . . in the case of communicable disease, courts have included in that class of persons at risk anyone who is physically intimate with the patient . . . Some states by statute require health care workers to counsel HIV-infected patients to take special precautions to avoid infecting others and to tell their sexual or needle sharing partners to seek testing, counseling and treatment. If patients indicate that they will not do so, the health care worker's obligation to warn others is defined by the law of the particular [state] (Furrow, 1995, pp. 152, 154).

Some states require that any instance of diarrhea and staphylococcal disease in infants be reported to the state epidemiology department. Communicable diseases may include tuberculosis, hanta virus, and whooping cough. Most states have enacted laws regarding mandatory reporting of such communicable diseases. For example, the New York State Sanitary Code, Chapter 1, Section 2.12 (1973), entitled "Reporting by others than physicians of cases of diseases presumably communicable," provides the following guidelines:

When no physician is in attendance it shall be the duty of the head of a private household or person in charge of any institution, school, hotel, boarding house, camp or vessel or any public health nurse or any other person having knowledge of an individual affected with any disease presumably communicable, to report immediately the name and address of such person to the city, council or district health officer (Pozgar, 1990, p. 141).

ANIMAL BITES

Many states, through animal control, have mandatory reporting of all animal bites. Rabies is the most serious potential outcome from animal bites, but infection is the most common complication (Callaham, 1978). Dog bites are more common than cat bites (Kizer, 1979). In more serious cases, where death or dismemberment has occurred, charges may be brought against the animal's owner (Borchelt, Lockwood, & Beck, 1983; Lauer, White, & Lauer, 1982; Pinckney & Kennedy, 1982; Wright, 1985). In treatment of dog bite wounds, recommendation is for the animal to be killed and tested as soon as possible, rather than holding the animal for observation ("Rabies Prevention," 1984).

BIRTHS AND DEATHS

Under state statutory law, all births and deaths must be reported. Births are of important significance for census reporting for states and for funding issues. The physician pronouncing a death must sign a death certificate (Pozgar, 1990, p. 142).

Death often occurs in emergency rooms, requiring health professionals to understand the many facets of this issue. From a legal standpoint, proper pronouncement, appropriate death notification, and management and delivery of the corpse are the main concerns (Pozgar, 1990, p. 160). Most states have provisions for qualified persons, in the absence of a physician, to pronounce death by following certain guidelines. Efforts should be taken to notify a physician by telephone or radio during the process. Some states also have nurse coroners who are legally qualified to pronounce death in the field. However, in a hospital emergency room, physicians pronounce death. Once death is pronounced, the nurse is usually responsible for thorough documentation of the final findings about the patient and the preparation of the body. If there is a concern that the death requires a medical examiner to investigate, additional care must be taken to include evidence that arrived with the patient, as well as all medical devices used while in the hospital (Pozgar, 1990, p. 142). This may include clothing, shoes, helmets, wallets, suitcases, nasogastric tubes, Foley catheters, chest tubes, tubes of blood drawn, bags of blood administered, and so on. Contact the medical examiner to determine how evidence should best be handled. Despite family's wishes, consent for an autopsy need not be obtained if the case is determined to be a coroner's case (Ford, 1987, p. 88).

Cases involving wrongful handling of dead bodies fall into four categories:

1. Mutilation of a body
2. Unauthorized autopsy
3. Wrongful detention
4. Miscellaneous wrongs, such as unauthorized sale, refusal or neglect in burial, and unauthorized use or publication of photographs taken after death (Pozgar, 1990, p. 160)

Respecting religious processes also falls into this category of issues. In the case of *Lott v. State* (1962), two bodies were mistagged, leaving a person of Catholic faith prepared for an Orthodox Jewish burial, and the person of Jewish faith prepared for a Catholic burial. The court held that the conduct was negligent, as it had resulted in mental anguish, for which liability was imposed.

SUSPICIOUS DEATHS

Suspicious deaths must be reported to the medical examiner's office for further investigation. Unnatural or violent deaths, occurring within 24 hours of discharge from a hospital, must be reported to the medical examiner (Pozgar, 1990, p. 142). This also includes deaths from what appears to be criminal activity. The medical examiner then makes the determination as to whether there is a need for an autopsy and investigation. If in doubt, it is always better to preserve the remains and evidence and to notify the examiner's office. Everything associated with the case needs to be considered as evidence from the scene and preserved for medical examiners and police officials. For example, evidence may include blankets wrapped around the person, vomitus, IV tubes, helmets, shoes torn off during the accident, articles imbedded in the person, impaling objects, and/or photographs from the accident scene. Today, forensic nurses are employed by police departments, emergency departments, and coroners' offices to assist in identifying, collecting, and preserving evidence. Forensic nurses may also be involved in the scene investigations and pronouncing deaths. Their ability to remain through the case from the beginning enables the forensic nurse to be available to testify if necessary.

FIREARM INJURIES

Gunshot wounds, inflicted by lethal weapons or by unlawful acts, require mandatory reporting. Some states include automobile accidents within their definition of lethal weapons. New York Statute 265.25, entitled "Certain Wounds to Be Reported," states:

Every case of a bullet wound, gunshot wound, powder burn or any other injury arising from or caused by the discharge of a gun or firearm, and every case of a wound that is likely to or may result in death and is actually or apparently inflicted by a knife, ice pick or other sharp or pointed instrument, shall be reported at once to the police authorities in the city, town or village where the person reported is located by the: a) physician attending or treating the case; or

b) manager, superintendent or other person in charge, whenever such case is treated in a hospital, sanitarium or other institution (Pozgar, 1990, p. 143).

CRIMINAL ACTS

Other criminal acts requiring mandatory reporting are attempted suicide, rape, assault, child molestation, or the unlawful dispensing or taking of narcotic drugs. Sometimes this information may be gathered under circumstances in which the communication may be considered privileged. Without the patient's expressed consent to disclose such information or without a statutory mandate that a report be made, it may be a violation of the patient's rights to report a suspected criminal act (Pozgar, 1990, p. 143).

THE SUSPECTED CRIMINAL PATIENT

Because of the nature of the emergency room, the ED is often the first point of entrance into the hospital for those who may be victims or perpetrators of criminal acts. Thus, the ED nurse may have the occasion to provide care for the patient who may be suspected of committing a crime. The nursing oath requires that the nurse provide care to all humans in need of attention regardless of race, creed, color, ethnicity, and socioeconomic background. The police, in an effort to gather evidence, may request the assistance of the ED nurse. If the patient is under arrest, the nurse can legally handle the belongings and take blood samples for evidence under the doctor's orders. If the patient is not under arrest, the nurse must make sure a valid search warrant is in effect before proceeding under the doctor's orders. Without such a warrant, the nurse may be sued for invasion of privacy as well as assault and battery if procedures are performed on behalf of the police.

The Fourth Amendment to the Constitution provides the right to be free of unreasonable search and seizure (Ford, 1987, p. 144). Even after conviction, the prisoner does not lose all rights, for the Eighth Amendment provides protection against any act that may be construed as "cruel and unusual punishment." Thus, the Eighth Amendment guarantees that prison officials and health care workers shall not deliberately ignore a prisoner's health care needs (Ford, 1987, p. 144).

The **exclusionary rule** stems from the Fourth Amendment's prohibition on unreasonable search and seizure. In the landmark case of *Mapp v. Ohio* (1961), the court held that (1) evidence obtained through an unlawful or unreasonable search cannot be used against the person whose rights the search violated; and (2) evidence in plain view could be confiscated, such as a weapon, drugs, or any item suspected of potential harm to others. Once confiscated, hospital officials and law enforcement officers must be notified immediately by the nurse. If evidence is confiscated without following the appropriate measures, such as without a search warrant, the evidence may not be admissible in a court of law. Further, the person collecting the evidence has the potential of being sued for invasion of privacy (Ford, 1987, p. 144).

In *State v. Perea* (1981), a nurse took the shirt of a suspect for safekeeping and later handed it to the police, even though it had not been requested. The court allowed the shirt to be admitted as evidence, for no governmental intrusion was involved and the suspect's rights had not been violated (Ford, 1987, p. 145).

In the case of *United States v. Winbush* (1970), the court ruled that evidence found through a routine search of an unconscious patient's pockets was admissible, because the purpose of the search was to obtain identification and medical information (Ford, 1987, p. 145).

In the case of *Commonwealth v. Storella* (1978), during a medically necessary procedure, a doctor removed a bullet from a patient. The doctor turned the bullet over to the police, and the court allowed the bullet to be admitted as evidence, because the doctor was acting according to good medical practice and not as a state agent. But anyone making searches for the sole purpose of obtaining evidence, especially at the request of the police, may be construed as becoming agents for the police (Ford, 1987, p. 145).

Opinions differ as to whether blood obtained without the consent of the patient can be admitted into a court of law. In *Scdhmerber v. California* (1966), the Supreme Court held that blood obtained without a warrant, incident to a lawful arrest, is not an unconstitutional search and seizure and is admissible evidence. Many courts have interpreted this decision to mean that a blood sample, to be admissible, must be obtained after the arrest and be drawn in a medically reasonable manner. But some courts also admit blood drawn for nontherapeutic reasons and voluntarily turned over to the police (*Turner v. State*, 1975).

Courts have ruled that blood samples were inadmissible in the following instances: (1) when police pinned a suspect to the floor while the blood was being drawn (*People v. Kraft*, 1970); (2) when a suspect's arm was broken while being twisted by a policeman, who was sitting on him to coerce consent to the blood sample (*State v. Riggins*, 1977); and (3) when obtained by untrained, nonhospital, personnel (*Rochin v. California*, 1952; a nasogastric tube was forced down a suspect to remove stomach contents).

Although in most instances a battery may be argued to have occurred if the provider has obtained a blood sample without the patient's consent, in some states an implied consent to provide a blood sample attaches when applying for a driver's license. In essence, the applicant consents to a blood alcohol test if arrested for drunken driving (Ford, 1987, p. 145).

The most important consideration before gathering any evidence is to consult state law, an enforcement officer, hospital policy, and/or a forensic expert, so no evidence is destroyed. Collection, preservation, and documentation all must follow precise steps, to maintain the chain of custody and the quality of the evidence, without violating rules of evidence governing its admissibility.

LIVING WILLS

The concept of individual instruction, or **advance directive**, as identified under the Uniform Health Care Decisions Act of 1994,

includes the following common terms encountered by health care providers: living will, do not resuscitate (DNR), euthanasia, right to die, and right to live (Furrow, 1995, p. 708). The very nature of issues related to advance directives brings constant legislative changes, which require providers to keep informed. The ED nurse may encounter a patient who has developed disabling, dysfunctional, or terminal illness and who may have requested that "no heroic measures" be taken. Providers who first encounter the patient must make the decision about what actions should be taken. Knowing individual state laws is critical in carrying out the wishes of those who do not want life-saving measures (Ford, 1987, p. 150).

If the patient has become incompetent, then a court-appointed or legal guardian, acting on behalf of the patient through a health care durable power of attorney, makes decisions on behalf of the patient (Furrow, 1995, p. 708). In the case of a person who is incompetent, the court intervenes appointing a guardian if (1) the physicians disagree on the prognosis, (2) the family members disagree on the wishes of the patient, (3) the patient's wishes cannot be known because he or she has always been incompetent, (4) evidence exists of wrongful motives or malpractice, or (5) no family member can serve as a guardian (Pozgar, 1990).

In 1976, California was the first state to enact what was called a **Natural Death Act**, or Living Will Act, which allowed competent persons to make life-saving decisions in advance of any situation in which they were unable to make independent decisions (Ford, 1987, p. 147). Through a **living will**, the patient gives the physician permission to withhold or discontinue treatment in advance, not leaving the decision to the family or health care team. Although a living will is considered legal in every state, it may not be legally binding in all states. Some states make living wills binding on doctors and impose penalties for noncompliance (Ford, 1987, p. 147). Hospital policy should follow individual state laws regarding living wills, for example (1) how they are implemented, (2) when and how they should be executed, (3) who must adhere to the will, (4) when the will applies, (5) what directives should be followed, (6) how long the will is valid, and (7) what documentation is required. Ethical dilemmas may arise if a person from a foreign country or a different state presents a living will in a state in which they are not recognized, for the second state may not have to honor the terms of the will (Ford, 1987, p. 156).

A living will may be invalidated when the patient asks for treatment that was refused under the terms of the living will (Ford, 1987, p. 157). The living will should be reviewed annually and re-signed each year, to indicate a continued awareness of the treatment decisions. In those states that recognize living wills, the family is unable to contradict the will unless it can be proven invalid (Ford, 1987, p. 157; Furrow, 1995, p. 710). A patient may request the nurse to assist in preparing or witnessing a living will (Ford, 1987, p. 157). If this occurs, the nurse should know individual state laws regarding participation in the execution of a living will. In addition, the nurse should be aware of hospital policy and discuss the patient's request with the nursing supervisor. If no restriction applies, there should be thorough documentation of the circumstances of the execution of the living will in the patient's chart.

Oral living wills may not be considered valid while a person is healthy, if any disagreement arises. Once a person is diagnosed with terminal illness, an oral request may be honored as long as the patient is still considered competent (Ford, 1987, p. 157). The oral living will may include the right to refuse treatment, including extraordinary means. If a patient makes such pronouncements to the nurse, thorough documentation should be made in the nurse's notes and notification of the physician should be made. Although specifically stated oral wills are not legally enforceable, a patient's right to refuse treatment is legally binding.

ORGAN DONATION

Organ donation is a serious concern of the health care industry. Originally, organ dona-

tions were considered experimental and there were few donors. Transplants have become a standard medical practice. With such success, potential recipients of organs may be counted in the thousands. Receiving organs, under the proper conditions with appropriate consent, remains the most difficult aspect of this science. Retrieving organs in a timely fashion, for proper preservation and transportation, is of the utmost concern. The emergency room is the primary area where a patient may be determined to be brain dead, about to die, or to have died, immediately presenting a potential candidate for organ donation. The need to preserve organs may require a health care worker to immediately approach family members regarding the potential for organ donation. Physicians usually make the request for organ donation, as they are best able to answer medical questions. A transplant coordinator may be involved but is usually not as available as the physician who has diagnosed the terminal condition or pronounced death.

Most states have enacted legislation to facilitate organ donations. All states have enacted the **Uniform Anatomical Gift Act**, which provides the following two mechanisms to donate organs: (1) a person 18 years or older may sign a card indicating a wish to be an organ donor (for example, on the back of a drivers license); and/or (2) a family member may provide authorization for organ donation by a family member by signing the appropriate document(s) (Pozgar, 1990, p. 166). However, if death occurs within 24 hours after admission to the hospital, the medical examiner must also be notified and sign a release for organ donation.

WORKPLACE VIOLENCE

Nurses working within emergency medical services are highly susceptible to violence (Pozzi, 1998), for the emergency department has one of the highest incidences of violence and abuse (Lanza, 1983). Emergency staff deal not only with the patient's volatile emotions, but also a dangerous combination of conditions including organic disorders, frustrations arising from long waiting periods, psychiatric emergencies, homicidal and suicidal patients, substance abusers, the flow of the general public, and distraught family members. Although measures to improve security and documentation have been implemented under the guidelines of the Occupational Safety and Health Administration (OSHA, 1996), many pitfalls remain. One of the most significant problems involves assisting health care providers to identify what constitutes workplace violence and abuse. Most people think of **workplace violence** as a disgruntled worker returning to cause harm to the boss or another coworker. But workplace violence also includes, but is not limited to, harassment, sexual gestures, threatening remarks, objects being thrown, spitting or hitting, and/or pulling away in anger. The majority of emergency department incidents stem from encounters with patients and their families.

Workplace violence can also include **horizontal violence,** demonstrated through acts of bullying, physicians demeaning nurses or throwing objects, actions that undermine a coworker, or threats (Spring & Stern, 1998). Violence is not necessarily overt, as when coworkers shoot one another; violence often takes place by more subtle yet very destructive methods. Horizontal violence is the most difficult situation to document, because reports of verbal confrontations are labeled "hearsay," and thus are inadmissible in court.

Fortunately, through education of health care personnel about horizontal violence, more employers are becoming aware of the issue (Queensland Nurses' Union, 1998). Hospitals are required to have policies on workplace violence, along with procedures for reporting its occurrence (OSHA, 1996). An **Employee Assistance Program (EAP)** can provide opportunities for employees to confide with counselors about abuses they have experienced in the workplace. Some hospitals have **Critical Incident Stress Management (CISM)** personnel, trained to offer additional assistance after incidents occur that are highly stressful, e.g., suicide of a patient. (For more information regarding the issues and laws related to violence in the workplace, refer to Chapter 24, Violence in Nursing.)

GOOD SAMARITAN

Nurses, physicians, emergency medical technicians (EMTs), physician's assistants, nurse practitioners, temporary nurses, traveling nurses, and flight nurses all may have opportunities to volunteer, subcontract, and/or represent their institution and/or employer at public events, carnivals, camps, resorts, and festivals. By doing so, providers may place themselves in situations for which they are inadequately prepared to manage emergencies or disasters. When faced with potentially unknown situations, emergency care providers should conduct prior assessment to ensure access to proper equipment, up-to-date medications, availability of telephones, methods to transport patients to safe areas through crowds, ability to treat more than one person, security support, hazardous plans control, evacuation plans, fire control, effective communications between other officials including security and fire control, and a safe weather-resistant building in which to work.

In the case of *Boccasil et al. v. Cajun Music Limited et al.* (1977), the wife of a patient alleged that: (1) the physician negligently and fatally delayed administration of epinephrine; and (2) that the nurse responded negligently to the medical emergency, by arriving at the scene without any medical equipment, thereby delaying the administration of epinephrine to the patient. Two separate judges held that the doctor and nurse were rendering gratuitous services and, therefore, were entitled to the protection of the Good Samaritan statutes (George, Quattrone, & Goldstone, 1998). Fortunately in this case, the court held that the two providers acted in good faith, within the realms of their education and training. Any difficulty the providers experienced with equipment or ability to provide emergency care was not relevant, because the plaintiff failed to establish a standard of care. If the plaintiff would have provided expert testimony to describe the standard and deviations that occurred, the judgment may have been different.

ADVANCED PRACTICE NURSES

Nurse practitioners, clinical nurse specialists, flight nurses, nurse-midwives, and forensic nurses have advanced the practice of ED nursing by obtaining specialized education and developing certification processes. Each one of these areas of advanced nursing maintains specific standards of practice developed from statutory laws, which have been written to establish the parameters or scope of ED practice. In addition, hospital policy and procedure, as often interpreted by the medical director, may dictate how advanced nursing is practiced within the boundaries of a particular hospital. The authorization for advanced practice nurses to write prescriptions is governed by the state's nurse practice act. Ultimately, writing prescriptions is limited to certain medications, but may require additional approval of the medical director when administered within the hospital setting.

The Emergency Nurses Association (ENA) has written guidelines establishing standards of care specific to emergency nursing. In addition, the ENA created the position of certified emergency room nurse, a certification administered by the Board of Certification for Emergency Nursing (BCEN). The purpose of such certification is to identify knowledge and skills by which safe and competent ED nursing practice can be measured. Flight and forensic nurses also have an association that has established specific standards of care for each area of advanced nursing practice. Flight nurses have a certification process similar to that of the ENA, whereas forensic nurses are still coordinating a certification process.

COMMON PITFALLS IN EMERGENCY DEPARTMENT NURSING PRACTICE

As previously stated, the emergency department is an area with one of the highest risks for professional malpractice within the health care system. Within the ED, triage is an extremely high-risk function, for decisions must be made rapidly upon patient arrival, in order to prioritize health care problems. Some of the most common errors in emergency departments occur within the triage decision-making processes. Choices must be made between treatment of patients with acute versus critical health care needs. Patients frequently believe that upon arrival at the emergency room their problems will be immediately addressed. However, patients frequently must wait while more acute patients receive and/or finish treatments or because there are few hospital beds in emergency departments. However, some patients may be unaware of the severity of their health care needs and politely wait in a long line, not asking for immediate help. This wait for emergency treatment is one of the most criticized problems of ED health care. Frequently, persons who monitor the waiting area are not trained health care providers. The wait also tends to intensify the feelings and reactions of patients. A "long wait" is speculated to be a leading cause of abusive and violent actions by patients and their families toward emergency health care providers.

Another pitfall of the ED is the treatment of the psychiatric patient. If disturbed or disruptive psychiatric patients are not sequestered, they may disrupt the ED with acting out behaviors. Inappropriate behavior tends to lower morale, interfere with medical care, and bring criticism on the hospital (Pegalis & Wachsman, 1982, p. 205).

Abuses that occur in an observation ward may include keeping patients who do not need observation, keeping patients too long, and/or indecision regarding diagnosis and treatment by the treatment team. Consequently, nurses become frustrated, in turn further affecting morale, patient turnover slows down, and patient frustration increases (Pegalis & Wachsman, 1982, p. 205).

Treatment can be inappropriate or dangerously delayed if there is no ready access to the patient's hospital records or the patient's history. Again, these delays increase the nurse's and the patient's frustration. But the most critical concern is the inappropriate treatment of a patient in need of emergency care, without a medical record to provide supportive information (Pegalis & Wachsman, 1982, p. 205).

Failure to provide paramedical staff to do technical tasks and failure to adjust the staffing schedule to the patient load have been determined to be two serious shortcomings that create patient frustration and ineffective turnaround of patients within the ED setting. With adequate staffing, there is ancillary staff to transport patients to areas of the hospital for medical tests, x-ray examinations, and blood work (Pegalis & Wachsman, 1982, p. 205). As managed care and census management have become more of a financial focus within hospitals, nursing staff have been exposed to a higher risk for malpractice. Maintaining an adequate number of well-trained nursing staff is critical to the continuous flow of patients through the ED.

ETHICAL CONSIDERATIONS

The burden of determining the extent of an emergency usually befalls the ED nurse. The ED nurse is often the first to assess patients, as triage is the most delicate and sensitive area of emergency nursing, leaving room for the most scrutiny and error. In the ER, quick nursing assessments must be detailed enough to distinguish and prioritize the most severe circumstances from minor or chronic complaints. The slightest error in decision-making can be irreversible and life-threatening. As noted previously, ER nursing carries a very high risk for malpractice, for the triage process is delegated to nurses who must demonstrate extraordinary skills, while receiving little legal support for errors in clinical judgment. Emergency departments continue to search for better procedures to more efficiently and effectively manage patient care, while minimizing legal risks.

Today telephone triage systems have been implemented as an additional method of providing "telehealth care" to patients. Via various communication systems, triage nurses are answering a variety of questions about patient health care, medications, and/or general health. These triage systems free hospitals, office physicians, and nurses to perform their duties; however, this freedom comes with legal risks. Those who participate in implementing a triage system have rigid guidelines or protocols to follow, including documentation procedures. Without the benefit of direct observation of the patient, the ability of the health care provider to holistically assess a patient is impossible. The patient is always reminded of the limitations of the telehealth triage process, and the "911" option must be offered during the beginning of the teleconsultation and/or triage process. Nurses must continue to follow hospital policies and procedures during the consultation and function within the scope of nursing practice to limit legal liability. (For more discussion on these issues, see Chapter 25, Telenursing.)

Nurses are often placed in ethical dilemmas. For example, a patient may make a sudden oral request during the last moments of consciousness regarding withholding life-sustaining treatment, without benefit of a witness. If family members disagree with the patient's requests and heroic measures are enacted, the resuscitated patient may have grounds to sue the nurse and/or doctor. To further complicate the situation, the nurse is simultaneously faced with the difficulty of obtaining a court-appointed guardian to make health care decisions, following the orders of the physician, and complying with hospital policy and procedure.

Floating nurses present another serious legal problem in the ED. With budget cuts and limited staff, hospitals frequently shift staff from one area to another to meet the demands of patient flow and care. But nursing practice within the ED is highly specialized, and nursing knowledge and skills must be comprehensive and adaptable to rapid changes in types and status of patients (Pegalis & Wachsman, 1982). Nurses from hospital units other than intensive care present a potential for serious legal liability, for they may be unable to function appropriately and in a timely manner during emergencies. If such a nurse must be placed in the emergency room during a crisis or serious staffing shortage, all precautions should be taken to place this nurse in areas compatible with training and experience. The floating nurse can be assigned tasks such as assisting with procedures, restocking, and/or tending to patients where care has been initiated, e.g., the patient waiting for laboratory results or a consult. If the health care system allows, the floating nurse should also "buddy" with a trained emergency nurse, assisting as needed.

RESEARCH SUGGESTIONS

Research in emergency medicine is critical. Accidents are a major cause of mortality. Nurses have become frustrated with managing the end product of accidents and have begun turning more focus on preventive measures. The ENA has taken a major step in promoting prevention with programs such as Safe and Sober, Safe Child Seat Program, Bicycle Helmet Programs, Gun Safety, Buckle Up with Sesame Street, and Injury Prevention.

More research is needed. The **ENA Code of Ethics** (ENA, 1989a) provides a distinctive set of ideals and standards of conduct regarding research activities. Prevention has become a more appropriate focus of emergency health care. Emergency nurses have a special credibility when speaking about seatbelts, drinking and driving, substance abuse, domestic violence, child abuse, and many other issues that relate to circumstances likely to lead to admission to the ED.

SUMMARY

The emergency department is one of the areas of the highest risk for charges of malpractice for any health care provider. The very nature of emergency health care problems provides a potential framework for miscommunication and error. Although the intent is to provide the best care to all persons, this goal is not always achieved. Antidumping laws prevent any person from being denied care regardless of race, nationality, and/or ability to pay. Patients must be treated and stabilized before being transported to another facility.

Nurses working in emergency departments are faced with a variety of ethical dilemmas, because of the advanced and often legally undefined nature of emergency nursing practice. As the law provides little support for emergency nurses and their extended skills, knowledge, and training, nurses must be sure to function within their scope of nursing practice. ED nurses have been found guilty of practicing outside their scope, regardless of the life-and-death decisions made while completing the nursing process. Ultimately, the ED nurse must consider the law and hospital policy and procedure before nursing interventions are implemented.

POINTS TO REMEMBER

- The scope of emergency nursing practice involves assessment, diagnosis, treatment, and evaluation of perceived, actual or potential, sudden or urgent, physical or psychosocial problems that are primarily episodic or acute and occur in a variety of settings.
- Because of the requirements of the Joint Commission on Accreditation of Healthcare Organizations (JCAHO), state laws, state licensing regulations, health department regulations, and an antidumping provision passed by Congress, hospitals no longer may turn away emergency room patients, but must provide at least minimal care to provide stabilization before transfer.
- ED nurses perform the function of initial screening, but the ultimate responsibility for the triage decisions remains with the senior resident.
- If there is reason to believe a patient discharge may be injurious to the health of the patient, the nurse has the duty to question the discharge.
- Restraining or detaining a patient inappropriately is false imprisonment.
- The rights and requests of a competent patient may not be disregarded, even if the

outcome of the refusal may be detrimental to health.

- Most states have statutorily imposed a specific mandatory obligation on nurses to report physically abused or neglected children.
- Mandatory laws requiring providers to report domestic violence to law enforcement officials have been ineffective in increasing referrals.
- The sexual assault nurse examiner (SANE) is a specially trained nurse who understands the issues and laws governing sexual assault and conducts specific forensic examinations and documentation designed for this emergency.
- Under state statutory law, all births and deaths must be reported.
- Gunshot wounds inflicted by lethal weapons or by unlawful acts require mandatory reporting.
- Other criminal acts requiring mandatory reporting include attempted suicide, rape, assault, child molestation, and the unlawful dispensing or taking of narcotic drugs.

REFERENCES

Abille v United States, 482 F. Supp. 703 (N.D. Cal. 1980).

Awkerman v Tri-County Orthopedic Group, 143 Mich. App. 722, 373 N.W. 2d 204 (1985).

Baldwin v Knight (569) S.W. 2d 450 (1978).

Big Town Nursing Home v Newman, 461 S.W. 2d 195 (Tex. Civ. App. 1970).

Boccasile et al v Cajun Music Limited et al, 694 A2d 686 (RI 1997).

Borchelt, P. L., Lockwood, R., & Beck, A. M. (1983). Attacks by packs of dogs involving predation on human beings. *Public Health Reports, 98,* 57–66.

Cal. Health & Safety Code § 7185-95 (West 1983).

Callaham, M. (1978). Treatment of common dog bites: Infection risk factors. *Journal of the American College of Emergency Practitioners, 7,* 83–87.

Carrow, D. M. (1980, January). *Rape: Guidelines for a community response* (pp. 130, 170, 253–255). Washington, DC: U.S. Department of Justice, Law Enforcement Assistance Administration, National Institute of Law Enforcement and Criminal Justice.

Carter v Cangello, 164 Cal. Rptr. 361 (Ct. App. 1980).

Citizens Hospital Association v Schoulin, 48 Ala. 101, 262 So. 2d 303 (1972).

Cline v Lund, 31 Cal. App. 3d 755; 107 Cal. Rptr. 629 (1973).

Commonwealth v Storella, 375 N.E. 2d 348 (Mass. App. Ct. 1978).

Darling v Charleston Community Hospital, 33 Ill. 2d 326; 211 N.E. 2d 253 (1965).

Emergency Nurses Association. (1989a). *Code of ethics.* Chicago: Author.

Emergency Nurses Association. (1989b). Scope of practice statement. *Journal of Emergency Nursing, 15*(4), 361.

Emergency Nurses Association. (1990). *Standards of emergency nursing practice.* St. Louis: Mosby–Year Book.

Erickson v Dilgard, 44 Misc. 2d 27, 252 N.Y. S.2d 705 (Sup.ct.1962).

Fjerstad v Knutson, 271 N.W.2d 8 (S.D. 1978).

Ford, R. D. (1987). *Nurse's legal handbook.* Springhouse, PA: Springhouse.

Furrow, B.R., Greaney, T.L., Johnson, S.H., Jost, T.S., Schwartz, R.L. (1995) *Health law.* St. Paul, MN: West Group.

George, J. E., Quattrone, M.S., Goldstone, M. (1998, October). Emergency nurses as good samaritans. *Journal of Emergency Nursing, 24*(5), 431.

Goff v Doctors General Hospital, 166 Cal. App. 2d 314, 333 P.2d 29 (1958).

Hemelt, M., & Mackert, M. (1982). *Dynamics of law in nursing and health care* (2nd ed.). Reston, VA: Reston Publishing.

Herr, R. D. (1998, October). Managed care and the emergency department: Nursing issues. *Journal of Emergency Nursing, 24*(5)406–411.

Hohenhaus, S. (1998, October). Sexual legislation and lessons learned. *Journal of Emergency Nursing, 24*(5), 463.

In re Estate Dorone, 524 A. 2d 452 (Pa.1987)

Johnstone, M. J. (1994). *Nursing and the injustices of the law.* Philadelphia: WB Saunders.

Kizer, K. W. (1979). Epidemiologic and clinical aspects of animal bite injuries. *Journal of the American College of Emergency Practitioners, 8,* 143–141.

Koeniguer v Eckrich, 422 N.W.2d 600 (S.D. 1988).

Kravis, T. C., Warner, C. G., et al. (1987). *Emergency medicine: A comprehensive review* (2nd ed.). Rockville, MD: Aspen Publication.

Lanza, M. (1983, January). The reactions of nursing staff to physical assault by a patient. *Hospital and Community Psychiatry, 34*(1), 44–47.

Lauer, E. A., White, W. C., & Lauer, B. A. (1982). Dog bites: A neglected problem in accident prevention. *American Journal of Disabilities in Children, 136,* 202–204.

Lott v State, 32 Misc.2d 296, 225 N.Y.S.2d 424 (Ct. Cl. 1962).

Mapp v Ohio, 367 U.S. 643 (1961).

Marks v Mandel, 477 So. 2d 1036 (Fla. Dist. Ct. App. 1985).

McLain, J. K. (1998). Research you should know (and do something) about. *Journal of Emergency Nursing, 24*(5)460–462.

Newberry, L. (1992). *Sheey's emergency nursing principals & practice* (3rd ed.). St. Louis: Mosby-Year Book.

Occupational Safety and Health Administration. (1996). *Guidelines for preventing workplace violence for health care workers and social service workers* (Publication No. 3148). Washington, DC: U.S. Department of Labor.

O'Connor v Donaldson, 422 U.S. 563 (1975).

Pegalis, S. E., & Wachsman, H. F. (1982). *American law of medical malpractice*. Rochester, NY: The Lawyers Co-Operative Publishing Company.

People v Kraft, 3 Cal. App. 3rd 890 (1970).

Pinckney, L. E., & Kennedy, L. A. (1982). Traumatic deaths from dog attacks in the United States. *Pediatrics, 69*,193–196.

Pozgar, G. (1990). *Legal aspects of health care administration* (4th ed.). Gaithersburg, MD: Aspen Publications.

Pozzi, C. (1998, August). Exposure of prehospital providers to violence and abuse. *Journal of Emergency Nursing*, 24(4)323.

Queensland Nurses' Union. (1998). Workplace bullying. *Queensland Nurses' Union Home Page*. www.qnu.org.au/safey.html

Rabies prevention. (1984). *Morbidity Mortality Weekly Reporter, 33*, 397.

Reporting by others than physicians of cases of diseases presumably communicable, New York State Sanitary Code, Chapter 1, § 2.12 (1973).

Rochin v State, 342 U.S. 165 (1952).

Sachs, C. J., Peek, C., Baraff, L. J., & Hasselblad, V. (1998). Failure of the mandatory domestic violence reporting law to increase medical facility referral to police. *Annotated Emergency Medicine, 311*, 488–494.

Sanchez v Bay General Hospital, 172 Cal. Rptr. 342 (Cal. Ct. App. 1981).

Schmerber v California, 384 U.S. 757 (1966).

Schloendorff v Society of New York Hospital, 211 N.Y. 125, 129, 105 N.E. 92, 93 (1914).

Spring, N. M. & Stern, M. B. (1998). Nurse abuse? Couldn't be! [On-line]. Nurse Advocate Web Site. Available: www.nurseadvocate.org/nurse_abuse.html

State v Perea, 95 N.M. 777 (1981, App.).

State v Riggins, 348 So. 2d 1209 (Fla. Dist. Ct. App. 1977).

Thomas v Corso, 265 Md. 84, 288 A.2d 379 (1972).

Toth v Community Hospital at Glen Cove, 239 N.E. 386, 292 N.Y.S. 2d 635 (Ct. App. 1968).

Turner v State, 258 Ark. 425 (1975).

United States v Winbash, 428 F.2d 357 (6th Cir. 1970).

Wickens, E. (1978). Textbook of emergency medical and emergency care as practiced at Massachusetts General Hospital. Baltimore: Williams and Wilkins.

Wilmington General Hospital v Manlove 54 Del 15, 174 A 2d 135 (1961, Sup).

Wright, J.C. (1985). Severe attacks by dogs: Characteristics of the dogs, the victims and the attack settings. *Public Health Reports, 100*, 55–61.

SUGGESTED READINGS

Gedde, L. (1998). *Medical device accidents*. Boca Raton, FL: CRC Press.

DiMaio, D., & DiMaio, V. (1993). *Forensic pathology*. Boca Raton, FL: CRC Press.

Flannery, R. (1995). *Violence In the workplace*. NY, NY: The Cross Roads Publishing Company.

Mitchell, J., & Bray, G. (1990). *Emergency services stress*. Englewood Cliffs, NJ: Prentice Hall.

Mitchell, J., & Everly, G. (1994). *Human elements training for emergency services, public safety and disaster personnel*. Ellicott City, MD: Chevron Publishing.

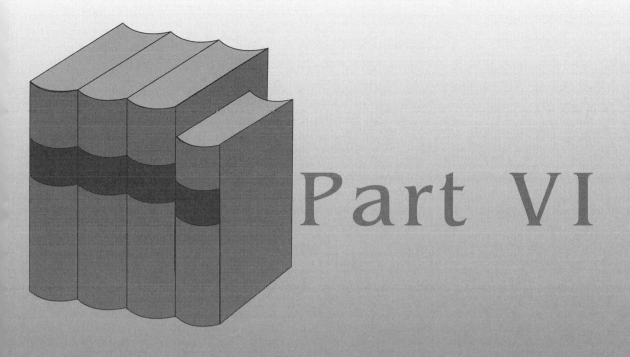

Part VI

NURSING LAW
AND
FORENSICS

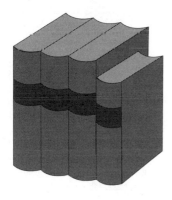

Chapter 22

FORENSIC NURSING

Barbara Scott Cammuso
Barbara Power Madden
Andrea J. Wallen

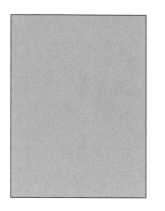

KEY WORDS

Americans with
  Disabilities Act of
  1990
Anti-Stalking Law
Bill of Rights
Chain of Custody
Conditions for
  Participation for
  Medicare and Medicaid
  Reimbursement
Consulting Experts
Credentialing
Criminal Justice
Elder Abuse Law
Evidence
Expert Forensic Nurse
  Witness
Forensic
Forensic Clients

Forensic Clinical Nurse
  Specialist
Forensic Nursing
Forensic Psychiatric
  Nurse
Forensic Sciences
Miranda Rights
Nurse Death Investigator
Nurse Practice Act
Obstruction of Justice
Sexual Assault Nurse
  Examiner (SANE)
Stalker
Testifying Witness
Uniform Controlled
  Substance Act
  of 1970
Violence Against Women
  Act of 1994

OBJECTIVES

After completion of this chapter, the reader will be
able to:
- Define the new specialty of forensic nursing and list
  some of its subspecialties.
- Identify selected federal and state statutes that have
  a forensic impact on nursing practice.
- Describe how the Bill of Rights and selected areas of
  common law influence how the nurse interacts with
  a forensic client.

- Describe regulations that may control the forensic nurse's role.
- Locate resources for professional standards and clinical practice guidelines used in forensic nursing practice.
- Differentiate between forensic issues that have an impact on the generalist's nursing practice and those that relate mainly to forensic specialty practice.
- Identify legal and ethical issues in forensic nursing that need further exploration and resolution.
- Explore nursing management issues related to the forensic area.
- Describe recommendations for improved interprofessional practice between nursing and the legal system.

INTRODUCTION— HISTORICAL PERSPECTIVE

The emergence of **forensic** nursing has gradually and steadily grown over the past years. Initially, nurses worked in well-known medicolegal settings, such as correctional settings, forensic psychiatric units, and coroners' offices. As far back as 1975, the chief medical examiner of Alberta, Canada, promoted the use of registered nurses as medical examiners' investigators (Lynch, 1993).

The role of the forensic nurse expanded to include many other settings, including emergency departments and courtrooms. A seminal nursing research study (Burgess & Holstrum, 1974) on rape trauma syndrome was a major factor in the development of the role of the sexual assault nurse examiner, the first nationally recognized forensic nurse role. In 1985, the U.S. Surgeon General's Workshop on Violence and Public Health focused on sexual and physical assault, homicide, and spousal abuse, which, together with the American Public Health Association's 1984 statement

that violence was a major public health issue, stimulated further development of nursing's role in this area. In 1991, the American Academy of Forensic Sciences accepted forensic nursing as a distinct discipline.

Subsequently, the first national meeting of sexual assault nurse examiners was held in Minneapolis, Minnesota, in 1992. This meeting evolved into the establishment of the International Association of Forensic Nurses (IAFN) under the initial presidency of Virginia A. Lynch, with the inclusion of nurses in other forensic roles (Ledray & Simmelink, 1997). The forensic nurse was accepted as a member of a distinct specialty by the American Nurses Association (ANA) in 1995, and the ANA, together with the IAFN, published the *Scope and Standards of Forensic Nursing Practice* in 1997. As stated in this document, the IAFN recognizes the ANA's role in defining the scope of nursing practice as a whole, but accepts accountability for defining, delineating the characteristics of, and establishing the scope of forensic nursing practice (IAFN & ANA, 1997).

DEFINITION OF FORENSIC NURSING

Forensic nursing is a professional specialty in which the specific focus of practice is the intersection of nursing and health care and the legal system. **Forensic nursing** is defined as:

The application of the forensic aspects of health care combined with the biopsychological education of the registered nurse in the scientific investigation and treatment of trauma and/or death related medical-legal issues (IAFN & ANA, 1997, p. 30).

Forensic nursing is an umbrella term encompassing a variety of more specific practice roles. Some of the subspecialty roles of the field are:

- Clinical forensic nurse specialists
- Forensic pediatric nurses
- Trauma nurses
- Forensic gerontology nurses
- Sexual assault nurse examiners
- Nurse attorneys
- Legal nurse consultants
- Transplant and organ bank nurses
- Forensic psychiatric nurses
- Correctional nurses
- Nurse death investigators/coroners
- Critical incident stress debriefer/bereavement counselor nurse
- Nurses, nurse educators, or nurse researchers specializing in practice involving crime or trauma
- Mass disaster team nurses

Forensic nurses provide nursing care to individuals, families, and groups in a variety of settings, which include hospitals, extended care facilities, homes, schools, police departments, correctional institutions, occupational facilities, legal offices, and medical examiner offices. In addition, they also practice as consultants to nursing, medical, and law-related agencies as well as providing expert court testimony. Further, forensic nurses are knowledgeable in the areas of evidence identification, collection, and preservation and death investigation. According to Lynch (1995, p. 41), "where health care interfaces with the law, forensic nurses are

being recognized as one solution in anti-violence strategies and as expert clinicians in the treatment of victims and perpetrators of human violence." Nurses are very familiar with the health care field, however, not as acquainted with the related fields of criminal justice, civil liability, and forensic science. **Criminal justice** encompasses the study of criminology, law enforcement, law adjudication, and corrections. Tort claims, such as personal injury or health care fraud, typically include knowledge of civil liability. **Forensic sciences** encompass a wide range of disciplines that relate to the resolution of legal matters (Eckert, 1992). Those that most directly apply to forensic nursing are chemistry, biology, toxicology, pathology, pharmacology, odontology, criminalistics, and psychology.

CONSTITUTIONAL LAW

The first ten amendments to the U.S. Constitution, collectively known as the **Bill of Rights**, are a particularly important part of the knowledge base of forensic nurses. When caring for clients who may be either victims or perpetrators of violence, nurses need to protect such rights as confidentiality and privacy, privilege against self-incrimination, protection from cruel and unusual punishment, protection from defamation of character, property rights, and equal protection under the law. They need also to be aware of the legal ramifications associated with warrants and warrantless searches, Miranda warnings, justifiable use of force, entrapment, and accessories before and after the fact.

STATUTORY LAW REGULATING FORENSIC NURSING PRACTICE

Forensic nursing is a relatively new area of nursing, and therefore there is a paucity of literature about statutory laws. The president of the IAFN affirms this information and states "that at this time there are no federal or state statutory laws regulating the actual practice of forensic nursing" (P. Seneski, personal communication, 1998). The practice of forensic nurses, as is the practice of all registered nurses and advanced practice nurses, is regulated by state nurse practice acts, which vary from state to state. A **nurse practice act** includes the following information: a definition of the scope of nursing practice, regulation of educational programs of nursing, rights of the nurse licensure, and the licensure requirements (ANA, 1990).

However, despite the lack of specific mention of the forensic nurse in the law, there are federal statutes affecting practice that lie within its domain, such as the **Violence Against Women Act of 1994**, which regulates and provides funding to states for domestic violence and sexual assault prevention, victim assistance, and prosecution of offenders; the **Americans with Disabilities Act of 1990**, which safeguards the rights of the disabled; and the **Uniform Controlled Substance Act of 1970**, which defines addiction, classifies drug categories, and requires the record-keeping and reporting necessary for drug diversion prevention and control. In relation to the last of these, forensic nurses are in the forefront of efforts to require classification of the "date rape" drugs, flunitrazepam (Rohypnol) and gamma hydroxybutyric acid (GBH).

On the state level, mandatory reporting laws are common. One example is the Massachusetts **Elder Abuse Law** (MGL. C19A, S14-26), which protects men and women, aged 60 and older, from actions that cause serious physical or emotional injury, caretaker neglect, and financial exploitation. According to Tatara (1995/1996), the types of agencies required to report elder abuse are adult protective services (APS), human service agencies, social service agencies, and law enforcement agencies. All 50 states have adult protective services, and if elder abuse is identified, the forensic nurse must report this finding. Similar provisions are in place for reporting child abuse, and there are varying requirements enacted by state legislatures regarding the mandatory reporting of abuse of the disabled, sexual assaults, and specific traumatic injuries.

Currently, all 50 states have anti-stalking laws, which the forensic nurse can use to counsel victims. California passed the first state **anti-stalking law** in 1990, which provides that

Both criminal and civil laws address stalking. According to California's criminal law, a **stalker** is someone who willfully, maliciously and repeatedly follows or harasses another (victim) and who makes a credible threat with the intent to place the victim or victim's immediate family in fear for their safety. The victim does not have to prove that the stalker had the intent to carry out the threat (California Penal Code, 1990).

COMMON LAW REGULATING FORENSIC NURSING PRACTICE

The authors conducted an extensive literature search was conducted, and no common law specifically addressing the specialty of forensic nursing was found. This is likely because the specialty only recently has been identified and defined. Common law regarding nursing practice is frequently noted within the area of malpractice. Some malpractice cases illustrate areas of forensic nursing practice. For example, in *Brennan v. Nussbaumer and Bible*, a 32-year-old Colorado woman claimed that her nurse therapist implanted false memories of sexual abuse, which led her to break off relations with her family. A psychiatrist involved in the client's 3-year medical treatment was also included in the suit. The jury returned a $120,000 verdict against the nurse.

Apart from the arena of malpractice suits, the area of common law most likely to be a regular part of forensic nurses' practice involves the recognition, collection, preservation, and documentation of evidentiary material, secondary to a crime or tort. The nurse's recognition of what, in any particular situation, constitutes useful and legal evidence, whether physical or spoken, is a basic part of forensic nursing education. **Evidence** includes pertinent information surrounding the client, the scene, or the suspect that might substantiate claims of innocence, guilt, or responsibility for outcomes. Collection requires knowledge of procedures for gathering evidence without contamination, without interfering with other aspects of the trauma or crime scene, and without jeopardizing the treatment of the client.

Preservation of evidence involves knowledge of the storage methods that best maintain different types of evidentiary material in a manner allowing accurate analysis by forensic scientists for use in court proceedings, as well as the procedures for establishing an ironclad **chain of custody** of such evidence from its collection to its ultimate end use in court. Forensic nurses' documentation, although not dissimilar to that necessary in all nursing specialty areas, is more likely to end up in court proceedings and thus will require closer attention to phraseology. It needs to be objective and factual, with perhaps more circumspection in stating the nurse's professional judgments than is customary in documenting care for the ill client. Forensic nurses should also avoid the error of slipping into police jargon or legal terminology, an occupational hazard for nurses who work closely with professionals in those fields. Documentation methods less common in regular nursing practice, such as photodocumentation, extensive body mapping, or colposcopy, may also be used in forensic nursing practice.

The situation dictates which of the four evidentiary elements (i.e., recognition, collection, preservation, or documentation) will predominate. A **sexual assault nurse examiner (SANE)**, for example, in most states implements a fairly standardized rape kit protocol for the recognition and collection of forensic specimens. With a willing client, then, the focus of the forensic nurse's legal concern becomes appropriate documentation of "excited utterances" and the preservation of the physical evidence through the chain of custody procedures. In other circumstances, such as the emergency department nurse receiving a police request to send blood for alcohol or drug testing against the expressed wishes of an injured and possibly intoxicated motor vehicle crash victim, the nurse's legal concerns may be more on the evidence collection itself. In this case, the forensic nurse should be aware that in *Schmerber v. California* (1966) the Supreme Court ruled that a nonvoluntary taking of a blood sample subsequent to a lawful arrest was not a violation of the self-incrimination privilege and could be entered as evidence in court.

Since the blood test evidence, although an incriminating product of compulsion was neither petitioner's testimony nor evidence related to some communicative act or writing by the petitioner, it was not inadmissible on privilege grounds (*Schmerber v. California*, 1966).

This evidence would "disappear" for judicial purposes if it were not permissible to acquire samples in timely fashion. However, it appears that opinions differ, often based on whether the blood sample was included within a medically necessary blood test battery rather than a separate intrusive measure such as stomach pumping.

Because common law is derived from decisions in court cases, testimony in and preparation for such cases are components of the forensic nursing role. Forensic nurses may serve as testifying witnesses, expert witnesses, and consulting experts. In the first of these, forensic nurses can reasonably expect to find themselves testifying in court, and therefore must familiarize themselves with the judicial system and procedures applicable in their state. They must also be very clear on the distinction between appropriate nursing actions in each of the three roles. As a **testifying witness**, the forensic nurse provides probative information about the facts of a particular case. Examples would be sexual assault nurse examiners who testify about their documentation on an assault victim, forensic psychiatric nurses involved in pretrial examination of defendants who testify about evaluations performed, or staff nurses describing activities surrounding the traumatic fall by an inpatient client. In all these cases, testifying nurses are dealing with matters of their direct knowledge from within professional nurse-client relationships. If not prevented by privilege, they may testify voluntarily or may be subpoenaed.

In contrast, forensic nurses serving as expert witnesses testify about standards of clinical nursing practice and state their opinions about whether nursing policies, procedures, or actions of individual nurses relevant to the judicial proceedings were appropriate and constitute acceptable professional or forensic nursing practice. In this case, the **expert forensic nurse witness** has no direct connection to or knowledge of the client and is basing testimony on extensive knowledge, experience, and education in the field of forensic nursing.

The forensic nurse's approach to these witness roles should be based on the different contexts. As a testifying witness, one only answers questions asked by the attorneys, usually without elaboration. Courtroom confrontation can be expected to focus on accuracy of factual memory, adequacy of documentation, and appropriateness of actions taken or not taken. As an expert witness, however, one attempts to provide a holistic picture of the practice arena in order to present the policy, procedure, or action in a broader professional context, thus often requiring elaboration (Shapiro, 1991). Courtroom confrontation can be expected to focus on adequacy of credentials as an "expert." Nurses holding themselves out as experts should be able to identify their competence and currency in a variety of ways: knowledge of current forensic nursing literature, active clinical forensic practice, forensic continuing education, research activity, publishing, teaching, consulting, membership in professional organizations, and peer review. At the present time, few forensic nurses, with the exception of sexual assault nurse examiners, have the opportunity to obtain specialty certification, another hallmark of expert practice. In both witness situations, forensic nurses would be wise to seek legal assistance prior to providing testimony.

As **consulting experts**, forensic nurses are not direct participants in court proceedings, but instead serve as experts in the medicolegal arena. They may work with attorneys to educate them on medical and health topics, or do research on and preparation for malpractice and medical fraud cases, divorce and custody proceedings, as well as for defending or prosecuting violence or trauma trials. They may also serve as consultants to agencies for the prevention and remediation of legal problems related to forensic situations. Evidence of their forensic expertise is similar to that of expert witnesses and may also include letters of reference from prior consultees.

STANDARDS REGULATING FORENSIC NURSING PRACTICE

GOVERNMENT REGULATION

Regulation of forensic nurses practicing in the role of the sexual assault nurse examiner is maintained at the state level and is still evolving. No state is known to have specifically incorporated this role into its nurse practice act. In some states, such as California, SANEs are employed by police departments or district attorneys' offices; in others, such as Massachusetts, they are certified by and under contract to the state department of public health to provide assault examinations. In yet others, they may function as independent practitioners in private practice, often in affiliation with or employed by a hospital emergency unit.

Roles in which forensic nurses are increasingly becoming involved but that at present have not adequately developed regulation or standards include death investigator, nurse coroner, and organ transplantation nurse, among others. States that mandate a medical examiner may have regulations that allow a nurse to serve as an assistant medical examiner or as a death investigator. Other states have coroner laws, which may not require any qualifications at all for the position. A number of states identify circumstances in which nurses may pronounce death and/or sign death certificates. Nurses knowledgeable in forensics must be familiar with their state's regulations regarding reportable cases of death, even if they do not have a relationship to the medical examiner's office. Situations commonly mandated to be reported include deaths not attributable to natural disease; sudden, unexpected deaths not attended by a physician; deaths within 24 hours of hospital admission; deaths caused or complicated by substance abuse; deaths in abortion, childbirth, or of those younger than 16; deaths while under anesthesia or police custody; and deaths apparently due to neglect or exposure.

Until 1998, each state had its own regulations regarding organ procurement and transplant. At that time, the Health Care Financing Administration issued **Conditions for Participation for Medicare and Medicaid Reimbursement**, which mandated hospitals to report every death and every severe neurological injury that may result in brain death to the regional organ procurement agency. Some states also require that all clients on entry into a hospital must be asked if they wish to be organ donors. Even when clients have indicated their desire to be organ donors, custom or state regulation may also require permission from the next of

kin. Clients' involvement with the medical examiner system does not automatically exclude organ harvesting, but may need to be explored. Forensic nurses should be able to educate other providers as well as family members about this new federal regulation and any applicable state regulations governing procurement.

NATIONAL NURSING ORGANIZATIONS: PROFESSIONAL STANDARDS

The standards set forth by the professional nursing association serve as the foundation for what the "competent and prudent nurse" should do or not do in many nursing situations. Therefore, as is true of all nurses, the forensic nurse needs to be very familiar with the general standards of practice promulgated by the American Nurses Associa-

---

BOX 22-1

EXCERPTS FROM THE *SCOPE AND STANDARDS OF FORENSIC NURSING PRACTICE*

Standard I. Assessment
  Criterion 5. The forensic nurse follows the chain of custody as indicated.
Standard II. Diagnosis
  Criterion 2. The forensic nurse identifies those diagnoses that are consistent with the findings of other forensic health care, law enforcement, and judicial professionals that will facilitate a controlled pathway throughout the judicial process.
Standard III. Outcome identification
  Criterion 4. Forensic outcomes include a time estimate and are documented as measurable goals, if applicable.
Standard IV. Planning
  Criterion 5. The plan of action provides for continuity of care by incorporating forensic teaching and learning principals [sic] into the overall plan of care.
Standard V. Implementation
  Criterion 2. Standardized care plans pertaining to forensic diagnoses are developed and available for use, if applicable.
Standard VI. Evaluation
  Criterion 2. Evaluation is used to revise forensic nursing diagnoses, outcomes and the plan of action as needed.

Source: IAFN & ANA, 1997, pp. 13–17.

tion (ANA, 1991). In addition, the IAFN joined with the ANA in the publication of the *Scope and Standards of Forensic Nursing Practice* (1997). This document not only serves as a helpful guide to development and implementation of forensic practice roles but also as a standard against which the actions of the forensic nurse may be measured in legal proceedings. Selected standards of care from this document are presented in Box 22–1 to illustrate relevant legal aspects. The IAFN has also published the *Sexual Assault Nurse Examiner Standards of Practice* in 1997 and had, as of 1998, a draft of standards for domestic violence practice.

Other widely accepted nursing protocols should also be reviewed for application to the forensic nurse's concerns. For example, *Nursing Outcomes Classification (NOC)* (Johnson & Maas, 1997) includes seven standardized outcomes and outcome indicators relating to abuse and neglect prevention and recovery, four related to alcohol and other drug abuse, four on safety knowledge, behavior, and status, as well as others on grief resolution, impulse control, parenting, social safety, and self-mutilation, and suicide restraint. Similarly, *Nursing Interventions Classification (NIC)* (McCloskey & Bulechek, 1996) describes related intervention activities appropriate for reaching these outcomes. Nurses, who do not intervene appropriately or do not document the outcomes of their forensic nursing interventions, using identified indicators when applicable, could be held liable for substandard practice.

CLINICAL PRACTICE GUIDELINES REGULATING FORENSIC NURSING PRACTICE

GOVERNMENTAL GUIDELINES

One of the stimuli for the development of the role of forensic nursing in the 1990s was the public health community's formal recognition of violence as a health issue and not simply a criminal justice one. This is well illustrated by the public health goals set in 1992 by the federal government in *Healthy People 2000* (U.S. Public Health Service, 1992). Box 22–2 includes 18 goals that specifically focus on forensic issues.

Another set of federal documents with which every nurse needs to be familiar are the guidelines for clinical practice and prevention. The guidelines of the Agency for Health Care Policy and Research (AHCPR) and the prevention guidelines of the Centers for Disease Control and Prevention (CDC) can assist prosecutors, plaintiffs, or defendants in a court of law, similarly to standards of the nursing profession. Practitioners in all health fields, under the legal mandate to act as competent and prudent care providers, are expected to know and to follow the care guidelines, or else be able to put forth cogent justification for not applying protocols in specific situations that end up in trial or litigation. Although there is nothing in the AHCPR guidelines targeted toward the specialty of forensic nursing specifically, recommendations for provider care of specific health conditions or populations may contain subrecommendations relevant to forensic nursing practice. One example is the recommendation in *Management of Cancer Pain* that "health care clinicians be aware of the unique needs and circumstances of clients from various ethnic and cultural backgrounds" (Carr et al., 1994, p. 139), with a note of concern about drug theft and violence in high-crime areas and their potential for impact on neighborhood pharmacies' practices of stocking opioid analgesics. This, in turn, will affect the ability of health care clinicians to develop effective treatment plans for local residents. A forensic nurse working with either substance abusers or crime perpetrators whose family members or neighbors are terminally ill or in chronic pain need to be cognizant of these issues. In addition, forensic nurses might serve as educators or consultants to community health or home care nurses to provide guidance or protocols for assessment of lethal weapons in the homes they visit (McClelland, Thompson, Prete, & Hatcher, 1996) and promote familiarity with state or local regulations regarding gun possession.

BOX 22-2

PUBLIC HEALTH GOALS FROM *HEALTHY PEOPLE 2000*

7.1	Reduce homicides.
7.2	Reduce suicides.
7.3	Reduce weapon-related violent deaths.
7.4	Reverse . . . the rising incidence of maltreatment of children younger than age 18.
7.5	Reduce physical abuse directed at women.
7.6	Reduce assault injuries among . . . [those] 12 and older.
7.7	Reduce rape and attempted rape of women.
7.8	Reduce . . . the incidence of injurious suicide attempts among adolescents.
7.9	Reduce . . . the incidence of physical fighting among adolescents.
7.10	Reduce . . . the incidence of weapon-carrying by adolescents.
7.11	Reduce . . . the proportion of people who possess weapons that are . . . dangerously available.
7.12	Extend [emergency department] protocols for routinely identifying, treating, and properly referring suicide attempts, victims of sexual assault, and victims of spouse, elder, and child abuse.
7.13	Extend . . . implementation of unexplained child deaths review systems.
7.14	Increase . . . [the] percent of children identified as neglected or physically or sexually abused [who] receive physical and mental evaluation with appropriate follow-up.
7.15	Reduce . . . the proportion of battered women and their children turned away from emergency housing.
7.16	Increase . . . the proportion of elementary and secondary schools that teach nonviolent conflict resolution skills.
7.17	Extend coordinated, comprehensive violence prevention programs to . . . jurisdictions with populations over 100,000.
7.18	Increase . . . officially established protocols . . . to facilitate identification and appropriate intervention to prevent suicide by jail inmates.

Source: United States Public Health Service, 1992.

In Massachusetts, for example, those under a restraining order for domestic violence must surrender their gun collections. Although the AHCPR is currently not publishing additional practice guidelines, forensic nurses will need to keep up to date with regard to any future clinical practice or prevention guidelines and review them for any legal implications applicable to their practice.

The official guidelines for primary care providers for prevention of common health problems have numerous clinical practice recommendations that relate to forensic nursing. Box 22–3 lists recommended pre-ventive activities applicable to forensic nursing in a variety of settings and roles.

INSTITUTIONAL PRACTICE GUIDELINES

The accreditation standards of the Joint Commission on the Accreditation of Healthcare Organizations (JCAHO) have begun to focus more heavily on forensic nursing issues, even though the term as such is not used. Box 22–4 provides examples from the 1997 standards that are of direct relevance

BOX 22-3

SELECTED RECOMMENDATIONS FROM THE REPORT OF THE U.S. PREVENTIVE HEALTH SERVICES TASK FORCE WITH APPLICATION TO IDENTIFIED FORENSIC NURSING ROLES

Nurses working in any setting, but particularly emergency or primary care should be:

- Including a few direct questions about abuse (physical violence or forced sexual activity) as part of the routine history. . . . All individuals who present with multiple injuries and an implausible explanation should be evaluated. . . . Suspected cases of abuse should receive proper documentation of the incident and physical findings (e.g., photographs, body maps); treatment of physical injuries; arrangements for counseling . . . and [referral agencies'] telephone numbers (p. 562).
- Screening to detect problem drinking and hazardous drinking is recommended for all adult and adolescent clients (pp. 575–576). [P]ersons who use occupant protection devices and avoid driving while alcohol or drug impaired are at significantly decreased risk of injury or death from motor vehicle crashes. . . . Counseling by clinicians to adopt these practices is effective in changing the behavior of motorists or passengers (p. 650).
- Counseling regarding other measures to prevent household and recreational injuries is recommended (p. 676).

Nurses working with adolescent or young adult populations, with the homeless, or in high-crime communities:

- In settings where the prevalence of violence is high, should ask adolescents and young adults about previous violent behavior or victimization, current alcohol and drug use, and the availability of handguns or other firearms. Clinicians should inform those identified as being at high risk for violence (p. 695).

Nurses working in substance abuse settings, forensic psychiatric units, or employee assistance programs, or dealing with survivors of those suffering violent or traumatic death:

- Should be alert to evidence of suicidal ideation when the history reveals risk factors for suicide, such as depression, alcohol or other drug abuse, other psychiatric disorder, prior attempted suicide, recent divorce, separation, unemployment, and recent bereavement (p. 551).

Source: Report of the U.S. Preventive Services Task Force, 1996.

to forensic nursing. As a result of the JCAHO standards, most hospitals have developed protocols for the assessment and referral of victims of violence, especially in the areas of domestic violence, sexual assault, and the care of prisoners within the emergency unit or hospital room. However, critical pathways for the care of clients with forensic involvement will need development.

ISSUES AND TRENDS

FORENSIC ISSUES IN EVERY NURSE'S PRACTICE

The U.S. legal system carefully protects the rights of individuals through specific evidentiary guidelines and governance of the actions of health care providers. Conse-

BOX 22-4

SELECTED STANDARDS FROM THE *COMPREHENSIVE ACCREDITATION MANUAL FOR HOSPITALS*

RI.1.2.4	The hospital addresses advanced directives; (1.2.5) . . . withholding resuscitative devices; (1.2.6) . . . forgoing or withholding life-sustaining treatment.
RI.2	The hospital has a policy for procuring and donation of organs and other tissues.
PE.1.8	Possible victims of abuse are identified using criteria developed by the hospital [further identified as physical assault, rape or other sexual molestation, domestic abuse, and abuse of elders and children].
PE.7	The special needs of patients who are receiving treatment for alcoholism or other drug dependencies are addressed by the assessment process.
TX.3.4	Preparing and dispensing medication(s) adhere to law, regulation, licensure, and professional standards of practice.
TX.7.1	Restraint or seclusion use within the organization is limited to those situations with adequate, appropriate clinical justification.
PI.3.3.1	Data on important processes and outcomes are also collected from autopsy results.
PI.4.5	The hospital initiates intensive assessment when statistical analysis detects undesirable variation in performance [adverse events, adverse reactions].
LD.1.1.3	The hospital plans for the appropriate care of patients under legal or correctional restrictions.
EC.1.3	A management plan addresses safety [accidents, occupational injury or illness, product recalls]; (1.4) . . . security; (1.5) . . . control of hazardous materials and waste; (1.7) . . . life safety [fire].
EC.2.11	Safety elements of the environment of care are maintained, tested, and inspected.
EC. 4. 21	Door locks and other structural restraints used are consistent with the hospital's mission and program goals.
HR.4.	The hospital orients and educates forensic staff [described as escorts or guards from jails, prisons, or military brigs].
MA.2.	The chief executive officer provides for compliance with applicable law and regulation.

Source: Joint Commission on the Accreditation of Healthcare Organizations, 1997.

quently, nurses in general practice are cognizant of individual client's rights in the context of their professional role as well as their professional accountability within state nurse practice acts. Forensic issues beyond these areas arise in every professional nursing practice setting, requiring nurses to broaden their scope of practice and think forensically. Making matters more complex, the United States is a litigious society, and nurses in the forensic area need to be aware of their responsibilities and liabilities in order to prevent potential problems.

Currently, nurses in general practice think and practice forensically only when faced with specific situations. They act in accordance with the law as mandated reporters for abuse and neglect of children, the elderly, or the cognitively impaired. Documentation of nursing care is done with the knowledge that information will sustain courtroom examination and scrutiny. Nurses protect clients' rights. However, advances in the forensic sciences will demand more of nurses in the future. For example, in DNA investigation, the emergency department nurse who discards items of clothing or carelessly handles specimens is not preserving DNA evidence properly. Can the nurse therefore be liable for destruction of evidence? If forensic photography is available to document injuries or care provided and is not used, is the nurse liable for inadequate documentation?

These questions illuminate issues that are still unfolding. As one example, a nursing newsletter (Doherty, 1998) reported three instances of civil suits against New Jersey nurses for failing to properly document and/or properly refer cases of child abuse, resulting in further injury to or death of the young clients. All nurses must realize that failure to act is tantamount to acting negligently. Although forensic nurses, by virtue of their presumed greater knowledge and skills, may be held to an even higher standard when their assessment, treatment, and referral skills do not adequately protect the victim of family violence, no nurse is "off the hook."

Nurses interact on a daily basis with individuals in numerous disciplines to provide effective client care. However, the relationships between the police, the judicial system, and nursing are unique because the intended outcome of interactions differs. Nurses relate to individuals as clients. The police officer may relate to these same individuals as victims, suspects, or alleged perpetrators. Likewise, the judicial system may relate to them as parties to an action, plaintiffs, or defendants. Interdisciplinary goals vary, producing situations where actions may be in conflict. Understanding the complexity of these relationships is important for all nurses. The *modus operandi* of the judicial system is very different from that of the health care system.

These interdisciplinary interactions sometimes flow smoothly, but, at other times, conflicts in goals can place the nurse in a challenging situation. Interventions in which the nurse participates may not, in reality, be for the client's benefit. Nursing actions may ultimately provide evidence that enables the courts to convict a client. The police officer, when investigating the white powder substance in the pocket of the driver in a car crash, is concerned about causes of the crash and preservation of possible evidence. The court system and the insurance company are interested in finding out who is responsible for the crash. The emergency department nurse is concerned about the effects of a possible drug dose on the client's health status and less concerned about the source or legality of the suspicious mix found in the client's pocket.

Similarly, the occupational health nurse is concerned with the prevention of occupational injuries through education of the players in the industrial system. However, in the event of an incident, the police and later the judicial system are concerned with identifying the party or agent responsible and ascertaining whether prudent precautions had been exercised. Collecting the suspicious medication or turning in significant information about an employer's noncompliance with safety regulations may not be advocating for the client.

At other times, interactions between the disciplines can flow smoothly, evolving into a relationship where all parties involved are collaborating to achieve mutual goals. Such collaborations have already been established. The sexual assault nurse examiner and the police department's rape response unit work as a team when a victim is brought to an emergency department. The **nurse death investigator** and the police collaboratively notify families of a sudden death. The **forensic psychiatric nurse** and the judicial system interact effectively in the process of determining whether a person is competent to stand trial.

As such forensic issues arise, nurses must become more sophisticated and educated about their forensic role and responsibilities. Interdisciplinary discussions to develop appropriate collaborative roles will need to occur over time, both reactively and proactively. These implications introduce numerous legal and ethical issues that professional nurses must be prepared to address.

These issues raise a number of questions for the profession. Does the nurse believe that the collection of evidence while caring for clients is part of professional practice? With regard to "damaging" information given to the nurse while the client is under the influence of a mind-altering substance (prescribed or illegal), are the client's statements admissible in court? When a home care nurse is visiting an elderly client's house, does he or she report the observation that the client's adult child is routinely selling drugs? If marijuana plants are growing in the client's home, does the nurse report it or look the other way? If an emergency department nurse were told by an injured automobile driver in confidence that he may have hit "something" or "someone," the nurse needs to know whether there is privileged communication for nurses under state law and, if not, should the nurse inform the police and violate confidentiality? Reporting a significant other as an abuser may stimulate that significant other to move the family or take the victim to another health care provider who is unaware of the forensic history. Has the nurse helped the victims by reporting abuse or further alienated them from the health care system?

Nurses should be aware that they may be subject to a criminal charge of **obstruction of justice** if they destroy evidence. They should consult with the legal representative at their institution to see whether there is a policy on evidence collection and, if so, what it is, or if not, whether one should be developed.

ISSUES FOR FORENSIC NURSES IN ADVANCED OR SPECIALTY PRACTICE

Advanced practice nurses who consider themselves to be **forensic clinical nurse specialists** (CNS) may come from diverse specialty areas. Nurses prepared at the master's level in areas such as critical care, family nurse practitioner, mental health, or gerontology who are caring for **forensic clients** in a variety of settings may identify themselves as forensic CNSs. Some of these nurses attend forensic continuing education, whereas others obtain a certificate in forensic nursing, as from Beth El College at the University of Colorado in Colorado Springs or Fitchburg State College in Massachusetts. New to the field are those nurses who are being educated in a formal graduate forensic nursing curriculum. Pioneering this move-

ment are the first graduates of this type from the Fitchburg State College program.

Forensic CNSs need to define their boundaries in relation to practitioners in other forensic disciplines. The culture, actions, and goals of police detectives and lawyers differ from those commonly found in professional nursing practice. The forensic CNS is knowledgeable about the legal system and in a position to anticipate when legal advice is needed, to gather information on a crime, and to collect pertinent evidence. When and how to engage in each of these actions must be decided after careful consideration of the legal and professional roles. Boundary issues develop whenever new interprofessional relationships are forged, and forensic CNSs must be aware of this dynamic so that relationships develop productively.

Forensic CNSs frequently find that the additional knowledge and expanded role place them in the position of inadvertently assuming the culture of other disciplines. As is the case with all interdisciplinary relationships, at times the boundaries of the nurse's professional behavior may be blurred. Care must be taken to clarify the relationship between the forensic CNS and the members of the criminal justice system. A forensic CNS who is consulting with the nursing staff about the care of an alleged perpetrator on a medical inpatient unit might be inclined to have the staff ask forensic questions when providing care. But these may be questions that should remain in the domain of the detective and answers that are not admissible in court because they were not preceded by **Miranda rights** (*Miranda v. Arizona*, 1966). The enthusiastic forensic CNS may also slip into the posture of providing in-depth legal advice to a client when a referral to a legal advisor would be in the client's best interest.

When interacting closely with another discipline, taking on the other's culture can also be a potential problem. When a nurse consistently interacts with the police, taking on the thinking, the language, or the behavior of the police officer may subtly occur. Clients may then be perceived only as victims or "perps." If the client is entering the health care system to receive quality health care, but the nurse takes on the posture and behaviors of law enforcement, then the client is in a relationship to the nurse to which he or she has not agreed. Conversely, if nurses are employed by the criminal justice system, they need to be very clear on what their job description entails and need to make this clear to the client and to interprofessional colleagues.

The current priorities for forensic CNSs are to define their role more clearly, develop appropriate credentialing, and articulate nursing accountability as this specialty practice develops. They may be guided in these tasks by the existing *Scope and Standards for Advanced Practice Registered Nursing* (ANA, 1996) as well as the *Scope and Standards for Forensic Nursing Practice* (IAFN & ANA, 1997). They have to keep in mind their original contract with the client and place their legal responsibilities in the context of this role and relationship. Those charting new water need to be critically involved with this process. Forensic CNSs have a challenging task because they are interfacing with very different systems.

Credentialing in the advanced role is a voluntary form of self-regulation that requires higher standards than licensure (Aiken & Catalano, 1994). At this time, certification through the American Nurses Credentialing Center is desirable but not available for forensic nurses at either the generalist or advanced practice level. All nurses must be aware of laws and regulations affecting their practice; however, advanced practice forensic nurses will have acquired education beyond the nursing norm on matters relating to criminal justice, liability, and forensic science. Even without formal credentialing, they may be held accountable to a higher standard for the legal aspects of their practice.

NURSING MANAGEMENT ISSUES

Institutional policies, procedures, and standards of practice need to be developed to reflect the generalist's professional responsibilities with regard to forensics, and knowledgeable nurses need to be involved in this process. Nursing management needs to ensure the provision of quality care for all clients, incorporating all responsibilities required by accreditation standards (see Box 22–4). Coupled with this knowledge of forensic issues, the development of procedures and policies must follow. It is not enough for the emergency room nurse to know how to care for the client; proper handling and preservation of evidence must be standard practice. It is not enough for the visiting nurse to report domestic violence on an elderly client; documentation of the abuse must be able to stand up in court. Likewise, it is not enough for the occupational health nurse to assess hazardous workplace situations; the legal rights of the workers must be incorporated into industrial procedures. As the field of forensic nursing develops, so must nursing management's response to such changes.

Managers must develop task groups to establish standards in a proactive rather than a reactive mode. The members of these teams must be selected with a careful eye on the interdisciplinary relationships. Involvement of police, detectives, lawyers, and hospital security as working members of the health care team is essential. Nurse managers must facilitate the participation of their staff nurses in such interdisciplinary collaboration. Alternate workload assignments and other types of support must be given for nursing staff to consult with members of the judicial system in their work environment. An example might be forensic psychiatric nurses working with the police department to develop policy and procedures for interacting with a psychotic or hallucinating person being transported to the hospital setting without injury to that person or to the officers.

Nursing management is mandated with monitoring and implementing domestic violence or sexual assault services or trauma evidence preservation procedures. Standards, policies, procedures, and appropriate forensic nursing outcomes must be developed. Failure to establish appropriate institutional protocols that are based on current scientific evidence and expert forensic opinion will leave the organization as well as its nurse managers open to litigation.

TRENDS

Technological advances in forensic investigation are developing rapidly, evolving into a precise and specific field. With the increased capacity of forensic scientists to investigate crime, implications exist for nurses. DNA coding sequences now in use are much more precise than hair, blood, and fingerprints were in the past. Think of the implications for nurses caring for victims or perpetrators of crime. As mentioned previously, the emergency room nurse who carelessly discards the victim's clothing may well be destroying potential evidence of DNA coding. When a trauma client dies in the hospital, nurses routinely remove tubing and make the person presentable for viewing by the family, but in doing so, may be inadvertently destroying evidence that the forensic pathologist can use to determine cause of death. The nurse in both these situations needs to think carefully about the care of the client and about the forensic ramifications. As the ability to investigate becomes more sophisticated, the trends for the practice of nursing will change.

Currently, there is much discussion regarding the registration of pedophiles and sexual predators and the extent of community notification. Ethical dilemmas can arise when nurses must prioritize the rights of the individual client versus the safety of the community in situations with evolving legal guidelines. For example, in many states, the school receives notification, but the statute is silent on what the school may do with that information. The school nurse who knows that a registered pedophile lives next door to a student may not be legally able to share this information with the student's parents because of the perpetrator's legal rights. How does this fit in with professional values of promoting student and community health and primary prevention?

Conflicts may arise between what nurses are legally mandated to do versus what they perceive as their ethical responsibilities. For example, the school nurse is a mandated reporter for maltreatment. However, reporting a family may alienate them, particularly if the abuse is sexual, and the nurse may be aware that child protection agencies in his or her state are grossly underfunded. The child may become lost in the system. In the meantime, the parents may become angry with the school for reporting them to the authorities and no longer perceive school staff as sources of support. Even though a mandated reporter, does the school nurse initially try to work with the family? Would this then leave him or her open to a charge of failure to follow the law? School nurses need to be involved in development of the school's policies and to become active politically to present issues to the general public and influence public policy.

RECOMMENDATIONS

EDUCATION

Educating nurses to be aware of potential forensic cases and how to interact more effectively is clearly indicated. There will be a need for formal and continuing education for nurses: attendance at conferences on forensic issues and nursing curricular enhancement at both undergraduate and graduate levels. Forensic content does not belong solely in the psychiatric course where it is too frequently placed. Content needs to be integrated into all clinical areas in order for students to appreciate that forensic issues occur in every clinical setting. In the maternity clinic, a pregnant mother arrives for an office visit with a black eye from "walking into the door" (for the 10th time). In the pediatric setting, an 8-year-old girl visits the school nurse's office with frequent unexplained urinary tract infections. In the college health office, a young student thinks it is all right for her boyfriend to control all her decisions and spy on her. Nursing students must be taught what to do when narcotics are disappearing on the acute medical-surgical unit. If these students are taught to think forensically throughout their education, forensic assessment will take its place beside physical, psychosocial, spiritual, and developmental assessments as an integral part of their critical thinking.

Specialty education in forensic nursing beyond the basic curriculum has yet to be standardized. More programs at the graduate and certificate level need to be developed. The IAFN is in the process of elaborating a core curriculum for the forensic specialty, which will not only serve as groundwork for educational offerings but also hasten the development of a national specialty certification. In addition, as at the undergraduate level, graduate nursing education in general should promote heightened awareness of the forensic implications of all areas of advanced practice.

COLLABORATION

The relationship between the legal, judicial, and nursing systems is complex. The formal education and professional socialization of nurses, police officers, and lawyers are inherently different. Collaborative relationships need to be nurtured. Nurses need to learn how the police officer or lawyer thinks and speaks. Nurses need to learn "legalese" and police language to be able to effectively converse with them on client issues. Although police officers learn principles of effective communication for interviewing and for defusing dangerous situations, caring is not the core of their profession as it is in nursing. Nurses need to educate the police about nursing roles in communication and advocacy, but they also need to be sensitive to circumstances where these nursing roles are perceived as counterproductive by other disciplines. For example, nurses are taught to be persistent in their advocacy efforts for clients. However, continuing to argue with an arresting officer or after a judicial decision has been made could well result in a breakdown in the collaborative relationship as well as a possible contempt of court or obstruction of justice charge. Realizing that at times their goals will be in conflict with those of the judicial system, they need to know how to decide when to insist and when to defer. Each profession acts and interacts with victims and perpetrators differently. "Turf" issues will arise, and nurses need to develop a cognitive awareness of the boundaries of others' turf and the best way to interact collaboratively in a given situation.

DOCUMENTATION

Nurses need to document based on a much more acute sense of the forensic issues. When forensic cases are identified, documentation should follow accepted forensic protocol. Forensic photography is admissible in court and is being increasingly used by forensic nurses to document injuries and care. Therefore, all nurses need to be taught the importance of forensic photography, and forensic nurses need to become proficient in its use. This documentation is especially useful in the emergency unit when potential forensic cases arrive. The age-old cliche that a picture is worth a thousand words is certainly true in the courtroom. Describing slash injuries in terms of millimeters and color in a narrative form palls when compared with the impact of a photograph of the same injuries properly lighted, measured, and related to the client's overall condition (Pasqualone, 1996).

RESEARCH

Knowledge in forensic nursing based on sound research methodology is only in its infancy, with existing studies concentrated mainly on the topic of abuse. An in-depth body of nursing knowledge on this and other forensic topics needs to be developed based on effective nursing interventions and outcomes. Currently, forensic nursing's scientific foundation draws heavily on research from the forensic sciences and related practice disciplines. Integration of this knowledge into a nursing framework via nursing research is needed for truly evidence-based forensic nursing practice. Lack of such a research base may create problems for forensic nurses serving as expert witnesses under the state and/or federal rules of evidence that require some test of reliability for knowledge and expert opinion.

MANAGEMENT

All areas of health care need to evaluate existing policies and procedures related to forensic issues, particularly in relation to the responsibilities of nurses. Hospital management needs to seek input from their local police when developing policies such as the disposition of suspicious pills. Home health agency administrators need to establish protocols for the visiting nurse who encounters more than casual use of street drugs in a client's home. School boards need to address the child protective agency collaboration necessary when the school nurse identifies a case of child abuse or neglect. It is crucial that forensically astute nurses serve on the interdisciplinary committees required to develop or to modify existing policies and procedures.

SUMMARY

In summary, nurses with an interest in crime proceedings and other aspects of the legal system now have a way to combine these two fields for the benefit of clients and society. Although only in its infancy, the field of forensic nursing offers new horizons for collaborative practice that can only be imagined.

POINTS TO REMEMBER

- Forensic nursing is a very new specialty that is still in the process of development and refinement.
- Forensic nursing is defined as the application of forensic aspects of health care combined with the biopsychological education of the registered nurse in the scientific investigation and treatment of trauma and/or death related medical legal issues (IAFN & ANA, 1997).
- There is little in the way of statutory laws regulating forensic nursing practice. Federal statutes affecting practice include the Violence Against Women Act, the Uniform Controlled Substance Act, and the Americans with Disabilities Act. State statutes include mandatory reporting and anti-stalking laws.
- Common law relating to forensic nursing may be found within the malpractice arena. In addition, case law relating to evidence and testimony and the constitutional rights of clients are areas of knowledge required in forensic nursing.
- Governmental regulations influence forensic nursing practice, particularly with re-

gard to sexual assault, child and elder abuse, death investigation, and organ donation.
- Professional nursing standards applicable to forensic nursing practice include the *Scope and Standards of Clinical Nursing Practice*, the *Scope and Standards of Forensic Nursing Practice*, the *Sexual Assault Nurse Examiner Standards of Practice*, the *Nursing Interventions Classification (NIC)*, and the *Nursing Outcomes Classification (NOC)*.
- Clinical practice guidelines applicable to forensic nursing practice may be found in *Healthy People 2000* and guideline publications from the Agency for Health Care Policy and Research and the U.S. Preventive Services Task Force.
- Institutional practice guidelines related to forensic issues have generally been developed according to the accreditation standards of the Joint Commission for the Accreditation of Healthcare Organizations.
- All nurses need to incorporate forensic issues into their critical thinking about client care. Examples include documentation, collection, and preservation of forensic evidence and protection of clients' rights in relation to the police or the judicial system.
- Nurse specialists in forensic nursing need to become involved in refining the definition of their role, clarifying interprofessional relationship and boundaries, and articulating their accountability for specialist practice.
- Forensic nurse specialists need to be leaders in developing credentialing standards for the specialty.
- Nurse managers must be proactive in development of policies and procedures related to forensic practice and in facilitation of nurse involvement with interprofessional collaboration.
- Forensic nurses need to keep current on advances in forensic science and relevant legal decisions that influence their practice.
- An ethical dilemma that arises in a number of forensic situations is the issue of the rights of the individual versus the safety of the community.

- Recommendations for improving forensic practice exist in documentation, collaboration, education, research, and management, both for generalist and specialist nursing practice.

REFERENCES

Aiken, T. D., & Catalano, J.T. (1994). *Legal, ethical and political issues in nursing*. Philadelphia: F.A. Davis.

American Nurses Association. (1990). *Suggested state legislation: Nurse practice act, nursing disciplinary diversion act, prescription authority act*. Kansas City, MO: Author.

American Nurses Association. (1991). *Scope and standards of clinical nursing practice*. Washington, DC: American Nurses Publishing.

American Nurses Association. (1996). *Scope and standards of advanced practice registered nursing*. Washington, DC: American Nurses Publishing.

Brennan v. Nussbaumer and Bible (Case No. 94-CV-2524).

Burgess, A. W., & Holstrum, L. L. (1974). Rape trauma syndrome. *American Journal of Psychiatry, 131*, 981–986.

California Penal Code (1990). 646.9 Retrieved February 1998 from the World Wide Web: http://www.ewss.com/fact 14.htm.

Carr, J., Payne, R. et al. (1994). *Management of cancer pain: Clinical practice guidelines No. 9*. AHCPR publication No. 94-0592. Rockville, MD: Agency for Health Care Policy and Research, U.S. Department of Health and Human Services.

Doherty, C. (1998). From the editor. On the edge. *The Official Newsletter of the International Association of Forensic Nurses, 4*(1), 2.

Eckert, W. G. (Ed.). (1992). *Introduction to forensic sciences* (2nd ed.). Boca Raton, FL: CRC Press.

International Association of Forensic Nurses. (1997). *Sexual assault nurse examiner standards of practice*. Thorofare, NJ: Author.

International Association of Forensic Nurses and American Nurses Association. (1997). *Scope and standards of forensic nursing practice*. Washington, DC: American Nurses Publishing.

Johnson, M., & Maas, M. (Eds.). (1997). *Nursing outcomes classifications (NOC)*. St. Louis: Mosby.

Joint Commission on the Accreditation of Healthcare Organizations. (1997). *Comprehensive accreditation manual for hospitals: The official handbook*. Oakbrook Terrace, IL: Author.

Ledray, L., & Simmelink, K. J. (1997). Efficacy of SANE evidence collection: A Minnesota study. *Journal of Emergency Nursing, 23*(1), 75–77.

Lynch, V. (1993). Forensic nursing: Diversity in education and practice. *Journal of Psychosocial Nursing and Mental Health Services, 31*(11), 7–11.

Lynch, V. (1995). Forensic nursing: An essential element in managing society's violence and victims. *American Society of Testing and Materials, 4*, 38–42.

McClelland, C., Thompson, P. A., Prete, S. M., & Hatcher, P. A. (1996). Assessing firearm safety in inner-city homes. *Nursing and Health Care: Perspectives on Community, 17*(4), pp. 174–178.

McCloskey, J. C., & Bulechek, G. M. (Eds.). (1996). *Nursing interventions classification (NIC)* (2nd ed.). St. Louis: Mosby.

Miranda v. Arizona, citation, 384 U.S. 436, 86 S.Ct. 1602, 16 L.Ed.2d 694 (1966).

Pasqualone, G. (1996). Forensic RNs as photographers: Documentation in the ED. *Journal of Psychosocial Nursing and Mental Health Services, 34*(10), 47–51.

Report of the U.S. Preventive Services Task Force: *Guide to clinical preventive services* (2nd ed.). (1996). Alexandria, VA: International Medical Publishing.

Schmerber v. California, 384 U.S. 757, 86 S. Ct. 1826 (1966).

Shapiro, D. L. (1991). *Forensic psychological assessment: An integrative approach*. Boston: Allyn & Bacon.

Tatara, T. (1995). An analysis of state laws addressing elder abuse, and exploitation. Massachusetts Elder Abuse Law, MGL. C19A, 214-26. B17.

Tatara, T. (1996). *Elder abuse in domestic settings*. Elder Abuse Information Series #3. Washington, DC: National Center on Elder Abuse.

The Uniform Controlled Substance Act of 1970, 21 U.S.C. § 802.

United States Public Health Service. (1992). *Healthy people 2000: National health promotion and disease prevention objectives*. Rockville, MD: U.S. Department of Health and Human Services.

SUGGESTED READINGS

State v. Perea, 95 N.M. 777, 626 P. 2d 851 (1981).

Massachusetts Elder Abuse Law, MGL C19A, S14-26 (1983).

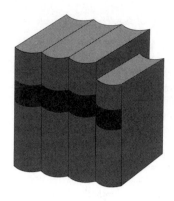

Chapter 23

LIFE CARE PLANNING

Doreen Casuto
Patricia McCollom

KEY
WORDS

American National Standards Institute (ANSI)	Conservator
	Fiduciary
	Guardian
Baclofen Pump	Life Care Plan
Blocked Account	Litigation
Bonded	Probate Court
Conclusions	Trust

OBJECTIVES

Upon completion of this chapter, the reader will be able to:
- Compare the definition of a life care plan with the definition of a nursing care plan.
- Discuss the components of a life care plan as used in patient and family education.
- Specify four types of records to be reviewed in preparation of a life care plan.
- Discuss four applications for a life care plan.

INTRODUCTION

A **life care plan** is a document generated by the nursing process that serves as an information management tool to identify complex needs of an individual in a clear and concise manner. First introduced into rehabilitation and legal literature in 1981, the term life care plan was identified as a component of rehabilitation evaluation (Weed, 1994). A life care plan was differentiated from discharge planning by its specification of associated costs for complex health care needs and inclusion of quality of life needs. Life care plans were used most frequently by attorneys dealing with personal injury **litigation** to identify future care costs as part of economic damages.

A definition of life care planning commonly accepted is:

A life care plan is a dynamic document based upon published standards of practice, comprehensive assessment, data analysis and research, which provides an organized, concise plan for current and future needs, with associated costs, for individuals who have experienced catastrophic injury or have chronic health needs (University of Florida/Intelicus, 1998).

This definition addresses the development of a life care plan as both individualized and research based and expands the life care plan beyond the courtroom into varying arenas.

Current applications for life care plans include:

- Insurance or reinsurance companies, to clarify potential costs in catastrophic or complex cases and to set reserves.
- Patients and families, to specify needs, suppliers, community resources, and expectations for health care needs.
- Health care facilities, to measure and evaluate treatment outcomes in specific populations.
- Elder care programs, to specify needs and services for individuals with chronic care needs.

417

- Schools for disabled students, to integrate health care needs into individualized education plans.

SCOPE OF PRACTICE

Nurses who prepare life care plans must recognize their obligation to first adhere to nursing standards, as developed by the American Nurses Association. The nursing process and nursing care plans provide a foundation for life care planning practice. However, life care planning is advanced practice characterized by broad clinical knowledge and expertise in current trends and research. It is collaborative in nature and includes the patient, family, care providers, and all parties concerned in coordinating, accessing, evaluating, and monitoring necessary services. As the transdisciplinary practice of life care planning continues to evolve, nurses will play a leadership role in the development of standards for practitioners and will promote collaboration and research.

LIFE CARE PLANNING PROCESS

REVIEW OF RECORDS

The review of records is the initial step in the life care planning process. Records hold valuable information about prior medical history, functional levels, and issues that have an impact on the individual's needs and, therefore, the life care plan. Often the individual referring the case for life care plan development is unaware of records that will be helpful to the life care planner. The following is a list of various types of records that should always be reviewed:

- *Past medical records:* provide insight into prior medical status, medications, frequency of visits, response to treatment, and compliance with recommendations.
- *Medical records from current incident:* emergency assessment, admission history, operative reports, consultant evaluations, imaging reports, laboratory results, therapies, nurses' notes, physician progress notes, and discharge summaries.
- *Rehabilitation records:* information about inpatient and outpatient care, initial and discharge summaries, interdisciplinary conferences, therapies, neuropsychological/psychological assessments and services, home evaluations, driving evaluations, as well as, physician reports and consultations.
- *Home health records:* details of home health services, which may include nursing assessments, nursing treatments, nursing assistant daily notes, therapy evaluations and treatments, and the plan of care established by assessment.
- *Physician records:* the physician records will include some information already included in the hospital records, but will also detail frequency of office visits, laboratory and x-ray reports, refills of prescriptions, and cancelled or missed appointments.
- *Psychological/neuropsychological evaluation:* information regarding testing, counseling, family support, and recommended interventions.
- *Developmental evaluation:* results of development evaluation for children.
- *School:* school records including standardized results, attendance, grade point average (GPA), and behavior.
- *Employment records:* regarding job performance, injuries, absence, attitude, and job description.
- *Interrogatories:* questions posed to the injured party and experts that deal with medical care, medications, equipment, services received, and costs.
- *Depositions:* injured individual and family, physicians, and other care providers or experts.
- *Bills:* costs incurred to date for medical care, equipment, and supplies.
- *Military records:* type of discharge, work assignments, and training.

A thorough review of the records will assist in identifying prior medical treatment and medications, need for assistance, bowel and/or bladder disturbances, and prior injuries and surgeries. Postinjury records supply the foundation for recommended future services, such as x-ray examinations, laboratory monitoring, or physician evaluations.

Physician records illustrate how often the person is examined, tests performed during the visit, medications prescribed, and their frequency and dosage. Follow-through by the patient can also be noted, such as frequently cancelled appointments and no-shows.

ASSESSMENT

The assessment is a vital component of data collection for the life care plan. The ideal situation is to complete the assessment in the home or residential setting, with a caretaker

included (McCollom, 1997). The person is in his or her usual environment, where he or she is more comfortable and the assessor can observe the person's functional status. The assessment interview provides an opportunity to observe the injured individual's understanding of his or her health status, the impact of the living environment on health, and interaction with significant other, family, or caretaker (Box 23–1).

Based on assessment, risk factors may then be identified for the individual, which equate to nursing diagnoses. The nurse life care planner should have specialized knowledge that enables detailed discussion of the individual risks associated with the injury and/or disability. Risk factors serve as a basis for **conclusions**, which are statements of long-term needs, supported by records, assessment, and communication with the

---

BOX 23-1

COMPONENTS OF ASSESSMENT

History
- Preexisting health status
- History of injury
- Surgeries, procedures, and treatment course
- Medical Diagnoses (as stated by treating physicians)
- Current Status
- Activities in a usual day
- Functional skills
- Self-care
    Cognition
    Communication
    Behavior
    Mobility
    Elimination
    Safety
    Community reentry efforts
- Nutrition status
- Medications

Psychosocial
- Living arrangements and family status
- Education
- Work history

Source: Used with permission of the Resource Associates, 1998 and P. McCollom, San Diego, CA.

treatment team and other experts. Examples of conclusion statements are:

- Mister X will require periodic, ongoing medical monitoring and prosthetic care for life as a result of bilateral below-the-knee amputations.
- Because of multiple life stresses, Mrs. Y should have access to counseling for adjustments to limitations and loss.

THE HOME VISIT

The level of mobility and function in the home setting provides essential information regarding need for assistive devices. During the assessment, the individual's current functional level can be evaluated and compared with the level portrayed in records. Often records are not current and are missing information regarding recent changes in abilities, hospitalizations, and current care providers. The opportunity to have the individual demonstrate transfer skills or ability to get in and out of the bathroom provides details regarding care needs often not adequately illustrated in the records and reports.

The home visit allows for identification of equipment available, the type and brand, the current usage, and status of the equipment. This information is necessary to identify how frequently equipment should be maintained and/or replaced. Often the individual is provided with equipment that is not used because of size, difficulty in use, and/or lack of understanding of how the equipment works. The location of equipment storage will provide information about use. The individual can demonstrate how and when the equipment is used and what would make it easier to use. Supplies, as well as packaging information, is often available to delineate vendors, type and amount of supplies provided, and frequency of delivery.

While the nurse is in the home, prescribed medications are reviewed. Access to medication containers allows the nurse to observe details regarding drug name, dosage, and physician who prescribed the drug. Further, the nurse can evaluate the person's understanding of the use of the medication and whether there is compliance with the prescription. The evaluation of the home itself is an important part of the review. Entrances and exits should be checked for ease of access and exit during emergency situations.

The layout of the home and the number of bedrooms and bathrooms provide information needed for potential live-in attendant care. The size of the bedroom may be an issue, if the individual uses a power chair or needs additional equipment such as Hoyer lifts or hospital beds. The placement of the bathroom and its accessibility can identify the need for modifications to allow for increased independence and safety issues. The kitchen and eating areas should also be evaluated. Whether or not the individual will be cooking, it is still important that he or she is able to access the kitchen, refrigerator, microwave, and eating area. If cooking is within the individual's ability or role, a more careful evaluation of layout and accessibility should be made. Space available for storage needs and access to storage should be considered, as well as which modifications have already been made and which have been planned. The American National Standards Institute (ANSI) has published accessibility standards, which serve as a resource to life care planners regarding accessibility needs.

The home visit provides an opportunity to meet the family and care providers. The family can provide information about routines and/or schedules. Plans for backup care providers and emergency situations can be discussed and reviewed. During the interview, observations can provide information about the relationship between the injured individual and the family. In this way, the life care planner can identify care needs and issues regarding relationships, dependence, independence, quality of life, and respite care. With information regarding the relationships within the family, it will be easier to identify the level of care needed, frequency of respite, and stability of the home or care situation. If the life care planner is unable to assess the individual at home, it is important to obtain the same information about the home, equipment, supplies, routines, and services.

OBSERVATION ALTERNATIVES

When preparing a life care plan for litigation and designated as a defense expert, the life care planner may be able to see the individual only in conjunction with an examination for independent medical evaluation. If that is the case, it is important that the life care planner speak with the attorney that retained him or her regarding restrictions that the plaintiff's attorney may have placed on during the physician's examination. Communication should take place with the physician who will be examining the patient prior to the appointment. Specific information needed should be discussed with the physician, to determine how best to obtain the data without interfering with the examination. Many physicians find that the questions asked by a life care planner enhance the information that they receive and are helpful in formulating their opinions.

If at all possible, it is helpful to observe the individual in different settings within the community. If a physician's appointment and/or clinic visit is scheduled, it will be helpful to attend. This contact provides the life care planner with an opportunity to meet the physician during a routine visit with the patient and to discuss patient and family concerns. Observation of the communication and relationship between the patient and/or family and the physician may provide information regarding the patient's or family's ability to advocate for their needs. Often they have difficulty understanding the treatment plan, and insufficient information and education has been provided to the family to ensure follow-through. Clarification of issues and care needs, as well as information obtained during the home visit, may be helpful for the physician in planning for or making recommendations for future care needs.

Having an opportunity to observe the individual in physical, occupational, or speech therapy provides information regarding commitment to the program, compliance with home therapy routines, response and effort during therapy sessions, as well as a chance to speak with the therapist. Information about frequency of therapies, communication among providers, evaluations, and goals and outcomes can be reviewed and discussed. The therapists are usually pleased to be included in the life care planning process and provide important information about the individual's needs for therapy and/or equipment. If the individual is receiving multiple therapies, it is important to communicate with each of the therapists involved in the treatment plan.

If the individual is attending school, it is helpful to go to the school. During the visit, observations can be made about the school itself, its layout, how the individual navigates around the campus, and the therapies and activities in which he or she is involved. Meeting with the teachers, therapists, and aides provides information about current functional levels, flexibility of the program, resources such as computers, and willingness to meet the individual needs of students. How the individual relates to peers, disabilities of others in the classroom, and the ratio of children to professional staff will assist in identification of placement needs and behavioral concerns. In addition to observation of the child in the school environment, an opportunity is provided, with appropriate consent, to review school reports and work.

COMMUNICATION WITH CARE PROVIDERS

The assessment is not complete unless communication occurs with physicians and other health care providers. These team members provide valuable information regarding how each views the injured individual and the support network. Often they have plans and goals and/or objectives that may not be documented in the records, but should be considered in preparing the life care plan. The physicians may prefer to discuss the care needs at an appointment with the injured individual or at a separate time when neither the patient nor the family is present.

Before the meeting with the physician and/or other care providers, it is important to identify the risks and care needs that have been associated with this individual's disability. Drafting issues and a list of concerns and questions is helpful in preparing for the discussion. The meeting with the physicians and/or care providers can be most effective if it is seen as a sharing opportunity for both parties. The life care planner may have had a chance to observe the individual in a variety of settings and frequently has communicated with other involved individuals. Providing information about observations and assessment while discussing the care needs promotes collaboration. A review of the current treatment should be discussed as well as plans for the future. Predictions for hospitalizations, potential surgeries, diagnostic workups, and orthotic and prosthetic needs should be discussed. It is important to determine whether these needs are likely to occur (probable, greater than 50 percent chance) or could occur (possible, less than 50 percent chance). After the meeting, it is helpful for the life care planner to prepare the recommendations from the discussion in writing for incorporation into the life care plan and for the physician's record. The plan can then be sent or faxed to the physician to re-review and comment on. This process allows both individuals to review communication and clarify any questions. The same technique can be used with other care providers, to enhance collaboration and communication.

INTEGRATION OF DATA

Once all information has been collected from records, home visits, and meetings, it is important to compile it in an organized fashion to ensure that issues and needs are not missed. Categorizing care needs as well as care issues is helpful in integrating the data obtained.

IDENTIFICATION OF NEEDS

By definition, a life care plan includes *all* the needs for an individual following injury or diagnosis of chronic health care conditions. Routine health care needs may be identified within the life care plan and noted as unrelated to injury. This allows use of the plan in various arenas beyond litigation,

such as patient or family teaching, discharge planning, or elder care.

The categories typically used in a life care plan are:

- *Preventive Medical Care:* physician visits, laboratory work, imaging studies, medications, therapies, x-ray examinations.
- *Surgery:* potential to occur is greater than 50 percent (e. g., removal of rods after initial injury, sphincterotomy for individual with bladder dyssynergy). Surgeries that are not probable, i.e., have less than a 50 percent chance for need, should not be included.
- *Hospitalization:* inpatient and emergency visits for falls or secondary effects of injuries and/or disability.
- *Therapy:* periodic evaluations and ongoing treatment. If there is significant treatment, it is important that any change in functional levels and improved independence be reflected in other areas of the plan.
- *Counseling:* services to address adjustment to disability for the individual and his or her significant other, family, and care providers. This should include evaluations, counseling, and behavioral intervention. Use of counseling services may be helpful in identifying strategies to change behavior or to improve compliance with home treatment programs.
- *Durable Medical Equipment:* mobility equipment such as wheelchairs, canes, walkers, beds, Hoyer lifts, and therapy equipment; prostheses and other equipment necessary for mobility and function following amputation.
- *Disposable Medical Supplies:* urinary, bowel, and skincare supplies; supplies for colostomy or ureterostomy.
- *Attendant Care Needs:* nursing care and supervision needed as a result of this injury, with resources for respite care. This area may include the costs associated with nursing case management services and guardian/conservator and attorney costs for the life of the individual, as appropriate.
- *Educational/Vocational:* additional services needed as a result of the injury, may include tutoring, additional educational testing, job placement, and vocational

counseling. At times, educational advocates are recommended to assist the school system in providing the needed benefits for the individual that are available but not routinely provided by the school systems. An educational advocate has the additional knowledge about the school system concerning what resources are available and how they can be obtained for a child. Sometimes the school system cannot meet the needs of the individual, and consideration should be given to the use of specialty or private schools. Children with dual disabilities, such as blindness and brain injury, often can best be served in a specialty or private school setting.

• *Transportation:* include adaptations to a car, such as hand controls, rear mirror enlargers, parking brake adapters, power lock downs and lifts, chair topers, or wheelchair racks. When the individual is dependent and the family cannot do car transfers, consideration should be given to use of a van. The van should be used for transportation of the individual and not as the family car. As the economist reviews the life care plan, the costs for routine vehicle transportation are subtracted from the van costs, because the need for transportation existed prior to the injury. Car phones should be considered for emergency use.

• *Housing Modifications:* accessibility needs for each individual, including wheelchair accessible bathrooms, two entrances/exits to the home for emergency evacuation, ramps, enlarged doorways, adaptations in the kitchen if the individual is able to be safe in his or her use of the kitchen, and air conditioning for individuals with temperature regulation loss. Security systems and automatic doors may be considered.

COMPONENTS ASSOCIATED WITH NEEDS

Needs should detail what care is required, the rationale and time frame for services, and should include frequency and cost of services. Resources providing for needs must be researched, and options for community services noted. For example, a guide dog or canine companion dog can be obtained at no cost, but the cost of food and veterinary care for the dog should be included in the care plan.

RESEARCH

Appropriate research methodology should be used in the development of cost projection for a life care plan. Research may include communication with manufacturers, physicians, facilities, and national research data banks.

Two research examples for life care planning are presented here.

BACLOFEN PUMP

The following is an excerpt from research gathered regarding the implementation and related expenses for a baclofen pump. The life care plan associated with this case was for an individual with quadriplegia suffering from unmanageable spasticity.

The **baclofen pump** is a method of controlling and managing a patient with spasticity of the extremities. Spasticity is caused by a decrease in GABA (γ-aminobutyric acid, a necessary acid). Some patients do well taking oral baclofen, but some patients with increased spasticity need more.

Baclofen is administered directly into the spinal fluid at a much lower concentration with a much more potent effect. The lower dosage eliminates potential side effects. The success rate with the baclofen pump has been very high because the pump is used only when there has been a demonstrated response to the medication when implemented on a trial basis.

Before the baclofen pump can be surgically placed, the individual must participate in a trial of intrathecal baclofen. The procedure involves a neurosurgeon, an anesthesiologist, and a 10-hour outpatient hospital visit. The anesthesiologist injects the baclofen into the spinal canal. The individual is then closely monitored for approximately 6 to 8 hours for response to the medication.

When the trial procedure has been tolerated with a good response, the next step is placement of an electronic pump to administer the baclofen. This procedure should be done at larger hospital centers that have resources and provide care for a high volume of patients with spinal cord injuries.

During surgery, the pump is implanted subcutaneously into the abdomen with a line that runs into the intrathecal canal to administer the baclofen. It is an involved procedure and may include a laminectomy. At minimum, an overnight stay is required.

After the pump has been implanted, maintenance care can often be completed by a local neurosurgeon. The pump must be reprogrammed, an electrical analysis completed, and medication refilled every 90 days.

Medication costs vary depending on dosage needed to manage spasms. The pump will need to be replaced approximately every 5 years.

Listed in Table 23–1 are charges associated with procedures for the baclofen pump in the Midwest.

COCHLEAR IMPLANTATION

The cochlear implant is an electronic device that stimulates the hearing nerves through electrical current. This enables individuals with profound hearing loss to receive sound. Part of the device, the internal components, is surgically implanted into the cochlea, and the implant is placed under the skin behind the ear. The external components, which include a speech processor and cable, are attached externally by way of a headpiece with magnet behind the ear. Sound waves are then picked up by the microphone attached to the headpiece and are converted into an electrical signal. The speech processor converts this signal into a coded signal that is transmitted across the skin to the implant. The signal causes impulses to be delivered to the brain, where they are interpreted as sound.

The following is an excerpt from a life care plan prepared in 1998 for a child with cochlear implants secondary to meningitis.

The child's x-rays showed evidence of ossification, or bone growth in the cochlea. She initially was fitted for 5 months with bilateral hearing aids to determine if she was a candidate for the implant. The physician recommended that only one ear be implanted so that as technology changed in the future, the other ear could be used. During the surgery, the physician was unable to implant all of the electrode array because of ossification, which resulted in reduced channels of stimulation. At the time the plan was prepared, the child was 7 years old and had the electronic device implanted for 1½ years.

A physician who specializes in cochlear implants will see children twice a year, adults 1 to 2 times per year. The costs associated with these visits are:

Initial evaluations @ $490
Follow-up visits @ $65 to $175
With diagnostic testing, every 2 to 5 years
  @ $500-$1000

The cochlear implant should be replaced or upgraded every 20 to 25 years. The prices associated with the implant are:

Implant Device	$25,000.00
Physician charge	$ 3,530.00
Anesthesia	$ 1,500.00
Hospital charges	$ 7,042.75

After the device is implanted, an audiologist works to program the implant to fit the individual needs of the patient. The initial costs are:

Programming/Remapping @ $125/hour, initially 2 to 3 hours for 2 to 4 times during the first year, and whenever the device is replaced or upgraded.

Summary of Potential Costs Following Cochlear Implant

- Programming/remapping in children should be planned approximately 2 to 4 times per year until the age of 18, and then 1 to 2 times per year.
- Speech therapy 1 to 2 times per week to assist them in maximizing the benefits of the implant. The sessions range in price from $90 to $120 per session.
- Testing of the individual's speech perception and auditory listening skills with the implant, twice a year with children, and

TABLE 23–1. TRIAL OF BACLOFEN PUMP IN THE MIDWEST

	Charge	Totals	Cost	Comments
TRIAL OF BACLOFEN	Physician charge Medication Outpatient charge (ave)		$ 748.00 250.00 1,915.00	
IMPLANTATION OF MEDTRONIC PUMP PROCEDURE				
Supplies	Medtronic pump Catheter	 Total charges for Supplies	9,862.50 442.50 10,305.00	Actual charges, January 1998, for a 2-day inpatient stay.
Physician charges	Neurosurgeon for pump and catheter placement Anesthesiology	 Total Physician Charges	3,040.00 1,054.00 4,094.00	
Facility Charges			5,564.42	Actual hospital facility charges from a January 1998 hospitalization for the usual 2-day stay. Includes 110 minutes operating room charges, medications, and additional supplies.
		Average Charge for Pump, Procedure, Supplies, and Facility	19,963.42	

(Continued)

TABLE 23–1. TRIAL OF BACLOFEN PUMP IN THE MIDWEST (Continued)

	Charge	Totals	Cost	Comments
Maintenance	Physician charge for evaluation and management		640.00	Performed every 90 days $160 × 4×/yr
	Refill and reprogram pump		600.00	Performed every 90 days $150 × 4×/yr
	Analysis		800.00	$200 × 4×/yr
	Medication		1,000.00	$250 × 4×/yr
		Annual Maintenance Charges	3,040.00	
Replacement of Pump	Pump		9,468.00	The pump would need to be replaced every 5 years. Charges based on 90th percentile of usual and customary billed charges. *Source:* Practice Management Information Corporation, Physician Fees, 1997.
	Catheter		570.00	May or may not need to be replaced.
	Physician charge Insertion of catheter		1,891.00 2,331.50	May or may not be charted at time of replacement.
	Facility charge		5,564.42 18,374.17	
	Average pump replacement charge			

Source: Reprinted with permission from The International Academy of Life Care Planners, 1998.

with adults one time per year, with approximately 6 to 10 tests each time at a cost per test of $60.

- A service contract for the speech processor and external equipment can be purchased after the initial 3-year warranty period. The cost of the service contract is $595 every 2 years.
- Insurance policy for loss or theft of the speech processor, which costs $135 per year.
- The speech processor should be upgraded every 5 years at a cost of $5000 to $6900.
- The headset with microphone, which includes the coil, magnet, microphone, and cables, should be replaced every 3 years at a cost of $360.
- Additional accessories that are needed:

> Telephone adaptor – $60.00
> Volume control for telephone – $60.00
> Dry pack to use with speech processor – $18.00
> Ear hooks – pack of 5 for $12.00
> Lapel clips – pack of 5 for $12.00
> Padded pouch – $30.00
> Coil – $60.00
> Magnet – $36.00
> Battery (double A) one per day – $19.12/month*

NURSING CARE OPTIONS

When preparing a life care plan, it is helpful to identify options for the provision of nursing care. This allows the family and patient the ability to make decisions in the future regarding the care that is most appropriate. Although the goal of rehabilitation for any individual is to be discharged home and remain there for the rest of his or her life, often it is not feasible or realistic. The families at times may feel guilty about these thoughts or concerns, and it is important to allay these fears by taking all these factors into account when preparing the life care plan (Table 23–2).

*Adapted and reprinted with permission from Casuto, 1998.

USES FOR LIFE CARE PLANS

FOR THE INSURANCE INDUSTRY

Lifetime needs assessments may be requested by an insurance company or reinsurance carrier to determine their exposure (anticipated costs) in a specific case. Both liability and workers' compensation payers find the information provided in a life care plan valuable. A life care plan identifies lifetime needs in a consistent, sequential manner and serves to provide accurate cost data for the payer. The needs and cost data are then reviewed by an actuary within the insurance company, and options for settlement are identified.

FOR LITIGATION

A life care plan offers a clear and concise presentation of current and future care needs with associated costs. It can be used for settlement purposes to provide a total dollar amount or as a section within the settlement brief. At trial, it can used by both the life care planner and the physicians as a teaching tool to educate the jury regarding the individual's status and specialized needs over his or her lifetime.

FOR PROBATE COURT

Probate court is the department of each county's superior court that deals with probate conservatorships, guardianships, and estates of people who have died. Probate courts have the legal right to make decisions about the individual's life and property. Cases involving a **guardian** or **conservator** are assigned to the probate court by the probate section of the superior court. In large counties, the probate court may be a separate department handling only probate issues, with either a judge or commissioner assigned to handle these cases (Judicial Council of California, 1992). Probate is the result of the outcome of litigation for minors or compromised adults. Probate court uses the

TABLE 23-2. LIFE CARE PLAN

This life care plan is for a 65-year-old man who had an anoxic episode during surgery. He is 6 feet 2 inches and weighs 215 pounds. As a result of the anoxia, he is currently in a subacute facility. He has a tracheostomy with copious secretions, is on gastrostomy tube feedings, is a brittle diabetic, and has hip and knee contractures on his right side. His wife is 55 years old and has a history of cardiac and back problems. They have four children who live in the area and are very supportive but are concerned about the effects of their father's needs on their mother's health. In discussion with all the family, the decision was made to include both alternatives for care, despite the plan for some initial rehabilitation intervention to decrease his care level.

Nursing Care	Frequency	Objective/Goal	Cost	Comment
Options: 1. Home with day or live-in licensed attendant	Ongoing	To provide nursing care, supervision, and assist with transportation	$26-$28/hour *OR* $257.50/day	*Agency* Cost/hour LVN, 16 hours/day *OR* Cost/day for live-in LVN
With respite care	6 weeks per year	To provide respite nursing care for hours of care provided by family	$26-$28/hour	Cost/hour LVN, 8 hours per day
2. Residential placement	Ongoing	To provide nursing care, supervision, and assist with transportation	$495/day	Cost per day, includes items from the plan
With weekends/weeks home to allow for family visits during holidays	6 weekends per year and 3 weeks	To allow for home care during stays at home	$26-$28/hour *OR* $257.50/day $371.25	Cost/hour LVN, 24 hours/day *OR* Cost/day for live-in LVN Cost/day for holding bed at X facility during trips home (75% of per diem bed rate for holding bed)

life care plan as a guide for budgeting and controlling the financial aspects of a trust.

FOR PATIENT AND FAMILY EDUCATION

Life care plans serve as excellent teaching tools for injured individuals and their families. Following catastrophic injury or a chronic diagnosis, the emotional upheaval and stress serve as barriers to learning. An individualized life care plan provides a reference resource for the individual and family regarding physician monitoring, equipment and supplies needed, providers, and community resources. Further, the life care plan can be used as an outcomes measurement tool by a facility to evaluate care, responses to treatment, and patient and family education. With conditions associated with aging, life care plans provide guidance and benchmarks for families regarding needs and care options.

FOR TRUST MANAGEMENT

When a **trust** is established, the law requires a **fiduciary** or guardian and attorney to:

- Analyze the goals of the trust in terms of what the trust will accomplish over the life of the individual.
- Develop, using the life care plan, a budget for expenditures, taking into account life expectancy or length of time the money will need to be used.
- Provide recommendations for the investment of the dollars: investment options, risk of investment, projected income, and tax consequences.
- Demonstrate that these investments will meet the ongoing and long-term needs of the individual, in terms of budget and life expectancy of the individual.

The judge then reviews the proposal and makes a determination of whether the investments are appropriate. This helps protect the fiduciary if there are financial problems in the future, such as poor investment income resulting in financial shortfall.

All guardians, fiduciaries, and family members should be **bonded**, or insured, if they will be managing the dollars. It is the court's decision whether or not the bonding is necessary, and they may at times waive the bond. Bonding protects the minor's or conservatee's money from inappropriate use or investment handling. "The bonding company reimburses the estate for any loss caused by the conserved's dishonesty or negligence, and the company then goes after the conserved to repay the loss" (Judicial Council of California, 1992). The court will initiate the bond; the estate is responsible for paying the bond's premium on an annual basis.

Example:

The parents of a child who obtained a large financial award from an injury suit could not qualify for a bond, and the court decided to waive the bond requirement. As a result, 16 years later, there were limited funds available to meet this young adult's needs. The family had inappropriately used the dollars, including moving three times, purchasing non–wheelchair accessible homes, and not having a vehicle that would safely transport the person within the community. None of the money could be retrieved and the court had little they could do to the parents, except taking over the deed for the house and placing it in the child's name. The system of requiring bonding prevents this from happening to other minors.

Example:

A child sustained significant injuries as a result of a vaccine. A life care plan was prepared for settlement purposes, and the child received a settlement as a result of an injury. The family was provided the life care plan with a variety of other documents but was never instructed about what the life care plan is and how it relates to the money awarded. The family was aware of the money, and it was deposited into a **blocked account** with the courts. The family used the money only for copayments for their insurance for their son or when the insurance denied the request for a physician's evaluation and/or treatment. For 10 years, the family continued to live in the same inadequate housing, attempting to make do with their own resources to cover the special needs of the child. Ten years after the award, the child was sent to an educational advocate for testing and evaluation. During the assessment, it was discovered that the family had received an award but had never had any education about how the money could be used and how to use the life care plan as a tool in the process. The educational advocate referred the family to a nurse case manager for assistance.

SUMMARY

A life care plan is a dynamic document based on published standards of practice, comprehensive assessment, data analysis and research, which provides an organized, concise plan for current and future needs, with associated costs, for individuals who have experienced catastrophic injury or have chronic health needs.

The transdisciplinary practice of life care planning is in evolution. Designed as a tool for litigation, the life care plans has developed a life of its own in nursing case management and outcome evaluation. If the life care plan is prepared only for purposes of litigation and is not used as a working document to assist the family and injured individual in obtaining the care and services needed, then significant dollars have been wasted and a valuable educational tool has been neglected. The life care plan is developed and prepared for the patient and the family; they have ownership of the plan. The plan is designed to promote the health and wellness through preventive health care of the individual, and access to the plan is vital to his or her well-being. Therefore, the role of the nurse life care planner may just begin with the end of a litigated case. The life care plan is a foundation for the case management process.

The professional nurse has unique skills for practice as a life care planner. With broad education, clinical, and community knowledge and research expertise, the nurse life care planner is able to assist the patient, family, and court system with coordination and implementation of a life care plan. Although the life care plan serves as a foundation for economic damages during litigation, a life care plan's implementation is its true measure of value.

POINTS TO REMEMBER

- Definition of a life care plan
- Transdisciplinary practice
- Practice in evolution
- Importance of review of varying records
- Assessment components
- Observations in alternative settings
- Research regarding options and costs
- Uses for life care plans
- Nurse's role in life care planning

REFERENCES

Casuto, D. (1998, July). Cochlear implant: Cost research. In P. McCollom (Ed.), *The Academy Letter, 1,* 2.

Judicial Council of California. (1992). *Handbook for conservators.* San Francisco: Author.

McCollom, P. (1997). Life care planning. In K. Johnson (Ed.), *Advance practice nursing in rehabilitation: A core curriculum* (pp. 251–255). Glenview, IL: ARN.

Resource Associates. (1998). *Assessment tool.* Author.

Spear, C. (1998, May). Baclofen pump: Cost research. In P. McCollom (Ed.), *The Academy Letter, 1,* 1.

University of Florida/Intelicus. (1998, April 3). 2nd Annual Life Care Planning Conference and the International Academy of Life Care Planners, Forensic Section Meeting, NARPPS Annual Conference, Colorado Springs, CO.

Weed, R. (1994). Life care plans: Expanding the horizons. *NARPPS Journal, 9*(2-3), 47–50.

SUGGESTED READINGS

McCollom, P. (1998). Life care planning. *Workers' Compensation Case Review, 4*(5), 70–72.

McCollom, P., & Sager, D. (1996). Case management. In S. Hoeman (Ed.), *Rehabilitation nursing process and application* (pp. 101–113). St. Louis: Mosby.

Week R. (Ed.). (1998). *Life care planning and case management handbook.* Boca Raton, FL: CRC Press.

Yudkoff, M. (1996). Working with nurse expert witnesses: Life care planning. In P. Iyer (Ed.), *Nursing malpractice* (pp. 829–834). Tucson, AZ: Lawyers and Judges Publishing Company.

Yudkoff, M. (1998). The life care planning expert. In J. Brewer-Bogart (Ed.), *Legal nurse consulting principles and practice* (pp. 657–686). Boca Raton, FL: CRC Press.

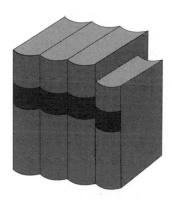

Chapter 24

VIOLENCE IN NURSING

Cheryl Pozzi

INTRODUCTION

This chapter analyzes the types of workplace violence nurses encounter, where violence occurs, and laws and regulations that protect nurses before and after becoming victims of violence. This chapter is also designed to educate the nurse about the incidence of violence and abuse in health care.

The problem of workplace violence was not clearly identified until the late 1980s. Because the problem has been recently identified, research is limited and laws are virtually nonexistent. Recognition of this type of violence is still in its infancy and desperately needs attention. Definitions of violence are varied, research has been singularly focused, and solutions provide protection rather than changing the actions of the perpetrator.

More nurses are being proactive, writing and reporting incidents, bringing criminal charges, pointing out various acts of harassment, coordinating charges with other nurses, and developing a no abuse and/or violence tolerance mode. Nurses realize that violence or abuse is not an act inflicted only by patients, but can be perpetrated by other nurses, physicians, administration, family members, and/or a third party. The history of nursing and the law is critical in demonstrating how violence among nurses began and why violence remains a crucial workplace issue today.

Discussions of workplace violence usually relate to a disgruntled employee returning to his or her place of employment after being fired and retaliating against fellow employees or supervisors with deadly force. Sensational acts of workplace violence involving multiple deaths in schoolyard and post office shootings often gain a great deal of media attention. Acts of violence have crept into our collective consciousness to such an extent that irrational, violent behavior is now commonly referred to as "going postal."

Unfortunately, the media often ignores the far more common acts of workplace violence, perhaps because these acts have become so prevalent as to not be newsworthy. The daily robbery and killing of a taxicab driver and the thousands of assaults on employees while at work tend to go without notice. Workers often pretend annoying behaviors do not exist, such as sexual remarks, shoving, demeaning comments from co-workers, and threats (Spring & Stern, 1998). In actuality, the majority of health care workers feel that tolerating abusive behaviors is a part of their job (Birkland, 1991; Lenehan, 1991; Occupational Safety and Health Administration [OSHA], 1996). Some nurses fear being told to deal with it or get out. Patients may spit, pull hair, pinch, scream obscenities, threaten to harm, throw food, grab any item as a potential weapon, ask for sexual favors, make sexual gestures, and so on. The patient's feelings of loss of control during an illness or injury may exacerbate stressful situations. Family members may also be guilty of abusive behaviors, perhaps more so because they are ambulatory and stressed over the illness of a family member. Patients and family often act out very differently from their norm during a crisis.

Psychiatric nurses have routinely confronted violent situations in the workplace. Regardless, nurses are not prepared for the violence they face in today's clinical settings. Nurses, as caregivers, are placed in an ethical dilemma when providing care to a physically or verbally abusive patient, for the nurse may have to choose between providing care or self-protection from harm. Role confusion and stress often cause nurses to retreat within rather than seek help from peers, management, or ethics committees available within the hospital organization. Psychiatric nurses often experience difficulty defining violence resulting from the patient's illness versus violence that is volitional or not illness based. Volitional violence is often either unreported or reported within a category of violence resulting from illness. The nurse rarely receives follow-up care for the emotional consequences of dealing with workplace violence.

On a peer level, workplace violence may occur when the nurse is abused by other nurses, physicians, and/or their employers (Spring & Stern, 1998). Nurses may ridicule each other publicly, in front of other nurses or patients. Nurses may be assigned the worst tasks or the most undesirable shifts, refused help with difficult tasks, and/or have questions for clarification answered in a demeaning manner. Graduate nurses may be treated very poorly and given the most difficult duties, as part of the traditional "initiation" other nurses had to endure. The problem of violence is not revealed or discussed with nurses who apply for nursing school or explained to nurses as a workplace hazard when applying for a job. Some physicians are still guilty of demeaning nurses, for example, throwing charts or surgical instruments, publicly screaming at nurses, making sexual comments, ridiculing the nurse who is unable to answer a difficult question, slamming telephones, insisting that nurses perform procedures that are out of their realm of practice, and intimidating those who question orders.

Although sexual harassment in the workplace is now illegal under federal law, these laws have not stopped its occurrence. Employers still pressure employees by granting job security and promotion in return for sexual favors, and staff and physicians often make sexual innuendoes. So when does lack of manners, common sense, and general courtesy become abuse? What is workplace violence?

DEFINITIONS

Defining violence in itself generates considerable discussion, for "the broader the definition, the more incidents will be captured" (Lipscomb & Love, 1992). Most think violence is an act that involves bodily harm to one person inflicted by another person. Few may think of actions or language that make a person uncomfortable in the workplace as a form of violence. *Webster's New World Dictionary* (1988) says the word **abuse** means "to hurt by treating badly; mistreat; injury, to use insulting comments, or bad language about or to; revile." *Random House College Dictionary* (1982) defines **violent** as "acting with or characterized by extreme force, characterized by injurious or destructive force, an unjust or unwarranted exertion of force or power, rough or immoderate vehemence as of feeling or language." *Black's Law Dictionary* (1979) defines **assault** as "any willful attempt to threaten and/or inflict injury upon the person of another, when coupled with the apparent ability to do so; and any intentional display of force, such as would give the victim reason to fear or expect immediate bodily harm."

Based on these definitions, an assault may be committed without actually touching, striking, or doing bodily harm to the other person. The Centers for Disease Control and Prevention (CDC) offers the following working definition of **workplace violence**: "violent acts, including physical assaults and threats of assaults, directed toward persons at work or on duty." California has been the most progressive state in developing guidelines specific to workplace violence. Cal/OSHA defined different types of workplace violence according to the following criteria:

The characteristics of the establishment affected, the profile and motive of the agent or assailant, and the preventive measures differ for each of the three major types of workplace violence events (State of California, Department of Industrial Relations, 1995).

In all three types of events, a human being, or **hazardous agent**, commits the assault. Box 24–1 lists the three types of workplace violence.

Those persons most at risk for *type I workplace violence* may be involved or located in any of the following situations: (1) working at a late night retail establishment; (2) employed as a taxicab driver; (3) employed as a security guard; (4) seeking money exchange, i.e., ATM machine; and/or (5) working as a single person or in a small number of persons at the employment site.

Those most at risk for *type II workplace violence* are: (1) service providers, (2) public safety and correctional personnel, (3) municipal bus or railway drivers, (4) health care and social service providers, (5) teachers, and (6) sales personnel.

Type II workplace violence may represent the most prevalent category of workplace violence resulting in physical injury.

Of increasing concern, though, are events involving assaults to the following type service providers: medical care providers in acute care hospitals, long term care facilities, outpatient clinics and home health agencies; mental health and psychiatric care providers in inpatient facilities, outpatient clinics, residential sites and home health agencies; alcohol and drug treatment providers; social welfare service providers in unemployment offices, welfare eligibility offices, homeless shelters, probation offices, and child welfare agencies; teaching, administrative and support staff in schools where students have a history of violent behavior (State of California, Department of Industrial Relations, 1995).

Those at most risk for *type III workplace violence* are a coworker, supervisor, or manager of a disgruntled or former employee and/or an employee involved in a domestic or romantic dispute. This group represents a much smaller proportion of injuries in California than those involved in types I and II workplace violence.

According to Cal/OSHA, "Some occupations and workplaces are at risk for more

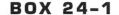

BOX 24-1

THREE TYPES OF WORKPLACE VIOLENCE

TYPE I:
The agent has no legitimate business relationship to the workplace and usually enters the affected workplace to commit a robbery or other criminal act.

TYPE II:
The agent is either the recipient or the object of a service provided by the affected workplace or the victim, e. g., the assailant is a current or former client, patient, customer, passenger, criminal suspect, inmate, or prisoner.

TYPE III:
The agent has some employment-related involvement with the affected workplace. Usually this involvement centers around an assault by a current or former employee, supervisor, or manager; by a current or former spouse or lover; a relative or friend; or some other person who has a dispute with an employee of the affected workplace.

Source: State of California, Department of Industrial Relations, 1995.

than one type of workplace violence event" (State of California, Department of Industrial Relations, 1995). Hospital emergency rooms, in addition to being at risk for type II events involving assaults by patients are also at risk for type I events. For example, gang members can enter a hospital emergency room to disrupt the medical care of a rival gang member who survived the initial attack, and in the process, the emergency room personnel may be physically harmed. Psychiatric settings are also the setting for multiple types of workplace violence, such as violent assaults by patients experiencing psychosis or under the influence of ingested chemicals and/or assault by family or others involved in domestic violence, placing staff at risk of being in crossfire. Soloff (1987) stated, "violence is endemic in the mental health treatment setting and constitutes a real and unacknowledged occupational hazard." (For the purpose of this chapter, the definitions of abuse, assault, and violence are defined within the parameters of the work environment.)

HISTORICAL OVERVIEW

In the health care industry, violence has increased in areas such as the emergency room, medical and surgical units, and community clinics. Violence has always been present in acute clinical environments and in psychiatric settings. Now with shorter lengths of stay, earlier discharges, and home health care, social workers and staff of emergency medical services (EMS) are at increased risk for exposure to violence. Nursing care presents challenges beyond the clinical care provided. Treatment plans must now consider risk for violence for both patients and staff.

As stated previously, workplace violence was unheard of until the 1980s. It was not that workplace violence had not occurred; rather, data collection had not established or defined the problem. The first real calculations of workplace deaths were not compiled until a survey of fatal occupational injuries, from 1980 to 1985, and another survey project of workplace-related homicides among health care workers, from 1980 to 1990 (Bell et al., 1990; Goodman, Jenkins, & Mercy, 1994). Both of these projects used information from death certificates compiled from the National Traumatic Occupational Fatality (NTOF) surveillance system. But the CDC questioned the validity and accuracy of the NTOF's statistics, concluding that the results were limited by the following variables on the death certificates: (1) there was often lack of detail to describe occupations within major industrial classifications; (2) the reporting of place of injury was not consistent or perhaps accurate; (3) there were no nationally standardized guidelines for completion of the work-related items; (4) accurate classifications of some occupations may have been difficult, because of ambiguity and potential misinterpretation of narrative entries; (5) precipitating events usually were not described; (6) exposure data needed to compute relevant risks were not available; (7) other relevant data sources on workplace deaths had not been linked into the data; (8) information on homicides in the U.S. population, from the National Center for Health Statistics (NCHS) vital statistics mortality data files, had not been compared with information on workplace homicide from NTOF; and (9) no national data source existed that allowed description of nonfatal injuries sustained as a result of violence in the workplace and also contained information on occupation, industry, and detailed circumstances of the event (CDC, 1992).

The NTOF data were not valid because the medical examiners and coroners did not use a standardized definition of an injury at work. The information on the death certificates was subject to individual interpretation by the certifier, and it did not include data on near-fatal or nonfatal incidents. Although the Occupational Health and Safety Administration (OSHA) had an established reporting mechanism in place for work-related injuries and workplace deaths, the OSHA 200 log did not include a mechanism to report deaths resulting from workplace violence. The same was true for assaultive injuries, with the surrounding circumstances of the incident documented in the narrative. But the manner and mechanism of death needed to be further explored, as the tabula-

tion system did not provide for documentation of narrative information. As a result of deficiencies in research, the actual number of workplace assaults and deaths has been very difficult to determine. According to reporting standards, OSHA does not require the reporting of harassment or abusive language; such a reporting requirement would expand the incidence of documented workplace violence into far greater numbers.

Knowledge of the history of nursing is important in appreciating the long-standing problem of the issue of violence in nursing. According to Gasparis (1990, p. 112), the demise of the Roman Catholic Church in England brought an end to the era of humanistic care of the sick. Subsequently, institutional care of the sick was provided by prostitutes, criminals, and alcoholics, whereas home care became the responsibility of the women of the family (Gasparis 1990, p. 112). Florence Nightingale (1867, p. 274) wrote that the nursing profession was initially viewed with a negative connotation, practiced by "those who were too old, too weak, too drunken, too dirty, too stolid, or too bad to do anything else."

According to Gasparis (1990, p. 112), during the Crimean War, Nightingale established the practice of nursing within the military system. Nightingale was a well-educated woman from the privileged class of England, with a commitment to return to society the good fortune she had received in her life and to dedicate her life to social reform at all levels. The British Army gave Nightingale the opportunity to implement her ideas on nursing, legitimizing meaningful health care work for the middle class woman. Rosenberg (1987, p. 217) presented the viewpoint that, at that time, people believed women were better suited for nursing because of their innate sensitivities, caring, reassurance to patients, and warmth. Gasparis (1990, p. 113) also noted the general feeling during that time period was "why train them [nurses] for something they innately know and do?" Smith summed up the general view of nursing during Nightingale's era in the following manner: "Nursing is as absolutely the peculiar province of women as any branch of housewifery. The qualities of a good nurse are vigilance, discretion, and gentleness; and these are her special qualities" (Smith, 1862, p. 149).

The first formal assignment for nurses met with ridicule by the British government. Nurses were not wanted and their services not valued. According to Gasparis (1990, p. 114), "It was here that nursing first experienced what would become a pattern of rejection, resistance, and scorn from the masculine medical and, ultimately, hospital establishment" (Gasparis, 1990, p. 114).

Even though Nightingale provided instruction for her nurses, she still did not treat them as equals and viewed them as the servant class, for according to Palmer 1984, p. 6, "She established hours of work comparable to those of servants in English households and recommended similar living conditions: small rooms with plain, simple furniture."

It was not until the Crimean War and World War I that society began to see any potential value in the career of nursing within organized health care. With each American war, the image of the nurse improved. By 1920, the majority of all nurses were working independently as private duty and contract nurses. Nurses had the freedom to accept assignments according to their own needs and schedules, for they could turn down assignments, choosing types of cases for which they would provide care, and take time off when they were too exhausted and/or had family needs (Gasparis, 1990, p. 116).

However, during the Great Depression, the public was unable to afford private duty nursing. Medical boards had been resentful of the nurse's ability to independently control assignments, and then "Suddenly nurses were dependent on the hospital structure for their very lives, exchanging services for food and lodging" (Gasparis, 1990, pp. 117, 118). According to Gasparis (1990, p. 118), the medical and administrative hierarchy gained control over nurses. Consequently, during the post–World War II period, nurses had to assume a second-class status, which led to subservience and various forms of abuse.

The education of nurses was abusive, as the training was similar to the workload found in a labor camp. According to Reverby (1987), nursing was an innate ability, so nurses spent tedious 12-hour days scrubbing floors and serving meals while attending serious contagious diseases. Many would fall ill themselves from the exhaustion and exposure, disabling and killing many students. Reverby (1987, p. 64) further noted, "Poor living conditions compounded the problem as nursing quarters were more barracks than homes."

Johnstone (1994, p. 79) also wrote of the early, abusive working conditions of nurses:

The early modern nurses were forced to endure exploitative work conditions characterized by employer demands to perform arduous duties, coupled with low pay, poor living conditions, long hours, and rigid discipline. Attempts to improve conditions met with stiff opposition from administrators on the grounds that it would not be "in the public interest" or "beneficial to the nurses themselves."

Nurses who dared to complain were severely abused or criticized and portrayed as "failed women," i.e., selfish, uncaring, disobedient, and disloyal (MacLean, 1903, p. 34). Nurses who would not comply with the demands of the health care system were abused, in the form of reprimands, whether they were a student nurse, who might be reprimanded by administration and/or physicians, or a nurse who might be reprimanded by other nurses and/or supervisors.

Gasparis (1990, p. 121) shared the point of view that nursing leadership feared ". . . too much education for nurses was not only unnecessary but dangerous, and would produce a generation of nurses who would not want to dirty their hands with the real stuff of nursing."

In the 1950s, a 2-year program for nurses was created. Gasparis (1990, p. 121) stated that the general population felt education for women was only for those who needed entertainment before their real job of marrying, having children, and keeping the house. Gasparis (1990, p. 122) also believed the nursing profession took a historical step backward when 2- and 3-year programs were created, without deciding how these different levels of nursing would be utilized. Diploma, associate degree, and baccalaureate nursing programs coexisted, thereby contributing to a differentiation of status and professionalism among nurses:

Though the intent may have been one of creating two levels of caregiver, the reality was the creation of a cheaper, quicker and less well-educated product. Nurses abused nurses, hospitals abused the nurses, and the stage was set for the scorn of the public" (Gasparis, 1990, p. 122).

Gasparis (1990, p. 122) further took the position that:

Nurses are and have been women who do women's work in a world where women and their work are of questionable value. Our society is still designed to overlook and devalue nurturing and caring based upon a patriarchal paradigm.

According to Johnstone (1994, p. 4), female physicians were quickly taught to adopt the patriarchal, paternalistic, and authoritarian values that are commonly associated with and upheld by the medical culture, which often resulted in female doctors treating nurses the way their male colleagues had historically treated nurses.

With the advent of the industrialization of the United States, unions had a significant impact on the delivery of health care, providing avenues for employees to deal with business and making changes in working conditions. In the early 1980s, nurses began joining unions at a rapid rate. Union organizations saw a golden opportunity to gain entry into an area that had previously been impenetrable. Under union organization, nurses were able to negotiate with hospital systems for better pay and working conditions, as well as to protect the profession from being replaced with nonprofessionals. A new stage had been set for nurses to develop a higher quality nursing profession. But unionization did not stop the workplace violence.

The logging industry was the first to contract with local hospitals, physicians, and clinics to provide an organized system of health care for its workers. Medicare followed a similar model for the care of those enrolled, and other insurance companies followed Medicare. The outcome of these actions was creation of the managed care organizations (MCOs), which dominate the health care industry today. MCOs contract with health care systems, formulating capitation rates for payment and controlling access to, and the duration of, care. As a consequence within the hospital system, the level of acuity has increased, because of the decreasing lengths of stay and the lowering of operational costs associated with direct patient care. The impact on nursing has been an increase in workload and a decrease in staff support and resources to perform the required care.

Corporate health care systems demand a profit margin, whereas nonprofit health care systems have the burden of caring for the uninsured, causing both to try to reduce expenses to gain profits. Thus, hospitals began seeking nonlicensed providers to perform nursing care for less pay, with the few nurses remaining placed at risk for injury and malpractice by being overworked. As history was once again repeating itself, minimizing the need and significance of the nursing profession, nurses sought the support of labor unions.

THE PROBLEM: WORKPLACE VIOLENCE

Because of the prevalence of workplace violence, efforts have increased to document, research, and analyze the problem. Research has revealed that workplace violence is a bigger problem than first believed. According to the CDC (1997), 20 workers are murdered and 18,000 are assaulted weekly while on duty. In 1994, the Bureau of Labor Statistics reported that homicide accounted for 16 percent of the 6588 traumatic work-related deaths in the United States, a figure that represents more than three workers killed every day in violent attacks (U.S. Department of Labor Statistics, 1995). The Department of Justice reports that in 1994 an estimated 1.4 million persons sought health care for assault-related injuries (U.S. Department of Justice, 1997). Violence has become known as the second leading cause of death in the workplace, with the first cause being transportation related (Jenkins, 1996).

Violence is rated the leading cause of workplace death among women (CDC,

1996). Health care workers, particularly psychiatric and emergency care nurses, are at the greatest risk for workplace assaults and violence (Castillo & Jenkins, 1994; Keep & Gilbert, 1992; Lipscomb & Love, 1992). In the United States, 106 health care workers were killed during incidents of occupational violence between 1980 and 1990. This figure included 27 pharmacists, 26 physicians, 18 registered nurses, 17 nurse's aides, and 18 other health care workers (Blair, 1997). The majority of nonfatal assaults occurred in the service industry, with 27 percent occurring in nursing homes, 13 percent in social services, and 11 percent in hospitals (CDC, 1997). Fatality figures were not compiled from one central source or database, as none existed. Information was gathered from death certificates, medical examiners' records, workers' compensation reports, and questionnaires (CDC, 1996). But domestic problems also spill over into the work environment. For example, an angry husband may approach his wife at her place of employment, thereby involving coworkers in acts of violence perpetrated in the workplace.

As for abusive behaviors and victimization, limited information is available in the criminal justice and public health literature regarding the nature and magnitude of nonfatal workplace violence (CDC, 1996). The possibility of victimization increases in a variety of settings, including employment situations (1) with routine face-to-face contact with large numbers of people, (2) involving the handling of money, (3) where employees work alone or in small numbers, (4) requiring working late into the evening, (5) in high crime areas, and/or (6) that require routine travel or do not have a single worksite (Castillo & Jenkins, 1994; CDC, 1992; Jenkins, Layne, & Kisner, 1992).

When individuals were asked if they reported workplace victimization to the police, 56 percent had not, with 40 percent of those stating the event in question was believed to be minor or a private matter (Bachman, 1994). The magnitude of the problem of workplace violence is most likely far greater than ever imagined, given the definitions of violence most researchers use, inconsistent reporting methods, and victims'

unwillingness to report such problems. Of great concern is the underreporting of violence and a persistent perception within the health care industry that assaults are a part of the job (Lanza & Campbell, 1991). The inability of law enforcement to reduce violent acts contributes to the belief that society is unable to do anything to prevent violence (Petrie & Garner, 1990). This attitude of helplessness encourages the public and government to believe that preventive measures are futile (Simonowitz, Rigdon, & Manning, 1997).

Media and journals rarely report stories of nurses being attacked at work, only reporting sensational stories, such as a nurse being seriously attacked in a parking lot. Many times these assaults in parking lots have not been depicted as workplace-related violence. Occasionally, the news media may report that a nurse was assaulted while at work in a psychiatric unit, or caught in the middle of a hate crime at an abortion clinic. Society expects certain professions to tolerate violent and abusive behaviors, because their professional environments are more prone to violence. Society places the burden of tolerance on the professional caregivers, expecting them to "deal" with violent behavior.

Emergency medical services (EMS) may include such providers as paramedics, emergency medical technicians, nurses, physicians, and physician's assistants. A study of violence in EMS providers revealed that although 91 percent had experienced some sort of violence within the past year, they had not been provided with training, equipment, or policies on how to handle a violent patient (Pozzi, 1998). Their basic training provides information on how to manage a patient with a medical condition that results in combativeness, such as a head injury, and how to restrain patients to protect themselves. But Pozzi (1998) found that employees felt they were not encouraged to report issues of abuse and felt dealing with abuse was an expected part of the job. Because EMS providers work in constantly changing and unpredictable environments, their risk of exposure to violence is high. Yet the EMS provider has even fewer resources for protection and assistance than do other providers within institutional environments. The most frightening factor that Pozzi (1998) discovered was that, given a violent situation and lack of training or proper tools, providers would resort to whatever means necessary in order to protect themselves, e. g., which may have included grabbing an ax off a fire truck. The potential for liability drastically broadens with that type of "resourcefulness."

The best example of professional preparedness in prevention of workplace violence is found in the training of law enforcement personnel. Police have an understanding that they may have to encounter an unpleasant, threatening, or hazardous situation many times within their day during their career. The police have been trained and provided with policies, procedures, and equipment to manage the situation. In turn, society realizes that there must be a basic respect for law enforcement in order for their services to be effective. Therefore, punishments for assaulting a police officer are greater than for assaulting a citizen. Health care workers face assaultive situations frequently, without the benefits of training, policies, procedures, or additional security support that police officers have received.

According to Nancy Purtell Director of Behavioral Health Services, of the University of New Mexico Mental Health Center:

In several communities throughout the country, police departments experience extensive training by the local behavioral health communities to effectively deal with individuals in a psychiatric crisis at risk for endangering themselves or someone else in the community. Many of these training programs are designed after the Crisis Intervention Training [CIT, 1996] model. CIT, which began in the Memphis Police Department, has spread to the Albuquerque Police Department, Portland Police Department and others (University of New Mexico Mental Health Center, 1998).

Ms. Purtell further noted:

The model of training merges clinical knowledge and tactical skills. The programs have resulted in fewer deaths of the mentally ill, fewer injuries and deaths to officers and more of the mentally ill being taken to hospitals for care instead of being arrested for minor crimes committed as a result of their mental illness (University of New Mexico Mental Health Center, 1998).

Psychiatric facilities have provided specialized training in hospitals, such as crisis prevention intervention (CPI, 1992). CPI provides organized training to staff with techniques to prevent injury to patients and staff, using verbal de-escalation techniques to avoid critical situations. If the situation advances to a critical issue of potential violence, the CPI technique provides basic protective strategies for staff and safe physical containment techniques for controlling the patient. In comparing CPI versus law enforcement training techniques, under CPI a hospital staff member is taught to accept the assault as a clinical situation, whereas the officer is taught and given the right to arrest and press criminal charges when assaulted.

Multiple ethical dilemmas face health care providers exposed to workplace violence, including a combination of lack of policies and procedures, threats of medical malpractice, minimal safety equipment, unclear direction from management, and lack of legislative initiative to provide legal support for their responses. Nurses often view filing complaints and/or pressing charges against patients as a beach of duty to provide care.

An even greater ethical dilemma often occurs when the complaint must be filed against a physician. Physicians are perceived as those who bring work to the hospital; therefore, because hospital administration does not want to alienate the physician, hospital staff are reluctant to complain for fear of being reprimanded or scolded.

Bandura (1973) suggests that aggressive behavior is learned by imitating familial, cultural, and media events. Berkowitz (1974) reported that lack of consequences following acts of violence tends to reinforce the behavior. Messer (1988) proposes that when violence is viewed as a normal problem-solving course of action, it does not stimulate guilt feelings and therefore becomes acceptable.

Additional problems from workplace violence encompass the feelings that arise in the victim as a result of assaultive behaviors. The feelings of animosity, fear, lowered self-esteem, decreased confidence, and self-blame can eventually lead to post-traumatic stress disorder (PTSD) (Lanza, 1993; Sonnenberg, 1988). Workplace violence leads to job dissatisfaction, frequent job turnover, poor performance, hostility toward patients, repressed anger, dysfunctional home situations, and/or alcoholism or drug abuse (Lanza, 1993; Mahoney, 1991). Box 24–2 lists the results of workplace violence. All the listed factors also cause nurses to develop job burnout, quitting their professions in favor of less stressful environments.

Workplace violence can be found in correctional nursing, home health care, pediatrics, operating rooms, obstetrics, delivery rooms, intensive care units, and/or general medical nursing units. High-risk patient care areas have begun taking precautions to reduce exposure to violence (Box 24–3).

Today the majority of health care organizations have comprehensive safety plans to address areas of risk for violence within the health care organization. Employers are also setting up systems to mediate problems between staff, regardless of the nature of the issue or complaint or the relationship between the parties. The plans have been developed from new laws, research, regulatory agencies, and professional standards that provide the foundation for the content and focus of the safety plan.

In psychiatric facilities, staff who have experienced violence from a psychiatric crisis situation are provided an opportunity to debrief. **Debriefing**, as defined in the *New Mexico Critical Incident Stress Management Team Basic Training Manual*, is "a structured process integrating crisis intervention techniques with education. It is a peer driven, clinical guided discussion of a traumatic event designed to mitigate or resolve the psychological distress associated with a critical incident or traumatic event" (Community Health Systems Division of the New Mexico Department of Health, 1996).

Debriefing allows staff to assess the critical event, evaluate their emotional response, and determine their current support needs. It also allows the staff to assess the team effort to contain the crisis and the final outcome of the event. Through this process, the organization is able to provide support for employees by identifying each individual's psychological and education needs. Additionally, the organization has an opportunity to troubleshoot if flaws are identified during the debriefing. Critical incident debriefing and review of each incident allows employees and the health care organization the opportunity to prevent employee and patient injuries and improve policies and procedures for handling future critical incidents.

BOX 24-2

RESULTS OF WORKPLACE VIOLENCE

Workplace violence may result in:
- Low morale among employees.
- Destruction of property.
- Expenses for health care for injured employees or clients.
- Poor image for the organization.
- Difficulty in recruiting and retaining staff.
- Costly absenteeism.
- Lost productivity.
- Higher insurance costs.
- Emotional trauma for other workers.
- Fear, defensiveness, and distraction for the assaulted employee.

Source: Adapted from Simonowitz et al., 1997.

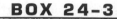

BOX 24-3

PRECAUTIONS TO REDUCE EXPOSURE TO VIOLENCE

- Place high security cameras and increase security personnel.
- Teach "verbal judo" to providers exposed to risk.
- Develop protocols for restraining patients.
- Place bulletproof glass in nurses' stations.
- Install emergency doors and entrances that prevent drive-through access from the outside.
- Install telephones with direct access to security.

THE LAW

Statutory law regulating violence within nursing practice is identified in civil and federal law, including the Civil Rights Act of 1964, Rehabilitation Act of 1973; Americans with Disabilities Act of 1990, the federal Occupational Safety and Health Administration (OSHA), state laws that regulate the Department of Public Safety and Workers' Compensation, and various state and federal laws that regulate mental health, labor practices, and tort claims. Understanding the extent of the laws as they apply to nursing practice is complex, requiring general knowledge of how these laws apply to the care of patients as well as to the nurse as the employee. No laws specifically address workplace violence toward, or abuse of, health care workers. No laws specifically regulate workplace violence, but indirectly regulate workplace violence in the following manner: acts of violence, such as murder, are classified as criminal acts; and acts or duties of the employer to protect, such as to provide a safe place to conduct work in accordance with the general duty clause, are classified under tort law. Depending on the severity of the act, violence may generally be categorized under laws governing one of the following: (1) hate crime, (2) domestic relations, (3) violent crime, (4) employment, (5) health and safety, (6) Federal Drug Administration, and/or (7) public safety.

HISTORICAL REVIEW OF THE LAW

In her book *Nursing and the Injustices of the Law*, Johnstone (1994) specifically addressed issues regarding the verbal and physical abuse of nurses by doctors, employers, and patients and the lack of law preventing such actions. Johnstone believes that the patriarchal and subordinate position of nurses in relation to hospital administrators and male physicians leaves nurses in powerless positions that the law, by omission, supports:

Whether male or female, a nurse still lacks legitimate authority as a nurse, and is legally bound to "obey" the lawful and reasonable orders of his or her superiors—the majority of whom are either directly or indirectly medical practitioners (Johnstone, 1994).

Sklar (1979) noted that, in difficult situations where a doctor insists on admitting a patient to an already overcrowded unit that is understaffed by nurses, nursing supervisors instruct nurses to cope and to "do the best you can." Peterson (1990) supports Sklar's point of view, noting that nurses are generally viewed only as employees who must work as directed.

Johnstone (1994, p. 8) contends that the rise in litigation against nurses is a reflection of nurses' being given increased responsibility rather than authority and of their being used increasingly as scapegoats by those who are more powerful and have competing interests at stake. Johnstone (1994) reported case after case in which nurses have been reprimanded, terminated, and even found guilty of manslaughter for refusing to carry out orders believed harmful to the patient. Courts often view a nurse's questioning of the doctor's orders as insubordination and disobedience (Johnstone, 1994). According to Johnstone (1994, p. 169), those who "exercise independent professional nursing judgment and who dare to evaluate and/or question a doctor's orders on the basis of their own independent professional nursing judgment run the very real risk of 'trespassing' on medical territory and of being censured accordingly."

COST OF VIOLENCE

Many states, as well as Washington, DC, identify acts of assault and violence as the leading cause of death in the workplace, over death by motor vehicle accidents (State of California, Department of Industrial Relations, 1995). Insurers report that more than 50 percent of their claims came from nonfatal assault in the health care industry ("Violence in Health Care," 1998). In 1995, 5500 workers' compensation claims were made for lost work time as a result of violence ("Violence in Health Care," 1998). These statistics do not include those who were assaulted and did not choose to report the incident or those who did report the incident but did not lose work time. According to the *Workplace Violence Reporter*, the number of assaults to health care workers "is way out of whack compared to all other occupations. The average number of work-related nonfatal assault injuries for all industries combined is 2.8 per 10,000. But looking at the nursing and personal care industry, the figure is 39.7 per 10,000" ("Violence in Health Care," 1998).

Claims paid for time taken off from work because of workplace violence–related injury, or for death benefits amount to $4.3 billion annually ("Violence in Health Care," 1998). If physical assault, emotional and mental distress, stalking, harassment, domestic violence, decreased productivity, and all other types of violence that can create lost work time were included, that figure would

be $36 billion annually ("Violence in Health Care," 1998). In Oregon, the average cost of a workers' compensation claim for violence was $8568 per injury. This figure does not include permanent total disability or fatality benefits, but only includes assaults accepted for workers' compensation claims (State of Oregon, Department of Consumer and Business Services, 1994).

EMPLOYER LIABILITY

DUTY TO PROVIDE A SAFE WORKPLACE

Ownership or control of the premises is required for imposition of premises liability. The employer owes a duty of ordinary care to protect visitors, including employees, against conditions that foreseeably pose an unreasonable risk of injury. The **general duty clause of the OSHA** (U.S.C. 29-654 (a)(l)) requires employers to provide a safe working environment (U.S. Department of Health and Human Services, 1993). According to Taylor (1995), "Negligence to protect against risk of violence also has been documented in worker's compensation and anti-discrimination laws, as well as union contracts."

The courts have identified the following key elements of the premises liability: (1) the owner/operator must have actual or constructive knowledge of the condition on the premises; (2) the condition posed must be an unreasonable risk of harm; (3) the owner/operator must not have exercised reasonable care to reduce or eliminate the risk; (4) the owner/operator's failure to use reasonable care must have proximately caused the plaintiff's injuries (see Amendment of the Uniform Jury Instructions for Civil Cases, cited in *Ford v. Board of County Commissioners*, 1996; and *Keetch v. Kroger Co.*, 1992).

The duty to provide a safe workplace requires the employer to protect or warn others from reasonably foreseeable harm and to warn of a known concealed danger. In *Coca v. Areco* (1962), the court held:

The proprietor of a place of business who holds it out to the public for entry for his business purposes is subject to liability to guests who are upon the premises and who are injured by the harmful acts of third persons if, by the exercise of reasonable care, the proprietor could have discovered that such acts were being done or about to be done, and could have protected against the injury by controlling the conduct of the other patron.

According to Buel (1995), in cases of domestic violence, an employer is more likely to know or suspect its possible occurrence than other, more random, incidents of workplace violence, for "the workplace often becomes the only place the assailant can locate and harm [the victim]." Duda (1997) also cautions, "Without knowledge about the signs of domestic violence, the risk of danger is magnified for the [victim] and the coworkers." The element of **foreseeability** requires only that the general danger, not the exact sequence of events that produced the harm, be foreseeable. The test for foreseeability has two prongs or two questions: (1) specifically, did the landowner or occupier realize or should he have realized the likelihood that such acts were occurring or about to occur; and (2) generally, did the landowner or occupier know or have reason to know from past experience of a likelihood of conduct on the part of a third person, which would endanger the safety of invitees? (*Guerrero v. Memorial Medical Center of East Texas*, 1997).

But *Guerrero* (1997) is a case that provides an example of an instance in which the hospital/employer was not held liable when an employee, while at work, was shot to death by an estranged husband. The employee had disclosed to the employer verbal abuse that she had been subject to, but had not informed the employer of the ongoing physical abuse. On the day of the employee's death, she had requested an escort from the parking lot when she arrived at work. Security personnel saw her estranged husband, asking him twice to leave the parking lot. The estranged husband appeared calm and made no threats to harm the employee. The estranged husband also did not give any indication to the employer that he was threatening, physically abusing, or seeking to harm the employee. Based on this set of facts, the court held that the hospital did not owe a duty to the employee, because the employer did not know and had no reason to know (1) that the estranged husband had been physically abusive or (2) was about to murder the employee (*Guerrero v. Memorial Medical Center of East Texas*, 1997).

Under this holding, if the employer has reason to suspect or know of the potential for workplace violence involving an employee, the employer has the duty to provide protection for the employee as well as third persons. And if a violent situation develops, the employer also has the duty to take reasonable steps to stop and/or control the incident, for example, by calling the police (*Barth v. Coleman*, 1994).

NEGLIGENCE

A claim for negligent hiring and/or retention is based on evidence of the following elements: (1) the employer was negligent in hiring or retaining the employee, that is, the employee was unfit, considering the nature of the employment and the risk posed to those with whom the employee would foreseeably associate, and the employer knew or should have known the employee was unfit; (2) there was a connection between the employer's business and the plaintiff; and (3) the negligent hiring or retention of the employee was the proximate cause of the individual's injury (*Akins v. Estes*, 1994; *Arrington v. Fields*, 1979; *Dieter v. Baker Service Tools*, 1987; *Doe v. Boys Clubs of Greater Dallas, Inc.*, 1994; *F&T Co. v. Woods*, 1979).

The New Mexico Supreme Court specifically equated the element of proximate cause with the element of foreseeability in *F&T Co. v. Woods* (1979), holding that the specific harm need not be foreseeable, but some general harm or consequence must be. Although negligent supervision or retention of an employee is similar in principle to negligent hiring, the focus is on the employer's post-hire actions. If an employer knows or should have known about an employee's violent propensities and fails to take reasonable action, the employer may be held liable.

Negligent retention is distinguished from

negligent hiring in that the former doctrine focuses on when the employer knew that an employee posed a threat to the safety of others and failed to provide protection, whereas the latter doctrine focuses on the employer's pre-employment investigation into the employee's background (*F&T Co. v. Woods*, 1979; *Los Ranchitos v. Tierra Grande, Inc.*, 1993; *Peek v. Equipment Services, Inc.*, 1995).

WORKERS' COMPENSATION

A 1992 study of violent acts that resulted in lost work days for health care providers indicated that 45 percent of injuries to health care providers were caused by patients, 31 percent by other persons, and 6 percent by coworkers or former coworkers. Of all non-fatal assaults, 64 percent occurred in service industries, 13 percent in social service agencies, 24 percent in nursing homes, and 11 percent in hospitals (BLS, 1994). A 1992 Washington State Psychiatric Facilities Survey studied two Washington state facilities, and revealed 50 percent of all workers' compensation claims from hospital employees were related to injuries from workplace assaults (BLS, 1994).

Workers' compensation provides the exclusive remedy to employees for disabling injuries incurred in the workplace "arising out of and in the course of employment" (*Gutierrez v. Artesia Public Schools*, 1978). When an injury does not fall within the Workers Compensation Act (WCA), its exclusivity provisions do not preclude recovery under other legal theories (*Sabella v. Manor Care, Inc.*, 1996). For example, under the terms of WCA, an injury must occur during the **course of employment**, meaning the injury must have occurred during the normal time, place, and/or circumstances of employment. In a previously discussed New Mexico case that did not fall under the terms of that state's WCA, an employee was shot to death while at work by the estranged husband of a coworker. The decedent had been involved in an affair with the wife of the estranged husband. Although the decedent was at his place of work, he was not working nor fulfilling his normal duties nor doing anything incidental to his work. The court held that with this set of facts the decedent was not injured in the "course of his employment" (*Gutierrez v. Artesia Public Schools*, 1978). But in another set of facts, a bank employee who was shot while delivering ransom money for release of his boss's wife was held to be acting within the course of employment and entitled to workers' compensation. The employee was handling money as he would within his banking role (*Jordan v. Farmers State Bank of Texas*, 1990).

Unpredictable behaviors encountered in the course of employment in health care facilities can also be dangerous, placing employees in situations of potential violence. Hospitals may encounter patients seeking drugs to support illegal habits. Hospitals are also known to be places where people in distress, distraught, or mentally ill are brought for purposes of treatment. Thus, the employer has prior knowledge that the employee will be working in an environment in which a hazardous condition may arise in the course of employment.

For the injury to arise out of the employment setting, it must be shown that the injury was caused by a risk that the employee was subjected to by employment (Gutierrez, 1975). In *Gutierrez v. Artesia Public Schools* (1978), the injury stemmed from a personal animosity between the decedent and the estranged husband and was not in any way related to the employment relationship. With issues involving domestic violence, the incidents are usually unrelated to the employment relationship, and WCA will not apply in most cases. However, the injured employee may file a claim against the employer under other legal theories, such as negligence and vicarious liability.

When injuries arise out of and in the course of employment, such as when one employee assaults another in a work-related matter, the exclusivity provisions of WCA may be waived only in cases where the employer had the intent to injure the employee. Thus, the **intentional assault exception** applies when an employer may be held liable for intentional torts that include an "actual intent to injure on the part of the employer" (*Gallegos v. Chastain*, 1981).

Goldberg (1997) compared remedies designed to curb violence in the United States and Great Britain. The comparative study contrasted these like nations' systems of compensation, safety, and tort laws and federal regulations for the purpose of assessing the effectiveness of these systems in deterring violence in the workplace. Goldberg (1997) reported:

Violence in the workplace, like other forms of violence, shows no signs of abatement—in fact, each new generation is immersed and indoctrinated into a culture of violence before its members ever set foot into a workplace as employees or customers.

Goldberg (1997) concluded that both systems of "compensation for American and British employees who are victims of criminal violence in the workplace is unsatisfactory." According to Goldberg (1997), the compensation systems did not get to the root cause of the violence or seek preventive measures; rather, they dealt with the aftermath of the violence. Goldberg (1997) disliked the punitive approach of seeking compensation for injury after the act of violence, as he viewed it as diminishing the intent of laws and regulations, which he believed were designed as preventive measures for containing violence in the workplace.

This study by Goldberg (1997) emphasizes the regulatory guidelines by which employers provide a safe work environment for employees in all industries: (1) OSHA regulations, within the United States; and (2) the Health and Safety Executive regulations, within the United Kingdom. These guidelines should have an enforcement strength for employers that is equitable for all industries and that supplements employers' efforts and should dramatically reduce the cost to employers, as well as reducing actual violence to employees.

The American Hospital Association was concerned that the OSHA Draft Guidelines for Workplace Prevention Programs for Health Care Workers, which recommended metal detectors within the workplace, were too costly because they "could cost . . . some $9000 to purchase each device and $100,000 to pay a guard to staff the devices on a continuous basis" (Goldberg, 1997). But as workers' compensation, Social Security, and health insurance plans place a greater financial burden on the employer, they are reluctant to spend more money for enhanced safety plans.

AMERICANS WITH DISABILITIES ACT

Employers may face liability under the Americans with Disabilities Act (ADA) when disciplining or terminating an employee's actual or threatening misconduct, if the employee's conduct can be attributed to a mental or psychological impairment. Under the provisions of ADA, if the employee makes a disability known to the employer, they must then provide reasonable accommodations to the worker, unless the individual poses a direct threat to the health and safety of others. The employer can dismiss or discipline the worker if the actual or threatened misconduct violates a workplace standard or is a direct threat, as defined under the ADA.

In a case involving ADA, the United States District Court of Minnesota ruled:

The Americans with Disabilities Act says an employer cannot discriminate against a qualified individual with a disability. A **disability** is a physical or mental impairment that substantially limits one or more major life activities. A **qualified individual** with a disability is a person who can, with or without reasonable accommodation, perform the essential functions of the job. Discrimination can include not making reasonable accommodation. By definition, reasonable accommodation does not impose an undue hardship or expense on the employer (D. Minn, 1997).

The Equal Employment Opportunity Commission (EEOC) regulations define the elements of the **direct threat standard** in the following manner:

- The employer must be prepared to show that there is significant risk of substantial harm.
- The threat must be imminent, based on the employee's current condition, and not speculation about the employee's future condition.
- The dangerousness of the employee must be based on an individual assessment of

that employee and on a reasonable medical judgment regarding the employee's condition.

- The potential for harm must be identified as significant and substantial and must be based on objective medical or other factual evidence regarding a particular individual.
- The duration of the risk must be assessed.
- The employer must determine whether the risk can be reduced or eliminated by some reasonable accommodation (EEOC, 1997).

If an employer takes action against a worker for violent conduct or for threatening violent conduct, and the employer is sued for disability discrimination under ADA, the employer may assert one or more of the following defenses: (1) the employee violated a workplace standard that is job-related for the position and consistent with business necessity; (2) the employee is unable to perform the essential functions of the job, and no reasonable accommodation exists that would enable the employee to perform the essential functions of the job; and/or (3) the employee would create a direct threat to the safety of himself or others, and no reasonable accommodation exists that would reduce or remove the danger. The mere possibility of future harm to an employee or others is not a defense under the ADA—the risk must be supported by objective evidence that is significant, specific, and current (Levin, 1995).

OCCUPATIONAL SAFETY AND HEALTH ADMINISTRATION

OSHA has traditionally been viewed as providing regulations for unsafe work practices, hazardous conditions, and exposure to hazardous chemicals or other agents. Statistics on violence in the workplace indicate that it is an increasing problem across America in all industries, in all ethnic groups, and for both sexes. Realizing that the basic regulations had not fully covered the issues of workplace violence, OSHA began working rapidly to create some guidelines for employers and workers to address the issue of workplace violence. Although these guidelines have been timely, they are only guidelines and do not carry any regulatory force behind them.

In 1996, the *Guidelines for Preventing Workplace Violence for Health Care Workers and Social Service Workers* were created by OSHA (OSHA, 1996). The guidelines define and describe the scope of workplace violence; however, the guidelines do not cover all aspects of workplace violence, for example, horizontal violence. **Horizontal violence** is vicious acts of abusiveness, sexual harassment, and throwing objects that occur among coworkers, yet frequently is interpreted as workplace violence ("Violence in Health Care," 1998). The guidelines contain suggestions on a written program, work site analysis, security provisions, hazard prevention, administrative controls, training, postincident response, record keeping, and evaluations. The guidelines also contain examples of an assault survey, policies, violence checklist, and incident report form. While the guidelines are not regulations, they benefit employers by providing a consistent method of managing the workplace violence and better documentation.

RECORDING REQUIREMENTS

According to Cal/OSHA Guidelines (State of California, Department of Industrial Relations, 1995, § 1430-1440), the following documentation of workplace violence is required to be recorded in the OSHA 200 log: loss of consciousness, restriction of work or motion, transfer to another job or termination of employment, and/or medical treatment beyond first aid. Reporting significant injuries such as assaults or homicide may be confusing to employers because they often represent a crime, which may result in a delay in reporting, as employers sort out their responsibility. Documentation of an incident does not necessarily imply that: (1) the employer or employee is at fault; (2) the injury or illness was compensable under Workers' Compensation; and/or (3) a violation of Title 8 Safety Order or a Penal Code section has occurred.

Employers are, however, required to file an Employer's Report of Occupational Injury or Illness for every injury or illness with the employer's Workers' Compensation insurer or with the Division of Labor Statistics and Research (DLSR). If the employer is self-insured, there may be additional documentation requirements for workplace violence beyond the OSHA 200 log (California Labor Code § 6409.1).

According to California Labor Code, § 6401.l(b):

In every case involving a serious injury or illness, or death, in addition to the report required by subdivision (a), a report shall be made immediately by the employer to the Division of Occupational Safety and Health by telephone or telegraph.

The term **serious injury or illness** is defined in California Labor Code § 6402(h) as "any injury or illness occurring in a place of employment . . . but does not include any injury, illness or death caused by the commission of a Penal Code violation." So, some employers may not report a death, as it may not be reportable to Cal/OSHA if it is caused by the commission of a penal code violation.

Similarly, Missouri's House Bill No. 153, § 1–7, establishes regulations designed to provide for protection from violence within hospitals, particularly emergency and trauma centers, to be monitored by the Department of Health's Hospital Safety Program. According to § 2.1 of this bill:

By July 1, 1998, all hospitals licensed pursuant to § 197.010 to 197.120, RSMo, shall conduct a security and safety assessment and, using the assessment, develop a safety plan with measures to protect personnel, patients and visitors from aggressive or violent behavior.

A significant part of the House Bill requires security training on the following topics:

General safety measures; personal safety measures; the assault cycle; aggression and violence predicting factors; obtaining patient history from a patient with violent behavior; characteristics of aggressive and violent patients and victims; verbal and physical maneuvers to diffuse and avoid violent behavior; strategies to avoid physical harm; restraint techniques; appropriate use of medication as chemical restraints; and any resources available to employees for coping with incidents of violence, including, but not limited to, critical incident stress debriefing or employee assistance programs.

These strong statements in the Missouri House Bill and by Cal/OSHA are becoming more common as various state departments of safety and local hospitals begin interpreting the application of OSHA guidelines within their organizations, to promote and provide for the safety of their employees, patients, and visitors.

Hospitals surveyed under the Joint Commission on Accreditation of Healthcare Organizations (JCAHO) incorporated many of the reporting requirements of OSHA, CDC, and others into the operational management of the care plans described in the chapter entitled "Environment of Care" in the *Joint Commission Comprehensive Accreditation Manual for Hospitals* (JCAHO, 1996). In this chapter, the term **environment** refers to:

Three basic components: building(s), equipment and people. Effective management of the environment of care includes using processes and activities to: a) reduce and control environmental hazards and risks; b) prevent accidents and injuries; and, c) maintain safe conditions for patients, visitors, and safety (JCAHO, 1996).

Data collection systems for safety concerns are identified with outcome measures demonstrating the organizational performance improvement activity. Incident reporting mechanisms require injuries of patients or staff with a moderate or severe rating to undergo further investigation. Outcomes of investigations trigger performance improvement activity and supervision by safety and risk management department personnel. Reporting, however, depends on employees' completing incident reports. As a result, some underreporting may exist because employees fear the focus will be placed on their job performance.

In 1996, the Legislature in the State of Washington considered a bill that would have forced all health care settings to develop workplace violence prevention plans as a condition of continuing licensing and certification (Washington State Bill 6643, 1996). This Senate Bill would have included security measures and policies aimed at spotting, managing, and responding to violence. The bill failed, but a legislative work group continues work on a revised bill, of which the outcome is currently unknown (Neurath, 1996).

California passed Assembly Bill No. 508 in February 1993 (amended in assembly April 22 and April 15, 1993), which included detailed information about violence and health care personnel. The bill basically identified emergency and psychiatric areas as problem areas, because of their frequent exposure and potential for violence. The Assembly Bill (1993) listed specific reporting, training, policy, staffing, physical layout, and security measures to be taken by various health care facilities for the protection of health care workers. Reporting requirements specified that any act of assault, as defined in § 240 of the California Penal Code, or battery, as defined in § 242 of the California Penal Code, against any on-duty hospital personnel shall be reported to local law enforcement within 72 hours of the incident. Any individual interfering with, or obstructing the reporting process, would be guilty of a misdemeanor.

INVESTIGATIONS

Cal/OSHA is required by California Labor Code § 6313(a):

To investigate all industrial accidents that are fatal to one or more employees or that result in a serious injury or serious exposure, unless the Division determines an investigation is unnecessary, in which case the Division shall summarize the facts indicating the accident need not be investigated and the means by which the facts were determined.

Because the California Labor Code, § 6302(h) excluded any injury or illness or death caused by the commission of a Penal Code violation from the definition of illness or injury, Cal/OSHA does not mandate a duty to respond to such accidents. But CAL/OSHA does have the authority to investigate any workplace accident on a discretionary basis, as provided by California Labor Code, § 6313(b):

The Division may investigate the causes of any other industrial accident or occupational illness that occurs within the state in any employment or

place of employment . . . and shall issue any orders necessary to eliminate the causes and prevent reoccurrence.

EVIDENCE SUPPORT

Nurses may face ostracism and reprisal from coworkers, staff from other departments, administration, and physicians after making charges against a patient, patient's family member, or other staff member. Although workplace violence has been listed as a zero tolerance issue in many workplaces, minor infractions are still tolerated. Those who dare to step out first with a complaint may find themselves with less support than expected. A good case example of this is a nurse who reported an abusive conversation between herself and a physician. She shared a taped conversation with the medical director who said he agreed verbal abuse should not be tolerated and he would take care of it, but did not. When she next went to the hospital administration, they did not follow through with any actions. The nurse retained an attorney, who then filed charges against the physician, winning the case, thus setting a strong precedence for nurses to prevent workplace violence (Ferguson, 1997).

According to Ferguson (1997), a successful outcome in a case involving workplace violence may depend on all or a combination of the following actions:

- Reporting the incident to law officials and/or seeking the guidance and counsel of an attorney.
- Keeping personal copies of evidence, such as tapes, paper work, photographs, and incident report forms submitted to the hospital, OSHA, police, and/or attorney, always storing the original evidence in a safe place outside of the workplace or with another trusted person.
- Taking the issue to the supervisor and/or through the chain of command, through the administrative hierarchy.
- Getting witness statements as soon as possible after the incident.
- Taking pictures of bruises, broken glasses, or torn clothes immediately after the incident.

- Asking a police officer to assist with photographs for evidence, because photography can be complicated, requiring advanced evidence of photography skills.
- Making a detailed report documenting all aspects of the event.
- Gathering items that may have been used as weapons, such as syringes, charts, surgical instruments, or anything thrown, involving the police if necessary, to secure these items as supportive evidence.
- Hiring a personal attorney rather than using the hospital attorney, for the hospital attorney represents and has the hospital's best interest in mind.
- Being proactive about the problem by seeking assistance, such as Critical Incident Stress Management (CISM) and legal support, counseling, or group support cumulative incidents as well as a single incident can cause post-traumatic stress symptoms.
- Confronting persons who are being abusive, in an attempt to de-escalate the situation or to let the perpetrator know the behavior will not be tolerated.

POSITION STATEMENTS

Nurses associations have developed position statements and/or news releases on violence in the workplace. For example, the Emergency Nurses Association (ENA) has written a position statement regarding violence toward health care workers (ENA, 1995). The ENA believes that health care organizations have a responsibility to provide a safe and secure environment for their employees and the public. The ENA also takes the position that emergency nurses have a right to take appropriate measures to protect themselves and their patients from injury caused by violent individuals present within the emergency setting:

ENA supports the concept of violence prevention and minimization of risk through the following measures: involvement with policy development for security issues; related education with communication techniques; education regarding gang culture; evacuation assessment skills; professional debriefing for those exposed to violence; use of

security personnel and structural/environmental controls for barriers against violence; legislation mandating use of safety controls and recognizing the rights of all involved; and collaboration with other organizations to promote safety for health care providers (ENA, 1995).

The Registered Nurses' Association of Nova Scotia (RNANS, 1997) *Position Statement on Violence in the Workplace* states that:

Violence or the threat of violence in the work place must not be tolerated under any circumstances . . . and that all workplaces implement a zero-tolerance policy towards violence in the workplace. . . . The registered nurse has a responsibility to prevent and reduce violence in the workplace in all practice domains . . . acknowledges that under-reporting of violent incidents is common.

A Canadian Nurses Association (CNA) news release condemned deliberate violence against health care workers including the death of a nurse from British Columbia working in Chechnya, who was one of six international aid workers (CNA, 1996).

CLINICAL PRACTICE GUIDELINES REGULATING VIOLENCE IN NURSING

The American Nurses Association (ANA) Standards of Clinical Nursing Practice and the Standards of Psychiatric-Mental Health Clinical Nursing Practice state:

Standards of Care pertain to professional nursing activities that are demonstrated by the nurse through the nursing process. These involve assessment, diagnosis, outcome, identification, planning, implementation, and evaluation. The nursing process is the foundation of clinical decision-making and encompasses all significant action taken by nurses in providing care to all clients (ANA).

Within these written standards, the nursing process focuses on the care of a patient in a disease process. Nursing care involves assessing physical and psychological symptoms; diagnosing the problem(s); identifying treatment outcomes, and identifying the treatment interventions; planning the course of care; implementing the plan; and evaluating the progress of the patient's course of treatment. If in any one of these segments of the nursing process the potential for violence is identified, preventive measures must be incorporated in the plan of care. To be successful in preventing violence, on behalf of the patient and the treating staff, knowledge of the types of preventive measures must be available through education programs and skills training. Most psychiatric and some medical facilities have established treatment protocols designed for critical incidents.

JCAHO has placed a significant focus on nursing practice standards related to the use of restraints and seclusion and management of the combative patient. Hospital standards of care related to restraints and/or seclusion do not address the potential for staff exposure to violence. Psychiatric facilities have mandatory training requirements for all personnel, with structured courses designed to maintain both patient and staff safety and care during a psychiatric crisis. Mandatory training provides health care workers with the necessary skills to prevent harm to the patient in crisis, while protecting themselves from injury. Many psychiatric facilities have trained staff in crisis techniques, also offering the training to personnel who work in high-risk areas in acute care hospitals, such as emergency rooms, and to security personnel. Crisis techniques give staff working in potentially violent areas tools for protection for self and others.

Prevention of violence is often the most successful tool. Hospital systems have created many means of prevention of violence, such as specific interventions identified in nursing policies and procedures and standards of practice that clearly define care and safety for patients at risk for injury. Patient rights advocates have increasingly required hospitals and health care organizations to monitor the use of restraints and/or seclusion to prevent violations of a patient's civil rights. Clinical procedures have to clearly outline a progressive plan, using the least restrictive means of care for patients at risk for harm to self and/or to others. Psychiatric facilities have in the past been most skilled at writing and implementing these least restrictive policies, because of the need to comply with the federal and state mental health codes. These codes govern health care workers' duties in the maintenance of patient rights, while caring for incompetent individuals.

The most recent JCAHO standards have emphasized the importance of standards applying to the care of patients in hospitals and clinics:

Staff roles and responsibilities in the use of special treatment procedures are identified for all appropriate disciplines. Restraint or seclusion may be used in response to emergent, dangerous behavior; addictive disorders; as an adjunct to planned care (JCAHO, 1996).

The emphasis on staff knowledge of these special crisis procedures is essential to their having the tools to protect patients and themselves in a violent situation. "Staff needs to be able to use restraint or seclusion when essential to protect patients from harming themselves, other patients, or staff" (JCAHO, 1996).

Clinical justification for the use of seclusion and restraints requires organizations to write clear policies and procedures, provide proper and adequate training for staff, and provide adequate support in the event a critical incident causes harm.

ETHICAL CONSIDERATIONS

JCAHO presents a compelling statement to hospital organizations about patient rights and organizational ethics, setting a standard that for most hospitals is a constant balancing act. According to JCAHO (1996):

Patients have a fundamental right to considerate care that safeguards their personal dignity and respects their culture, psychosocial, and spiritual values. These values often influence patients' perceptions of care and illness. Understanding and respecting these values guide the provider in meeting the patients' care needs and preferences.

Nurses are advocates for patients, thus, volitional acts of violence against a nurse by a patient are confusing for the nurse. Appropriate safeguards for self-protection may not be taken by the nurse if the patient's actions are misread by the nurse.

Further, staff may ignore the needs of patients who have demonstrated behaviors that are difficult to manage. For example, confused patients may act out without fully understanding what they are doing, whereas other patients may knowingly be demanding, hostile, and abusive. Hostile actions may alienate, frighten, or frustrate the caregiver; so when the patient's call light goes on, there may be an extended time before it is answered. Also, nurses may avoid patients when family members are visiting, because family members may be abusive or overly demanding. Such avoidance may impede the patient's treatment plan or facilitate complications in patient care, because managing the patient's adversative behavior was not appropriately included in the plan of care.

Nurses also face an ethical dilemma when reporting the abusive and/or violent patient or family member to an authority figure. Nurses need to understand that beyond guidelines established in hospital policy and procedure, workers' compensation, and/or OSHA, charges can be brought not only against the perpetrator but also the employer if necessary.

Nurses must also be aware that the patient may bring charges against them for abusive acts, for example, restraining and medicating the patient after the medication has been refused. Misunderstanding policies and procedures regarding restraints opens the nurse to charges of abusive treatment, false imprisonment, and/or violation of a patient's civil rights.

Nurses must be alert to patient care avoidance, for this avoidance may become generalized to patients with a certain diagnosis with whom the nurse has had previous negative experience. In certain sections of the country, avoidance may also be directed toward certain ethnic groups in the form of prejudice. For example, if a hospital tends to receive a large majority of a certain ethnic group involved in violent crimes, gangs, drug trade, and violent behavior in the hospital, then generalizations may be made that persons of that ethnicity tend to be violent. These generalizations may impede the care provided to the patient from that ethnic group.

MALPRACTICE CONSIDERATIONS

Health care professionals have a duty to comply with appropriate standards of practice. In crisis situations, nurses must be aware of not only patient but employee rights and the practice standards that govern the decision-making process. Crisis events that are well documented prevent the nurse, hospital, or other practitioners from unnecessary involvement in litigation, as long as policy and procedure, as well as practice standards, were maintained.

FUTURE RESEARCH CONSIDERATIONS

Many agencies conduct research into workplace violence. However, violence toward health care workers still remains the least studied and documented, even though it is one of the most prevalent forms of workplace violence. Research studies should be conducted on the roadblocks that exist, which prevent adequate reporting of violent acts, and the reason charges are not pursued against perpetrators of violence within the health care industry. Thorough research of actual assault cases may also lead to a variety of answers, for documentation of real cases in any significant quantity is difficult to find. Most research has involved surveying persons who are recalling violence that has occurred. Although recall is helpful in identifying the issue of violence, recalled information may be exaggerated or diminished over time. Research regarding patients who were involved in the incidents may be useful in attempting to determine whether there was something the health care worker did or said that the patient perceived as provoking the violent response.

Few articles have been written about nurse-to-nurse abuse or physician-to-nurse abuse, both noted to be ongoing problems. These types of abuse may require detailed research and investigations to ascertain the extent of the problem. Observations have been made regarding environmental factors that may contribute to violent behavior, including decreased services to the poor and ill, early release of patients from mental health facilities without proper follow-up, ease in obtaining weapons, and increased use of violence to solve problems. Other issues to research may include the history of violence as a means of controlling or intimidating others; violence related to cultural or religious differences; fear or anger at the caregiver for denial of wishes, wants, or needs; poor management styles; and failure to respect and understand the needs of employees (Simonowitz et al., 1997).

SUMMARY

Violence toward health care workers is reaching significant proportions. The reasons for this rise in violence is debatable; the fact that violence exists is not. History has shown that violence is growing and becoming an accepted part of the health care industry, with nurses consistently facing violence in daily nursing duties. Those outside the nursing profession are unaware of how much violence nurses meet on a regular basis in treating patients.

Legislation is needed to provide support for health care workers in preventing workplace violence, for example, making violence toward health care personnel as great an offense as violence against law enforcement personnel. But currently, legislation specific to violence against health care workers is trivial to nonexistent. Hospitals and health care facilities are taking more aggressive actions to provide protection and security measures to improve the situation and provide a means of prevention. In controlled environments, prevention measures are much easier to manage. However, for those who work in prehospital care, prevention measures are harder to provide. For the health care provider, the first line of defense is becoming educated and learning to manage violent situations. The most important measures must provide procedures for reporting the violent incident and debriefing support for all persons involved. Too often, health care workers minimize the occurrence of such incidents without understanding the long-term implications of violence for themselves, other health professionals, and society. Legislation must create stronger consequences for workplace violence, which may occur only with better reporting and support from nursing organizations.

POINTS TO REMEMBER

- Under the provisions of the Americans with Disabilities Act, if the employee makes a disability known to the employer, reasonable accommodations must be provided to the worker, unless the individual poses a direct threat to the health and safety of others.
- Psychiatric nurses routinely confront violent situations in the workplace.
- On a peer level, workplace violence occurs when a nurse is abused by other nurses, physicians, and/or their employers.
- Although sexual harassment in the workplace is now illegal under federal law, these laws have not stopped its occurrence.
- In type II workplace violence, the agent is either the recipient or the object of a service provided by the affected workplace or the victim, e. g., the assailant is a current or former client, patient, customer, passenger, criminal suspect, inmate, or prisoner.
- Health care providers are at risk for type II workplace violence.
- During the Crimean War and World War I, society first began to see potential value in the career of nursing within organized health care.
- With the advent of the industrialization of the United States, unions had a significant impact on the delivery of health care, providing avenues for employees to deal with business and making changes in working conditions.
- In the early 1980s, nurses began joining unions at a rapid rate.
- The logging industry was the first to contract with local hospitals, physicians,

and clinics to provide an organized system of health care for its workers.

- According to the CDC (1997), 20 workers are murdered and 18,000 are assaulted weekly while on duty.
- Violence has become known as the second leading cause of death in the workplace, with the first cause being transportation related.
- Violence is rated the leading cause of workplace death among women.
- Health care workers, particularly psychiatric and emergency care nurses, are at the greatest risk for workplace assaults and violence.
- The best example of professional preparedness in prevention of workplace violence is found in the training of law enforcement personnel.
- No laws specifically address workplace violence toward, or abuse of, health care workers.
- Insurers report that more than 50 percent of their claims came from nonfatal assault in the health care industry.
- The average number of work-related nonfatal assault injuries in the personal care industry is 39.7 per 10,000.
- Ownership or control of the premises is required for imposition of premises liability.
- The employer owes a duty of ordinary care to protect visitors, including employees, against conditions that foreseeably pose an unreasonable risk of injury.
- If the employer has reason to suspect or know of the potential for workplace violence involving an employee, the employer has the duty to provide protection for the employee as well as third parties.
- Workers' compensation provides the exclusive remedy to employees for disabling injuries incurred in the workplace.
- When an injury does not fall within the Workers' Compensation Act (WCA), its exclusivity provisions do not preclude recovery under other legal theories.
- Under the Americans with Disabilities Act, discrimination can include not making reasonable accommodation.
- Under the Americans with Disabilities Act, a reasonable accommodation for a dis-

abled worker may not impose an undue hardship or expense on the employer.
- The standard of care in psychiatric facilities is the least restrictive environment.

REFERENCES

Akins v. Estes, 888 S.W.2d 35 (Tex. App.-Amarillo 1994).

Arrington v. Fields, 578 S.W.2d 173, 178 (Tex. Civ. App.-Tyler 1979, writ ref'd n.r.e.).

Bachman, R. (1994). Violence and theft in the workplace. In *U.S. Department of Justice crime data brief* (NCJ-148199). Washington, DC: U.S. Government Printing Office.

Bandura, A. (1973). *Aggression: A social learning analysis.* Englewood Cliffs, NJ: Prentice Hall.

Barth v. Coleman, 118 N.M. 878 P.2d 319 (1994).

Bell, C., Stout, N., Bender, T., Conroy, C., Crouse, W., & Myers, J. (1990, June 13). Fatal occupational injuries in the United States, 1980 through 1985. *Journal of the American Medical Association, 263*(22), 3047–3050.

Berkowitz, L. (1974). Some determinants of impulsive aggression: Role of mediated association with reinforcement of aggression. *Psychology Review, 81,* 165–176.

Birkland, P. (1991). Violence and assault: Part of the job? [Guest editorial]. *Journal of Emergency Nurses, 17*(5), 267–268.

Black's Law Dictionary (5th ed., p. 105). (1979). St. Paul, MN: West Publishing.

Blair, D. (1997, April). Violence in the health service. *The Safety & Health Practitioner,* pp. 20–24.

Buel, S. (1995). *Domestic violence: More prevalent than you think* [Video]. Wilkes-Barre, PA: Wyeth-Ayerst Laboratories Public Library Network and Karol Media.

Bullock v. Parkchester General Hospital, 3 App Div 2d 254, 160 NYS2d 117, affd 4 NY2d 894, 174 NYS2d 471, 150 NE2d 772, 1957.

Canadian Nurses Association. (1996, December 18). *National nursing association condemns violence against health care workers.* Ottawa: Author.

Castillo, D. N., & Jenkins, L. E. (1994, February). Industries and occupations at high risk for work related homicide. *Journal of Occupational Medicine, 36*(2), 125–132.

Centers for Disease Control. (1992, September). *Homicide in U.S. workplaces: A strategy for prevention and research* (Pub. No. 92-103). Washington, DC: U.S. Department of Health and Human Services, National Institute for Occupational Safety and Health.

Centers for Disease Control. (1993, December). *Homicide in the workplace* (Doc. # 705003). Washington, DC: U.S. Department of Health and Human Services, National Institute for Occupational Safety and Health.

Centers for Disease Control and Prevention. (1996, June). *Violence in the workplace: Risk factors and strategies* (Current Intelligence Bulletin 57). Washington, DC: U.S. Department of Health and Human Services, National Institute for Occupational Safety and Health.

Centers for Disease Control and Prevention. (1997, June). *NIOSH facts: Violence in the workplace* (Pub. No. 96-100 Doc. 705002). Washington, DC: U.S. Department of Health and Human Services, National Institute for Occupational Safety and Health.

Cleary, D. M. (1975). A non strike for patient care. *Modern Healthcare, 3*(6), 42–44.

Coca v. Areceo 71 N.M. 186, 189, 376 P.2d 970, 973 (1962).

Coleman v. Mercy Hospital, Inc. So.2d 91 (Fla.App. 3 Dist 1979).

Community Health Systems Division of the New Mexico Department of Health. (1996). *New Mexico critical incident stress management team basic training manual*. Sante Fe, NM: Author.

Crisis Intervention Training (CIT). Seminar presented by the Albuquerque Police Department and the University of New Mexico Health Sciences Center at the University Health Center in April, 1996.

Crisis Prevention Intervention. Seminar presented at Brookfield, Wisconsin, in 1992.

Czubinsky v. Doctors Hospital, 188 Cal.Rptr.685 (App 1983).

Daley v. St. Agnes Hospital, Inc 490 F Supp 1309 (1983).

Dieter v. Baker Services Tools, 739 S.W.2d 405, 408 (Tex. App.-Corpus Christi 1987).

Doe v. Boys Clubs of Greater Dallas, Inc., 868 S.W.2d 942, 950 (Tex. App.-Amarillo 1994).

Donnelly, G., Mengel, A., & King, E. (1975). The anatomy of a conflict. *Supervisor Nurse, 6*(11), 28–38.

Duda, R. (1997, December). Workplace domestic violence: Intervention through program and policy development. *American Association of Occupational Health Nurses Journal, 5*(12), 619–623.

Emergency Nursing Association. (1995). *Position statement* (Revised). Park Ridge, IL: Author.

Equal Employment Opportunity Commission. (1997a, March 27). *Guidelines on psychiatric disabilities and the American with Disabilities Act*. Washington, DC: Author.

Equal Employment Opportunity Commission. (1997b). *Technical assistance manual* (pp. 10–11). Washington, DC: Author.

F&T Co. v. Woods, 92 N.M. 697, 594 P.2d 745 (1979).

Ferguson, S. (1997, Winter). Dissection of a verbal abuser. *Revolution-The Journal of Nurse Empowerment*, pp. 19–22.

Flannery, R. (1995). *Violence in the workplace*. New York: Crossroad Press.

Flinders Medical Center Incorporated v Tingay (appeal) case (1984) 51(1) IRSA 1 (Print No 4/1984, No 108 of 1983).

Floyd v. Willacy County Hospital District, 706 SW 2d 731 (Tex. App 13 Dist 1986).

Ford v. Board of County Commissioners, 188 N.M. 134, 897 P.2d 766 (1994).

Gallegos v. Chastain, 95 N.M. 551, 553, 624 P.2d 60, 63 (Ct.App. 1981).

Gasparis, L. (1990). *Nurse abuse: Impact and resolution*. New York: Power Publications.

Goldberg, R. S. (1997). 397 victims of criminal violence in the workplace: An assessment of remedies in the United States and Great Britain. *Comparative Labor Law Journal, 18*, 397.

Goodman, R., Jenkins, L., & Mercy, J. (1994, December 7). Workplace-related homicides among health care workers in the United States, 1980 through 1990. *Journal of the American Medical Association, 272*(21), 1686–1688.

Guerrero v. Memorial Medical Center of East Texas, 938 S.W.2d 789 (Tex. App.-Beaumont 1997).

Gutierrez v. Artesia Public Schools, 92 N.M. 112, 114; 583 P.2d 476, 478 (Ct. App. 1978).

Hanewinckel v. St. Paul's Property and Liability, 611 So.2d 174 (La.App. 5th Cir. 1992, writ denied) 614 So.2d 65 (La. 1993).

Hospital of St. Vincent of Paul v. Thompson, 116 Va. 101, 81 S.E. 13, 18, 51 L.R.A., N.S., 1025.

House Bill No. 153, 89th General Assembly, State of Missouri, 1997.

W. Guy Hudson and Grandview Osteopathic Hospital, Plaintiffs in error v. Zona Blanchard, 294 P.2d 544 (Okl. Sup.Ct. 1956).

Hunter, G. (1984, July). Nurse gets $8000.00 settlement. *The Advertiser (Adelaide)*, p. 24.

Jenkins, E. L. (1996). Workplace homicide: Industries and occupations at high risk. *Occupational Medicine State of Art Reviews, 11*(2), 219–225.

Jenkins, E. L. , Layne, L. A., & Kisner, S. M. (1992, May). Homicide in the workplace: The US experience, 1980-1988. *American Association of Occupational Health Nurses, 40*(5), 215–218.

Johnston, R. (1979, May). Nurses and job satisfaction: A review of some research findings. *Australian News Journal, 5*(11), 23–27.

Johnstone, M. J. (1994). *Nursing and injustices of the law*. Sydney, Australia: Bailliere Tindall.

Joint Commission on Accreditation of Healthcare Organizations. (1995). *Accreditation manual for hospitals*. Oakbrook, IL: Author.

Joint Commission on Accreditation of Healthcare Organizations. (1996). *Joint Commission comprehensive accreditation manual for hospitals* (pp. EC1, RI-1, TX-7). Oakbrook, IL: Author.

Jones, M. (1985). Patient violence: Report of 200 incidents. *Journal of Psychosocial Nursing and Mental Health Service, 23*(6), 12–17.

Jordan v. Farmers State Bank of Texas, 791 S.W.2d 1 (Mo.Ct.App. 1990).

Keep, N., & Gilbert, P. (1992). California Emergency Nurses Association's informal survey of violence in California emergency departments. *Journal of Emergency Nursing, 18*, 433–442.

Keetch v. Kroger Co., 845 S.W.2d 262, 264 (Tex. 1992).

Lanza, M. (1993, January). The reactions of a nursing staff to physical assault by a patient. *Hospital and Community Psychiatry, 34*(1), 44–47.

Lanza, M., & Campbell, D. (1991). Patient assault: A comparison study of reporting methods. *Journal of Nursing Quality Assurance, 5*, 60–68.

Lenehan, G. (1991). Notes on the "Violence in the emergency department" theme issue. *Journal of Emergency Nursing, 17*(5), 263–264.

Levin, R. L. (1995). Workplace violence: Navigating through the minefield of legal liability. *Lab Law, 2*(2) at 178.

Lipscomb, J., & Love, C. (1992, May). Violence toward health care workers: An emergency occupational hazard. *American Association of Occupational Health Nurses Journal, 40*(5), 219–226.

Los Ranchitos v. Tierra Grande, Inc., 116 N.M. 222, 861 P.2d 263 (Ct. App. 1993).

Lowery-Palmer, A. (1982). The cultural basis of political behavior in two groups: Nurses and political activists. In J. Muff (Ed.), *Socialization, sexism, and stereotyping: Women's issues in nursing* (pp. 189–202). St. Louis: C.V. Mosby.

Lungsford v. Board of Nurse Examiners, 684 S.W.2d 391 (Tex. App. 3 Dist. 1983).

Lybecker, C. (1998). *Violence against nurses: A silent epidemic* [On-line]. Available: http://www.nurseadvocate.org

MacLean, M. (1903, June 24). Lecture by Miss MacLean to the nurses of the Victorian Trained Nurses' Association. *Una, 1*(2), 34–35.

Mahoney, B. (1991). The extent, nature, and response to victimization of emergency nurses in Pennsylvania. *Journal of Emergency Nursing, 7*(5), 282–294.

Matter of the Amendment of the Uniform Jury Instructions for Civil Cases Vol.35, No.6, SBB 6 (1996).

Memorial Hospital v Oakes, Adm'x, 200 Va. 878, 108 S.E.2d 388.

Messer, S. (1988). Research on cultural and socioeconomic factors in criminal violence. *Psychiatry Clinics of North America, 11*, 511–525.

Mundy v Department of Health, 620 So.2d 811 (La. 1993).

Neurath, P. (1996, September 6). Violence stalks the health care field: Nurses, social workers in Washington more likely to be attacked than police officers or jailers. *Puget Sound Business Journal* [On-line]. Available: www.ameity.com/seatttle/stories/09/696/focus1

Nightingale, F. (1867). Suggestions on the subject of providing, training and organizing nurses for the sick and poor in workhouse infirmaries. Reprinted in L. R.

Seymer (Ed.), *Selected writings of Florence Nightingale*. New York: Macmillan.

Nurses and workplace violence. [On-line]. Available: http://www.nurseadvocate.org

Occupational and Health Safety Administration: General Duties Clause, U.S.C. § 29–654(a)(1) 1970.

Occupational Safety and Health Act in Title 29 Code of Federal Regulations, Part 1904 (BLS, 1986a).

Occupational Safety and Health Administration. (1996). *Guidelines for preventing workplace violence for health care workers and social service workers* (Publication No. 3148). Washington, DC: U.S. Department of Labor.

Palmer, I. S. (1984, July/August). Nightingale revisited: Pages from nursing history. *Nursing Outlook*.

Peek v. Equipment Services, Inc., 906 S.W.2d 529 (Tex. App.-San Antonio 1995).

Peterson, R. L. (1990, February). *Nurses Act review: Industrial implications*. Seminar presented at Australian Nursing Federation (Victorian Branch), Prince Henry Hospital, Melbourne.

Petrie, C., & Garner, J. (1990). Is violence preventable? In D. Besharov (Ed.), *Family violence: Research and public policy issues*. Washington, DC: AEI Press.

Pozzi, C. (1998, August). Exposure of prehospital providers to violence and abuse. *Journal of Emergency Nursing, 24*(4), 320–323.

Random House college dictionary (Revised Edition, p. 1469). (1982). New York: Random House.

Registered Nurses' Association of Nova Scotia. (1997, June). *Position statement on violence in the workplace*. Dartmouth, NS: Board of Directors.

Reverby, S. (1987). *Ordered to care: The dilemma of American nursing* (pp. 1850–1945). New York: Cambridge University Press.

Roanoke Hospital Association v. Jeane Franklin Hayes 133 S.E.2d 559(Va.Sup Ct App. 1963).

Rosenberg, C. E. (1987). *The care of strangers: The rise of America's hospital system*. New York: Basic Books.

Ryan, J., & Poster, E. (1989). The assaulted nurse: Short term and long term responses. *Archives of Psychiatric Nursing, 3*(6), 323–331.

Sabella v. Manor Care, Inc., 121 N.M. 596, 599, 915 P.2d 901, 905 (1996).

Simonowitz, J., Rigdon, J., & Manning, J. (1997, June). Workplace violence: Prevention efforts by the occupational heath nurse. *Journal of the American Association of Occupational Health Nurses, 45*(6), 305–318.

Sklar, C. (1979, February). You and the law—On trial! *Canadian Nurse, 75*(2), 8–10.

Smith, S. (1862, September 13). Female nurses in hospitals. *American Medical Times*, p. 5.

Soloff, P. H. (1987). Emergency management of violent patients. In R. E. Hales & A. J. Frances (Eds.), *Psychiatry Update: American Association Annual Review* (Vol. 6). Washington, DC: American Psychiatric President.

Sonnenberg, S. (1988, December). Victims of violence

and post traumatic stress disorder. *Psychiatric Clinic of North America, 11*(4), 581 590.

Spring, N. M., & Stern, M. B. (1998). Nurse abuse? Couldn't be! *Nurse Advocate Web Page* [On-line]. Available: http://www.nurseadvocate.org/nurse_abuse.html

Stake v. Woman's Division of Christian Service, 73 N.M. 303, 387, P.2d 871 (1963).

Stanely, L. (1979, March). Doctors: What to do when the MD is wrong. *Registered Nurse, 42*(3), 22–30.

State of California, Department of Industrial Relations, Division of Occupational Safety and Health. (1995, March 30). *Cal/OSHA guidelines for workplace security* (Revised, pp. 7–9). Sacramento, CA: Author.

State of Oregon, Department of Consumer and Business Services. (1994). *Violence in the workplace, Oregon, 1988 to 1992: A special study of workers' compensation claims caused by violent acts.* Salem, OR: Information Management Division.

Taylor, R. (1995). *The rockem-sockem workplace* [On-line]. Available: http://www.ecovote.org/fund/workplace/

Turner v. Jordan, 957 S.W.2d 815 (Tenn., 1997).

University of New Mexico Mental Health Center. (1998). Interview with Nancy Purtell, Director of Behavioral Health Services, Albuquerque, NM.

U.S. Department of Health and Human Services. (September, 1993). *Preventing homicides in the workplace* (Publication No. 93-109). Cincinnati, OH: Author.

U.S. Department of Justice. (1997, August). *Violence-related injuries treated in hospital emergency departments* (NCJ-156921). Washington, DC: Author.

U.S. Department of Labor Statistics. (1995). *Census of fatal occupational injuries: 1994* (News Bulletin 95-288). Washington, DC: Author.

Violence in health care profession enormous and costly problem. (1998, May). *Workplace Violence Reporter, 4*(5), 1.

Walker v. Memorial Hospital, 187 Va. 5, 7; 45 S.E.2d 898.

Webster's new world dictionary (3rd. ed., p. 6). (1988). New York: Simon and Schuster.

Workplace violence: Navigating through the minefield of legal liability. *Labor Law, 2*(2), 178.

SUGGESTED READINGS

Callahan, R., & Callahan, J. (1996). *Thought field therapy and trauma: Treatment and theory.* La Quita, CA: Thought Field Therapy Training Center. [On-line]. Available: http://www.tftrx.com

Carmel, H., & Hunter, M. (1989). Staff injuries from inpatient violence. *Hospital and Community Psychiatry, 40*(1), 41–46.

Castillo, D. N. (1994). Non-fatal violence in the workplace: Directions for the future research. In *Questions and answers in lethal and non-lethal violence.* Proceedings of the Third Annual Workshop of Homicide Research Working Group, Washington, DC, National Institute of Justice.

Mitchell, J., & Bray, G. (1990). *Emergency services stress: Guidelines for preserving the health and careers of emergency services personnel.* Englewood Cliffs, NJ: Prentice-Hall.

Upledger, J. (1997). *Your inner physician and you.* Berkeley, CA: North Atlantic Books.

Upledger, J., & Vredevoogd, J. (1983). *Craniosacral therapy.* Seattle, WA: Eastland Press.

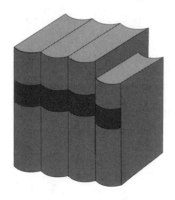

Chapter 25

TELENURSING

Mary E. O'Keefe

ETHICAL CONSIDERATIONS AND CONFLICTS
RECOMMENDATIONS FOR RESEARCH AND
MALPRACTICE PREVENTION
RESEARCH
MALPRACTICE PREVENTION
Potential Malpractice Issues
Strategies to Prevent Malpractice
Protected Delivery of Electronic Documents
Informed Consent Regarding Telenursing
Confidentiality
SUMMARY
POINTS TO REMEMBER
REFERENCES
INTERNET RESOURCES
SUGGESTED READINGS

KEY WORDS

Cellular Pirates	On-line Service
Civil Remedies	Otherwise Privileged
Core Requirements	Party States
Cybercare	Patient
Decryption	PDF Files
Demand Management	Pecuniary Damages
Electronic Media	Peripherals
Encryption	Person
E-Zine	Police Power Doctrine
Hacking	Public-Key Encryption
Health Care	Reasonableness
Health Care Communications	Remote State
Health Care Information	Sniffing
Health Care Provider	Spoofing
Home State	Stark Amendment Violation
Host State	Telecommunications
Malice	Telemedicine
Multistate Licensure Compact	Telenursing
Multistate Licensure Privilege	Telepathology
Mutual Recognition Model	Teleradiology
National Council of State Boards of Nursing (NCSBN)	Valid Disclosure
	Virtual Nursing
	Waive
	Willful Disclosure
	Wire Communication

459

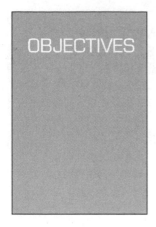

OBJECTIVES

Upon completion of this chapter, the reader will be able to:

- Discuss the definitions of telenursing.
- Identify duties to reasonably protect the confidentiality of health care information under the Uniform Health Care Information Act.
- Discuss the right to privacy during telephone communications.
- Discuss the right to privacy during computer communications.
- Identify legal issues and trends in telenursing.
- Identify research issues and trends in telenursing.

INTRODUCTION

Telehealth speeds access to health care in city and rural areas. In mid-1997, the Office of Rural Health Policy, U.S. Department of Health and Human Services, reported that 416 rural hospitals have functioning telehealth programs while 564 facilities are in the planning stages to establish a telehealth program (Grande, 1997, pp. 59–60).

Telehealth is a combination of telemedicine and telenursing (Tabone, 1997). The American Nurses Association (ANA) defines telehealth as the delivery of health care, removing time and distance barriers, via electronic media (ANA, 1997a; Walker, 1997). The ANA then defines telenursing as a form of telehealth, with "the focus on nursing via telecommunications" (ANA, 1997a; Walker, 1997).

"Telenursing is any nursing at a distance, mediated in whole or in part through electronic means" (Yensen, 1996, p. 213). Nurses who participate in telenursing participate in **demand management**, because these nurses are asked by the patients to help them manage their decisions in self-care and to decide when to physically enter the health care system. Through telenursing, nurses respond to demands from patients for assistance in the management of their health care needs relative to safety, confidentiality, ethical issues, logistics of care, and access and application to the health care system (Tabone, 1997).

The purpose of this chapter is to assist the nurse in preventing malpractice, avoiding legal risks, and reducing liability by becoming "telenursing literate" (Abke & Mouse-Young, 1997, p. 3).

HISTORICAL PERSPECTIVE

For years, telephone conversations have occurred between nursing health care providers (the terms *nurse* and *provider* are used interchangeably in this chapter) and colleagues for years, but no particular terminology was used to describe this practice (Yensen, 1996, p. 213). With the advent of new technology, the practice of health care has moved to a variety of other electronic media. The electronic practice of health care, encompasses telemedicine and telenursing, and is labeled telehealth.

Telenursing evolved from, and derives its definition from, previous definitions of telemedicine. Before the advent of telenursing, the American Medical Association (AMA) Council on Medical Education defined **telemedicine** as "the provision of health-care consultation and education using telecommunication networks to communicate information . . . [and] . . . medical practices across distance via communications and interactive video technology" (Abke & Mouse-Young, 1997, p. 3).

Granade (1997, pp. 59–60) defined telemedicine as "the use of communications technology to transmit health information from one location to the other" (Telemedicine Research Center, 1997). The ANA defines telemedicine as a subset of telehealth, including teledermatology and telepsychiatry (ANA, 1997a; Walker, 1997). Telemedicine also includes the transmission of radiographic (**teleradiology**) and pathology images (**telepathology**). Telenursing involves telemetry and telephone triage (Granade, 1997).

The most simplified, comprehensive definition of telemedicine has been identified by Abke and Mouse-Young (1997, p. 3): "telemedicine is purely a transfer of medical data, medical information, and medical expertise between two points—point A and point B." The definition of telemedicine may be paraphrased to formulate a comprehensive definition of **telenursing**, which is the electronic transfer of nursing data, nursing information, and nursing expertise between two points. According to Gobis (1997, p. 14), telenursing encompasses the "practice of nursing by an electronic medium, such as telephone, facsimile, Internet, computerized health care systems, diagnostic and video imaging, or video-conferencing."

PRACTICE GUIDELINES IN TELENURSING

The benefits of telenursing have been many and varied. Benefits of telenursing to the profession include the development of nursing skills and opportunities. These benefits to nursing provides: (1) an ongoing update of skills, through electronic nursing rounds or case conferences; (2) reduction of professional isolation; (3) easy access to pharmacology resources and literature; (4) promotion of consultation and corroboration with colleagues; and (5) permission for the nurse practitioner to assess the patient in the patient's environment (Abke & Mouse-Young, 1997, p. 4).

The hospital benefits by providing more cost efficient and effective patient care. These benefits are demonstrated as: (1) a reduction in emergency room visits, as a result of an increase in home health monitoring via telephone, (2) an efficient expansion of the duties and responsibilities of the home health care practitioner, and (3) maintenance of the socioeconomic viability of rural hospitals, as they are able to retain patients (Abke & Mouse-Young, 1997, p. 4).

Ultimately, insurance companies are the greatest beneficiaries. Insurance companies benefit by: (1) decreasing administrative costs, (2) reducing duplication of services, and (3) more efficiently using nursing resources (Abke & Mouse-Young, 1997, p. 4).

The transmittal of health care information is subject to a variety of state and federal laws and regulations. On the federal level, one of the laws regulating the utilization of health care information via telenursing is the Uniform Health Care Information Act (UHCIA, 1997). There is nothing written in the nursing or legal literature regarding the application of the UHCIA to telenursing. Therefore, the definitions and principles of the UHCIA that are applicable to telenursing are taken from a standard legal reference, American Jurisprudence Second Supplement.

UNIFORM HEALTH CARE INFORMATION ACT

The provisions of the Uniform Health Care Information Act (UHCIA, 1997) govern the flow of health care information. Under the UHCIA, **health care** is any care, service, or procedure administered by the provider, such as diagnosis, treatment, and maintenance of the patient's physical or mental condition, and/or that affects the structure and/or any function of the body (Physicians & Surgeons, Etc. (a), 1999; UHCIA, 1997, § 1–101, 1–102).

PATIENT HEALTH CARE INFORMATION

The federal government passed the UHCIA for the purpose of protecting health care information. **Health care information** is:

any information, whether oral or recorded in any form or medium [emphasis added], that identifies or can readily be associated with the identity of a patient and relates to the patient's health-care. The term includes any record of disclosure of health-care information" (Physicians & Surgeons, Etc (a), 1999; UHCIA, 1997, § 1–101, 1–102).

The government has a public interest in ensuring the patient's right to confidentiality or privacy, even when the health care information is held by someone other than the patient (the terms *confidentiality* and *privacy* will be used interchangeably). Under the terms of the UHCIA, the **patient** is the person who receives health care and who has received health care, including the deceased. Further, a **person** may be: (1) an individual, or a patient; (2) a legal or commercial entity, such as a health care provider; or (3) a government entity or agency, such as a managed care organization or correctional facility (Physicians & Surgeons, Etc (a), 1999; UHCIA, 1997, § 1–101, 1–102).

To maintain the patient's trust and confidence, the provider must have rules ensuring that health care information is not improperly disclosed. The UHCIA defines a **health care provider** as a person licensed, certified, or authorized by law to provide health care in the ordinary course of business or practice of their profession, such as a nurse (Physicians & Surgeons, Etc. (a), 1999; UHCIA, 1997, sections 1–101, 1–102). The health care information of the patient must be protected because it is personal and sensitive and, if improperly used or released by the provider, may result in significant harm to the patient's interests in privacy, health care, or other interests (Physicians & Surgeons, Etc (a), 1999; UHCIA, 1997, § 1–101, 1–102).

According to the UHCIA, patients must have access to health care information to allow the patient to make informed decisions to provide informed consent and correct inaccurate or incomplete information that may be in the medical records. The movement of patients and health care information has also compelled the need for uniform laws, because of: (1) the movement occurring across state lines, (2) the access and exchange of health care information between providers from central data banks, and (3) the developing trend toward multistate providers (Physicians & Surgeons, Etc (a), 1999; UHCIA, 1997, § 1–101, 1–102). The terms of the UHCIA also identify the legal implications of transmittal of health care information while practicing telenursing.

LEGAL IMPLICATIONS OF THE UHCIA

The legal implications of telenursing are well identified within the provisions of the UHCIA. Primarily, the legal implications of telenursing fall under the categories of the: (1) standard for disclosure, which is that of reasonableness; (2) nurse's potential for civil and criminal liability, including damages; and (3) elements necessary in order for the nurse to obtain a valid disclosure authorization from the patient.

STANDARD OF REASONABLENESS

The standard that the provider must follow under the UHCIA (Physicians & Surgeons, Etc (a), 1999; UHCIA 1997, § 7-101) to protect the confidentiality of health care information is that of **reasonableness**. Failure by the nurse and/or health care provider to use reasonable safeguards to secure the confidentiality of all health care information that is maintained or accessed may result in criminal and/or civil liability and penalties under the UHCIA (Physicians & Surgeons, Etc (a), 1999; UHCIA 1997, § 8-101). For example, the nurse may be found guilty of a misdemeanor and/or may be punished by a fine not exceeding $10,000 and/or imprisonment for a period not exceeding 1 year for conviction of: (1) **willful disclosure** of health care information, a penalty which may be applied in instances when the nurse knew or should have known that the disclosure was prohibited; (2) presenting a certification or disclosure authorization to obtain health care information from another provider, known to be false; and/or (3) examining and/or obtaining health care information from another provider by bribery, theft, or misrepresentation of identity (Physicians & Surgeons, Etc (a), 1999; UHCIA 1997, § 8-101).

The appropriate law enforcement agency may maintain a civil action against the nurse to enforce the terms of the UHCIA (Physicians & Surgeons, Etc (a), 1999; UHCIA 1997, § 8-102). The **civil remedies**, or judicial relief, available to the patient under the UHCIA (Physicians & Surgeons, Etc (a), 1999; UHCIA 1997, § 8-103) include the patient's right to maintain the following legal actions against the nurse: (1) a court order requiring the nurse to comply with the confidentiality provisions of the UHCIA; (2) recovery of **pecuniary damages**, or the amount of losses sustained by the patient because of the violation of confidentiality; and (3) if the nurse acted with **malice**, that is by actions that were willful or grossly negligent, the patient may recover an amount up to $5000 in excess of pecuniary damages. However, a nurse who relies in good faith on a disclosure authorization is not liable for disclosures made in reliance on that certification (Physicians, & Surgeons, Etc., 1999; UHCIA, 1997, § 8-103).

VALID DISCLOSURE UNDER THE UHCIA

Under the general provisions of the UHCIA, the nurse has a **valid disclosure** for release of health care information only with the written authorization of the patient. Without written disclosure, the nurse may not disclose the patient's health care information, because oral permission does not result in a valid disclosure. Further, the provider must maintain for 3 years a record of all those persons who have examined, in whole or in part, a patient's health care information. This record of disclosure must include the name, address, affiliation, persons receiving or examining the information, date of receipt or examination, and a description of the infor-

mation disclosed (Physicians, & Surgeons, Etc., 1999; UHCIA, 1997, § 2-101).

In order for the nurse to disclose the patient's health care information under the UHCIA, a valid disclosure authorization by the patient must be: (1) written, dated, and signed by the patient; (2) specify the type or nature of information to be disclosed; and (3) identify the person to whom the health care information will be disclosed. The provider must keep the authorization or revocation with the patient's health care information from which the disclosures were made (Physicians, & Surgeons, Etc., 1999; UHCIA, 1997, § 2-102).

The nurse must observe specific restrictions in the disclosure of the patient's health care information. For example, the signing of the disclosure does not waive any other rights the patient may have under law, such as right to confidentiality of records not specifically disclosed. Nor does the authorization permit disclosure of health care information received by the provider more than 6 months from the date of the signing of the disclosure (Physicians, & Surgeons, Etc., 1999; UHCIA, 1997, § 2-102).

The patient may revoke the health care information disclosure authorization any time, unless the disclosure is necessary to ensure payment to the provider for health care already delivered, or other substantial action has been taken in reliance on the health care information, such as the initiation of a lawsuit based on the information. As noted previously, the patient cannot maintain a claim against the nurse for good faith reliance on a disclosure that was withdrawn without notice (Physicians, & Surgeons, Etc., 1999; UHCIA, 1997, § 2-103).

Health care information may be disclosed by the provider, without authorization by the patient, in specific situations identified under state law. For example, the provider may disclose without authorization health care information by the patient to the extent that a recipient needs to know the health care information. The provider may need to have access to the health care information for directory information, unless the patient specifies otherwise. Or disclosure may be made by the provider as required by law, such as reporting information regarding communicable disease to health authorities to protect the public, or a psychiatric profile of an inmate to law enforcement agencies (Physicians, & Surgeons, Etc., 1999; UHCIA, 1997, § 2-104).

Or, a provider in response to a compulsory civil process or discovery in any judicial, legislative, or administrative proceeding, may disclose health care information in the specific instances identified under state law.

RIGHT TO PRIVACY AND ELECTRONIC MEDIA

The federal government, through the UHCIA, regulates the use and access to health care information. But the federal government has developed another set of regulations to control **health care communications**, that is health care information being electronically wired by the provider. These regulations are designed to guarantee the patient's right to privacy of health care communications when telenursing is practiced via electronic media.

Telenursing involves point-to-point contact between peers, nurse and patients, consumers, nursing educators and students, and patients within support groups. This point-to-point contact is made through a variety of **electronic media**, including but not limited to telephone, radio, television, electronic networks such as the Internet and intranets, fax, voice mail, and pagers (Yensen, 1996, p. 213).

These communication media facilitate and expand the nurse's ability to provide patient care, through (1) teleconferencing, (2) telephone triage, (3) telecollaboration, and (4) retrieving health care records and information from databases via voice-activated technology.

The computer and telephone are two forms of electronic media used for health care communications. Health care information transmitted electronically via these media becomes an electronic form of communications. Therefore, the UHCIA governs the right to privacy of electronic forms of health care information transmitted via the electronic media, such as computer and telephone.

Use of the computer and telephone to transmit health care information has an impact on the nurse-patient relationship, because the nurse has a duty to reasonably protect the privacy of the patient's health care information. The ANA defines the electronic communications of health care information as **telecommunications** (ANA, 1997a; Walker 1997). The privacy of health care communications transmitted via computer and telephone across state lines is also governed by the UHCIA, which guarantees the patient the right to confidentiality of medical records, except in certain instances that are often not well defined. In general, patients do not **waive**, or give up the right to, the privilege of confidentiality in all health care information simply because of a signature on a disclosure authorization.

Electronic health care information is a wire communication under the Federal Wiretap Statutes (1993, § 2510[1]), a **wire communication** is defined as:

Any [health care] communication made in whole or in part through the use of facilities for the transmission of communications by the aid of wire, cable, or the like connection between the point of origin and the point of reception furnished or operated by any person engaged as a common carrier in providing or operating such facilities for the transmission of interstate or foreign communications.

Nurses transmit health care information routinely via telephone and computer. The original and most common method of transmitting health care information used by the nurse over decades has been via the telephone.

RIGHT TO PRIVACY VIA THE TELEPHONE

Under the Federal Wiretap Statutes, a telephone conversation falls under the category of a wireless communication (*Forsyth v. Barr*, 1994). Thus, wiring health care information via a telephone does not likely result in a waiver of the privilege of confidentiality by the patient. Federal Wiretap Statutes expressly provide that an available privilege is not waived with interception of a telephone communication, whether or not (1) it is being transmitted over land-based telephone lines, a cordless telephone, or a cellular telephone; (2) the transmission contains voice or data, such as facsimile; and/or (3) the interception is intentional or inadvertent or even unauthorized (Hricik, 1997, p. 106).

Although the UHCIA statutes have not been thoroughly tested, it seems highly unlikely that the interception of wired health care communications would have an impact on an otherwise valid claim of confidentiality by the patient. Telephonic health care communications, including voice and facsimile, may be **otherwise privileged**, or categorized as privileged by other characteristics than just being a private communication (Hricik, 1997, p. 106; *United States v. Turner*, 1975/1976). Historically, Congress intended to subordinate the law in the interest of preserving and creating otherwise privileged communications in four relationships: (1) physician-patient, (2) lawyer-client, (3) clergyman-confidant, and (4) husband-wife (Hricik, 1997, p. 106; Senate Report No. 1097, 1968).

In general, the provisions of federal law stipulate that confidential health care communications do not lose their privilege because they are intercepted. The interception of health care communications would not impact on an otherwise valid claim of confidentiality by the patient (Hricik, 1997, p. 106; *United States v. Turner*, 1975/1976).

The threshold issues for the nurse in electronically transmitting health care information include the following considerations: (1) is the health care communication otherwise privileged under state law; and/or (2) do the UHCIA and Federal Wiretap Statutes apply under federal law? As a general principle, under both state and federal law, the patient does not waive the right to the confidentiality of his or her health care information if it is intercepted or reviewed while being electronically wired.

The disclosure of even unprivileged information by the provider can cause harm to the patient. Under the administrative law of the state boards of nursing, the nurse has a duty in general to protect the confidentiality of all information regarding the patient. Therefore, absent the patient's consent or legal exception, the transmission of any information regarding the patient may violate the nurse's duty of confidentiality to the patient (Hricik, 1997, p. 106).

Objectively, telephone communications are not often inadvertently overheard or misdirected. Equipment used to intercept land-based telephone calls is illegal to possess. Telephone communications can also be intercepted by unauthorized listening, such as picking up the extension of the telephone. Regular landline communications made by the provider regarding the patient's health care information are confidential. These conversations are made under circumstances where confidentiality is reasonably ensured and there exists a reasonable expectation of privacy for the patient (Hricik, 1997, p. 106).

The confidentiality of health care communications is not guaranteed on land-based telephones. But health care communications of the provider are subject to the protection provided under the Fourth Amendment, that is, protection from unreasonable search and seizure (Hricik, 1997, p. 107; *Katz v. United States*, 1967). Federal statutes protect the provider's land-based telephone communications against interception, preventing the waiver of an otherwise available privilege to the patient (Federal Wiretap Statute of 1968, § 2517(4); Hricik, 1997, p. 107).

Federal Wiretap Statutes provide a remedy of civil damages to the patient if the oral health care communication of the provider is intercepted, disclosed, and/or intentionally used and criminal penalties for intentional interception of healthcare communications (Federal Wiretap Statute of 1968, § 2520(a) and § 2511, respectively; Hricik, 1997, p. 107).

Further, if the provider's health care communications are illegally intercepted, they cannot be admitted as evidence in any proceeding, whether or not the information is privileged (Federal Wiretap Statute of 1968, § 2515; Hricik, 1997, p. 107). Even with the actual risk of misdirection or interception, the discussion of the patient's confidential health care information by the provider during a land-based telephone call does not result in a violation of the provider's duty of confidentiality to the patient. The patient's expectation of confidentiality need not be guaranteed or an absolute expectation. The patient's expectation of confidentiality of his or her health care communications need only be a "reasonable" expectation (Hricik, 1997, p. 107).

RIGHT TO PRIVACY VIA THE CORDLESS TELEPHONE

A technological distinction exists between telephone communications conducted via a cordless rather than a land-based telephone. A broadcast of the provider's communication is made between the handset and the base station of the cordless telephone. According to *United States v. Smith* (1992/1993, p. 177), the cordless telephone actually uses a radio signal. A cordless telephone consists of a base unit, which is attached to the land-based telephone line. A mobile unit transmits the radio signals that carry the provider's health care communications to and from a base unit (Hricik, 1997, p. 107).

Under the 1992 Amendments to the Federal Wiretap Statutes, cordless telephone communications are protected to the same degree as land-based telephone communications. The fact that the cordless telephone broadcasts health care communications over FM radio frequencies does not destroy the patient's reasonable expectation of confidentiality. With either innocent or intentional interception of the provider's health care communications, the patient's privilege is not lost (Federal Wiretap Statutes of 1968, 1992 Amendments, § 2510(1) and § 2512(a); Hricik, 1997, p. 108).

In summary, unintended interceptions of cordless health care communications can occur through devices such as other cordless telephones, FM radios, and baby monitors. But under federal criminal and civil law, intercepted cordless telephone communications cannot be introduced into evidence, even though there is no privilege of patient confidentiality. Whether or not to discuss a confidential health care communication over a cordless telephone then becomes an issue of balancing the risks of harm versus the

benefits to the patient. When the risk of disclosure of the health care information would cause greater harm than benefit to the patient, the provider should make the cordless telephone call only after the patient has been informed of the potential risks of disclosure of the health care communication and agreed in writing to allow the provider to make the cordless transmission regarding their health care (Hricik, 1997, p. 108).

RIGHT TO PRIVACY VIA THE CELLULAR TELEPHONE

Cellular telephones are similar to cordless telephones because they broadcast the provider's health care communications to a receiving station, which in turn transmits the communication over a land-based telephone line. But the provider's cellular telephone communication is not as easily intercepted as a cordless telephone communication.

Cellular telephones do not transmit the provider's health care communications within a frequency range capable of inadvertent interception by airway users, cordless telephones, or listeners of FM radio (Hricik, 1997, p. 108). Cellular telephone communications are commonly intercepted inadvertently by other cellular telephone users. Scanners can intercept cellular telephone communications. Scanners purchased before 1993 are still legal. **Cellular pirates** use scanners and other technology to intercept and sell telephone health care communications (Hricik, 1997, p. 108).

Since 1986, cellular telephone communications have the same legal protection and right to privacy as land-based telephone communications. Thus, interception of the provider's cellular telephone health care communications is a federal crime, and the patient's privilege of confidentiality is not lost. Considering the ease with which the provider's cellular telephone communications are intercepted by other cellular telephones, the provider must also weigh the risks of harm versus benefits to the patient of disclosure using this type of health care communications. Again, when the risk of harm is greater than the benefit to the patient, the provider should make the cellular communication only after the patient has been informed of the potential risks of disclosure of the health care communication and agreed in writing to allow the provider to make the cordless transmission regarding his or her health care (Hricik, 1997, pp. 109–110).

LEGAL IMPLICATIONS OF TELENURSING

Because there are no reported legal cases involving telenursing practice, Gobis (1997, pp. 8–10) drew analogies from four telemedicine malpractice claims based on telehealth issues related to failure to properly diagnose a medical condition and failure to promptly examine a patient with a life-threatening condition.

On analyzing these telehealth cases, Gobis (1997, p. 10), a nurse-attorney, concluded courts are willing to find that a duty is owed by the provider to the patient, even though health care is provided over the telephone. Gobis further concluded that the scenario in which telehealth is provided is analogous to the scenario in which telenursing is provided, in the following manner, as nurses: (1) give advice; (2) have direct contact, through verbal interaction, with the patient; (3) refer patients to treating providers, if the patient's symptoms and/or treatment can wait until the next day; (4) refer patients to emergency facilities for urgent symptoms and/or treatment; (5) have access to the patient's health care information; (6) share control of the course of treatment with the patient; and (7) charge for their services.

Gobis (1997, p. 10) summarized her opinion by stating that the courts are likely to find that nurses who give telephone advice owe a duty to the patient and could be held liable for negligence and/or malpractice. Gobis (1997) also analyzed telemedicine cases involving patient relationships.

The issue of whether or not a consultation between a treating provider and a specialist/consultant establishes a provider-patient relationship is a frequently litigated issue (Gobis, 1997, pp. 10–13). The majority opinion of the court is that:

Telephone consultations in which the consultant does not examine or speak with the patient do not create a sufficient tie between the consultant and the patient to form a [provider]-patient relationship. . . . "The majority of jurisdictions have determined that a [provider-provider] consultation which involves an informal opinion or recommendations is insufficient to establish a duty on the part of the consultant" (Gobis, 1997, pp. 10, 12).

But other case law also exists that holds that a provider-patient relationship can be established even though the provider had no contact with the patient. Based on these cases, Gobis (1997, p. 12) concluded that in analogous situations, the determination of the existence of a nurse-patient relationship may depend on whether the patient: (1) obtained and/or relied on the nurse's health care advice; (2) received health care advice or just an informal opinion or a recommendation; (3) had direct contact from the nurse; (4) was examined by the nurse; (5) was referred for teleconsultation or treatment; (6) had the health care records examined by the nurse; (7) was charged for telenursing services by the nurse; and/or (8) was receiving treatment under the control of the nurse.

RIGHT TO PRIVACY VIA COMPUTER

As communication technologies have advanced, nurses have used other media in addition to the telephone to transmit health care information. Since the mid-1980s, nursing practice has evolved into the era of telenursing via the computer.

According to Yensen (1996, p. 213), electronic media through which the computer wires health care communications include: (1) intranets, or local area networks, such as those within hospitals; and (2) Internets, or wide area networks, such as a global network. An on-line Internet or intranet service provides wire communications, as defined under the Federal Wiretap Statutes (Federal Wiretap Statutes, 1992, § 2510(1); Hricik, 1997, p. 112). A number of privacy issues arise in relation to the transmitting of the patient's health care communications via the computer. These issues involve the wiring of health care communications (1) directly from provider to provider, (2) via private networks or intranets, (3) via semi-public networks, and/or (4) via the Internet.

PROVIDER-PROVIDER HEALTH CARE COMMUNICATIONS

Provider-to-provider health care communications commonly are wired or transmitted via an intranet within the employer's individual organizational network. Nurses use intranets for access to: (1) policies and procedures, (2) care maps, (3) clinical protocols, (4) standards of care, (5) formularies, (6) drug databases, (7) nursing knowledge bases, and (8) decision support systems (Yensen, 1996, p. 214).

Within the provider's intranet network exists a reasonable expectation of privacy. But within the provider's Internet network, which communicates health care information directly over land-based telephone lines, the reasonable expectation of privacy is not lost (Hricik, 1997, p. 110; Jarvis & Tellman, 1996).

For example, a fax sent via computer or telephone between two providers containing health care information is an electronic digital communication sent over a land-based telephone line, subject to a right of confidentiality or privacy by the patient. Even the possibility that the fax may be misdirected by the provider does not destroy the patient's right to claim the privilege of confidentiality. According to Hricik (1997, p. 110), the patient's digital health care communications transmitted by the provider over a land-based telephone line in whatever form has the same right to privacy as oral health care communications transmitted over a land-based telephone line.

PRIVATE NETWORK HEALTH CARE COMMUNICATIONS

As discussed previously, private network wiring or communicating of health care information is an everyday occurrence within the provider's organization. These health care communications, usually wired via e-mail with or without attachments, are entirely over land-based telephone lines located within the internal structure of the provider's organization. Even if requiring outside telephone lines to reach outlying sites of the provider, these health care communications are clearly made with a reasonable expectation of privacy by the provider and are subject to the privacy rights of the patient (Hricik, 1997, p. 110).

SEMI-PUBLIC NETWORK PASSWORD–PROTECTED ENCRYPTED HEALTH CARE COMMUNICATION

Under the UHCIA, if the provider transmits health care information via computer over an external e-mail network with reasonable security, then the health care communications are subject to a reasonable expectation of confidentiality by the patient (Jarvis & Tellman, 1996; *National Emp. Serv. Corp. v. Liberty Mut. Ins. Co.*, 1994; *State v. Canady*, 1995.) Secure networks may include, for example, Prodigy, Earthlink, AT&T, America Online, or Microsoft Network. The basic distinction between internal and external semi-public on-line service is that anyone who pays may have access to the on-line service (Hricik, 1997, p. 110).

A legal distinction exists between internal and external computer networks. Providers who have access to a private network are bound by a duty of confidentiality to the employer. Thus, inadvertent or intentional interception or transmission of health care communications over an internal computer network has no effect on the patient's right to privacy and claim of privilege of confidentiality (Hricik, 1997, p. 111).

Those who are paid members of a semi-private on-line service do not have a duty of confidentiality to the provider or sender of the health care information transmitted via e-mail. But, under the Fourth Amendment, what a provider wants to keep confidential, even on a computer network with public access, may be constitutionally protected

(Hricik, 1997, p. 111; *Katz v. United States*, 1967).

The court in *United States v. Maxwell* (1995) applied the *Katz* (1967) principle, holding that an e-mail stored in a semi-public on-line service, such as America Online, was subject to a reasonable expectation of privacy. The court reasoned:

[The provider and/or patient] clearly had an objective expectation of privacy in those [health care communications] stored in computers which he alone could retrieve through the use of his own assigned password. Similarly, [the provider and/or patient] had an objective expectation of privacy with regard to messages he transmitted electronically to other [providers within] the service who also had individually assigned passwords. Unlike [health care communications] by cordless telephones, or calls made to a telephone with six extensions, or telephone calls which may be answered by anyone at the other end of the line, there was virtually no risk that [the provider's] computer transmission could be received by anyone other than the intended recipients (see also, Hricik, 1997, p. 111).

Under the *Maxwell* (1995) holding, the provider who is a subscriber to semi-public on-line service can send health care communications to another provider who accesses the same on-line service with a password and have a reasonable expectation of privacy in the patient's health care information. But there is contrary court ruling regarding the expectation of privacy in communications transmitted between providers on semi-public on-line services (see also, Hricik, 1997, p. 111).

In a case from which principles of disciplinary law may be applied analogously to potential state nursing board actions against the nurse-provider, a state bar association's ethics committee analyzed whether or not a lawyer could provide legal advice over an on-line service without violating the duty of confidentiality, absent consent of the client. The professional disciplinary committee reasoned that adequate information must be obtained to identify a client and make a complete inquiry into the issues. The disciplinary committee further reasoned that, even if privileged communications are transmitted via private electronic mail rather than

through public notices on electronic bulletin boards, by the very nature of an on-line service, the system operators may gain access to any of the client communications occurring within the on-line service. The disciplinary committee offered the opinion that the client's confidentiality must be maintained when any communications are wired via electronic media, unless the client has given a written waiver of the right to confidentiality (Hricik, 1997, pp. 111–112; South Carolina Bar Advisory Op., 1995).

Although the on-line operator has access to every e-mail sent by the provider, under federal law it is unlawful for the operator to read every e-mail. Operators of electronic communication services may intercept communications only to protect the rights or property of the on-line service. But that on-line service cannot observe or randomly monitor health care communications, except for mechanical or service quality control purposes (Federal Wiretap Statutes, 1968, § 2511 (2)(a)(i); Hricik, 1997, p. 112].

Two federal laws are applicable to health care communications wired via semi-public network and password-protected on-line services. First, under the Federal Wiretap Statutes (1968/1992, § 2510 *et seq.*), operators in an **on-line service**, which is an electronic Internet communication service, may observe or randomly monitor health care messages *only* for mechanical or service quality control checks. According to one could not imagine a situation in which the monitored health care information would need to be disclosed by the operator for the protection of the rights or property of the on-line service purposes (Hricik, 1997, p. 112).

Second, under the UHCIA, health care information is any form or medium of information, oral or recorded, that can identify or is associated with the patient and relates to his or her health care (Physicians & Surgeons, Etc. (a), 1999; UHCIA, 1997, § 1-102). This definition clearly covers the electronic form of health care communications wired by the provider over an on-line service and, thus, would also be subject to a right to privacy by the patient under the UHCIA.

INTERNET HEALTH CARE COMMUNICATIONS

The Internet was developed in response to an experimental project of the Department of Defense. The Internet is currently a collection of more than 50,000 networks, which link 9 million computers in 90 countries, of which 40 million people have access to its information and tools (Hricik, 1997, p. 112, citing *Shea on Behalf of American Reporters v. Reno*, 1996).

A distinction exists between the mechanism for sending an electronic communication between a provider's computer to a password-protected mailbox and one sent over the Internet. The e-mail sent over the Internet:

. . . goes from the [provider's] computer [via a land-based telephone line] through several intermediate computers—each of which is owned by third parties—before reaching the recipient's mailbox. In addition, the [health care] e-mail can be replicated and split into separate "packets" of information as it is being transmitted: thus multiple copies can exist at any given time, but they may each be but a portion of the whole (Hricik, 1997, p. 112).

The purpose of breaking the health care information down into separate packets is to ensure that, even if part of the Internet is damaged by enemy attack, the message will get through (Hricik, 1997, p. 112; Jarvis & Telleman, 1996; and *Shea on Behalf of American Reporters v. Reno*, 1996).

Although a nurse-provider may have a host computer with a unique Internet address, that host computer will not be the only computer that has access to the information highway. The electronic health care information will not go directly from the provider's host to the recipient's host computer. The health care communication may be sent through as many as a dozen routers, or computers owned by third parties, which help distribute the health care communications via the Internet (Hricik, 1997, p. 114). [As with cellular and cordless telephone communication, the electronic health care communication is broadcast over the Internet and may also be intercepted while temporarily stored in any router.] But as previously noted, the Internet router may only observe and monitor the health care communication for mechanical or service quality control checks (Federal Wiretap Statutes, 1968, § 2511(2)(a)(i); Hricik, 1997, p. 114).

Further, the provider must analyze the nature of the health care communication to assess whether there exists a reasonable expectation of privacy by the patient. The health care communication is wired through land-based telephone lines to the intermediate computers or routers. When wired, the same laws that protect land-based telephone calls protect health care communications. Interception of an Internet health care communication also requires a wiretap. Thus, the security of a health care communication wired over the Internet via telephone lines has the same expectation of privacy as an ordinary phone call (Hricik, 1997, p. 114, citing, Gidari, 1996; *State v. Cartson*, 1996).

ENCRYPTED MESSAGES

The major difference between electronic messages wired via the Internet and land-based telephone lines is that the health care communication may be accessed while stored in the router's computer. According to the holding in *United State vs. Maxwell* (1995), an encrypted health care communication wired over the Internet would most likely be subject to a reasonable expectation of privacy (Bensinger, 1996; Hricik, 1997, p. 114).

Encryption is an electronic technology by which the provider electronically locks or encrypts the health care communication and the receiver has the electronic key to open the message by **decryption**. The most common form is **public-key encryption**, which simply means the decryption key is kept secret by the receiver of the health care communication. But the encryption key is made public and may be posted on the Internet or given to the provider by diskette or e-mail (Bensinger, 1996; Hricik, 1997, p. 114).

According to Hricik (1997, p. 114), if a provider wires an encrypted health care communication over the Internet, and reasonably believes that only the intended recipient has a key to decode the message, then the patient about whom the encrypted communication is the subject has a reasonable expectation of privacy in the wired information. In general, encrypted Internet health care communications retain a privilege of confidentiality.

ISSUES AND TRENDS

According to Anders (1997), telenursing triage is growing at a rate of 25 percent per year (see also, Horton, 1997). The interest in learning and sharing information about telenursing is also growing. The American Academy of Ambulatory Care Nursing has developed its own Internet **e-zine**, or electronic magazine, entitled *Telephone Nursing Telezine* (Horton, 1997; Webster, 1996). A review of the nursing and legal literature revealed a wide variety of legal issues and trends in telenursing, whose answers will be of interest to the nurse as health care provider. These issues related primarily to the subject of nursing licensure.

NURSING ISSUES

Under the **police power doctrine** found in the Tenth Amendment, the states are given the authority to regulate health care for the safety and security of their citizens (Gobis, 1997, p. 13). But telenursing envisions a country with no state lines. This vision of nursing practice creates actual and potential telenursing licensure and/or regulation issues (Gobis, 1997, pp. 14-16).

Horton (1997) is of the opinion that professional nursing organizations and regulatory agencies should implement core requirements in telenursing practice, as suggested by Simpson (1997). These **core requirements** would be defined as standards for telenursing practice, which would "blend the scopes of practice across state boundaries" (Horton, 1997).

Nurse practice acts do not specifically address the use of the telephone to provide nursing care. A few of the state boards of nursing have offered opinions that telephone advice and triage are encompassed within the scope of nursing practice. The Wisconsin State Board of Nursing, for example, is of the opinion that telephone triage must be conducted according to a protocol or standing order that provides for the supervision by a physician, dentist, or podiatrist and that would involve nursing, but not medical, diagnosis. In contrast, the Emergency Nurses Association has developed a position statement that states that emergency room (ER) nurses should not render telephone diagnosis or treatment (Gobis, 1997, pp. 7–8).

Gobis (1997, p. 8) is of the opinion that:

A quality assurance program should be utilized to ensure quality control of telephone triage. . . . [I]t is widely recognized that the use of the telephone in providing nursing advice falls within the scope of nursing practice. All states and many professional organizations agree that *if nursing services are provided, the practice constitutes nursing . . . how nursing services are delivered makes no difference . . . nursing advice provided in-person, by telephone, or electronically constitutes the practice of nursing* [emphasis added].

LICENSURE FOR TELENURSING PRACTICE

Congress passed the Telecommunications Reform Act of 1996 (TRA) in an effort to develop: (1) standards for telehealth practice, (2) policies for reimbursement, and (3) an infrastructure within which to practice telehealth (Board of Nurse Examiners of the State of Texas, 1998a). No state legislatures have passed statutes to specifically control telenursing (Gobis, 1997, pp. 13–14).

Since the TRA was passed, a number of nursing organizations have been involved in defining telenursing practice. Other organizations have assembled task forces to address this issue. One of these organizations, the **National Council of State Boards of Nursing** (NCSBN), is not only studying the issue but drafting model rules to regulate nursing practice across state lines (Gobis, 1997, pp. 13–14). The NCSBN has been exploring multistate licensure through endorsement (Grande, 1997, p. 60).

The NCSBN is a nonprofit organization composed of the boards of nursing from the 50 states, the District of Columbia, and the five territories of the United States. The trends in telehealth have prompted the NCSBN to examine barriers to practicing nursing across state lines and improve access to care for the patient/consumer (Board of Nurse Examiners of the State of Texas, 1998a).

The NCSBN recognizes that the practice of nursing via electronic means (that is, telenursing) is the practice of nursing across state lines. Nursing practice across state lines is defined as occurring:

... when a nurse in one state crosses a state line to practice or when, through telecommunications technology, the nurse teaches nursing, consults with other providers or directly communicates with clients and their families in another state (Board of Nurse Examiners of the State of Texas, 1998a).

Citing the Executive Summary of the Telemedicine Report to Congress, Horton (1997) identifies two alternatives to multistate licensure. The **mutual recognition model**, is a method through which the **host state,** or the state in which the patient resides and/or the nurse's services will be provided, agrees to legally recognize the standards under which the nurse practices telenursing. After 3 years of study, the nursing regulation model recommended by the Task Force was the mutual recognition model. The NCSBN adopted the model in August 1997, and an interstate compact to implement the model, in December 1997. The compact was implemented in January of 2000, when the NCSBN data bank became operational.

TELENURSING ACROSS STATE LINES

Grande (1997, p. 60) points out that the nurse who staffs a telephone advice line, for a hospital network or managed care organization with a multistate network, provides nursing care to patients in states in which they are not licensed. As there is no law regulating telenursing, Grande (1997) suggests that the nurse practicing nursing across state lines may want to consider one or all of the following actions to prevent disciplinary actions: (1) obtaining licenses in states in which the patients are located, (2) consulting the state licensure board for a written opinion on the scope of practice relative to telenursing, (3) consulting the employer's policy and procedure manual on nursing licensure, and (4) consulting the employer's legal counsel about the issue, obtaining a written opinion.

Multistate Licensure Compact

The **multistate licensure compact** is a contract between states and is the mechanism by which the mutual recognition model will be implemented by the NCSBN to provide telenursing across state lines (Texas Nurses Association, 1998a, p. 5). Those states that are members of the compact are called **party states**. Under the compact, the nurse's state of residence—the state that will grant the license, set the licensure standards, and take disciplinary action under that license—is referred to as the **home state**. A **multistate licensure privilege** is the authority to practice in any of the party states (Texas Nurses Association, 1998a, p. 5).

According to the Texas Nurses Association (1998a, p. 5), the practice of nursing occurs where the patient or recipient of nursing services is located. The practice standards are set in the **remote state**, or any state in which the nurse practices other than the home state. As there are no uniform standards between states for recognition of advanced practice nurses, the multistate licensure compact will not include these professional nurses (Texas Nurses Association, 1998a).

IMPLEMENTING ORDERS FROM OUT-OF-STATE PHYSICIANS

Grande (1997, p. 60) also poses the question of the nurse's legal liability for implementing orders from an out-of-state physician. Grand (1997, p. 60) again suggests that the nurse should follow the same preventive measures as the nurse practicing telenursing across state lines, including reviewing any attorney general's opinions on the issue.

The attorney general of the state of Mississippi has determined that, before physicians that are licensed out-of-state may give orders they must also be licensed by the state of Mississippi. The attorney general did not address the liability of the nurse who does or does not follow such orders (Grande, 1997, p. 60).

TELENURSING STANDARDS

The ANA has identified other telenursing issues that will need to be considered, including: (1) how the scope of nursing practice will be changed or expanded; (2) whether the standards of clinical practice will need to be revised; (3) how the lack of personal contact will change the nurse-patient relationship; (4) what education is needed in the use of telecommunication equipment; and (5) the development of practice guidelines (Walker, 1997). The rapidly growing amount of legislation has only increased the number of legal issues that have been raised relative to telehealth. Many of these legal issues are specific to telenursing.

LEGAL ISSUES

Hricik (1997, p. 114) posed the following series of legal questions, in an effort to provide direction for the development of guidelines for the regulation of provider and patient privacy rights, when wiring health care communications via the Internet.

Are unencrypted Internet e-mail messages confidential? No independent opinion exists on this issue within the nursing profession regarding the confidentiality of unencrypted Internet health care communications. Therefore, nursing may look to opinions rendered related to this issue in other professions. An opinion on this issue was examined by Hricik (1997) from within the legal profession, discussing the Iowa Bar Association's (IBA) disciplinary committee's opinion that

unencrypted electronic messages regarding clients should not be sent over the Internet (Hricik, 1997, p. 114; citing the Iowa Bar Association Formal Opinion of 1996.

The IBA held the view that:

Pure inter-exchange of information or . . . communication with clients . . . is an exception . . . but with sensitive material . . . must have written acknowledgment by [the] client . . . which . . . includes consent for communication . . . on the Internet or non-secure intranet or other forms of proprietary networks, or it must be encrypted or protected by passwords/firewall or other generally acceptable equivalent security system (Hricik, 1997, p. 114).

In looking for an answer to this issue, one may consider, as did the IBA, the Federal Wiretap Statutes, which specify that intercepted otherwise privileged electronic health care communications do not lose their privileged character (Federal Wiretap Statutes, 1968/1992, § 2517(4); Hricik, 1997, p. 115).

Is misdirected e-mail regarding the patient's health care confidential? Misdirection of electronic health care communications does occur over the Internet, an occurrence that federal statutes do not specifically address. A relevant factor to consider in answering this issue is the fact that a misdirected fax regarding the patient's health care, which is wired over telephone lines, does not lose its privilege of confidentiality. Therefore, one may argue that if e-mail is misdirected, because it is also wired over telephone lines, the patient likewise does not lose his or her privilege of confidentiality (Hricik, 1997, p. 115).

Does intercepted e-mail regarding the patient's health care retain its privilege of confidentiality? Electronic health care communications can be intercepted through **hacking**, which encompasses: (1) **sniffing**, or capturing health care information as it travels through the intermediate or router's computer; or (2) **spoofing**, which is programming a router's computer to act as the recipient host (Hricik, 1997, p 115; Jones, 1997).

Hacking is a felony, because the provider's

e-mail regarding the patient is intercepted for purposes other than for mechanical or service quality control checks (Hricik, 1997, p. 116; Federal Wiretap Statutes, 18 U.S.C. § 2517[12]). In answering this issue of whether or not intercepted e-mail is confidential, nursing may look to an analysis by Girardi (1996):

Interception of [health care] communications over the Internet or over the phone should not result in a waiver of the . . . privilege [of confidentiality, as] . . . there is no waiver of privilege when a thief steals a document out of a file cabinet, and likewise no waiver when the file is in digital form and the break-in occurs through the phone line.

ETHICAL CONSIDERATIONS AND CONFLICTS

Telenursing has escalated in the past years without ethical or legal guidance. Telenursing has been conducted through electronic technologies, including satellite, telephone systems, and the Internet (Board of Nurse Examiners of the State of Texas, 1998a), without benefit of established standards of telenursing care. Within these electronic media, Yensen (1996, p. 213) views telenursing as a subset of **virtual nursing**, a type of nursing that is role-played or simulated. Tabone (1997) also describes telenursing as the age of **cybercare**, as nursing care is provided in cyberspace.

When telenursing provides simulated nursing care, it adds the dimensions of distance, electronic media, and mediation. Although telenursing removes the dimensions of the personal closeness and physical contact within which nursing is traditionally practiced, this distance results in increasing patient autonomy. Telenursing also remains a simple and inexpensive mechanism to guarantee distributive justice, providing nursing care and health care information to a wide number of patients in a number of states.

The greatest ethical dilemma that the nurse faces in telenursing is related to the issue of the right to privacy of the patient's health care information. An ongoing challenge to nursing will be to maintain standards of nursing practice, while providing for the confidentiality of the patient's health care information (Yensen, 1996, p. 214).

RECOMMENDATIONS FOR RESEARCH AND MALPRACTICE PREVENTION

The review of the nursing and legal literature raises a number of key areas for research and malpractice prevention. The purpose of this section is to identify present and future research issues for telenursing and ideas for malpractice prevention.

RESEARCH

As telenursing is a new concept, minimal research has been conducted to measure its effect on the delivery and outcome of health care services. A promising application of telehealth is the use of two-way videos. The provider and patient can interact with one another face to face while miles apart, via cameras mounted on top of their computers. Interactive videos work along the same principles, except the communication is wired via two-way cable television (Grande, 1997, pp. 59–60).

Peripherals are diagnostic equipment, such as the stethoscope or otoscope, that may be used to monitor the patient via the telehealth network. Peripherals provide for wire transmission of diagnostic sounds and images. Peripherals are typically used to transmit health care information by two methods. The first method allows the nurse to watch patients perform self-care, such as take their blood pressure, change a dressing, or give themselves intravenous therapy. The second method allows the nurse to do a hands-on assessment while transmitting the images and information to the physician in another location (Grande, 1997, pp. 59–60). Peripherals and interactive videos are commonly used in home telenursing.

Wootten, Loane, Mair, Allen, Doolittle, Begley, McLernan, Moutray, & Harrison (1998) conducted a joint United States and United Kingdom study of home telenursing (US/UK Study). An abstraction instrument, tested in the United States, was used to review nursing notes for patients nursed at home in both the United States and the United Kingdom. Of the 1700 cases of home nursing care, 906 were in the United States and 839 in the United Kingdom.

Preliminary data suggested that the following percentage of home nursing visits could have been conducted via telenursing: (1) United States, 45 percent; and (2) United Kingdom, 15 percent. Pilot trials also revealed that even low-quality videos would have been useful in home nursing visits in either Kansas City or Belfast. The preliminary findings of the US/UK Study indicated that telenursing could potentially play a significant role in the effectiveness and efficiency of delivery of home health nursing care. Further studies are warranted to monitor the effectiveness of this type of home health care telenursing program (Wootten, Loane, Mair, Allen, Doolittle, Begley, McLernan, Moutray, & Harrison, 1998).

The University of Kansas Medical Center and Kendallwood Hospice in Kansas City collaborated on a pilot study of telenursing for the terminally ill, via the public telephone network (UKMC/KH Study). Interactive video was placed in the homes of six terminally ill patients and three nurses who received the after-hours calls. For two separate 3-month periods, data regarding interactive patterns was gathered. Video assessments were conducted by the nurse to determine whether the patient needed an in-person visit. The results of the UKMC/KH Study suggested a general satisfaction with telenursing, by both patients and caregivers, especially those patients in a rural setting, who lived a long way from the nurse's base station, and in an urban setting, who lived in an area that was unsafe at nighttime. Again, further study is warranted to determine the effectiveness of the use of telenursing with the terminally ill patient (Doolittle, Yaezel, Otto, & Clemens, 1998).

The University of Kansas Medical Center (UKMC) conducted a study of a home telenursing project directed towards elderly individuals (UKMC Study). The project nurses used telenursing "cockpits" at three different sites to provide home health nursing services. Video pictures were transmitted via a cable television–based interactive video system. The interviews were conducted of patients receiving telenursing, in the following two phases: (1) phase 1, interviews of the 22 new patients; and (2) phase II, interviews of the nine remaining subjects still receiving telenursing. The patients did not express any worry, excitement, or difficulties with the electronics. Nor did telenursing have any negative effects on communication. The results of the UKMC Study suggested a need to clearly define the purpose and goals of telenursing and to replicate the study to determine the effectiveness of telenursing with elderly populations (Whitten, Mair, & Collins, 1997).

The European Union, Eductra, has designed Project Telenurse, which is being developed internationally. This is a 30-month project, begun in January 1996, for the purposes of: (1) developing standardized nursing care for wards, hospitals, regions, and countries; (2) promoting the use of these standards in Europe and internationally; and (3) utilizing the developing International Classification for Nursing Practice (ICNP) as a clinical information and data gathering source (Yensen, 1996, p. 214).

A North American telenursing research project is also being developed at Montana State University. This project is a clinical telenursing project, designed by Dr. Clarann Weinert, to care for cancer patients (Yensen, 1996, p. 214).

MALPRACTICE PREVENTION

Telenursing has been developed without legal or ethical guidance, and thus is an area of nursing practice with the potential of high legal risk. To prevent nursing malpractice, the nurse must be aware of legal issues that may potentially interfere with the success of telenursing and specific strategies to prevent malpractice in telenursing.

POTENTIAL MALPRACTICE ISSUES

Abke and Mouse-Young (1997) identified a variety of legal issues that may potentially interfere with the success of telehealth and leave the nurse open to a suit for malpractice. For example, the authors ask the question: What protocol should the nurse utilize when referring a patient to a teleconsultant? Through development of a protocol, the referring nurse will be aware of the credentials of the teleconsultant. Further, the referral will explicitly outline the roles of the referral nurse and the teleconsultant, so that there is collaboration in meeting the patient's needs.

The nurse must be aware not to commit a **Stark Amendment violation**. Violations of the Stark Amendment occur when the provider invests in a telehealth project and the provider furnishes telecommunication equipment to smaller facilities. Both situations could be interpreted as inducing referrals to the provider (Abke & Mouse-Young, 1997).

The telenursing practice must have established emergency measures. The provider has a duty to develop, and test periodically, emergency backup transmission plans. Backup measures must be developed in the event of equipment failure, weather interference, or other factors that may result in a foreseeable impact on the electronic transmission of health care information. If no emergency backup plan is in place, and interference occurs with resulting damages to the patient, the provider may be sued for medical negligence (Abke & Mouse-Young, 1997).

The nurse must provide the patient with informed consent. California currently requires physicians to obtain both verbal and written consent before providing health care via telemedicine. Because telenursing is an experimental form of nursing, nurses may be held to a higher standard in obtaining informed consent to provide treatment and/or wiring electronic health care information (Abke & Mouse-Young, 1997).

As noted previously, nurses must provide for the patient's confidentiality in the wiring of health care information. States are not uniform in their confidentiality laws relating to the transfer of health care information. Nurse-providers either treating patients or wiring electronic health care information must be aware of the law and risks related to the patient's privacy rights in patient treatment and health care information (Abke & Mouse-Young, 1997, p. 6).

STRATEGIES TO PREVENT MALPRACTICE

A number of preventive strategies have been identified by Abke and Mouse-Young (1997, p. 6) which the nurse may institute in order to prevent malpractice and reduce legal liability in the high-risk area of telenursing. These preventive strategies or remedies may include:

- Actively working with professional nursing organizations to promote uniform opinions and standards in telenursing.
- Providing patients with informed consent, so they are aware of all providers treating them.
- Clarifying individual responsibilities with all providers, so the patient does not "fall through the cracks" of the health care system.
- Providing a system to verify and document the quality and qualifications of the provider and the health care information.
- Defining goals and specifying health care services that are lacking, with ongoing evaluation of whether either can reasonably be provided.
- Providing ongoing evaluation of telenursing services, to ensure quality of patient care.
- Primarily, if the nurse questions the quality of the teleconsultation or ability to consult with a particular set of symptoms, referring the patient for a face-to-face consultation with the appropriate provider (Abke & Mouse-Young, 1997, p. 6).

PROTECTED DELIVERY OF ELECTRONIC DOCUMENTS

According to Harrison (1998, p. 476), the nurse may use a variety of precautions to protect health care databases and communications from damage while on the hard drive or invasion from either viruses or hackers. For example, the nurse may use utilities programs, which are designed to promote uninterrupted operation under Windows software, including Symantec Norton Utilities, Crash Guard Delux, and Cybermedia First Aid. Also, a variety of antivirus software is available, including Dr. Solomon's Antivirus Toolkit, Symantec Norton Anti-Virus, or Cybermedia Guard Dog. The provider should also be aware that databases on the hard drive and any important files should be backed up and stored on a network or zip drive on a regular basis (Harrison, 1998, p. 476).

Encryption software, which maintains the right to privacy of the patient's health care information, includes Eudora Pro and Adobe System's Acrobat. Acrobat uses a portable document format for its files, called **PDF files**. Acrobat has the unique capability of allowing for the encrypting and decrypting of electronic health care information in PDF files, in any format, on any web browser, or with any software application. Its counterpart, Acrobat Reader, is available free of charge on-line (may be downloaded from http://www.adobe.com). PDF files are widely used in the federal government and are being considered as the Federal Information Processing Standard and the standard of the National Archive Record Administration (Harrison, 1998).

INFORMED CONSENT REGARDING TELENURSING

The nurse must inform the patient about the risks and benefits regarding telenursing so that the patient can make an informed decision as to whether or not to use this technology. The nurse should explain, for example, that: (1) the diagnosis is based upon a wired image, which may not be visualized as clearly by the provider as it would be face-to-face with the human eye; (2) the provider may diagnose only with the eyes and ears, not with other vital means of diagnosis such as touch and smell; but (3) the patient need not travel a long distance

to receive care from the nurse (Granade, 1997, p. 60).

States that currently require informed consent, both written and verbal, before providing nonemergency care include California and Arizona. In California, the provider in charge of patient care must give oral and written information regarding: (1) risks and benefits; (2) access to information that is wired by the provider; and (3) privacy rights, that is, the health care communication will be protected by existing confidentiality rules (Granade, 1997, pp. 60–61).

Granade (1997) also recommends that when giving informed consent a nurse should: (1) check state law to determine the legal elements; (2) consult the policy and procedure manual to determine the employer's criteria; and (3) document that informed consent has been obtained and that the patient understands the plan of care (Granade, 1997, p. 61).

As further protection against a malpractice and/or disciplinary action, the nurse should: (1) document actions and assessments when assisting another provider during a telehealth procedure, especially if relying on the senses to make a diagnosis; (2) chart what the patient says, what is seen, and instruction given; (3) preserve all health care communications, including telemetry or videotapes, in the patient's charts; and (4) establish and follow standard protocols and/or standing orders (Granade, 1997, pp. 61–62).

CONFIDENTIALITY

Confidentiality may be reasonably maintained through the following precautions: (1) using fiberoptic lines, as opposed to copper lines, to wire health care communications, because they are more difficult to tap; (2) using encryption technology to wire health care communications; (3) verifying the authenticity before responding to a health care communication; (4) during a teleconsultation, informing the patient of other providers present; (5) establishing and following policy for storing data gathered during telenursing consultation; (6) keeping videotapes, audiotapes, backup computer discs, and any other data for the same amount of time that paper records must be preserved; and (7) staying current with laws regulating telenursing, through regular literature review and seminars that provide legal updates on the subject (Granade, 1997, p. 62).

SUMMARY

Telenursing is defined as the electronic transfer of nursing data, nursing information, and nursing expertise between two points. Under the Uniform Health Care Information Act, the nurse must reasonably protect the confidentiality of health care information. The patient's rights to privacy during telephone and computer communications have been identified under the Federal Wiretap Statutes and the Uniform Health Care Information Act. There are several legal issues and trends in telenursing, including: (1) licensure for telenursing practice, (2) telenursing across state lines, and (3) implementation of orders from out-of-state physicians. [Because telenursing is such a new concept, further research to measure its effectiveness in the delivery and outcome of health care services is needed as well as development of specific strategies for malpractice prevention.]

POINTS TO REMEMBER

- Telenursing is a subset of telehealth.
- Telenursing is the electronic transfer of nursing data, nursing information, and nursing expertise between two points.
- The Uniform Health Care Information Act (UHCIA, 1997) controls and protects the flow of health care information within telenursing practice.
- Under the UHCIA (1997), the standard that the nurse must follow in protecting the health care information of the patient is that of reasonableness.
- Under the UHCIA (1997), civil and criminal remedies are available to patients for violation of their right to confidentiality of health care information.

- Federal Wiretap Statutes (1968/1992) control the right to privacy of the patient when wiring health care information over regular, cordless, or cellular telephone lines.
- Federal Wiretap Statutes (1968/1992) control the right to privacy of the patient when wiring health care information via computer.
- The nurse may reasonably provide for the confidentiality of health care communications when wired via computer through encryption.
- No laws exist that regulate telenursing practice across state lines.

REFERENCES

Abke, A., & Mouse-Young, D. (1997, Fall). Telemedicine: New technology = new questions = new exposures. *Journal of Risk Management, 17*(4), 3–6.

American Nurses Association. (1997a, April). Telehealth: A tool for nursing practice. *Nursing Trends & Issues, 2*, 2.

American Nurses Association. (1997b). Telehealth legislation—1997. *State legislative trends and analysis* (pp. 39–40). Special report to the 1997 House of Delegates, No. 97-STA-07. Washington, DC: Author.

Anders, G. (1997, February). How nurses take calls and control the care of patients from afar. *The Wall Street Journal*, pp. A1, A6.

Bensinger, P. (1996, May). *Can the decrepit encrypt?* ABA 22nd National Conference on Professional Responsibility in Chicago, IL.

Board of Nurse Examiners of the State of Texas. (1998a, July). Multistate regulation of nursing. *RN Update, 29*(3), 1.

Board of Nurse Examiners of the State of Texas. (1998b, July). Multi-state regulation: The mutual recognition model. *RN Update, 29*(3), 9-10.

Doolittle, G. C., Yaezel, A., Otto, F., & Clemens, C. (1998). Hospice care using home-based telemedicine systems. *Journal of Telemedicine and Telecare, 4*(1), 53-89.

Federal Wiretap Statutes of 1968/1992; Wire and Electronic Communications Interception and Interception of Oral Communications, 18 U.S.C. S. §§ 2510 *et seq.*

Forsyth v. Barr, 19 F. 3d 1527, 1534 (5th Cir. 1994).

Girardi, A. (1996, February). Privilege and confidentiality. *Computer, 13*(2), 133.

Gobis, L. (1997). Telenursing: Nursing by telephone across state lines. *Journal of Nursing Law, 3*(3), 7–17.

Granade, P. (1997, July). The brave new world of telemedicine. *RN*, 59–62.

Harrison, A. (1998, May) Delivery of electronic documents. *Texas Bar Journal, 61*(5), 476–478.

Horton, M.C. (1997). Letters: Licensure and Telehealth *Nursing Management 28* (6), 10.

Hricik, D. (1997, February). Confidentiality issues and privileges in high-tech communications. *Texas Bar Journal, 60*(2), 104–119.

Jarvis, P., & Tellman, B. (1996, May). *High-tech ethics and malpractice issues.* 22nd National Conference on Professional Responsibility, Chicago, IL.

Jones, R. (1997). *Client confidentiality: A lawyer's duties with regard to Internet e-mail* [On-line]. Available: http://www.kuesterlaw.com.

Mortensen, R., & Neilsen, G. (1994). Telenursing: European classification of nursing practice with regard to patient problems, nursing interventions, and patient outcomes, including educational measures. *Computer Methods & Programs in Biomedicine, 45*, 171–173.

Multistate Licensure Compac. [On-line]. Available: www.ncsbn.org

National Emp. Serv. Corp. v. Liberty Mut. Ins. Co., 3 Mass. L. Rptr. 221 (Mass. Super. Ct. 1994).

Office of Rural Health Policy, U.S. Department of Health and Human Services. (1997, February). *Exploratory evaluation of rural applications of telemedicine.* Rockville, MD.: Author.

Physician's, Surgeons Etc. (a): Uniform Health Care Information Act. In *American Jurisprudence Trials Supplement* (2nd ed.) (Vol. 61, Section 165.3). (1999). St. Paul, MN: West Publishing.

Physician's, Surgeons Etc. (b): Authorization of disclosure under the Uniform Health Care Information Act. In *American Jurisprudence Trials Supplement* (2nd ed.) (Vol. 61, Section 171.5). (1999). West Publishing.

Project Telenurse [On-line]. Available: http://www.dihnr@inrt.uni-c.dk.

Senate Report Number 1097, 90th Congress, 2nd Session 100 (1968) (reprinted in 1968 U.S.C.C. & A.N. 2112, 2189).

Shea on Behalf of American Reporters v. Reno, 930 F. Supp, 916, 925 (S.D.N.Y. 1996) 1966.

South Carolina Bar Advisory Op. 94-27 (January 1995).

State v. Canady, 460 S.E.2d 677 (W. VA. 1995).

State v. Cartson, 913 P. 2d 709 (Ore. 1996).

Tabone, S. (1997, Sept.). Mapping the telehealth maze. *Texas Nurse, 71*(8), 12.

Telemedicine Research Center. (1997). *What is telemedicine?* Portland, OR.: Author.

Texas Nurses Association. (1998a, November/December). Questions and answers about multistate licensure compact. *Texas Nursing*, p. 5.

Texas Nurses Association. (1998b, November/December). Texas moves toward multistate nurse licensure legislation in 1999. *Texas Nursing*, pp. 4, 11.

Uniform Health Care Information Act, § 1-101 *et seq.* (1997).

United States v. Maxwell, 43 Fed. R. Serv. 24 (U.S.A.F. Ct. Crim. App. 1995).

United States v. Smith, 978 F. 2d 171 (5th Cir. 1992), cert. denied, 113 S. Ct. 1620 (1993).

United States v. Turner, 528 F. 2d 143, 155 (9th Cir. 1975), cert. denied, 96 S. Ct. 426 (1976).

Walker, J. (1997, October). Telehealth: A complex issue being addressed by state and federal governments. *AORN Journal, 66*(4), 709–712.

Webster, K. (1996, August). A newsletter for and about telephone nursing services. *Telephone Nursing Telezine* [Online]. Available: http://www.ally.ios.com/~webster/tntaug96.html.

Whitten, P., Mair, F., & Collins, B. (1997) Home telenursing in Kansas: Patients' perceptions of uses and benefits. *Journal of Telemedicine and Telecare, 3*(1), 67–69.

Wootten, R., Loane, M., Mair, F., Allen, A., Doolittle, G., Begley, M., McLernan, A., Moutray, N., & Harrisson, S. (1998). A joint US-UK study of home telenursing. *Journal of Telemedicine and Telecare, 4*(1), 83–85.

Yensen, J. (1996, July/August). Telenursing, virtual nursing, and beyond. *Computers In Nursing, 14*(4), 213–214.

SUGGESTED READINGS

Katz v. United States, 389 U.S. 347 (1967).

Milholland, K. (1995). Telehealth, telenursing, telewhat? *American Nurse, 27*, 13.

INTERNET RESOURCES

EDUCATRA guidelines. [On-line]. Available: http://www. mi.rulimburg.nl.0f:/educatra/guidelin.html

Executive summary, telemedicine report to Congress. (1997, January 31). [On-line]. Available: http://www.ntia.doc.gov/reports/telemed/execsum.htm

Health Policy Tracking Service home page. [On-line]. Available: http://www.hpts.org/

International TeleNurses Association. [On-line]. Available: http://www.itna@listserv.bcm.tmc.edu

National Council of State Boards of Nursing Home Page. [On-line]. Available: http://www.ncsbn.org/files/newsreleases/nr970825. html

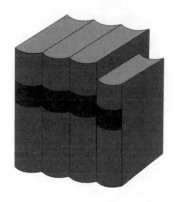

Chapter 26

CORRECTIONAL NURSING

Mary E. O'Keefe

(continued)

KEY WORDS

Actual Knowledge
Actual Intent
Administrative Law
Affirmative Defense
Amnesty International
Compensatory Damages
Cruel and Unusual
  Punishment
Culpability
Defenses
Deliberate Deprivation
Deliberate Indifference
Discretionary Decisions
Distinguish
Ethical Dilemma
Federal Common Law
Good Faith
Habeas Corpus
Hands-on Policy
Holding
Immunity
Intentional Injury
Keep-locking
Malice
Mere Possibility
Minimally Adequate
Multidisciplinary
  Treatment Team
  (MDTT)

Negligence
Nonmaleficence
Practical Constraints
Prima Facie Case
Provider
Punitive Damages
Qualified Immunity
Reckless Disregard
Recklessness
Respondeat Superior
Serious Medical Need
Situational Right to
  Privacy
Standard of Reasonable
  Care
Standard of Review
Statutory Law
Tort
Totality of the
  Circumstances Test
Totality of Conditions
  Test
Use of Force
Waive

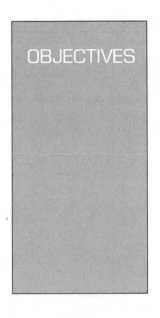
Upon completion of this chapter, the reader will be able to:

- Discuss the constitutional, statutory, and common law under which the rights of inmates have been established.
- List specific rights guaranteed to inmates under constitutional, federal, and state law.
- Identify the standards of care that guide nursing practice within a correctional facility.
- Identify duties that the nurse, as provider and member of the multidisciplinary treatment team, has to the inmate.
- Analyze legal and ethical issues relevant to the nurse in avoiding legal risks, preventing malpractice, and reducing liability while practicing within a correctional facility.

INTRODUCTION

The laws affecting correctional nursing have been, and are, dynamic in interpretation and application. These laws are dynamic in interpretation because they are constantly evolving from a combination of constitutional, federal, and state laws, which are applied and reinterpreted by the courts on an almost daily basis. Laws affecting correctional nursing are dynamic in application because the individual correctional facility is allowed wide discretion when interpreting and implementing these regulations, which are designed to provide for the security, diagnosis, and treatment of prisoners.

HISTORICAL PERSPECTIVE

Historically, the administration of the criminal justice system has been a function of both state and federal agencies. Since 1930, the Bureau of Prisons has administered the federal prisons and correctional systems (Humphrey, 1981). Before the 1970s, the judicial system maintained a **hands-on policy** regarding prison administration, placing the laws regulating correctional facilities within the authority of the legislative and executive branches of the state and federal governments (*Procunier v. Martinez*, 1974).

Since the 1970s, inmates have filed a record number of lawsuits against everyone involved in their security, diagnosis, and treatment within the correctional system. Ultimately, these lawsuits have established prisoners' rights under constitutional, federal, and state law.

MULTIDISCIPLINARY TREATMENT TEAM

The authority overseeing the administration of inmates' rights within the correctional facility is the multidisciplinary treatment team. Currently, nurses function within the correctional setting as a coprovider within the **multidisciplinary treatment team (MDTT)**, a team of professionals that monitors and determines all aspects of the security, diagnosis, treatment, and rights of the inmate, through a shared decision-making process. The MDTT is composed of everyone who provides care to the inmate, including but not limited to the nurse, treating physician, psychiatrist, psychologist, social worker, recreational therapist, and security officers. (Members of the MDTT are referred to individually as a **provider**, and collectively as providers, coproviders, or members of the MDTT.) The term *provider* also encompasses all those who are representatives of, and supervised by, the warden or any of the government entities controlling the correctional system on the state or federal level. In summary, all persons who participate in shared decision-making regarding the security, diagnosis, treatment, and rights of the inmate are providers and members of the MDTT.

The provider, as member of the MDTT, shares the development of the inmate's treatment plan and participates in subsequent treatment reviews and decisions. The treatment plan encompasses not only the inmate's right to health care, but also governs all other rights and privileges that the inmate is allowed to receive within the correctional system.

Gobis (1997, p. 8) proposes that "if nursing services are provided, the practice constitutes nursing. . . . [H]ow nursing service is delivered makes no difference. . . . [N]ursing advice provided . . . constitutes nursing." Nurses, as members of the MDTT, provide advice on all aspects of care, including not only the diagnosis and treatment, but also the level of security and other rights granted to the inmate. Therefore, if the nurse provides advice to the MDTT, then this practice constitutes nursing.

Participation in the MDTT places the nurse in a high-risk category for legal liability. The nurse participates in shared decision-making on a global variety of inmates' rights, and these decisions require knowledge of more than just the law regulating the inmate's rights to health care. Case law addressing legal issues regarding the nurse within the MDTT is basically nonexistent. Case law concerning health care claims against nurses by inmates is cited throughout this chapter. But more frequently cited, as they are more common, will be older, analogous, landmark cases concerning inmate's claims against the nurse's coprovider within the MDTT. These cases are analogous because they identify decisions regarding health care made by the nurse's coproviders as members of the MDTT. The purpose of citing these analogous cases will be to identify the court's decisions identifying duties the nurse's coproviders have to the inmate and to relate these duties to the nurse as a shared decision-maker and coprovider within the MDTT.

The purpose of this chapter is to facilitate the nurse's decision-making functions within the MDTT, by providing information on (1) the law under which the MDTT is directed to provide for the rights of the total inmate population; (2) the professional standards under which the nurse as provider is directed to furnish the individual inmate's health care needs; (3) the individual inmate's rights, guaranteed by constitutional, statutory, and common law (Penal and Correctional, 1987/1998); and ultimately, (4) the nurse's duties as a member of the MDTT.

THE LAW

In order to avoid legal risks and prevent malpractice suits, the provider must be aware of not only the basic rights of prisoners but also the laws under which prisoner's rights have been defined. The purpose of this section is to discuss and identify: (1) the constitutional, federal, and state law under which prisoners' rights have been mandated; and (2) analogous case law, which further defines the rights of prisoners and corresponding duties of all providers as members of the MDTT within the correctional system.

CONSTITUTIONAL LAW

The prison population is the only population in the United States guaranteed health care, under the Eighth Amendment to the Constitution. The inmate's right to receive health care and the provider's obligation to render health care for those being punished by incarceration have been well established via the Eighth Amendment and federal common law (Penal and Correctional, 1987/1998). This section discusses standards of care for prisoners, which have been identified under the Eighth Amendment, including the general standard (cruel and unusual punishment) and the health care standard (deliberate indifference).

EIGHTH AMENDMENT STANDARD: CRUEL AND UNUSUAL PUNISHMENT

Under the Eighth Amendment, the general standard the courts utilize for assessing liability for the outcome of the care and treatment of the inmate is whether or not the action or inaction by the provider resulted in cruel and unusual punishment (Box 26–1).

By definition, application of the standard of **cruel and unusual punishment** means that the court asks the question: Is the action or inaction of the provider of such a cruel and unusual nature that its effect on the inmate serves (1) to deny a constitutional right, (2) to inflict further penalty on the inmate over and above that imposed by law, and (3) results in the unnecessary or wanton infliction of pain on the inmate?

Examples of actions or inactions resulting in cruel and unusual punishment to the inmate are many and varied in federal common law. In the landmark health care case *Estelle v. Gamble* (1976), the U.S. Supreme Court held that failure to provide inmates with necessary health care was an example of cruel and unusual punishment under the Eighth Amendment. The Supreme Court theorized that inmates, by reason of deprivation of their freedom or liberty, cannot provide for or have access to health care. In this landmark case, the Supreme Court established the standard for identifying the type of behavior the provider must demonstrate in denying health care, which results in liability for cruel and unusual punishment to the inmate.

CONSTITUTIONAL HEALTH CARE STANDARD: DELIBERATE INDIFFERENCE

The Supreme Court held that the behavior of the provider, in denying health care, must evidence deliberate indifference (*Estelle v. Gamble*, 1976). **Deliberate indifference** within the correctional setting encompasses an intentional disregard of the inmate's constitutional right to health care. In *Estelle v. Gamble* (1976), a Texas prison inmate alleged that providers violated the cruel and unusual punishment clause of the Eighth Amendment by failing to provide the inmate with adequate health care when the prisoner sustained a back injury while performing prison work. In this precedent-setting case, the Supreme Court held that providers have a duty to ensure health care for inmates with serious medical needs, defining failure to do so as deliberate indifference. The court defined **serious medical need** as "one that has been diagnosed by a physician as mandating treatment or one that is so obvious that even a lay person could easily recognize the necessity for a doctor's attention" (*Hendrix v. Faulkner*, 1981). According to *Estelle v. Gamble* (1976), deliberate indifference to a prisoner's serious medical needs constitutes cruel and

BOX 26-1

U.S.C.A. CONSTITUTION AMENDMENT EIGHT

The nurse's general duties to the inmate, as a provider within the MDTT, are founded within the terms of the Eighth Amendment of the Constitution. The standard of care that must be rendered to the inmate by providers is defined within the Eighth Amendment as follows:

"Excessive bail shall not be required, nor excessive fines imposed, nor cruel and unusual punishment inflicted."

unusual punishment under the Eighth Amendment, giving rise to a civil rights claim against the provider under the Civil Rights Act of 1871 (Box 26–2).

The Supreme Court in *Estelle* (1976) further defined deliberate indifference as the provider's (1) failure to respond to the inmate's serious health care needs, (2) intentional denial or delay of the inmate's access to health care, and/or (3) interference with the inmate's health care once it has been prescribed.

Health care provided to the inmate must be not only adequate, but reasonably intended to satisfy health care needs (*Crawford v. Loving*, 1979). Medical care must be comparable in quality and availability to that which is obtainable by the general public in the area in which the correctional facility is located (*Barnes v. Government of Virgin Islands*, 1976).

In summary, under constitutional law, the provider's deliberate indifference to an inmate's serious medical needs leads to cruel and unusual punishment, a civil rights violation under federal law. The nurse, as a provider within the MDTT, has a constitutional duty to render health care to the inmate, for failure to do so results in cruel and unusual punishment to the prisoner, under the court's holding in *Estelle v. Gamble* (1976).

FEDERAL COMMON LAW

Many other rights of inmates, and corresponding duties of providers, have been identified under federal common law. Under federal common law, inmates or any type of detainee have a right to sue the federal government, correctional facility or authority, or any providers, individually or as a member of a MDTT. The purpose of this section is to discuss (1) the prisoner's right to sue under civil rights acts, (2) the prisoner's rights to sue under federal common law, (3) a theory of provider liability, labeled *respondeat superior*, and (4) a provider defense, labeled qualified immunity.

PRISONER'S RIGHT TO SUE UNDER CIVIL RIGHTS ACTS

The federal government, through legislation, has expanded prisoners' rights to sue under various civil rights acts. The specific elements necessary for proving a civil rights violation of the inmate's right to health care has been established under federal common law. In one such case, a California inmate alleged that he received improper and inadequate treatment by the provider subsequent to a fracture of the left side of his face, which resulted in permanent loss of vision and

BOX 26-2

CIVIL RIGHTS ACT OF 1871 (42 U.S.C.A. 1983 *et seq.*)

The nurse's duty to protect the civil rights of the inmate, as a provider within the MDTT, is guided by the standard specified in the following statutory language:

"Every person who, under color of any statute, ordinance, regulation, custom, or usage of any State or Territory, subjects, or causes to be subjected, any citizen of the United States or other person within the jurisdiction thereof to the deprivation of any rights, privileges, or immunities secured by the Constitution and laws, shall be liable to the party injured in an action at law, suit in equity, or other proper proceeding for redress."

disfigurement. The California federal court held that an inmate can show a violation of right to health care by proving: (1) an acute physical condition, (2) an urgent need for health care, (3) a failure or refusal of the provider to deliver that health care, (4) a tangible or real residual injury or lasting harm to the inmate caused by failure of the provider to render health care, and (5) that the acts or inactions of the provider occurred under circumstances that would shock the judicial conscience (*Mayfield v. Craven*, 1969). (Terms such as *shock*, unless otherwise defined, take on their common sense, customary dictionary definition; that is, the behavior would disturb or disgust the court or the average juror.)

As noted previously, there are few reported cases involving civil rights claims by prisoners against nurse-providers. But as inmates usually file their own lawsuits and quite artfully draw from analogous case law, in future lawsuits against nurses, the courts will most likely apply the principles of law derived from the court's previous decisions involving claims against the nurse's coproviders within the MDTT. Prisoners are well aware that their right to sue under federal common law is unquestioned and well established.

PRISONER'S RIGHT TO SUE UNDER FEDERAL COMMON LAW

The prisoner's right to sue has been well established under federal common law. **Federal common law** refers to federal court holdings or decisions that become commonly held or repeated decisions in similar cases in other federal courts in other jurisdictions or locations. A federal court, in *Hampton v. Holmesburg Prison Officials* (1976), clearly defined types of actions an inmate may bring against providers. A prisoner's legal actions under federal common law usually arise under (1) a **habeas corpus** action, which is a claim regarding wrongful incarceration; (2) a **tort** action, which is a claim for malpractice, negligence, and/or damages; and/or (3) a civil rights actions (Penal and Correctional, 1987/1998). One standard commonly used by the courts to review the facts in these legal actions is called totality of the circumstances.

Standard of Review of Lawsuits: Totality of the Circumstances

Lawsuits involving the civil rights of prisoners are subject to a specific **standard of review**, or method by which the court analyzes all the facts of the case. The standard of review for the judicial system, in determining whether or not the prisoner's civil rights are being or have been violated by the provider, is based on the **totality of the circumstances test**. By definition, this test or standard calls for the court to consider all the facts surrounding the inmate's circumstances within the entire prison system, versus analyzing the facts simply from the viewpoint of the individual inmate or correctional facility (*Ramos v. Lamm*, 1980).

In *Cody v. Hillard* (1984), a class action suit, prison inmates claimed that the conditions and practices of their confinement within the correctional facility were cruel and unusual punishment. Using the totality of the circumstances standard, the federal court agreed with the inmates. The court held that a confinement is cruel and unusual punishment when there exists: (1) bad or unhealthy environmental conditions in cells, halls, kitchen, and food storage areas; (2) double-celling of inmates in single-cell accommodations; and/or (3) failure to provide needed health, dental, psychiatric, and psychological care (*Cody v. Hillard*, 1984).

When analyzing the totality of the conditions of confinement within the correctional facility, the courts may also look at some of the following parameters within which the provider, individually and as a member of the MDTT, makes decisions to provide for the security, diagnosis, and treatment of the inmate: (1) the setting, for example, questioning whether it is a minimum security facility or a maximum security facility in which the physically assaultive mentally ill are confined; (2) the diagnosis, including the acuity of the prisoner's symptoms, the overall condition, and willingness to cooperate; and/or (3) the provider's relationship within the MDTT with security, including security's willingness to respond in emergency situations (*Cody v. Hillard*, 1984).

However, there are instances in which a constitutional deprivation may be established in a singular or specific instance, such as any infringement by the MDTT on the inmate's right to have access to court (*Johnson v. Avery*, 1969). Although untested, the courts may also look to the totality of the circumstances created by the effect of decisions made by the MDTT. For example, did the decision of the MDTT to deny the previously suicidal inmate the right to have a pencil in his cell for safety and security reasons ultimately have the effect of: (1) denying the right to communicate with an attorney, and (2) therefore denying access to court?

Theory of Provider Liability: *Respondeat Superior*

One theory of liability under which the correctional facility may be held responsible for acts or inactions of the providers that deny the inmate's rights, is the theory or doctrine of *respondeat superior*. Simply defined, this doctrine means that the prison system can be held liable for the acts or inactions of the provider only if the prison administration knew, or should have known, of the negligent acts of the provider and/or MDTT. In *Layne v. Vizant* (1981), the First Circuit court held that "a director and warden may be parties to such a suit under the theory of *Respondeat Superior*, and may demonstrate deliberate indifference, for example, by interfering with the inmate's [health] care."

In essence, the doctrine of *respondeat superior* is available for prisoners' claims of violation of civil rights by a warden as a member of the MDTT, if the administration of the correctional facility either directed or participated in the violation at issue, along with individual providers or others within the MDTT. If the warden or his or her representative function as active members of the MDTT, then the courts could assume

actual knowledge, that is active agreement and participation in the actions or inactions of the MDTT that served to deny the inmate's rights. The warden, individual provider, and/or the MDTT may become defendants to an inmate's lawsuit. As defendants, providers seek **defenses** to the lawsuit, or theories by which they may prove they are not liable for the inmate's claims.

Provider Defense: Federal Government Immunity

One defense that may be available to the provider is that of immunity. The defense of **immunity** means the right to be free of any type of claim, including liability. The defense of immunity is an **affirmative defense**, meaning the burden is on the provider to come forward to claim and prove the right to the immunity defense (*Thompson v. Burke*, 1977).

In a landmark case on the issue of immunity, *Procunier v. Navarette* (1978), a California inmate claimed that providers negligently and inadvertently interfered with a constitutional right and failed to properly train providers in rendering the constitutional right. The Court held the immunity defense was available to the MDTT if (1) the inmate's constitutional rights were clearly established at the time of the alleged action or inaction by the MDTT; (2) the MDTT did not know of the inmate's rights; (3) the MDTT did not and could not have known their conduct deprived the inmate of a constitutional right; and/or (4) the MDTT acted without malicious intention to cause deprivation of guaranteed rights of the inmate (*Procunier v. Navarette*, 1978).

Defense of Qualified Immunity

The type of immunity available to the provider in suits by prisoners under federal law is known as qualified immunity. According to the holding in *Procunier v. Navarette*, (1978), " [Providers] are entitled to qualified, rather than absolute immunity, in good-faith fulfillment of their responsibilities" (see also, *Wood v. Strickland*, 1975). As nurses may be sued as individual providers by an inmate, certain federal statutes and common law have created a qualified immunity, providing the nurse with a defense to lawsuits initiated by the inmate. Having a **qualified immunity** simply means that the provider is immune from prosecution or suit by the inmate if evidence is provided that the actions or inactions at issue were performed in **good faith**. By definition, good faith actions or inactions of the provider are those sincerely believed to be in the best interest of the inmate. The goal of qualified immunity is to allow the MDTT to "exercise their discretion without fear of reprisal by the inmate" (*Wood v. Strickland*, 1975).

The court in *Procunier v. Navarette* (1978) held that when the provider commits an **intentional injury**, the consequences of the action or inaction are intended; that is, there is an intent by the provider to deprive the inmate of a constitutional right or cause other injury. **Negligence** is not sufficient to raise a constitutional issue, as this term implies that although the provider subjected the inmate to an unreasonable risk or loss of a civil right, the provider did not mean the harm or injury that in fact resulted (*Procunier v. Navarette*, 1978).

In summary, under the immunity defense, the provider may claim the actions, inactions, or decisions at issue, whether made as an individual provider or as a member of the MDTT, were performed with the good faith belief that the intervention(s) was in the best interest of the inmate.

Inmate's Right to Damages under Federal Law

The provider, who cannot prove good faith when denying a civil right may be liable for damages under federal law. The inmate may be able to recover damages from the provider if successful in a civil rights claim. According to the holding in *Wellman v. Faulkner* (1983), "To recover damages under 42 U.S.C.A. 1983, the inmate must establish the [MDTT's] personal responsibility for the claimed deprivation of a constitutional right" (see also, *Duncan v. Duckworth*, 1981, p. 655). The personal responsibility require-

ment may be satisfied in instances in which (1) the provider acted, or failed to act, with a deliberate or reckless disregard of the inmate's constitutional rights; or (2) the acts or inactions causing the deprivation of a constitutional right resulted from direction by the MDTT, or with their knowledge and consent (see also, *Crowder v. Lash*, 1982). In summary, the test to determine whether or not the inmate can recover money damages from the provider under a civil rights claim is wrongful intent and/or culpable negligence (*Owens-El v. Robinson*, 1978).

STATE LAW

The nurse's practice, individually and as a member of the MDTT within a correctional facility, is governed not only by federal law but also by state law. The purpose of this section is to discuss: (1) state statutory laws regulating nursing as a provider of care within a correctional facility, and (2) the inmate's right to sue under state law.

STATE STATUTORY LAW

Under state **statutory law**, the laws developed by the state legislature, the state reinforces federal statutes governing prisoners' rights. For example, the federal civil rights statutes, referred to in previous sections as 42 U.S.C.A. 1983 (Box 26–2), became the law of the state when the state legislature passed and enacted the same civil rights statute. Thus, civil rights guaranteed to a prisoner via the passage of 42 U.S.C.A. 1983 became implemented and guaranteed to the prisoner on the state level as a corresponding state civil rights law.

The nurse's duty to render the care guaranteed to inmates by federal and state civil rights laws is governed by various state **administrative laws**, or regulations designed to control professional licensing agencies, including: (1) the state board of nursing, which regulates and controls nursing license and practice; (2) the state board of health, which regulates and controls health care practices of the providers within the correctional facility; and (3) the prison board, which regulates and controls the functioning of the correctional facility. As the nurse's practice is governed by all these state administrative agencies, the prisoner's right to sue the nurse as provider falls under not only federal law but also under state law.

RIGHT TO SUE UNDER STATE LAW

Inmates, or any other type of detainee, have a right to sue the state government, correctional facility or authority, or any employee or health care provider under state law. Prisoners' actions under state law may arise under: (1) civil rights claims, (2) habeas corpus actions; and (3) common law tort actions, through which inmates have a right to bring suits for negligence and malpractice in state court. These tort claims, or civil wrongs, are usually related to, for example, negligent acts by unlicensed providers, acts of malpractice by licensed providers, failure of providers to give informed consent, and for resulting damages to the inmate.

As demonstrated by the federal case law previously cited, a federal court will intervene in the administration of health care services to an inmate only to correct a violation of a constitutional dimension, such as a violation of the civil right to health care or an Eighth Amendment violation (*Burks v. Teasdale*, 1980). Negligence and medical malpractice issues are left to the state courts.

Medical Malpractice versus Civil Rights Issues

The federal courts will not intervene in mere inmate allegations of negligence or mistake on the part of the health care provider (*Bowring v. Godwin*, 1977). Such cases are state or malpractice issues, and the federal courts try civil rights violations.

For example, a Pennsylvania inmate was told by the prison ophthalmologist that he must have eye surgery or lose his vision. The inmate was not transferred to the hospital, but continued to be treated with eye drops by a provider. The inmate lost the vision in both eyes and brought action against the MDTT and his ophthalmologist, claiming they had violated his civil rights by not providing him adequate health care treatment. But the Pennsylvania Court held that this was malpractice and did not become a violation of the prisoner's constitutional rights simply because the patient was a prisoner (*Parilla v. Cuyler*, 1978). Thus, the inmate had a cause of action for malpractice in the state court, but not automatically a cause of action for violation of civil rights in federal court, just because he was an inmate.

A **prima facie case** of civil rights violation—or classic, textbook case with all the elements of deliberate indifference—did not occur in the landmark case on inmate health care, entitled *Estelle v. Gamble* (1976). In this Supreme Court case, the inmate had been treated by health care providers on 17 occasions over a 3-month period following a injury. Because the inmate had received health care treatment, the legal issue was not whether a civil rights violation had occurred under federal law in the form of denial of health care, but whether malpractice had occurred under state law. The *Estelle* (1976) court theorized that the health care provider's failure to use additional diagnostic techniques or other forms of treatment was a matter of health care judgment by the provider and, as their failures were a potential breach of duty, a malpractice issue.

Inmate's Right to Compensatory and Punitive Damages under State Law

Under a state common law tort action, a civil action for harm done to the plaintiff, an inmate may be able to recover both compensatory and punitive damages from the provider (Penal & Correctional, 1987/1988). An inmate may file a claim for **compensatory damages**, claiming the amount of money the inmate asserts will be just compensation for the monetary loss that will be, or has been, incurred because of the provider's wrongful action or inaction. Compensatory damages may include recovery for loss of: (1) present and future wages; (2) pain and suffering; and/or (3) past, present, and future medical expenses. Damage to the inmate is often hard to prove, or may be minimal to nothing, for the prisoner's medical expenses are paid by the state or federal government and the prisoner is not employed, so has no loss of wages.

Because the correctional facility is a government entity, the amounts of damage that can be paid to the prisoner are usually subject to a statutory limit. For example, in some jurisdictions the amounts of damages that may be recovered are limited to a cap of $100,000 per incident. But if the provider is held individually or personally liable, there is no comparable statutory limit regarding monetary liability.

The inmate may also claim **punitive damages**, claiming an amount of money that would punish the MDTT or provider, if the wrongful act was held by the court to have been performed with **malice**, or intent to cause the inmate harm.

In summary, it is clear that the nurse, if sued by the inmate individually and/or as a member of the MDTT: (1) has the same duty to the inmate as identified for coproviders within the MDTT, under the corresponding standards of care, as previously defined under both federal and state constitutional, statutory, and common laws; (2) is subject to suit by inmates under both federal and state law; and (3) may be subject, as an individual provider and as a member of the MDTT, to the payment of both compensatory and punitive damages. The legal risks apparent to the provider through an inmate's lawsuit only make more evident the need to avoid legal risks, prevent malpractice suits, and reduce liability through greater awareness of prisoners' rights.

PRISONERS' RIGHTS

As a provider and member of the MDTT, the nurse is called upon, on a regular basis, to participate in shared decisions regarding the prisoner's access to a variety of rights within the correctional system. Generally, along with the right to sue, prisoners have a right to (1) visitation by their families, attorney, and friends; (2) association with other inmates; (3) use of the mail, unless it must be restricted for special previewing precautions; (4) freedom of religious expression and practice of religion; (5) legal services, such as a lawyer to represent the inmate during any criminal proceeding; and (6) access to the judicial system, such as the right to a law library and legal publications (Penal & Correctional 1987/1988). The purpose of this section is to discuss the prisoner's basic rights relative to: (1) privacy; (2) protection from violence, suicide, or self-inflicted harm and risk of disease; and (3) as previously identified, health care.

RIGHT TO PRIVACY

The prisoner's right to privacy has been reviewed and limited in a variety of federal cases directed at health care issues relevant to the nurse as provider. In one case involving the issue of privacy, a male inmate claimed that a female nurse violated his privacy rights simply by dispensing medications in his cell block (*Robbins v. South et al.*, 1984). The Montana District Court held that the prisoner's privacy rights were not violated, because a prisoner does not possess the same privacy rights as the ordinary citizen. The inmate has a **situational right to privacy**, which is limited by the fact that the inmate is incarcerated and is subject to the discretion or decision-making authority of the MDTT. For example, the MDTT may restrict the inmate's privacy in order to protect the inmate from self-harm, by searching the cell for weapons or drugs, and/or protect others, by searching the inmate's cell for weapons.

Most state legislatures have written statutes that provide almost unlimited access to any type or form of information about the inmate, including medical and/or psychiatric information. But constitutional, federal, or state laws do not clearly identify the parameters of the inmate's right to privacy, nor the provider's corresponding duty to protect that right to privacy. The issue of inmate privacy is a gray area, which makes any decision of the MDTT impinging on privacy rights legally risky and a potential for civil rights and/or malpractice claims by the inmate. Providers must, therefore, cope with the inmate's dynamic and situational right to privacy. As noted previously, it is within the MDTT's discretion to limit the inmate's right to privacy based on a duty to protect the inmate from harm.

RIGHT TO PROTECTION

The nurse, individually and as a member of the MDTT within the correctional facility, must to be aware of the rights of prisoners and the legal risks of **discretionary decisions**, or those subject to the judgment of the MDTT, limiting constitutionally protected rights. The provider's duties are frequently centered on the prisoner's rights to certain types of protection. Specifically, the inmate has a right to protection from: (1) violence, (2) suicide and other self-inflicted harm, and (3) unreasonable risk of disease.

RIGHT TO PROTECTION FROM VIOLENCE

The duty to protect the inmate is based on statutory and constitutional law. In *Alberti v. Heard* (1984), an inmate filed suit claiming that the staffing patterns at Harris County Jail, Houston, Texas, resulted in too few providers to protect the inmates from one another, making the jails unsafe for the inmates. Inmates testified about graphic examples of rape, assault, and other acts of violence, so widespread that the situation clearly established the inability of the existing providers to protect the inmates.

The *Alberti* (1984) court held that, in order to guarantee prisoners protection from violence, the MDTT is required to:

- Provide an adequate inmate/provider ratio. Although the inmate/provider ratio in *Alberti* (1984) met the minimum jail standards of the State of Texas, the court held that one statewide staffing pattern could not be used to staff all types of correctional facilities, when the pattern resulted in an inadequate number of providers.

- Supervise inmates on a continuing basis.
- Provide a call system available to be used by inmates to communicate emergency situations to the provider, which allows for immediate response time.
- Alter the monitoring of cells, so that inmates cannot predict when the provider will return.
- Assign the various levels of security risk inmates to specific, segregated, uncrowded areas. All levels of security risk inmates cannot be assigned to, and crowded into, the same area.
- Provide adequate sleeping areas. Inmates cannot be forced to sleep on floors, tables, and next to toilets.

The Texas court held that the lack of one or any combination of these conditions may be such deliberate indifference by the provider as to result in cruel and unusual punishment to the inmate (*Alberti v. Heard*, 1984). Thus, the courts used Eighth Amendment standards to measure the provider's compliance with the duty to protect the inmate.

EIGHTH AMENDMENT STANDARDS FOR DETERMINING DUTY TO PROTECT

No independent standard exists by which the courts may measure the provider's efforts to protect the prisoner from violence, except the previously identified Eighth Amendment standards. Under these standards, the court asks the question: Are the threats or acts of violence (1) cruel and unusual punishment (*Capps v. Atiyeh*, 1982); (2) deliberate indifference (*Lewis El v. O'Leary*, 1986), and/or (3) deliberate deprivation (*Little v. Walker*, 1977).

Failure to Protect As Cruel and Unusual Punishment

A group of Oregon prisoners brought a class action suit in which they challenged their living conditions. Inmates claimed the conditions were so crowded that they were likely to cause mental and physical deterioration of the inmates. In this instance, the Oregon court held that ordinarily a court might order providers to protect the inmates from other providers. But this court did not order providers to protect the inmates from other providers, who had stripped the inmates of clothing and bedding and held inmates that way overnight. According to the Oregon court, these acts by providers did not show a pattern of brutality, nor were they cruel and unusual punishment (*Capps v. Atiyeh*, 1982).

This Oregon case clearly identified a duty of the nurse and all the members of the MDTT to protect and provide adequate living conditions, including food service, for the inmates. But this holding again leaves the issue of the inmates right to privacy unclear and confusing. In this case, although the inmates had a constitutional right to privacy, they could also be stripped by the provider and left naked, all in the interest of security (*Capps v. Atiyeh*, 1982). Other courts, when analyzing the provider's behaviors related to duty to protect, look to the standard of deliberate indifference and whether the provider's actions and/or inactions resulted in the cruel and unusual punishment.

Failure to Protect
As Deliberate Indifference

An Illinois inmate filed suit claiming that providers acted with deliberate indifference in response to anonymous threats made against the inmate (*Lewis El v. O'Leary*, 1986). The inmate, who was unprotected by providers, was attacked and repeatedly stabbed. The Illinois Court held a provider's deliberate indifference to an inmate's need for protection constitutes cruel and unusual punishment, actionable under the Eighth Amendment (see also, *Little v. Walker*, 1977).

When assessing the provider's efforts to protect the inmate from violence, the standard of deliberate indifference encompasses several types of **culpability**, or guilt. For example, the provider acts with **reckless disregard** when ignoring a substantial risk of danger to the inmate that is either known or would be apparent to a reasonable provider in the same position (*Lewis El v. O'Leary*, 1986).

Recklessness is characterized by highly unreasonable conduct, or a gross departure from ordinary care by the provider, in a situation where a high degree of danger to the inmate is apparent (*Benson v. Cady*, 1985; *Lewis El v. O'Leary*, 1986). The provider who is simply negligent by failing to take reasonable steps to protect an inmate is not liable under the Eighth Amendment for a civil rights violation (*Davidson v. Cannon*, 1986; *Lewis El v. O'Leary*, 1986).

In *Lewis El v. O'Leary* (1986), on two occasions, upon hearing anonymous threats to this Illinois inmate's life, the provider immediately approached the inmate to determine whether the threat had substance. The inmate voiced no concern, implying only a **mere possibility,** or slightest chance, that he would be the subject of violence. Upon his assault, the Illinois court held that the provider's inactions were not reckless, because they were based on the inmate's lack of concern for his safety.

Failure to Protect
As Deliberate Deprivation

The provider's failure to protect the inmate may also violate the Eighth Amendment standard called deliberate deprivation. The term **deliberate deprivation** of protection from violence concerns the intentional removal or denial of that right by the provider. In a related case, to avoid gang-affiliated and violence-prone inmates, an inmate chose to be placed in segregation-safekeeping or isolation (*Little v. Walker*, 1977). Within that setting, providers made no distinction between disciplinary and protective segregatees, denying the inmate basic freedoms, including exercise, religion, and speech. Gang-affiliated inmates served these inmates their meals without provider supervision and forced inmates to perform unnatural sexual acts in order to get their meals. Rebellious inmates took over the isolation area and over a 9-hour period repeatedly raped inmates kept there. After the rebellion, providers continued to house inmates in the same area with their attackers. The inmates filed a civil rights lawsuit, claiming the constant, repeated physical attacks and sexual assaults by other inmates, with no reasonable protection by providers, were cruel and unusual punishment under the Eighth Amendment. The federal court supported the inmate's claims, holding that in this instance:

- The sexual abuse the inmates received in isolation, in general, was cruel and unusual punishment.
- Failure of the MDTT to implement measures to protect the inmates was incompatible with an inmate's constitutional rights to protection, which resulted in the inmates' being forced to endure sexual attacks contrary to "the evolving standards of decency that marks the progress of a maturing society . . . [or]. . . involve the unnecessary or wanton infliction of pain" (*Estelle v. Gamble*, 1976, p. 102; *Little v. Walker*, 1977).

The term *deliberate deprivation* denotes two types of culpability by the provider: actual intent and/or recklessness (*Kimbrough v. O'Neil*, 1976; *Little v. Walker*, 1977). **Actual intent** by the provider encompasses both a special intent to deprive the inmate of his or her constitutional rights as well as a general intent, whose natural consequences deprive the inmate of rights (*Little v. Walker*, 1977; *Monroe v. Pape*, 1961). Recklessness follows an objective or observable standard, specifically, "whether the conduct is with such disregard of the [inmate's] clearly established constitutional rights that [the] action cannot reasonably be characterized as being in good faith" (*Little v. Walker*, 1977; *Wood v. Strickland*, 1975).

In summary, to claim an Eighth Amendment civil rights violation based on deliberate indifference, the courts have held a sufficient foundation may be established by providing evidence of either actual intent or recklessness by the provider (*Estelle v. Gamble*, 1976, p. 105; *Little v. Walker*, 1977).

These cases involving nursing coproviders reveal that the nurse's analogous decisions and actions, individually or as a coprovider within the MDTT, may also constitute deliberate deprivation of the inmate's right to protection if the following elements are present: (1) a special intent by the provider to deprive the inmate of the constitutional right to protection, such as denying access to protection when there is a serious threat; and/or (2) a general intent by the provider to deprive the inmate through the natural consequences of decisions, such as deprivation of protection by denying the inmate the mechanism to ask for protection. Ultimately, these cases reaffirm the inmate's right to, and providers' duty to render, protection from sexual assault.

RIGHT TO PROTECTION FROM SEXUAL ASSAULT

Prisoners have a right to be free of sexual assault by other prisoners (*Ramos v. Lamm*, 1980). Providers have a duty to assess the mental status of the inmate to determine his or her ability to self-protect. The provider must then report to the MDTT the special needs the inmate has for protection. The provider may have a higher duty to protect the mentally challenged inmate, who may be unable to understand or express the extent of the abuse he or she has been experiencing.

The mentally challenged prisoner is only one type of inmate who requires close observation and special protection from inmates and/or other providers in order to ensure that the standard for protection from sexual assault is maintained. For example, an Alabama inmate witnessed the mass homosexual rape of his cellmate while in a prison diagnostic center. He reported the names of the offenders to providers, became known as a "snitch," and was constantly exposed to threats of violence by other inmates. He was placed in a minimum-security facility, and because he was an irritation to providers, always asking for headache medication and wandering at night, he was moved back to the general population. On the day he arrived back in the general population, he was murdered. The Alabama Court held the prisoner's right to protection from violence included the right to be secure from constant threats of violence from either prisoners or providers, and he should have been given ongoing protection by providers because of the constant threats to his life (*Gullatte v. Potts*, 1981).

In a similar case, inmates at El Paso County Jail initiated a class action suit regarding conditions of prison life. The Texas Court held that the primary responsibility of the prison system "is to protect society from those considered dangerous." But state and prison officials, as members of the MDTT, have a corresponding duty to take reasonable steps to ensure that prisoners are free from threats or acts of violence from other prisoners and/or providers (Prison (a), 1987; *Smith v. Sullivan*, 1977).

The courts support the MDTT in enforcement of what might otherwise be classified as harsh security measures, when they are designed to protect the inmate. For example, subsequent to a series of assaults on inmates by other inmates in a New York prison, the warden declared a state of emergency and completely locked down the prison. The MDTT had confined every prisoner to their cell or transported them to special lockdown areas, called **keep-locking**. The New York Court supported the provider's actions and held that the method(s) by which protection is given to those prisoners who are at risk for assault is left to the discretion and judgment of the MDTT (*Gilliard v. Oswald*, 1977).

RIGHT TO PROTECTION FROM PROVIDERS

The courts also recognize that there are situations that require protection of the inmate from the providers. As noted previously, not only must the MDTT take steps to protect prisoners who are reasonably in danger of being victimized by fellow prisoners, but also inmates who may be victims of violence by providers (*Toussant v. McCarthy*, 1984). A group of California inmates brought a claim protesting the conditions of their confinement in segregation (Box 26–3). The California District Court held that the following practices by the MDTT may demonstrate deliberate indifference to the duty to protect inmates from threats or actual violence, if they coexist in areas in which a high level of violence is likely: (1) an inadequate number of providers; (2) a failure to segregate hardened, violent inmates from younger inmates; and (3) physical facilities that do not facilitate the detection of violence by providers (*Toussant v. McCarthy*, 1984).

The duty of the provider to report acts, or threatened acts, of violence against the inmate must he based on established policy and procedure within the correctional facility. Providers have a duty, under statutory law, to report any harmful acts or threats made to the safety of the inmate. The MDTT must take immediate steps to investigate and discipline any provider who inflicts harm on or threatens an inmate.

RIGHTS IN PROTECTIVE CUSTODY VERSUS GENERAL POPULATION

The inmate in the general population has the same right to protection by the provider, and may have to be placed in protective custody to do so. But the prisoner's right to protection from violence is not dependent on whether the prisoner is in protective custody. In *Bishop v. McCoy* (1984), a West Virginia prisoner challenged the conditions of his custody. The prisoner had been placed in protective custody subsequent to breaking up a fight while in the general population and providing the MDTT with information regarding the fight.

The West Virginia court held that the prisoner had a right to be reasonably protected from constant threats of violence and sexual assaults. The court realized the need to segregate the violent from the nonviolent inmate. The court held that the prisoner did not have to be assaulted before a need for segregation into protective custody was apparent. The following two conditions must be met prior to inmate segregation: (1) there must be a pervasive risk to the inmate from other inmates while in the general population, and (2) the MDTT must have been exercising reasonable efforts to prevent in-

BOX 26-3

SUMMARY OF HOLDINGS
IN *TOUSSAINT V. MCCARTHY* (1984)

All the following rights, guaranteed to the inmate under the Eighth Amendment, must be provided by the MDTT:
- Adequate heat, lighting and ventilation
- Plumbing, a basic aspect of sanitation
- An environment that is reasonably free of excessive noise
- Electrical wiring that is not a fire hazard
- An opportunity to have clean clothing
- Reasonably clean, sanitary bedding
- Hot running water
- A reasonable number of showers per week
- Environments free of standing water, fungus, and mold
- A sanitary environment free of rats, birds, mice, and cockroaches
- Food stored, prepared, and served under sanitary conditions
- Confinement in cells that are not small and cramped and/or is not indefinite, allowing for reasonable exercise periods

The following are privileges that are not guaranteed to the inmate under the Eighth Amendment, and may be denied by the MDTT:
- Visits
- Use of the telephone
- Activity programs

tentional harm or risk of harm to the inmate while in the general population (*Bishop v. McCoy*, 1984).

Courts look to the frequency of the attacks on the inmate as part of the previously cited *totality of the circumstances* test in determining the provider's duty to protect. A group of Wisconsin prisoners was immediately moved from one protective unit to another, subsequent to an attack by another prisoner. The petitioning inmates claimed that they feared for their lives when they had to return to their previous unit in the general population for showers three times a week. The court held that the MDTT had not violated the prisoners' right to protection by deciding to return the inmates to the general population. The Wisconsin court further held that isolated instances of attacks on prisoners do not rise to the level of a civil rights violation of duty to protect, without a showing of an inability or unwillingness of the MDTT to

prevent the attack(s) or the recurrence of attack(s) (*Ballard v. Elsea*, 1980).

Prisoners often attack one another spontaneously, whether placed in a common day room or exercise area. But a prisoner attacked does not automatically have a civil rights claim, even if the provider has just removed the attacker's handcuffs immediately prior to the attack (*Massey v. Smith*, 1983). For example, an Indiana inmate, upon entering a day room, was attacked spontaneously by a prisoner who had been placed there while waiting to be assigned to a cell. The providers immediately broke up the attack. The attacking inmate was subsequently assigned to a psychiatric unit.

The Indiana court held that the test of whether or not an act or inaction by the provider is a violation of the Eighth Amendment prohibition against punishments or conditions that result in the unnecessary or wanton infliction of pain is: Were reasonable steps taken by the provider to prevent the pervasive risk of harm to the inmate? (*Massey v. Smith*, 1983). Thus, reasonable steps must be taken by the MDTT to prevent the pervasive risk of harm to the inmate, by staffing with sufficient levels of providers with appropriate supervisory techniques, to protect prisoners from any source or variety of violence (*Alberti v. Heard*, 1984).

It is clear from the holdings in these cases that the nurse, individually and as a coprovider within the MDTT, has a duty to protect the inmate against violence, under the Constitution, specifically the Eighth Amendment, and common law. Failure of the nurse to meet the duty to protect the inmate against violence or threats of violence is deliberate indifference to the safety and security of the inmate under the Eighth Amendment and results in cruel and unusual punishment.

The nurse has a duty to protect the inmate from other inmates as well as other providers within the MDTT. The duty of the MDTT to protect the inmate from violence exists whether there is a mere possibility of it occurring or whether the inmate is in protective custody or the general population. The provider's duty to protect may rise to a higher level if: (1) the inmate is very young, (2) there is an inadequate number of providers, (3) violent inmates are not segregated but intermingled among the inmates, and/or (4) the physical layout of the facility does not facilitate detection of violence. As noted previously, the provider's failure to ensure the inmate protection from violence may be deliberate indifference.

RIGHT TO PROTECTION FROM SUICIDE AND OTHER SELF-INFLICTED HARM

Prisoners have a right to, and providers have a duty to ensure, protection from suicide and other self-inflicted harm (*Kanayurak v. North Slope Borough*, 1984, pp. 898–899). The parents of an inmate in Houston, Texas, sued various providers when their son hanged himself in a solitary cell within a few hours of arrest. The Texas court held that providers have a duty to protect inmates from self-injury (*Patridge v. Two Unknown Police Officers of City of Houston*, 1985). No medical distinction was held to exist under the Eighth Amendment between right to medical, psychological, or psychiatric care. "Treatment of mentally disturbed [suicidal] inmates is a 'serious medical need' under *Estelle* [1976]."

In another case on this point, *Kanayurak v. North Slope Borough* (1984), an Alaskan inmate was taken into protective custody with a blood alcohol level of 0.246 percent. The inmate began yelling, asking someone to locate her children. The providers were aware that the inmate had experienced the following recent crises: one son had been stabbed to death 4 months earlier; a second son had burned to death in a fire 2 months earlier; 2 to 3 months earlier the victim had been divorced; and 2 to 3 weeks earlier the victim's mother had died. The providers closed the door to the cell area to muffle the noise made by the inmate. A video monitor provided a view of the cell area of the inmate, although the monitor in the inmate's cell was partially blocked by a metal bar. As only the inmate's legs were visible, she appeared to be sitting, when actually she had hanged herself.

The Alaska court held that the following set of facts are notice to a provider that an inmate is so intoxicated as to be unable to exercise due care to self-remove from apparent or imminent danger: (1) high blood alcohol level, (2) slurred speech, and/or (3) difficulty walking, such as having to physically self-support (*Kanayurak v. North Slope Borough*, 1984, pp. 898–899).

The duty to prevent suicide exists whether an expert provider has declared the prisoner to be mentally incapacitated or intoxicated. In *Pretty on Top v. City of Hardin* (1979), an inmate from Montana was observed drinking and was arrested for having an open bottle in public. Although he had been drinking, the inmate seemed to have control of his body, as he did not stagger and was coherent. Because the jail he was placed in was used mainly for detoxification, minimum supervision was maintained by the MDTT. The inmate was observed each day by the provider, who reported that his demeanor, attitude, and activities were normal. Four days after his arrest, the inmate committed suicide, by stabbing himself in the throat, neck, and chest with a wooden knife. None of the providers knew how he obtained the knife.

The Montana court held that the:

"[Provider] is not liable to a prisoner in his keeping for injuries resulting from the prisoner's own intentional conduct. . . . Absent some possible special circumstances a [provider] is under no duty to prevent the latter from taking his own life.

Special circumstances, which elevate the duty of care of the provider, occur once the provider knows, or has reason to know, of the suicidal tendencies. The Montana court held that a provider has notice of suicidal tendencies when the inmate: (1) has a history of mental or emotional disease, (2) had previously attempted suicide, and (3) had been observed to have abnormal conduct and demeanor (*Pretty on Top v. City of Hardin*, 1979).

Standard for Protection from Self-Inflicted Harm: Reasonable Care

The standard used to judge whether or not the inmate has been provided protection from suicide by the MDTT is that of the **standard of reasonable care**. This standard means that if the provider has knowledge of or reason to believe the prisoner might inflict self-harm, a duty arises to exercise reasonable care to prevent such harm (*Sudderth v. White*, 1981).

A case in point involves a Kentucky inmate who was a university student, who was arrested, incarcerated, and subsequently committed suicide by hanging himself (*Sudderth v. White, 1981*). The providers had been told to watch the boy as he might try to commit suicide. A member of the MDTT warned other providers to "check on him every now and then through the night." The Kentucky court held there was evidence that providers knew the prisoner was suicidal because the providers had seen the cuts on the prisoner's hands and wrists, which were still healing, and because the inmate had been previously examined by providers,

and transferred to the hospital for treatment, because he was in poor physical condition.

The courts must take into consideration the prisoner's mental and physical condition in determining whether or not the provider has breached the duty to exercise reasonable care to prevent self-harm (*Sudderth v. White*, 1981). For example, if the inmate has self-inflicted an injury and is bleeding profusely the nurse may not be allowed to intervene because the inmate has refused to give up the object or weapon, which may be used in turn to harm or threaten the providers. The inmate may literally bleed to death before a provider intervenes and is allowed into the cell to administer emergency care. In this instance, the court looks to the totality of the circumstances, including the prisoner's violent mental and physical nature and willingness to injure others, in determining whether or not the providers exercised reasonable care in either preventing the inmate from self-inflicting the initial injury or disarming the inmate, in order to protect the providers from injury, before health care is rendered.

Providers do not deprive a prisoner of his or her civil rights when treating the inmate's suicide attempt, real or feigned, as an actual attempt. In *Lee v. Downs* (1979), a Virginia inmate, after a threat from other inmates, was moved to maximum security, where in a feigned attempt at suicide, she was found later with an electrical cord around her neck. She was taken to the prison clinic, where 4 days later she feigned another attempt, removing her paper gown and setting it on fire. The female providers, taking her suicide threats seriously, were assisted by two male security guards in performing a vaginal examination to search for more matches.

The Virginia court held that the body cavity search was reasonable, because providers had to search for other materials by which the inmate might inflict self-harm. The presence of male guards is warranted during a body cavity search of a female when the inmate: (1) is large and strong, (2) had resisted arrest before, and (3) had attempted to inflict self-harm before. But, the Virginia court held that forcing a female to disrobe in front of male guards is cruel and unusual punishment when: (1) the inmate would have voluntarily removed her clothes if the guards would have left the room; and (2) there was no policy that provided that the female prisoner did not have to disrobe in front of male guards in the absence of necessity (*Lee v. Downs*, 1979).

Providers may have a higher duty to prevent the suicide of those who are medically trained. Providers cannot arbitrarily ignore or disregard threats of a prisoner known to have substantial medical training and who is threatening suicide by a feasible method. In *Matje v. Leis* (1983), the family of an Ohio inmate brought suit claiming that inadequate supervision of an inmate, a registered nurse, had resulted in her suicide. The family claimed inadequate custodial care. The Ohio court established the standard that applied in determining adequate custodial care of the suicidal inmate, looking to the "reasonableness of the [provider's] conduct in light of what they knew about the inmate."

Suicidal threats must be responded to in a manner consistent with the correctional facility's policy and procedure. Although there is no duty to prevent a suicide, when a suicide is reasonably foreseeable, the provider should follow reasonable procedures sufficient to prevent the suicide (*Vienneau v. Shanks*, 1977). Reading the prisoner's mail may not be a reasonable method of preventing suicide. A Wisconsin pretrial detainee, who had attempted suicide, sought to stop providers from reading all her nonlegal mail. The Wisconsin court held that the prisoner's right to not have her mail read is a First Amendment right. The MDTT is required to exercise control over a detainee's environment in such a way as to prevent self-harm. The Wisconsin court held that the MDTT had means other than reading the inmate's mail to protect her, which included isolation, constant observation, control of cell contents, and periodic searches (*Vienneau v. Shanks*, 1977).

Providers may not reasonably deprive an inmate of a bed, toilet, and sink in an effort to prevent suicide (*Attorney General v. Sheriff of Worcester County*, 1980). The Worcester County Jail, in Massachusetts, contained seven isolation units that did not contain a toilet, sink, or raised bed. Each contained a hole in the floor, covered with a grating, which could be flushed outside the cell. A public health requirement stated that every inmate's cell must contain a bed, toilet, and sink. The correctional facility intended to install a toilet, sink, or raised bed in six of the units, keeping the seventh as before for temporary confinement of suicidal patients. The Massachusetts court held that a toilet, sink, or raised bed contributes to the health and sanitation in the cell and access to these facilities must be provided by the MDTT. As evidence was provided that revealed that indestructible toilet, sink, or bed units existed, which could not be used by the inmate to self-injure, the Massachusetts court held that these were valid requirements in every cell (*Attorney General v. Sheriff of Worcester County*, 1980).

Inmates who demonstrate extremely suicidal behavior are usually placed in isolation, which may be a security room containing nothing. The criteria and procedure for putting the inmate in isolation must be clearly identified according to the facility's policy and procedure. Also, policy and procedure must be established that clearly inform the MDTT when the inmate may have access to a toilet and running water and inform the inmate of the behavior that must be demonstrated in order to be removed from isolation.

Forcing Treatment to Prevent Bodily Harm

Policy and procedures must also be established regarding instances when the MDTT may force treatment. In general, courts have allowed providers to force treatment on inmates to prevent bodily harm. In one such case, a New York inmate went on a hunger strike to protest prison conditions on behalf of the other prisoners and to demonstrate his unwillingness to testify in an upcoming court proceeding. In this instance, the New York court allowed providers to force-feed the inmate to prevent self-inflicted harm. The court would not allow self-inflicted harm designed to prevent the inmate from testifying in an upcoming court proceeding in which he did not want to testify (*In re Sanchez*, 1983).

The provider's legitimate interest in preventing the prisoner's suicide exists even if the prisoner claims suicide is protected as a freedom of expression under the First Amendment (*Von Holden v. Chapman*, 1982). Mark David Chapman, serving a sentence for killing John Lennon, the former Beatle, refused to eat as he intended to commit suicide by starvation. Chapman claimed his right to commit suicide was a protected expression under the First Amendment. The MDTT at the psychiatric center where Chapman was in custody applied for an order granting permission to force-feed the inmate. The New York court held that, although Chapman's status as a prisoner severely limited his constitutional privileges, "the right to privacy does not include the right to commit suicide." The court further held that a prisoner may starve to death who is sane and rational and under a death sentence (*Von Holden v. Chapman*, 1982; *Zant v. Prevatte*, 1982).

Prison facilities must have a written policy and procedure regarding when and how to compel the inmate's cooperation in any type of treatment. For example, when compelling an inmate to take any type of psychoactive mediation for mental illness, the provider must make sure there is documentation that without this medication the inmate: (1) is likely to cause serious harm to the self or others, and (2) will suffer severe and abnormal mental, emotional, and physical distress. Documentation must indicate that these conditions are imminent or immediate. The order to medicate must be given by two physicians, one being a psychiatrist, with the order being valid for one dose only. In an emergency, the order to compel medication may be given by one physician; but within 48 hours, the determination to force medicate must be made by two physicians.

This series of cases identifies the duties of the nurse, as an individual provider and as a member of the MDTT, to protect the inmate from self-inflicted injury such as suicide. The nurse has no duty to prevent suicide. The standard applicable in the duty to protect is that of reasonable care, requiring the provider to pose the question: Does the provider or the MDTT have knowledge of, or reason to believe, the prisoner might inflict self-harm? When determining whether the nurse acted in a reasonable manner, the courts will most likely look to the prisoner's mental and physical health profile.

Prisoners do not have a constitutional right to commit suicide. But the provider may choose not to intervene in a prisoner's suicide if the prisoner is sane and rational and under a death sentence or dying.

Finally, body cavity searches are reasonable if the provider is looking for a device with which the inmate may inflict self-harm. The courts have also provided legal support by which the MDTT can make decisions to force-feed the inmate to prevent self-harm and compel cooperation in treatment.

RIGHT TO PROTECTION FROM UNREASONABLE RISK OF DISEASE

The conditions of the correctional facility must be such that the prisoner is not unreasonably exposed to the risk of disease (*Grubbs v. Bradley*, 1982). Prisoners brought a class action suit in 12 of Tennessee's adult penal facilities, claiming living conditions within the institutions were cruel and unusual punishment. The Tennessee court used the **totality of conditions test** to determine whether the conditions of confinement had caused unreasonable exposure of inmates to the risk of disease, by posing the following questions:

- Were prison conditions unsanitary, exposing the inmate to an unreasonable risk of disease?
- Was shelter adequate, including minimally adequate living space; for example, adequate ventilation, sanitation, bedding, hygienic materials, and utilities?
- Was housing adequate, with comfortable temperatures or without loud noise, absent extreme conditions that would endanger the inmate's health?
- Had providers demonstrated a pattern of conduct that amounted to a denial of medical care through systematic and gross deficiencies in staffing, facilities, equipment, or procedures?

According to *Grubbs v. Bradley* (1982), the fact that inmates degenerate psychologically and physically as a result of incarceration is not evidence that the providers have violated the inmates' civil rights through inadequate conditions of confinement. But if conditions within the correctional facility are so bad that serious psychological and physiological deterioration in the inmate is inevitable, then those conditions are a violation of the inmate's civil rights.

In summary, the following types of confinement and patterns of practice by providers constitute cruel and unusual punishment, as these conditions deny the inmate the right to reasonable protection from disease: (1) double-celling of inmates; (2) confining inmates in cells without running water for more than 1 week; (3) confining inmates in cells unfit for human habitation; (4) unsanitary conditions in food storage, preparation, and service areas; (5) failure to protect inmates from violent attacks; (6) failure to provide minimally adequate care; and (6) confinement of inmates in segregation status for more than 1 week without exercise (*Grubbs v. Bradley*, 1982).

Segregation of Inmates with Communicable Disease

Another series of cases held that providers have a duty to protect inmates from the spread of contagious or communicable disease, such as acquired immunodeficiency syndrome (AIDS) and tuberculosis (TB). In *LaRocca v. Dalsheim* (1983), a New York inmate sought the removal of all inmates suffering from AIDS, demanding their transferal to a hospital for treatment. The New York court held that the MDTT acted correctly in segregating AIDS inmates, to prevent its spread through sexual coercion. But as the inmates with AIDS were segregated, they did not have to be removed to a hospital, so long as providers maintained precautions for other communicable diseases, such as hepatitis B.

In a supporting case, the court held that the MDTT could maintain a separate ward for prisoners with contagious disease (*Laa-*

man v. Helgemoe, 1977). The court held that a prisoner within the general population found to be infected or contagious should be segregated or isolated to a separate unit or facility. Further, those having contracted contagious or communicable diseases had to be given the proper treatments for their diagnosis (*Smith v. Sullivan*, 1977).

An Oklahoma inmate was placed in a prison cell with three other prisoners, one of which had smallpox. The inmate brought an action claiming a civil rights violation for failure to provide necessary protection from risk of disease. The Oklahoma court held that a provider must be called to attend a sick prisoner. As noted previously, prisoners with contagious diseases must be isolated and have no contact with other prisoners. But, the Oklahoma court held, for the provider to fail to provide isolation is negligence and not deliberate indifference to the health care needs of the inmate placed in the cell with the sick prisoner (*Hunt v. Rowton*, 1930).

The MDTT continuously makes determinations on the environmental conditions to which the inmate will be subjected. Placing the inmate in a condition that poses an unreasonable risk of serious damage to his or her future health may demonstrate deliberate indifference, for example, through exposing the inmate to environmental tobacco smoke. In *Helling v. McKinney, Nev.* (1993), a Nevada inmate filed suit claiming that being assigned to a cell with an inmate who smoked five packs of cigarettes a day was a health risk and was cruel and unusual punishment, violating his Eighth Amendment rights. The court agreed, stating that the health risk posed formed the basis of a valid civil rights claim against providers for failing to protect the inmate from unreasonable risk of disease.

In a related case, a Texas inmate brought a civil rights action, claiming that when the providers placed him in a jail cell with an AIDS patient, they violated his constitutional right to be free from risk of exposure to disease. The Texas court held that placing an inmate in a cell with another inmate who has tested positive for AIDS did not equal deliberate indifference, where the inmate did not contend there are any activities that could pose serious risk of AIDS transmission, such as through sexual contact or intravenous drug use (*Welch v. Sheriff, Lubbock County*, 1990).

Examination and Testing for Communicable Disease

Inmates need not be routinely examined by providers to prevent unreasonable risk of exposure to disease. Incoming prisoners do not need to "be given a [health care] examination within 36 hours of incarceration in the absence of reasonable grounds to suspect that an inmate requires such examination to protect himself and others" (*Estelle v. Gamble*, 1976). In some jurisdictions, instances that violate required standards of adequate health care services include those in which inmates: (1) with contagious or communicable disease, such as scabies or gonorrhea, are incarcerated and left in the midst of the inmate population; or (2) are without medical attention for an unreasonable amount of time, up to a month or more (*Smith v. Sullivan*, 1977).

The failure of providers to test inmates routinely for contagious disease has not been held to be deliberate indifference. In *Feigley v. Fulcomer* (1989), a Pennsylvania inmate brought suit claiming that providers were not adequately protecting him from HIV, violating his civil rights. The Pennsylvania court held:

- Failure of providers to immediately and automatically segregate inmates who test positive for HIV or have any stage of AIDS is not a violation of civil rights.
- To hold the MDTT liable for failure to protect, under the doctrine of *respondeat superior*, the inmate must prove: (1) the MDTT had knowledge of and condoned the behavior of providers who failed to prevent homosexual conduct and intravenous drug use, or (2) the MDTT failed to train providers regarding preventing the spread of HIV in the prison population.

A prisoner in the Nevada State Prison was forced to submit to a blood test for AIDS, which was drawn by nurses, under threat by the guards of being shot with a "taser" gun. The Nevada court held that prisoners do not forfeit all constitutional rights to refuse health care testing, although inmates' "Constitutional rights are subject to substantial limitations and restrictions in order to allow [providers] to achieve legitimate correctional goals and maintain institutional security" (*Walker v. Sumner*, 1990). But the seizure of an inmate's blood specimen without explanation by the provider is unconstitutional. The inmate's civil rights are violated even if such an act was in response to concern of the MDTT for the potential spread of AIDS and the resulting welfare of the staff, citizens, and the prison community (*Bell v. Wolfish*, 1979; *Walker v. Sumner*, 1990). However, if an active case of tuberculosis is detected in the prison population, the MDTT may compel inmates to submit to tuberculosis testing (*Langston v. Commissioner of Correction*, 1993).

RIGHT TO PROTECTION OF THE PROVIDER FROM INMATE VIOLENCE AND FALSE CLAIMS

Providers must protect themselves from acts of violence. An unarmed provider has no duty as a matter of law to intervene physically in a prison fight, which may ultimately cause the provider serious injury and/or worsen the situation or even jeopardize the safety of the prisoners (*Arnold v. Jones*, 1989). Although this type of situation is rare, interventions into the physical fights of prisoners are a function of security services and not a function of a nurse-provider. Nurses must remember in the prison setting their security is a priority also, and they should let security forces physically protect not only the inmate, but also the nurse from the inmate, when appropriate. For example, in maximum security cell blocks, pairs of nurses with security guards must shield themselves behind shatterproof screens when they enter the cell block area to dispense medications, an entourage that must be formed by and for providers to ensure safety for one another.

The MDTT must take preventive measures to ensure that the inmate does not make false accusations of abuse and/or civil rights deprivation against the individual providers when intervening in threatened acts of violence. The MDTT must have established policies and procedures for provider interventions into situations in which the inmate is uncooperative and must be physically restrained. These procedures ideally involve the use of teams of providers with video cameras that intervene and secure the inmate who is uncooperative in their treatment regimen or whose behavior is escalating to a level that threatens the safety of the individual provider, other members of the MDTT, and/or other inmates. After such an intervention, and to avoid legal risk and/or reduce legal liability, the team of providers who have intervened must be sure to document in the inmate's chart: (1) the cause of the event, (2) the progression of the event; (3) the intervention of the security officers; (4) the providers involved; (5) a complete head-to-toe assessment of the physical status of the patient, focusing on injuries, bruises, or cuts, and finally; (6) head-to-toe photographs of the inmate, to provide an immediate record of the inmate's physical condition, as the inmate may self-injure to bolster claims of provider abuse.

RIGHT TO PROTECTION OF THE COMMUNITY FROM INMATE VIOLENCE

The MDTT has a duty to protect the community outside the correctional facility and avoid legal risks and liability, for example, by being vigilant in helping to prevent the wrongful parole of an inmate. In one case on this point, the estate of a woman, kidnapped and murdered by a Massachusetts inmate while on furlough who had previously threatened her life, brought suit against a number of providers, including the medical director and two assistants at a state hospital for wrongfully paroling an inmate (*Estate of Gilmore v. Buckley*, 1985). The estate of the deceased woman claimed, although the parole board had denied the inmate parole, the information and supporting documentation sent to the correctional facility by the MDTT via interdepartmental mail never reached the furlough administrator. The Massachusetts court would have held deliberate indifference to the deceased woman's constitutional rights with evidence that the MDTT knew, or should have known, that the breakdown in communication was likely to occur and would have resulted in the wrongful parole and furlough of the inmate (*Estate of Gilmore v. Buckley*, 1985).

The previously cited and discussed cases support the conclusion that the nurse, as an individual and a coprovider within the MDTT, has a duty to protect the inmate from risk of exposure to communicable disease. Further, providers may compel testing for specific communicable diseases only when that disease is actively detected within the prison population.

RIGHT TO HEALTH CARE

As stated previously, prisoners have a constitutional right to needed health care (Prisons (b) 1987/1998; *Estelle v. Gamble*, 1976). A corresponding duty of the provider exists to deliver reasonable health care to inmates. The MDTT's failure to provide prisoners with reasonable health care is a violation of their constitutional rights and cruel and unusual punishment under the Eighth Amendment of the Constitution (*Estelle v. Gamble*, 1976). Specific standards have been established that guide the provider in rendering minimum acceptable nursing care (Box 26–4).

NURSING STANDARDS OF CARE

Nursing practice within correctional facilities is subject to a variety of standards of care for prisoners, for not only health care but also all aspects of prison life. These health care standards have evolved since approximately the 1960s, under the guidance of a variety of organizations that have been working closely with this special population.

The American Nurses Association Standards for Nursing Practice in Correctional Facilities (ANA, 1985) defined nursing practice within a correctional facility in the following manner:

BOX 26-4

SUMMARY OF HOLDINGS FROM *HINES V. ANDERSON* (1977)

The following decisions from *Hines v. Anderson* (1977) **distinguish** or clarify some inmates' rights to health care provided by one court, of which the provider and/or MDTT must be aware:

- The inmate's right to receive necessary and adequate health care; treatment need not include purely elective surgery or treatment.
- The administration of methadone in a drug maintenance program is not required.
- On admission, inmates must receive physical and psychological examinations, and the results noted on their charts.
- Indigent inmates must be provided prosthetic devices, such as artificial limbs, eyeglasses, false eyes, dentures, braces, casts, and crutches. Prosthetic devices may be provided for cosmetic reasons only if the attending physician determines they are necessary for psychological purposes.
- Inmates should have an opportunity to participate in mass inoculation programs that have been instituted by governmental agencies for the public.
- Each inmate released after incarceration for 1 year or longer, on reasonable request, should be given a free physical examination.
- Inmates have a right to be treated at the prison health care facility, at their personal expense, by a private health care provider. If the provider is located elsewhere, the inmate must pay the expense of guards and transportation to see the provider.
- Sick call should be held on a daily basis.
- As far as feasible, no person who is inmate should be a health care provider.
- Other providers cannot override the judgment and orders of health care providers within the MDTT regarding health care needs.
- The Department of Health must conduct an annual inspection of the correctional facility.
- No inmate shall be transferred back to the prison from a hospital facility while they have a continuing health care need, unless the inmate specifically asks for the transfer.
- A prescribed diet shall be provided as ordered by the MDTT.
- Psychologists shall make rounds on all inmates a minimum of every 2 weeks, to observe and inquire into the mental health needs and status of all inmates.
- Inmates cannot be denied health care because they cannot, orally or in writing, describe their problem.
- Inmates shall not be denied health care or attention while in lock-up. They will be provided a health care request form, and a health care provider will visit the inmate the same day.
- Health care providers must meet criteria for their job descriptions in order to be employed as such.
- Inmates who evidence, or are diagnosed with, a contagious disease: (1) shall be segregated from other inmates, (2) shall not participate in providing health care, and (3) shall not work in food or clothing areas of the prison.

The major thrust of nursing care in correctional settings is the provision of primary care services for the population from the time of entry into the system, through transfers to other institutions, to final release from custody. Primary health services in this field include the use of all aspects of the nursing process in carrying out screening activities, providing direct health care services, analyzing individual health behaviors, teaching, counseling, and assisting individuals in assuming responsibility for their own health to the best of their ability, knowledge and circumstances (ANA, 1985).

The correctional nurse is primarily held to the legal definition of nursing practice in the state of license. But as the ANA Standards are a national professional statement of not only desired, but also expected, nursing practice within a correctional facility, they are standards for which the correctional nurse may be held accountable by the legal system.

CONSTITUTIONAL STANDARD OF REASONABLE HEALTH CARE

The health care provided must be reasonable in light of all the circumstances surrounding the illness and incarceration of the inmate (*Isaac v. U.S.*, 1979). By *reasonable health care* the courts mean the prisoner has a right to receive health care under circumstances that any reasonable person would seek health care (*Brewer v. Perrin*, 1984).

Right to Health Care under the Standard of Reasonableness

The duty to provide reasonable health care arises because a prisoner is completely dependent on providers for health care (*Laaman v. Helgemoe*, 1977). The prisoner's loss of liberty prevents his or her ability to meet or attend to specific or unique personal health care needs (*United States v. Bundy*, 1983). For example, in *Bundy* (1983), an inmate asked the court for a reduction in her sentence because her arthritic condition had worsened during incarceration and she was not receiving adequate health care. The federal court held that the MDTT must have

adequate providers to render the proper treatments, for example, for treatment of arthritis. Even contracting out health care (for example, to a regional medical facility to provide unique health care services) does not relieve the facility's MDTT from their duty to ensure reasonable health care within the correctional facility (Prisons (c) 1987-1998 § 89).

The right to reasonable health care includes psychiatric care. A Virginia inmate told providers he was under psychiatric care and needed psychiatric help. Arresting officers told the inmate he would receive psychiatric treatment after he withdrew his request for counsel and confessed to the charges against him. The Virginia court held the acts of the arresting officer unconstitutional, as prisoners have a right to health care and providers who have custody have a duty to procure that health care (*Vinnedge v. Gibbs*, 1977).

The prisoner's health care must be reasonably designed to meet both routine and emergency health care needs (*Laaman v. Helgemoe*, 1977). It is reasonable that mobility-impaired inmates are provided with wheelchairs and/or other mobility aids (*Casey v. Lewis*, 1991). An inmate need not be in a wheelchair to be declared handicapped. An inmate brought a class action suit challenging prison policies in the Arizona Department of Corrections. The Arizona court held that prisoners who are HIV positive are handicapped as defined under the Rehabilitation Act of 1973. Thus, discrimination is not allowed against inmates with HIV diagnosis under this 1973 act (*Casey v. Lewis*, 1991.

A New York inmate brought suit, claiming providers were negligent in their failure to provide health care until 3 days after his symptoms of stomach pain began. The court held that, under the Federal Torts Claim Act, the United States may be held liable to an inmate for negligent failure to provide reasonable medical care. The New York court then awarded the prisoner only $1000, for approximately 3 days of pain and suffering (*Isaac v. U.S.*, 1979).

In *Brewer v. Perrin* (1984), a 15-year-old Michigan inmate was arrested after coming home drunk and chasing his brother around the neighborhood with a butcher knife.

Providers knew the arrestee was a juvenile. He fought, kicked, and screamed on the ride down to the police station. The juvenile was placed in a cell especially designed for juveniles, with audio but no video monitoring. Although a detoxification cell was available (with soft surfaces and no bars and that was observable from the security corridor), prison policy required the inmate be placed in the cell for juveniles. Providers turned off the sound monitoring system because the juvenile continued shouting and screaming. Providers checked the juvenile only once in 1½ hours. The juvenile used his shirt to hang himself.

The Michigan court held that reasonable health care encompasses not only serious physical needs, but also serious psychological needs (see also, *Bowring v. Godwin*, 1977; and *Inmates of the Allegheny County Jail v. Pierce*, 1979). The court held that the providers in *Brewer* (1984) should have known by his behavior that the juvenile inmate needed psychiatric attention. The court further held providers demonstrated deliberate indifference when they failed to: (1) consider that a juvenile inmate sobering up can become very depressed; (2) immediately take the juvenile before the probate court, as is usually ordered by state statute; and (3) monitor the juvenile in his cell (*Brewer v. Perrin*, 1984).

A MDTT that allows a nonphysician to perform surgery during nonemergency situations in hospital prisons exhibits gross deliberate indifference (*Burks v. Teasdale*, 1980). But other nonemergency health care needs of inmates may be routinely screened and cared for by physician's assistants and nurse practitioners.

The MDTT demonstrates deliberate indifference when prisoners are not able to make their health care problems known or do not have access to providers who are competent to deal with their health care needs. According to the courts, access to incompetent providers is meaningless, and in essence, no health care has been provided (*Hoptowitt v. Ray*, 1982).

A group of inmates brought a claim against the MDTT at the Washington State Penitentiary, alleging that certain conditions within the correctional facility were not

reasonable and constituted cruel and unusual punishment, including overcrowding, high levels of violence, and inadequate medical care. The Hoptowitt (1982) court held:

- It is reasonable to withhold rehabilitation, including educational, recreational, and vocational programs, as inmates have no constitutional right to these health care services.
- Isolation doors, which are closed metal doors, are unreasonable and are cruel and unusual punishment as this type of door does not allow in fresh air or light, and may be mentally and physically damaging to the inmate.
- Deprivation of adequate food, clothing, shelter, sanitation, medical care, and personal safety to the inmate while in isolation is unreasonable and constitutes cruel and unusual punishment.
- The longer the deprivation by the provider, the more unreasonable, and the closer the deprivation comes to infliction of pain on the inmate. In an actual emergency, the MDTT may be more restrictive and suspend certain services to the inmate. But the more basic the need, the less amount of time the MDTT can reasonably withhold it from the inmate, such as emergency health care.

Unless there are aggravating circumstances, a prisoner's dissatisfaction with the effectiveness of health care treatment and outcome is not grounds for a civil rights claim. In *Sowell v. Israel* (1980), the prisoner slipped and fell while assigned to a kitchen job. He was assigned to a "sick cell," where he was examined by both doctors and nurses and given a treatment regimen of moist heat and a lumbar corset. Although the court recognized the inmate's dissatisfaction with the course and outcome of his treatment, the court held that providers did not demonstrate deliberate indifference to his health care needs simply because of the inmate's dissatisfaction with treatment.

In *Turner v. Plageman* (1976), an inmate in a correctional unit argued that he had received improper health care treatment when he complained of headaches and dizziness. Because he had no fever, providers ordered him to return to work. The court held that refusing to grant a prisoner's request to be absent from work owing to headaches and dizziness, and subsequently punishing him for failure to return to work, was not so serious and unreasonable as to constitute a violation of the prisoner's constitutional rights.

Health care must be provided when necessary (*Hunt v. Rowton*, 1930). Mere slowness in providing health care to the inmate may not be deliberate indifference, but unreasonable delay in providing health care is a constitutional violation of the prisoner's civil rights (see also, *Estelle v. Gamble*, 1976). The courts will look to a wide variety of surrounding circumstances in analyzing the reasonableness of delay of health care, including but not limited to: (1) acuity of the condition of the inmate; (2) level of security precautions required by this inmate; (3) physical location of any specialized health care services that may be necessary for the inmate, for example, dialyses; (4) availability of the type of health care specialist necessary to treat the inmate; and (5) availability of, and time required to travel to, the location at which health care will be provided. Along with assessing the reasonableness of health care, the courts also analyze the adequacy of health care (*Hunt v. Rowton*, 1930).

ADEQUACY OF HEALTH CARE

The adequacy of health care is the quality of health care rendered by the provider and/or the MDTT. Correctional facilities designed to meet inmates' health care needs must be sufficient to serve adequately those health care needs (*Laaman v. Helgemoe*, 1977). Federal and state case law has defined what constitutes reasonable or adequate health care. For example, a Rhode Island inmate underwent surgery while incarcerated at a correctional facility. On return to prison, the inmate was placed in a punitive segregation unit to complete a disciplinary action. The primary provider recommended a shower and change of surgical dressings three times a day. The inmate was supplied with bandages and

taught to change his own dressings, that is, he was taught self-care, although occasionally the provider would help him with the procedure. He sometimes was allowed to shower only once a day. He developed an infection in the surgical wound and filed a civil rights action against the MDTT, claiming inadequate health care (*DesRosiers v. Moran*, 1991).

When the adequacy or quality of health care in a correctional facility is evaluated, the (*DesRosiers*, 1991) court held that the **practical constraints** facing the providers, or limitations in ability to provide care, should be analyzed. The court held that the failure of the nurses to change the inmate's bandages three times a day was not deliberate indifference. The court reasoned, because of the practical constraints of the provider, the inmate was taught to change his own bandages. He had ready access to supplies and never complained of problems in doing so. The court held that there was no evidence that providers knew infection would result if the inmate showered less often (*DesRosiers v. Moran*, 1991).

The adequacy of health care of prisoners and prison conditions must also be evaluated against a background of the history of inmate violence (*Bruscino v. Carlson*, 1988). An inmate incarcerated in the U.S. Penitentiary located in Marion, Illinois, a maximum security facility designed to be the successor to Alcatraz, filed a civil rights claim against providers regarding the inadequacy of health care. As a level 6 federal prison (security rating from 1 to 6, with six having the highest security), this facility housed approximately 300 of the most dangerous and violent prisoners and state prisoners too violent to handle. The Illinois court held that the MDTT in such a maximum security facility may arbitrarily determine whether to provide prisoners with privileges amounting to more than reasonably adequate food, clothing, shelter, sanitation, medical care, and personal safety (*Green v. McKaskle*, 1986).

Providers need not establish a system of routine examination of inmates (*Smith v. Sullivan*, 1977). But there must be a system in place to provide health care for prisoners who become ill when providers are not on duty (*Hines v. Anderson*, 1977). The inmate in *Hines* (1977) brought a class action suit under the theory that health care and facilities at the Minnesota State Prison violated civil rights, as there was no system to provide health care when providers were off duty. The Minnesota Court held that providers must ensure that the rights as stated in the Patient Bill of Rights are also made available to inmates who receive health care treatment within the correctional facility.

Florida courts have held that inadequate health care treatment existed when there was inadequate means of communication between inmates and the MDTT by which the need for health care was made known. In addition, the Florida court held that there were inadequate health care services if there were deficiencies in such health care services as laboratory or x-ray equipment or therapists and there was no formal arrangement for emergency services. The Florida court ordered, along with correction of inadequate services, a formal contract with a hospital emergency room within close proximity to ensure these services (*Miller v. Carson*, 1975).

In another suit brought by inmates in Florida, to alleviate inadequate health care caused by overcrowding, the Florida court held that deliberate indifference to health care needs of prisoners may also be shown if: (1) adequate health care is denied as a result of prison overcrowding, with resulting inability of the provider to assess for or intervene in health care needs; or (2) simply because the MDTT failed to appropriate sufficient amounts of money to provide the necessary health care (*Costello v. Wainwright*, 1976).

Box 26–5 summarizes court decisions identifying inmates' rights for various types of health care services.

BOX 26-5

HOLDINGS RELATIVE TO HEALTH CARE SCREENING, MEDICATIONS, ABORTION, AND DENTAL CARE

The following is a summary of court decisions that identify inmates' rights to health care screening, medications, abortion, and dental care, of which the provider and/or MDTT must be aware:

- **Health Care Screening**: Necessary and qualified providers who are trained to identify and cope with healthcare emergencies must be available to the inmate at all times (*Laaman v. Helgemoe*, 1977). Health care screening of new inmates must be performed by providers who are qualified to perform such assessments (*Cody v. Hillard*, 1984).
- **Medications**: Medications cannot be prescribed at the convenience of the MDTT. Medications can be prescribed only as part of an individual treatment plan. Further, psychotropic medications can be prescribed for the inmate only after examination by a physician (*Jackson v. Hendrick*, 1974).
- **Abortion**: The correctional facility may have a responsibility to pay for health care expenses related to non therapeutic abortions performed on the inmate. Requiring inmates to obtain their own financing before having the procedure performed may be unconstitutional (*Monmouth County Correctional Institutional Inmates v. Lanzaro*, 1987).
- **Dental Care**: Prisoners have a right to reasonable dental care (*Laaman v. Helgemoe*, 1977). But reasonable delay in dental care, up to 90 days, may not rise to the level of a constitutional violation (*Robbins v. South et al.*, 1984).

FINANCIAL RESPONSIBILITY FOR HEALTH CARE

Generally, the MDTT must realize that the correctional facility is responsible for the allocation, cost, and delivery of the health care required by prisoners (*Wilkinson v. State*, 1983). Health care may include the right to and costs of having a specific provider. In *Wilkinson v. State* (1983), a pregnant inmate, who was soon to give birth, was sentenced to serve 10 years at a women's correctional facility. The inmate's testimony at the sentencing hearing indicated a strong relationship with her provider of prenatal care. The Montana court allowed the inmate to stay at the county jail and give birth at the county hospital, and the state correctional agency was ordered to pay for the costs.

The court in another jurisdiction rendered a contrary holding. An Oklahoma inmate injured his back while in maximum security. He disagreed with the diagnosis and prescribed treatment of two providers who examined him, and he requested to see a specific provider in the Oklahoma area who was in private practice. The Oklahoma court held that an inmate has no right to a particular course of treatment or a particular provider (*McCraken v. Jones*, 1977).

A correctional system cannot be held financially liable for providing treatment to the inmate for a lifetime for an illness it did not cause (*Commonwealth v. Lyles*, 1983). A Pennsylvania inmate, who escaped from a correctional facility, sustained multiple gunshot wounds, which resulted in permanent paraplegia, and subsequently was recaptured. The Pennsylvania court held that the inmate, upon release, could not hold the state responsible for these costs for a lifetime because they had occurred during an attempted escape. But, the MDTT must be aware that an inmate who received dialysis or insulin therapy prior to incarceration must be provided such treatment during his or her entire incarceration, at the expense of the state (*Commonwealth v. Lyles*, 1983).

An inmate who is serving a sentence and is then involuntarily committed and/or transferred to a psychiatric hospital by the correctional facility is not responsible for the cost of the psychiatric care, nor is the family (*Matter of Commitment of F.H.*, 1992). A New Jersey inmate was sentenced to a term in an adult diagnostic and treatment center for having committed a sex crime. After a suicide attempt, he was involuntarily committed by the acting warden to an adult forensic unit. A lien was subsequently placed against the inmate's property in the full amount of his psychiatric care. The New Jersey court held that the inmate's psychiatric care would be paid by the state, whether psychiatric treatment was voluntarily sought or involuntary commitment or treatment ordered by the MDTT (*Matter of Commitment of F.H.*, 1992).

An inmate involved in an automobile injury while on furlough from a state correctional facility remains in custody of the state, and the state is responsible for the cost of the injury. In the Texas case of *Bryson v. State* (1990), an inmate had been on a 3-day furlough to seek employment prior to parole, when he was in an automobile accident. He was then taken to a university medical center for treatment. The prisoner was paroled while undergoing treatment at the medical center. The Texas court held that the inmate's health care bill would be paid at the medical center. The court reasoned that the inmate was not receiving the ideal type of assessment and treatment by the providers at the correctional facility. The prison should have provided for a variety of opinions regarding the health care needed and health care by an interdisciplinary treatment team, such as a MDTT (*Bryson v. State*, 1990).

DIVERGENCE OF OPINION ON TREATMENT PLAN

As in most groups with a variety of opinions on health care treatment, the MDTT may not agree on the course of therapy for the inmate, resulting in a divergence of opinion on the appropriate treatment plan. The following case is an example. A North Carolina inmate claimed to be a member of a certain Jewish sect and wished to abide by their laws. The prisoner claimed that as a result of the provider's failure to give him proper food and treatment, his health had been impaired. The MDTT disagreed on the management of his care. The North Carolina court held that, when there exists a complete divergence of opinion as to the inmate's physical and psychological condition, the MDTT may be compelled to grant the inmate a furlough. This furlough would be at the inmate's expense, in order to obtain another opinion as to the exact nature and appropriate treatment (*Prushinowski v. Hambrick*, 1983).

RIGHT TO REFUSE TREATMENT

Regardless of the standards, rules, and regulations the MDTT must follow, the courts have affirmed a prisoner's right to refuse life-sustaining treatment (Penal & Correctional (a): 1987/1998). But an inmate may have no protected liberty interest in not participating in or refusing a treatment program. For example, inmates may be required to attend educational programs for prisoners who are sex offenders if they have refused other forms of health care treatment (*Sundby v. Fiedler*, 1993). The courts have also preserved the right of the inmate to **waive**, that is refuse, relinquish, or forgo treatment.

Waiver of Treatment

If an inmate waives treatment, the duty of the MDTT to treat is discharged, negating the possibility of the inmate's filing a lawsuit under the deliberate indifference standard. In *Thor v. Superior Court* (1993), a California inmate jumped or fell from a prison wall, fracturing cervical vertebrae and becoming a quadriplegic. After the fall, the inmate's providers alleged that the inmate had intermittently refused to eat and had a substantial risk of death, and they asked for a tube to be inserted to feed and medicate the inmate.

The California court in Thor (1993) held:

A competent, informed adult has a fundamental right of self-determination to refuse or demand the withdrawal of medical treatment . . . irrespective of personal consequences . . . in the absence of evidence demonstrating a threat to institutional security or public safety, . . . [the members of the MDTT] . . . have no affirmative duty to administer

such treatment and may not deny a person incarcerated in state prison this freedom of choice.

In general the MDTT must have established policy and procedure regarding follow-up care and documentation in response to an inmate's waiver or refusal of any type of health care, whether the refusal is of life-sustaining treatment or daily medications. The inmate usually provides a written waiver of treatment on a form standardized by the correctional facility. The nurse is usually the member of the MDTT who obtains the signature of the inmate on the written waiver. The records of all waivers must be kept on the inmate's chart.

Involuntary Treatment

The provider must carefully follow prison policy and procedure when participating in any intervention in which the inmate participates involuntarily. Most psychiatric correctional facilities require the videotaping of involuntary interventions, as it requires **use of force**, which is *any* touching of the inmate.

An inmate may be compelled to undergo involuntary treatment when such measures are reasonably required to protect the prisoner or fellow inmates from substantial possibility of harm. For example, the involuntary treatment of an inmate with psychotropic medications is warranted, over the objection of the prisoner, when psychotic behavior is a threat to the safety and/or security of the inmates and/or providers (*Sconier v. Jarvis*, 1978).

But a provider may not medicate a death row prisoner with antipsychotic drugs against his or her will in order to carry out a death sentence. In *State v. Perry* (1992), a Louisiana inmate had a history of mental illness, having been diagnosed with schizophrenia in 1983. He was in and out of mental hospitals, having escaped twice. His parents made him sleep in a shed behind their house because of his disruptive conduct. The inmate was sentenced to death for murdering his mother, father, nephew, and two cousins in a murder episode in 1983. A psychiatric expert, in determining the inmate's competency, assisted the Louisiana court in concluding that the inmate was competent for execution only when maintained on antipsychotic medications, specifically Haldol. The Louisiana court further cited the U.S. Supreme Court in holding that sentencing a prisoner who is insane to the death penalty is prohibited by the Eighth and Fourteenth Amendments (see also, *Ford v. Wainwright*, 1986).

A New Jersey inmate, and other prisoners within the New Jersey prison system, filed a complaint against a provider within the MDTT, seeking to prevent this provider from treating prisoners and seeking damages for injuries resulting from the provider's conduct. The inmate, who had a chronic ear infection, was allergic to penicillin and feared that an ear cleansing solution prescribed by the provider might contain penicillin. The provider refused to tell the inmate the ingredients of the ear wash. The New Jersey court held that, although professional medical and nursing judgment is presumed valid in a decision to compel the inmate to involuntary treatment, the inmate retains a limited right to refuse health care treatment and a related right to be informed of the proposed treatment and viable alternatives (*White v. Napoleon*, 1990). Failure to provide informed consent regarding treatment may amount to medical experimentation.

Medical Experimentation

Constitutional challenges to medical experimentation by the MDTT have been based on the inmate's right to freedom from intrusions into the privacy of the mind and body under the First, Third, Fourth, Ninth, and Fourteenth Amendments (*Roe v. Wade*, 1973). Inmates are often involved in medical experimentation in two contexts. First, the prisoner may volunteer to participate in drug-related research by the provider within the correctional facility, receiving compensation for acting as a "human guinea pig." Second, as a result of decisions of the MDTT to use experimental drugs to modify the inmate's behavior, experimentation in behavior modification often takes place in what may ultimately be a scientifically unapproved and unsound manner (Penal & Correc-

tional (c): 1987/1998). In this latter instance, if the inmate does not have informed consent, such medical experimentation by the MDTT could constitute a violation of the Eighth Amendment prohibition against cruel and unusual punishment.

Further, unauthorized experimentation by the MDTT could also be a violation of the inmate's rights under the First and Fourteenth Amendments, for these amendments guarantee a right to be free from interference with one's thoughts and sensations. In *Mackey v. Procunier* (1973), an inmate in a California correctional facility, with his consent, underwent shock treatment. The inmate complained that without his permission he was given succinylcholine, a relaxant, which he characterized as a "breath-stopping" and as a paralyzing "fright drug."

The California court in *Mackey* (1973) held that the MDTT had been engaged in experimentation with the "relaxant" on fully conscious inmates, actions specifically not recommended in the use of this drug. According to the court, being given a "fright drug" without inmate consent evidenced cruel and unusual punishment, or "impermissible tinkering with the mental processes." These acts are specifically forbidden by the First and Fourteenth Amendments. The Mackey (1973) Court further held that the inmate had been subjected to experimentation without his consent.

RIGHT TO HEALTH CARE UNDER THE STANDARD OF DELIBERATE INDIFFERENCE

Analysis of rights to health care also fall under the constitutional standard of deliberate indifference (*Mackey v. Procunier*, 1973). As noted previously, an inmate who is a victim of deliberate indifference to serious medical needs has grounds for a case of an Eighth Amendment civil rights violation based on denial of health care treatment. The federal courts are quick to point out that when establishing deliberate indifference "an accidental or inadvertent failure to provide adequate care will not suffice for [civil rights] purposes" (*Layne v. Vizant*, 1981).

According to *Burks v. Teasdale* (1980), to prove deliberate indifference, plaintiffs must provide evidence either of a "series of incidents closely related in time . . . [that] may disclose a pattern of conduct amounting to deliberate indifference to medical needs of prisoners" and/or that "the [health care] facilities were so wholly inadequate that suffering would be inevitable." (See Boxes 26–6 and 26–7 for examples of situations that do and do not meet the conditions of deliberate indifference.)

A civil rights action brought by Indiana prison inmates challenged conditions of confinement at the state prison (*Wellman v. Faulkner*, 1983). The Indiana court held that deliberate indifference to serious health care needs can be proven with evidence of repeated negligent acts that disclose a pattern of conduct by the MDTT and/or systematic and gross deficiencies in staffing, facilities, equipment, or procedures, which effectively results in the denial by the MDTT of access to adequate health care by the inmate (see also, *Ramos v. Lamm*, 1980, p. 575).

The *Wellman* (1983) court held that the following examples are evidence of general deficiencies sufficient to establish deliberate indifference to serious health care needs: (1) use of providers who are recent immigrants, do not have full use of the English language, and cannot effectively communicate with the inmates; (2) understaffing of the psychiatric care component of the health care system, including situations in which there is no provider with a psychiatric specialization and no prospect of providing one; (3) numerous cases of health care maltreatment, including failure to treat stomach disorders, painful abscesses, or an apparent heart attack, and/or provide dental care; and (4) failure to provide necessary health care supplies, for example, forcing inmates to reuse colostomy bags (*Wellman v. Faulkner*, 1983).

An Illinois inmate claimed he was subject to cruel and unusual punishment when denied health care treatment for two infected toes (*Andrews v. Glenn*, 1991). The inmate signed up for sick call for the purpose of having his toes treated. He reported late to the nurse for treatment, so was asked to return the next day. The nurse then referred

BOX 26-6

NURSING CARE THAT IS NOT DELIBERATE INDIFFERENCE

The courts have held that the following examples of inmate health care by the nurse are *not* examples of deliberate indifference:

- Refusing to help a prisoner apply external medication because of other nursing duties (*Sires v. Birman*, 1987).
- Refusing to treat a patient for a preexisting injury, because the state is not responsible for injuries occurring prior to incarceration (*Watson v. Carton*, 1993)
- Delaying treatment of cuts and bruises for 14 hours after arrest, when such injuries were not serious and the delay did not exacerbate the injuries (*Martin v. Gentile*, 1988)
- Failing to provide physical therapy for an inmate with a broken wrist, after the therapy had been prescribed (*Warren v. Missouri*, 1993)
- Failing to administer a precise, prescribed dosage of medication to an inmate with diagnosed coronary artery disease, a diagnosis that qualifies as a serious medical condition (*Brewer v. Blackwell*, 1993)
- Failing to quarantine an inmate infected with tuberculosis, when inmates were screened but no other steps were taken to prevent the spread of tuberculosis (*Blumhagen v. Sabes*, 1993)

BOX 26-7

NURSING CARE THAT IS DELIBERATE INDIFFERENCE

The courts have held that the following examples of inmate health care by the provider *are* examples of deliberate indifference:

- Delaying for 2 years scheduling surgery to repair broken pins in a hip (*Hathaway v. Coughlin*, 1988)
- Failing to ensure proper hiring, supervision, and/or training of providers assigned to perform treatments (*Simpkins v. Bellevue Hospital*, 1993)
- Depriving a transsexual inmate of estrogen therapy, when the inmate had undergone therapy for 17 years, as well as undergone surgery to enhance appearance as a female, and deprivation of estrogen would reverse years of healing medical treatment (*Phillips v. Michigan Dept. of Corrections*, 1990)
- Refusing to continue treatment of serious chronic urinary infections over a 5-month period, the result of which was complete urinary dysfunction requiring constant catheterization (*Wood v. Sun*, 1988)

the inmate for examination by the doctor in 3 days. The nurse reported that the foot condition was not serious. The Illinois court held that the following three conditions must be met when determining whether or not the provider demonstrated deliberate indifference to a serious medical need: (1) a serious health care problem, (2) a substantial potential for harm to the inmate if the health care is denied or delayed by the provider, and (3) the harm to the inmate actually results from the delay or denial by the provider (see also, *Thomas v. Pate*, 1974).

A class action suit was brought by inmates of the Monmouth County Correctional Institution challenging the policies and practices of the MDTT, claiming they denied pregnant inmates access to, and funding for, abortions (*Monmouth County Correctional Institutional Inmates v. Lanzaro*, 1987). The New Jersey Court held that the MDTT's requirement that inmates finance their own abortions was unconstitutional, as this policy restricted the inmate's right to choose abortion. The court also held that the following practices by the MDTT constituted deliberate indifference: (1) the requirement that the inmate obtain a court-ordered release as a precondition to obtaining an abortion, and (2) the failure to minimize delay in accessing abortion ser-

vices for the inmate. The Monmouth (1987) court also held that for a condition to be a serious health care need it did not have to be an abnormal medical condition.

A paraplegic Kansas inmate filed a civil rights action against providers, claiming that confinement without proper medical care was cruel and unusual punishment, in violation of the Eighth Amendment (*Lee v. McManus*, 1982). The paraplegic inmate sought injunctive relief, "to prevent further denial of [health] care prescribed for him by [the provider] specialists who had treated him for his paraplegia." The inmate was injured and became a paraplegic when a provider injured his spine. As a result of the paraplegia, the inmate suffered a neurogenic bowel and bladder (no control), loss of skin sensation with a very deep decubitus ulcer (bedsore), and abnormal reflexes, or spasticity, of the lower limbs, causing stiffening of the joints. Without further health care attention, the inmate's potential complications included kidney damage, infection, and joint contractures (*Lee v. McManus*, 1982).

On discharge from the health care facility at which he was treated, the inmate was prescribed, but did not receive, the following care and treatment by the MDTT: (1) daily range of motion exercises, the lack of which caused the joints to become stiffened and more spastic; (2) biweekly catheter replacement, having it changed only once when it came out by accident; (3) stool softeners, suppositories, or assistance with the commode, the lack of which caused the inmate to be forced to defecate in bed; (4) daily fluid intake of 3000 cc, of which he received only a pitcher of water a day; and (5) daily changing of bandages, which were actually changed only twice in a month (*Lee v. McManus*, 1982).

In response to the paraplegic inmate's claims, the *Lee* (1982) court held that deliberate indifference to plaintiff's serious health care needs may be shown when providers have prevented the inmate from receiving recommended treatment (see also, *Ramos v.*

Lamm, 1980). When a paraplegic inmate has unique health care needs, providers have a duty to investigate and take affirmative action to meet those unique health care needs (*Lee v. McManus*, 1982).

The *Lee* court (1982, p. 391) further held that deliberate indifference by the provider may be shown through testimony of a health care expert that the plaintiff had serious medical needs and the defendant had shown deliberate indifference to those health care needs. Plaintiff's expert testified that if the paraplegic inmate did not receive immediate and continuous health care treatment, he would suffer irreparable harm (*Lee v. McManus*, 1982).

Box 26–8 lists examples of nursing care that is in violation of an inmate's Eighth Amendment rights.

BOX 26-8

NURSING CARE THAT IS CRUEL AND UNUSUAL PUNISHMENT

The following care of the inmate by the Provider has been held to violate the inmate's Eighth Amendment civil rights and to be cruel and unusual punishment:

- Forcibly treating an inmate with an intramuscular injection of a major tranquilizer, without prior assessment by a provider (*Knecht v. Gillman*, 1973)
- Failing to properly observe and/or communicate with inmates who have serious health care needs (*Todaro v. Ward*, 1977)
- Failing to properly screen/assess the inmate (*Todaro v. Ward*, 1977)
- Denying the inmate access to a physician (*Todaro v. Ward*, 1977)
- Failing to write policies and procedures for nursing care (*Lightfoot v. Walker*, 1980)
- Improperly executing standing orders (*Knecht v. Gillman*, 1973)
- Giving a juvenile inmate an injection of a central nervous system depressant in retaliation for undesirable behavior (*Nelson v. Heyne*, 1974)
- Prescribing and administering controlled substances without consultation with, or authorization from, a physician (*Knecht v. Gillman*, 1973)
- Failing to respond to inmates' health care needs in relation to an addiction (*Palmigiano v. Garrahy*, 1977)
- Using restraints, isolation, and tranquilizing drugs as antitherapeutic, punitive measures (*Knecht v. Gillman*, 1973)
- Failing to develop quality assurance measures (*Lightfoot v. Walker*, 1980)
- Being disorganized, inaccurate, and unprofessional in record keeping (*Burks v. Teasdale*, 1980)

Right to Health Care of a Pretrial Detainee

The sentenced inmate is not the only prisoner who has a right to health care under the Eighth Amendment. The right to health care also extends to the pretrial detainee. In *Holly v. Rampone* (1979), a Pennsylvania pretrial detainee informed a member of the MDTT upon arrival at the prison that he was a heroin addict, his last drug use had been approximately 8 hours earlier, and he needed health care. The inmate was informed that there was no methadone program. The inmate experienced withdrawal symptoms. The inmate was seen by a provider who could not prescribe methadone, but he was told he would be put on the waiting list to see a provider with prescriptive authority in approximately 4 days. On the day that the inmate saw the provider with prescriptive authority, he asked for and was denied an eye examination to replace eyeglasses damaged during his arrest. About 3 weeks later the inmate fell, he alleged, as a result of the absence of eyeglasses. The inmate was again examined by the same provider, asked for and was refused an x-ray examination. The Pennsylvania inmate claimed that he had sustained permanent injury to his back from the fall, caused by lack of eyeglasses. The inmate brought suit claiming his Eighth and Fourteenth Amendment rights had been violated by the MDTT (*Holly v. Rampone*, 1979).

The *Holly* (1979) court held that an inmate has no constitutional right to x-ray or other diagnostic tests if only the inmate feels such tests are necessary for diagnosis of an injury (see also, *Estelle v. Gamble*, 1976, p. 98). A prisoner cannot be the final judge of what health care treatment is necessary (see also, *Fore v. Goodwin*, 1976). Although there may be a more effective treatment, an inmate cannot sustain a civil rights action against the provider for improper health care treatment in this instance (see also, *United States v. County of Philadelphia*, 1969).

The *Holly* (1979) court also held that prison literature must forewarn inmates seeking treatment for ordinary problems, such as an eye examination, that they may experience a delay in examination and treatment if there are a large number of requests for the same treatment received from other inmates. The Pennsylvania court held that the MDTT's denial of an examination for the unsentenced inmate was not punishment in the constitutional sense (see also, *Bell v. Wolfish*, 1979). The MDTT's policy to provide only emergency medical care to unsentenced inmates or detainees was held by the Pennsylvania court to be reasonable. The court concluded that the length of detention of the unsentenced inmate is unknown; therefore, there was not deprivation of health care, because there was an alternative, justified purpose to which the denial of less than emergency health care was rationally connected (see also, *Bell v. Wolfish*, 1979, pp. 1873–1874).

In *Estelle v. Gamble* (1976), the Supreme Court held that action or inaction by providers must offend the "evolving standards of decency" in order to be deliberate indifference. The court noted that the providers in that care *Holly* (1979) had responded to the inmate's health care needs with timely treatment, in compliance with the standards of decency. The *Holly* (1979) court further held that the inmate could not prove an element of *Estelle* (1976) "[w]here the plaintiff has received some care, [as] inadequacy or impropriety of the care that was given will not support [a claim of deliberate indifference]" (see also, *Roach v. Kligman*, 1976).

As a pretrial detainee, an inmate's right to health care rises to a higher level than simply to be free of cruel and unusual punishment. A detainee has a right to be free from any punishment (*Bell v. Wolfish*, 1979). As noted previously, a restriction on the health care of a pretrial detainee must serve a legitimate government interest or it will amount to punishment (*Holly v. Rampone*, 1979, pp. 1873–1874).

In summary, restriction of health care imposed on a pretrial detainee that is arbitrary or purposeless may be inferred to amount to punishment. But not every condition or disability imposed by the provider that results in discomfort for the inmate should be described as punishment. Unless the providers express an intent to punish, in determining whether or not treatment or lack thereof is cruel and unusual, the question is: (1) whether there is an alternative purpose to which the health care restriction may rationally be connected, and (2) whether the health care restriction appears excessive in relation to the alternative purpose assigned to it (*Holly v. Rampone*, 1979; *Kennedy v. Mendoza-Martinez*, 1963). Juvenile detainees also have a right to a specific type of health care.

RIGHT TO MENTAL HEALTH CARE

Inmates have a right to treatment for psychiatric and psychological problems, and the MDTT has a duty to provide psychiatric care (*Laaman v. Helgemoe*, 1977). The prison psychiatric services must be **minimally adequate**, or of a standard or quality designed to meet the prisoner's basic mental health needs. "When inmates with serious mental ill[ness] are effectively prevented from being diagnosed and treated by qualified professionals, the system of care does not meet the constitutional requirements set forth by [*Estelle v. Gamble*, 1976]" (*Laaman v. Helgemoe*, 1977).

Pennsylvania courts have held that the absence of psychiatric nurses created unnecessary problems for prisoners who had mental health needs. In *Owens-El v. Robinson* (1978), a Pennsylvania inmate filed suit claiming that conditions of psychiatric treatment at the Allegheny County Jail violated the constitutional rights of the inmates because they were denied psychiatric care. The Pennsylvania court held that the equal protection clause of the Fourteenth Amendment was violated when methadone treatment was provided to only those inmates who lived inside the county in which the jail was located.

In determining whether or not an inmate is entitled to psychological or psychiatric treatment, the court will hold a hearing to determine whether the inmate has a qualified mental illness. In *Bowring v. Godwin* (1977), a Virginia inmate was denied parole based on "the results of a psychological evaluation indicating that '[the inmate] would not successfully complete a parole period'." The inmate claimed that, because a

psychological evaluation, diagnosis, and treatment were part of the criteria for his parole, the provider had a duty to furnish him with a diagnosis and corresponding treatment, so that he could potentially be paroled. The Virginia court held that "prisoners are guaranteed the provision of life's basic necessities for the period of their confinement." The MDTT must provide adequate food, clothing, shelter, and reasonable health care (see also, *Estelle v. Gamble*, 1976). The court further held that no distinction existed between a prisoner's right to health care for physical needs and psychological care for psychiatric needs (*Bowring v. Godwin*, 1977).

According to *Bowring* (1977), an inmate is entitled to psychiatric care if a health care provider, exercising ordinary care and skill at the time of the observation, determines: (1) the inmate's symptoms evidence serious disease or injury; (2) the disease or injury is curable or may be substantially alleviated; and (3) the inmate would be substantially harmed by delay or denial of treatment. But the court in Bowring (1977) limited treatment by the MDTT to what is reasonable in cost and time. The test of whether or not health care is reasonable and should be delivered by the MDTT is one of *medical necessity*. This court held one of the primary purposes and goals of incarceration is rehabilitation, even though not specifically mandated by the Constitution. The court noted that the provider must diagnose a mental illness before the inmate's right to treatment exists (*Bowring v. Godwin*, 1977).

Boxes 26–9 and 26–10 discuss the criteria used in determining the right to and appropriateness of psychiatric care for inmates.

Rights Related to Restraints, Isolation, and Segregation

While treating the inmate with a mental illness, the MDTT is often faced with the need to assess the inmate's rights regarding restraints, isolation, and segregation. These are well-recognized mechanisms used by the MDTT in the discipline of inmates. The nurse-provider may be placed in the dilemma of functioning in, or choosing be-

BOX 26-9

CRITERIA FOR DETERMINING THE INMATE'S RIGHT TO PSYCHOLOGICAL AND/OR PSYCHIATRIC TREATMENT

The following criteria may be used by the MDTT to determine whether or not an inmate is entitled to psychological or psychiatric treatment. A qualified health care provider, exercising ordinary skill and care at the time of observation, must conclude with reasonable medical certainty:

- The inmate's symptoms evidence a serious disease or injury;
- The disease or injury is curable or may be substantially alleviated; and
- The potential for harm to the prisoner by reason of delay or the denial of the psychiatric care would be substantial (Penal & Correctional (b), 1987/1998.

tween, discipline and health care roles when these disciplinary devices are used. Inmates have brought many claims against members of the MDTT for inhumane use of these mechanisms.

Mentally ill prisoners may be subjected to the use of seclusion and restraints for health care purposes only. In *Burks v. Teasdale* (1980), Missouri inmates initiated a class action suit against the Missouri State Penitentiary, complaining of overcrowding and unsanitary conditions and challenging the constitutionality of their psychiatric care. The Missouri court held that "the Constitutional rights of inmates are to be scrupulously observed [by the MDTT]." In this instance, the court held inmate transfer practices denied psychiatric care when: (1) inmates were referred back to the correctional facility against medical advice, as they were subject to unnecessary pain and suffering, and (2) inmates experienced unnecessary delay prior to transfer and/or referral to psychiatric institutions, because of delays by the MDTT in obtaining custody personnel who would aid in the prisoner transfer (*Burks v. Teasdale*, 1980).

Another federal court has held that placing an inmate in a bare concrete cell, without mattress, blanket, or heat and with a toilet with a hole in the floor, is cruel and unusual punishment (*Davis v. Smith et al.*, 1981). The 8th Circuit Court further held that "abuses, degradation and denial of basic amenities of life cannot be tolerated within any lawful confinement."

Generally, the MDTT has a strong interest in segregating mentally disturbed inmates, and separate facilities and/or treatment may be required. In *Finney v. Mabry* (1982), an Arkansas inmate brought a class action suit, which challenged the constitutionality of conditions in the Arkansas Department of Corrections. The Arkansas court held that it is unconstitutional to use unauthorized providers as actual security officers, with power over other inmates, and the use of verbal abuse, cursing, or racial slurs by providers on any inmate cannot be tolerated.

Drug and Alcohol Treatment

An inmate has a right to treatment for drug- and alcohol-related problems. But, as noted previously, there is no duty to provide the inmate with methadone treatment (*Walker v. Fayette County*, 1979). For example, in Washington, inmates have a right to be treated for alcoholism, but the treatment need not be individualized, such as one-to-one counseling with a therapist, if it includes a variety of

BOX 26-10

CRITERIA FOR DETERMINING THE APPROPRIATENESS OF PSYCHIATRIC CARE

According to the U.S. Court of Appeals of the Ninth Circuit in *Gates v. Shinn* (1996), the courts may use some, or all, of the following criteria to determine whether the inmate has received appropriate psychiatric care from the provider:

- The avoidance of "egregious or flagrant conditions" that would violate the inmate's right to psychiatric care
- The level of care at other state psychiatric facilities
- The level of care at other federal psychiatric facilities
- Recommendations of a health care treatise on psychiatric care
- Published standards of a professional psychiatric association
- Malpractice standards
- Recommendations of the treating doctor
- Recommendations of the chief psychiatrist
- Standards of comparable treatment of a private medical insurer
- Provisions commonly inserted into health maintenance organization (HMO) contracts
- Accreditation standards of a professional board.

programs such as Alcoholics Anonymous (*Aripa v. Department of Social and Health Services*, 1978). Washington inmates were routinely encouraged to participate in 12-step programs such as Narcotics Anonymous or Alcohol Anonymous, organized by lay or clergy representatives or volunteers.

RIGHTS OF JUVENILE DETAINEES

Juvenile detainees or inmates have the same basic rights as adult detainees or inmates. The laws of the state in which the correctional facility holding the juvenile is located generally governs the rights of juvenile detainees or inmates.

Amnesty International, a nongovernmental international human rights organization, released a report in November 1998 that voiced the belief that the United States has violated international human rights treaties by the treatment of children within the U.S. courts and prison systems. Specifically, the Amnesty Report faults the U.S. juvenile justice system for: (1) sentencing juveniles to

life in prison; (2) treating juveniles as adults; (3) failing to provide adequate care; (4) failing to provide adequate protection; (5) confining juveniles for minor crimes; and (6) sentencing juveniles to the death penalty (Meisler, 1998).

LIFE PRISON TERMS

The Amnesty Report cites the state of California for sentencing juveniles younger than age 18 to life without parole. Currently, there are 14 prisoners serving life terms in California prisons who were sentenced when they were younger than age 18. According to Amnesty International, this practice by the State of California violates a treaty signed and ratified by the United States, entitled the International Covenant on Civil and Political Rights (Meisler, 1998).

CERTIFICATION AS AN ADULT

Amnesty International is also concerned by the tendency of many states to have juveniles certified, and tried, as adults. The Amnesty Report estimated that 200,000 children are certified and prosecuted as adults every year; 7000 children are held in adult jails pending trial; and 11,000 children are currently serving sentences in adult prison or similar correctional centers (Meisler, 1998).

ADEQUATE CARE AND PROTECTION

The Amnesty Report has also issued a strong indictment against the level of care and protection received by juveniles within the U.S. prison system. Their indictment is supported by the U.S. Justice Department, which in November 1998 filed suit against the State of Louisiana for failure to provide adequate care to 1750 children confined within its correctional system. In their suit, the U.S. Justice Department accused the State of Louisiana of subjecting juveniles to a substantial risk of serious harm from juvenile-on-juvenile assaults, use of excessive force and abuse by staff, and inadequate suicide prevention (Meisler, 1998).

Guards in South Carolina were accused by Amnesty International of punching, kicking, and choking children in their custody and spraying them with chemicals. Guards in Kentucky were accused of using stun guns and pepper spray to break up fights between the juveniles (Meisler, 1998).

According to the Amnesty Report, guards at the Arizona Boys Ranch were accused in the death of a 16-year-old male juvenile. These guards were charged with placing the juvenile in solitary confinement for a total of 8 days in February 1998, forcing him to do pushups when he complained he was too sick to exercise. Nicholas Contraras died in March 1998 while doing these forced pushups (Meisler, 1998).

CONFINEMENT FOR MINOR CRIMES

The first U.S. juvenile court was established in 1899 by the State of Illinois. The Illinois model was adopted by every other state. But according to Amnesty International, the Illinois model has been weakened in the past two decades by a growing rate of juvenile

crime, a demand for retribution, an increased number of juvenile criminals, and an inadequate number of facilities for their confinement (Meisler, 1998).

According to the Amnesty Report, juveniles are placed in correctional facilities for minor crimes. In a 1997 survey in Georgia, Amnesty International identified juveniles confined for a variety of minor infractions including: (1) a 14-year-old, confined for painting graffiti on a wall; (2) an 11-year-old, confined for threatening his teacher; (3) a 16-year-old, confined for disobeying her father by throwing items in her room and not attending school; (4) a 13-year-old, confined for stealing $127 from her mother; and (5) other juveniles for swearing at their teacher (Meisler, 1998).

THE DEATH PENALTY

The Amnesty Report also voices a concern about juveniles being executed for crimes committed when they were younger than age 18. According to the Report, two juveniles were executed in 1998, and 70 similar juvenile prisoners are on death row awaiting execution. Although execution of juveniles is specifically prohibited by the Covenant, the United States also specifically filed a reservation against any terms banning juvenile executions (Meisler, 1998).

ISSUES AND TRENDS

The purpose of this section is to identify issues and trends within correctional nursing. Issues and trends are discussed according to those identified as arising from the correctional law affecting nursing practice and those identified within correctional nursing practice.

THE LAW

As noted at the beginning of this chapter, correctional law is continuously evolving and being tested by the penal system and its consumer, the prisoner, specifically in relation to prisoner's rights. Future legal issues in correctional nursing may include: (1) right to access medical care outside the prison at the inmate's own expense, (2) right to an abortion within the correctional facility, (3) rights of infants born in prison to receive health and foster care, and (4) right to keep, adopt, and/or place the children of inmates.

In the past, lawsuits have been the mechanism for changing and controlling not only health care practice within the correctional system but all other inmate issues and rights (Northrop & Kelly, 1987, pp. 264–265). Currently the trend may be toward the use of alternate dispute resolution within the prison system to settle all types of inmate/provider disputes (see Chapter 15, Alternate Dispute Resolution in Nursing, for a discussion of this issue).

At the present time, of foremost consideration is the trend in the correctional system toward privatization of prison health care. Currently, state and federal governments, through their departments of corrections, the Federal Bureau of Prisons, and the U.S. Department of Justice, are responsible for the administration of most correctional facilities. County, city, or local sheriff's departments also administer local correctional facilities. The current trend toward privatization is specifically geared toward creating for-profit prisons administered by private corporations and contracting out health services to private groups.

The nurse employed by a privatized correctional facility has unique legal responsibilities, for the type of employer affects the type of legal relationship the nurse has with the prisoner (Northrop & Kelly, 1987, p. 254). For example, the nurse employed by the privately run prison is not sheltered against inmate lawsuits under the defenses of qualified and sovereign immunity, as previously discussed.

CORRECTIONAL NURSING PRACTICE

The scope of nursing practice within the correctional facility is dynamic. Issues within correctional nursing practice fall under the categories of: (1) general nursing practice, (2) advanced nursing practice, and (3) nursing administration.

GENERAL NURSING PRACTICE

In general nursing practice, the problem of staffing a correctional facility is never ending and difficult to meet. Nurses often find themselves subject to fabricated complaints and/or extreme verbal abuse and threats (Northrop & Kelly, 1987, p. 257). Nurses are forced to work with staff who are not well trained and/or inadequate in number (*Collins v. Schoenfield*, 1972). The federal courts have held that the use of inmates who are not nurses to provide nursing care to other inmates is an example of cruel and unusual punishment, a violation of the prisoner's Eighth Amendment rights (*Burks v. Teasdale*, 1980). According to *Gates v. Collier* (1974), the correctional facility may only use trained and competent inmate personnel to supplement prison staff.

Nurses are needed with expertise in psychiatric, community health, medical-surgical, and emergency room nursing. In a crisis situation, such as prisoner(s) spontaneously acting out physically and/or verbally, the nurse may be called on to demonstrate all these skills simultaneously. Nurses in correctional facilities must also be provided with continuing education. The federal courts have held that if a health care worker has no continuing education in general, but more specifically, no continuing education in cardiopulmonary resuscitation and emergency care, this is an example of cruel and unusual punishment, in violation of the prisoner's Eighth Amendment rights (*Palmigiano v. Garrahy, 1977*).

ADVANCED PRACTICE NURSING

Advanced practice nurses, who are nurse practitioners and/or clinical specialists in the areas of psychiatric-mental health, primary care, obstetrics and gynecology, and pediatrics, are needed in correctional facilities. Nurses are often found in situations where they are forced to prescribe medications (*Collins v. Schoenfield*, 1972). As the advanced practice nurse may be given prescriptive authority, the availability of prison health services would be further enhanced by the use of the advanced practice nurse in the clinical area and to screen those psychiatric inmates who cannot be safely brought out of their cell.

NURSING MANAGEMENT

The administration of correctional facilities is the overall responsibility of the government. But, nurses trained in management skills are needed to deal with competing non–health care institutional concerns, which often arise within the structure of the MDTT. Sources of competition are mostly found and played out within the decision-making process of the MDTT. Decisions are often made that place the nurse in an ethical dilemma.

ETHICAL CONSIDERATIONS AND CONFLICTS

An **ethical dilemma** by its very nature is a choice between two or more undesirable alternatives. Often a basic conflict exists between the mission, philosophy, and roles of the various types of providers within the MDTT. Because of core differences, the provider is frequently pressured to compromise ethical principles in a wide variety of situations (Northrop & Kelly, 1987, p. 263). Refer to Chapter 4, Ethics in Nursing, for an ethical framework within which the nurse may analyze and attempt to resolve these ethical dilemmas.

The purpose of this section is to discuss ethical issues related to: (1) punishing versus rewarding crime, (2) health care versus security functions, (3) prenatal and postnatal issues, and (4) reporting abuse of inmates versus denial of protection by coproviders.

PUNISHING VERSUS REWARDING CRIME

Because of the focus on prison reform, the ethical dilemma regarding the function and purpose of the MDTT and/or correctional system continues. The question repeatedly argued within the MDTT is whether the focus of the MDTT should be that of punishing the inmate or should the focus be

on rehabilitation, which opponents view as rewarding the crime. The theoretical justification for punishment of prisoners within the penal system include retribution, deterrence, and isolation (Palmer, 1985). The theoretical justification for rehabilitation of prisoners is based on the provider's basic duty to provide care to the inmate, including beneficence and nonmaleficence.

The nurse continuously encounters the ethical dilemma of **nonmaleficence**, or not causing harm, in a system that, by its nature, is designed to punish. The ANA Standards (ANA, 1985) specifically exclude the nurse's involvement in the correctional facility setting in security functions, including disciplinary committees or functions, and direct or indirect participation in lethal injections.

HEALTH CARE VERSUS SECURITY FUNCTIONS

Within the MDTT, the nurse is constantly faced with the need to balance security versus health care needs of the prisoner. The prison administration is responsible for maintaining internal order, discipline, security, and rehabilitation. The MDTT is oriented toward the dangerousness of a prisoner, whereas the nurse is oriented toward the inmate's health and illness. Although the nurse is responsible for providing health care services and thus rehabilitation, the nurse shares in the decisions to provide, while not actually physically providing, overall security.

The nurse is involved with security roles within the MDTT. For example, an inmate who is injured requires sutures. The suturing equipment should not be left within an inmate's reach, because the inmate might take the equipment, such as sutures, scalpel, or forceps, to use as a potential future weapon. This may be considered only a safety issue in a hospital, but it is a security issue in a prison.

Further, the nurse as a member of the MDTT, is involved in security functions, by participating in decisions about the level of security and freedom that the inmate may have. For example, the MDTT may place a prisoner under strict security. Then over a period of time, the nurse and other members of the MDTT may decide to grant the prisoner more privileges, up to level 5, having maximum privileges.

Nurses must be aware of the nature of the population with which they work and be knowledgeable about the need for, functioning of, and access to the security system, although not physically participating in the security role.

PRENATAL AND POSTNATAL ISSUES

Prenatal and postnatal ethical issues, which arise in correctional facilities, primarily are centered around vaginal searches and the right to keep an infant in prison. As previously noted, the ANA Standards (ANA, 1985) exclude the nurse's involvement in the correctional facility setting in the physical aspect of security functions, including body cavity, strip, or vaginal searches. The ethical issue arises because vaginal searches create a risk of harm through potential infection to the pregnant inmate; yet failure to do a vaginal search may allow the inmate to hide a weapon that may be used to harm others.

In a majority of states, an inmate who becomes a mother is separated from her infant within 48 hours (Norz, 1989). A New York court affirmed the MDTT's right to determine that the best interest of the child would be served by not permitting the mother to keep her child with her in prison (*Bailey v. Lombard*, 1973). Providers faced with a similar dilemma, such as the mother who wishes to keep her child with her in prison, may turn to these New York guidelines for determining the best interest of the child in such a situation.

The New York court's guidelines, cited in *Bailey* (1973), call for the MDTT to assess: (1) the facilities for the care of the child, with a focus on his or her well-being or safety; (2) the parenting skills and psychological health of the mother; (3) any psychological reports of the mother; (4) the offense with which the mother is charged, and its relation to parenting skills; and (5) the length of sentence, the sterility of the environment,

and the ultimate effect on the child (Norz, 1989, pp. 70–71).

REPORTING ABUSE OF INMATES VERSUS DENIAL OF PROTECTION BY COPROVIDERS

According to the ANA Standards (ANA, 1985), the nurse must report any harmful and/or inappropriate behavior by anyone against the inmate. But an unwritten code often exists within the correctional facility that dictates that members of the MDTT will not report a coprovider for inflicting harm on an inmate. Consequently, the nurse may be caught between the choice of: (1) not reporting the harmful behavior, and violating professional legal and ethical standards; or (2) reporting the harmful behavior, and being found in a life-threatening situation, physically unprotected by other members of the MDTT.

RECOMMENDATIONS FOR RESEARCH AND MALPRACTICE PREVENTION

The purpose of this section is to recommend research in which the provider may participate within the correctional facility, malpractice prevention techniques, and methods of correctional advocacy.

RESEARCH

Minimal research exists regarding correctional systems, especially the functioning and contribution of nurses within the system (Northrop, 1985, pp. 264–265). The newsletter *Parameters, Guidelines and Protocols* is "a monthly publication reviewing legal decisions, legislation and related developments involving practice guidelines" (Advisory Board, 1996). *Parameters* has reported that the governmental entity Agency for Health Care Policy and Research (AHCPR) accepts proposals to fund evidence-based practice centers (EPCs) in order "to strengthen the scientific evidence base of health care organizations." The function of an EPC within a correctional facility would be to produce evidence-based reports and assessments of the effectiveness of nurses and available policies, procedures, and technology within correctional facilities. The correctional facility's EPC could "provide the organization with a scientific foundation upon which clinical practice guidelines, performance measures and quality improvement tools can be developed" (Advisory Board, December 1996).

The EPC could produce evidenced-based reports that are scientifically developed, related to, for example: (1) the functioning and contribution of providers within the correctional system; or (2) the development of protocols for analyzing specific issues, such as prenatal and postnatal care, for the purpose of determining the best interest of the child within the correctional facility. The EPC could also specifically address: (1) the positive and negative effects on the child of staying with the mother within the prison system; and (2) the positive and negative effects on the child of being placed in foster care.

MALPRACTICE PREVENTION

Prevention of malpractice encompasses consideration and knowledge of all of the previously cited law, applicable standards, and the rights of prisoners. Further, because of the volumes of new cases filed by prisoners each year, and the resulting volumes of court decisions, the provider must keep abreast of evolving law, standards, and rights of the prison population. The previously discussed creation of an EPC would provide the correctional facility with a scientific foundation on which clinical practice guidelines, performance measures, and quality improvement tools could be developed, thus further preventing, and decreasing, the possibility of prisoner claims against the health providers.

CORRECTIONAL ADVOCACY

Prisons have dramatically changed for the better. We have all seen the media portrayal of prison life, including amenities such as color television and gymnasiums with exercise equipment. But that is the exception, for in some states, prisons are not even air-conditioned. Communities often need to be aware of the true nature of prison structure and functioning in order to reduce their fears of its inhabitants and unrealistic assessment of their amenities.

Nurses need to be more involved in correctional advocacy within the community where the institution is located. Nurses can make the community aware of the type and amount of health care available to, and needed by, the inmate through community education programs.

Graduate level nurses, such as psychiatric nurse practitioners, are desperately needed. But undergraduate schools of nursing, in states with high prison populations, also have an obligation to (1) provide a knowledge base that will increase the undergraduate and graduate nurse's ability to provide services to inmates; (2) provide clinical experiences within correctional facilities for the nursing student; and (3) improve the skills and technology available to nurses working within the correctional system. The education and role of the correctional nurse must become as dynamic as the law that governs correctional nursing practice.

SUMMARY

The rights of inmates have been established by constitutional, statutory, and common laws, including: (1) the basic rights of privacy; (2) protection from violence, suicide or self-inflicted harm, and risk of disease; and (3) health care.

The correctional nurses are primarily held to the legal definition of nursing practice as defined by state law. However, the American Nurses Association has published Standards for Nursing Practice in Correctional Facilities, and various other professional organizations related to the correctional system have formulated guidelines for the health care needs of inmates. All these standards are based on the constitutional standard of care, which is reasonableness.

The correctional nurse functions as a

coprovider on the multidisciplinary treatment team (MDTT), which is composed of all those who provide care to the inmate. The MDTT has the responsibility for development of treatment plans, while ensuring the constitutional rights of inmates. The nurse's failure to meet a duty to the inmate and/or interference with the inmate's rights can result in legal liability based on such constitutional tests as cruel and unusual punishment, deliberate indifference, and/or deliberate deprivation. The case law determining the interpretation and application of these principles is constantly evolving, and the nurse-provider must stay abreast of these developments as a way of ensuring adherence to applicable laws as well as avoiding malpractice liability.

Legal and ethical issues relevant to nursing practice within a correctional facility point out the conflicts that can exist between the security and punishment functions of the facility and the nursing focus on provision of health care.

POINTS TO REMEMBER

- The administration of the criminal justice system is a function of both state and federal agencies.
- Nurses function as providers within a multidisciplinary treatment team (MDTT).
- The MDTT's obligation to provide health care for those whom it is punishing by incarceration is established under the Eighth Amendment of the Constitution.
- Federal and state governments have further provided many rights for prisoners under statutory and common law, based on civil rights acts and constitutional law.
- Under constitutional law, the provider's deliberate indifference to an inmate's serious medical need leads to cruel and unusual punishment, a civil rights violation under federal law.
- An inmate can prove a violation by the provider of the inmate's civil right to health care with evidence of: (1) an acute physical condition, (2) an urgent need for health care, (3) a failure or refusal of the provider to deliver that health care, (4) a

tangible or real residual injury or lasting harm to the inmate caused by failure of the provider to render health care, and (5) acts or inactions of the provider that occurred under circumstances that would shock the judicial conscience.
- Under federal common law, the totality of the circumstances tests the standard of review for the judicial system in determining whether or not the prisoner's civil rights have been violated by the provider.
- The correctional facility may be found liable for negligent acts of the MDTT, and/or the individual provider, under the doctrine of *respondeat superior,* if the facility knew or should have known of these negligent acts.
- Inmates or any type of detainee have a right to sue the federal government, correctional facility, or providers, individually or as members of the MDTT.
- Inmates have a right to receive both compensatory and punitive damages.
- The nurse is primarily held to the definition of nursing practice and the standards of care within the jurisdiction of practice.
- Prisoners have a right to: (1) visitation by their families, attorney, and friends; (2) association with other inmates; (3) use of the mail, unless it must be restricted for special previewing precautions; (4) freedom of religious expression and practice of religion; (5) legal services, such as a lawyer to represent the inmate during any criminal proceeding; and (6) access to the judicial system, such as the right to a law library and legal publications.
- Prisoners have a right to certain types of protection, which specifically include the right to protection from violence, right to protection from suicide and other self-inflicted harm, and right to protection from unreasonable risk of disease.
- In general, prisoners have a constitutional right to health care.
- The provider has a corresponding duty to render to the prisoner reasonable health care.
- At a minimum constitutional level, the care the inmate receives from the provider must not evidence deliberate indifference to the inmate's serious medical needs (that is, the deliberate indifference standard) or

result in cruel or unusual punishment, under the Eighth Amendment.

- The health care provided must be reasonable in light of all the circumstances surrounding the illness and incarceration.
- Inmates have a right to treatment for psychiatric and psychological problems, and the MDTT has a duty to provide psychiatric health care.
- Generally, the correctional facility is responsible for health care costs incurred by prisoners while incarcerated.
- Unauthorized health care experimentation is a violation of the inmate's rights under the First and Fourteenth Amendments, as inmates have a right to be free from "interference with one's thoughts and sensations."
- The state in which the correctional facility holding the juvenile is located generally governs the rights of juvenile detainees.

REFERENCES

Advisory Board. (1996, December). *Parameters, Guidelines and Protocols, 2(12).*

Alberti v. Heard, 600 F. Supp. 443 (D.C. Tex. 1984), stay denied 606 F. Supp. 478, affirmed 790 F.2d 1220.

American Nurses Association. (1985). *American Nurses Association standards for nursing practice in correctional facilities.* Kansas City, MO: Author.

Andrews v. Glenn, 768 F. Supp. 668 (C.D. Ill. 1991).

Aripa v. Department of Social and Health Services, 588 P.2d 185, 91 Wash.2d 135 (Wash. 1978).

Arnold v. Jones, 891 F.2d 1370 (C.A.8 Iowa 1989), reh. den.

Attorney General v. Sheriff of Worcester County, 413 N.E.2d 722, 382 Mass. 57 (1980).

Bailey v. Lombard, 101 Misc.2d 439, 441, 347 N.Y.S.2d 872, 876 (Sup. Ct. 1973).

Ballard v. Elsea, 502 F. Supp. 105 (D.C. Wis. 1980).

Barnes v. Government of Virgin Islands, 415 F. Supp. 1218 (D.V. Virgin Islands, 1976).

Bell v. Wolfish, 441 U.S. 520, 545-47, 99 S.Ct. 1861, 1877, 60 L.Ed.2d 447 (1979).

Benson v. Cady, 761 F.2d 335, 339 (7th Cir. 1985).

Bishop v. McCoy, 323 S.E.2d 140 (W.Va. 1984).

Blumhagen v. Sabes, 834 F. Supp. 1347 (D.C. Wyo. 1993).

Bowring v. Godwin, 551 F.2d 44 (C.A. Va. 1977).

Brewer v. Blackwell, 836 F. Supp. 631 (S.D. Io. 1993).

Brewer v. Perrin, 349 N.W.2d 198, 132 Mich. App. 520 (1984).

Bruscino v. Carlson, 854 F.2d 162 (1988), rehearing denied, certioari denied, 109 S.Ct. 3193, 491 U.S. 907, 105 L.Ed.2d 701.

Burks v. Teasdale, 492 F. Supp. 650 (D.C. Mo. 1980).

Capps v. Atiyeh, 559 F. Supp. 894 (D.C. Or. 1982).

Casey v. Lewis, 773 F. Supp. 1356 (D. Ariz. 1991).

Civil Rights Act of 1871, 42 U.S.C.A. 1983 *et seq.*

Cody v. Hillard, 599 F. Supp. 1025 (D.C. S.D. 1984).

Collins v. Schoenfield, 344 F. Supp. 257 (D. Md. 1972).

Commonwealth v. Lyles, 464 A.2d 712, 77 Pa. Cmwlth. 15 (Pa. 1983).

Costello v. Wainwright, 525 F.2d 1239 (C.A.5 Fla. 1976), on reh., 539 F.2d 547 (C.A.5 Fla. 1976), reversed on other grounds, 430 U.S. 325, 51 L.Ed2d 372, 97 S.Ct. 1191, on remand, 553 F.2d 506 (C.A.5 Fla. 1977).

Crawford v. Loving, 84 F.R.D. 80 (D.C. Va. 1979).

Crowder v. Lash, 687 F.2d 996, 1005 (7th Cir. 1982).

Davidson v. Cannon, 106 S.Ct 668, 88 L.Ed.2d 677 (U.S. 1986).

Davis v. Smith et al., 638 F.2d 66 (8th Cir. 1981).

DesRosiers v. Moran 949 F.2d.15 (R.I. 1991).

Duncan v. Duckworth, 644 F.2d 653 (7th Cir. 1981).

Estate of Gilmore v. Buckley, 608 F. Supp. 554, 560 (D.C. Mass. 1985).

Estelle v. Gamble, 429 U.S. 97 (1976), 50 L.Ed.2d 251, 97 S.Ct.285, rehearing denied, 429 U.S. 1066, 50 L.Ed.2d 785, 97 S.Ct. 798, and on remand, (C.A.5 Tex.) 554 F.2d 653, rehearing denied, (C.A.5 Tex.) 559 F.2d 1217, and certioari denied, 434 U.S. 974, 54 L.Ed.2d 465, 98 S.Ct. 530.

Feigley v. Fulcomer, 720 F. Supp. 475 (M.D. Pa. 1989).

Finney v. Mabry, 534 F. Supp. 102 (D.C. Ark. 1982).

Ford v. Wainwright, 477 U.S. 399, 106 S.Ct. 2595, 91 L.Ed.2d 335 (1986).

Fore v. Goodwin, 407 F. Supp. 1145 (D. Ca. 1976).

Gates v. Collier, 349 7. Supp. 881 (DC Miss., 1974).

Gates v. Shim, No. 94-17146 (9th Cir. 1996).

Gilliard v. Oswald, 552 F.2d 456 (C.A. N.Y. 1977), rehearing denied, 557 F.2d 359.

Gobis, L. (1997). Telenursing: Nursing by Telephone Across State Lines. *Journal of Nursing law, 3(3),* 7-17.

Green v. McKaskle, 788 F.2d 1116 (C.A.5 Tex. 1986).

Grubbs v. Bradley, 552 F. Supp. 1052 (D.C. Tenn. 1982).

Gullatte v. Potts, 654 F.2d 1007 (C.A. Ala. 1981).

Hampton v. Holmesburg Prison Officials, 546 F.2d 1077 (3rd Cir. 1976).

Hathaway v. Coughlin, 841 F.2d 48 (C.A.2 N.Y. 1988).

Hendrix v. Faulkner, 525 F. Supp. 435, 454 (N.D. Ind., 1981).

Helling v. McKinney, 113 S.Ct. 2475 (1993), 509 U.S. 25, 125 L.Ed.22, on remand, 5 F.3d 365.

Hines v. Anderson, 39 F. Supp. 12 (D.C. Minn. 1977).

Holly v. Rampone, 476 F. Supp. 226, 231 (D.C. Pa. 1979).

Hoptowitt v. Ray, 682 F.2d 1237 (C.A. Wash. 1982), appeal after remand, 753 F.2d 779.

Hunt v. Rowton, 288 P. 342, 143 Okl. 181 (1930).

Inmates of the Allegheny County Jail v. Pierce, 612 F.2d 754 (1979).

In re Sanchez, 577 F. Supp. 7 (D.C. N.Y. 1983).

Isaac v. U.S., 490 F. Supp. 613 (D.C. N.Y. 1979).

Jackson v. Hendrick, 321 A.2d 603 (Pa. 1974).

Johnson v. Avery, 393 U.S. 483, 89 S.Ct. 747, 21 L.Ed.2d 718 (1969).

Kanayurak v. North Slope Borough, 677 P.2d 893 (Alaska 1984).

Kennedy v. Mendoza-Martinez, 372 U.S. 144, 168-9, 83 S.Ct. 554, 567-8, 9 L.Ed.2d 644 (1963).

Kimbrough v. O'Neil, 545 F.2d 1059, 1061 and n. 4 (7th Cir. 1976) (en banc).

Knecht v. Gillman, 488 F.2d 1136 (8th Cir. 1973).

Laaman v. Helgemoe, 437 F. Supp. 269 (D.C. N.H. 1977).

Langston v. Commissioner of Correction, 614 N.E.2d 1002, 34 Mass. App. Ct. 564, review denied, 618 N.E.2d 71, 416 Mass. 1101 (1993).

LaRocca v. Dalsheim, 467 N.Y.S.2d 302, 120 Misc.2d 697 (1983).

Layne v. Vizant, 657 F.2d 468 (1st Cir. 1981).

Lee v. Downs, 470 F. Supp. 188 (D.C. Va. 1979), aff'd., 641 F.2d 1117.

Lee v. McManus, 543 F. Supp. 386, 391 (D.C. Kan., 1982).

Lewis El v. O'Leary, 631 F. Supp. 60, 61 (ND. Ill. 1986).

Lightfoot v. Walker, 486 F. Supp. 504 (S.D. Ill. 1980).

Little v. Walker, 552 F.2d 193,197 (7th Cir. 1977), certiori denied, 435 U.S. 932, 98 S.Ct. 1507, 55 L.Ed.2d 530 (1977).

Mackey v. Procunier, 477 F.2d 877 (C.A.9 Cal. 1973).

Martin v. Gentile, 849 F.2d 865 (C.A.4 Md. 1988).

Massey v. Smith, 555 F. Supp. 743 (D.C. Ind. 1983).

Matje v. Leis, 571 F. Supp. 918 (S.C. Ohio 1983).

Matter of Commitment of F.H., 6120 A.2d 882, 258 N.J.Sup. 532 (1992).

Mayfield v. Craven, 299 F. Supp. 1111 (E.D.Ca. 1969), aff'd., 433 F.2d 873 (C.A.9 Ca. 1969).

McCraken v. Jones, 562 F.2d 22 (C.A. Okl. 1977), cert. den., 98 S.Ct. 1474, 435 U.S. 917, L.Ed.2d 509.

Meisler, S. (1998, November 18). Report cites abuses against jailed youths: Group says U.S. violates international law. *Houston Chronicle*, p. 5A.

Miller v. Carson, 401 F. Supp. 835 (M.D. Fla. 1975).

Monmouth County Correctional Institutional Inmates v. Lanzaro, 834 F.2d 326 (C.A.3 N.J. 1987), certiori denied, 108 S.Ct. 1731, 486 U.S. 1006, 100 L.Ed.2d 195.

Monroe v. Pape, 365 U.S. 167, 187, 207, 81 S.Ct. 473, 5 L.Ed2d 492 (1961).

Nelson v. Heyne, 491 F.2d 353 (7th Cir. 1974).

Norris v. Frame, 585 F.2d 1183, 1189 (3d Cir. 1978).

Northrop, C. & Kelly, M. (1987). Nursing practice in correctional facilities. In C. Northrop, *Legal issues in nursing.* St. Louis, MO: CV Mosby.

Norz, F. (1989). Prenatal and postnatal rights of incarcerated mothers. *Columbia Human Rights Law Review, 29,* S-55, S-58.

Owens-El v. Robinson, 442 F. Supp. 1368 (D.C. Pa. 1978).

Palmigiano v. Garrahy, 443 F. Supp. 956 (D. R.I. 1977).

Parilla v. Cuyler, 447 F. Supp. 363 (D.C. Pa. 1978).

Patridge v. Two Unknown Police Officers of City of Houston, 751 F.2d 1448, 1453 (C.A. Tex. 1985).

Penal and Correctional (a): Medical care for inmates. Generally. In *American Jurisprudence* (Volume 60, Section 91). (1987; Supplement 1998). Rochester, NY: Lawyers Cooperative Publishing.

Penal and Correctional (b): Medical care for inmates. Addictive drug maintenance programs; methadone. In *American Jurisprudence* (Volume 60, Section 95). (1987; Supplement 1998). Rochester, NY: Lawyers Cooperative Publishing.

Penal and Correctional (c): Medical care for inmates. Medical experimentation. In *American Jurisprudence* (Volume 60, Section 97). (1987; Supplement 1998). Rochester, NY: Lawyers Cooperative Publishing.

Phillips v. Michigan Dept. of Corrections, 731 F. Supp. 792 (W.D. Mich 1990).

Pretty on Top v. City of Hardin, 597 P.2d 58, 182 Mont. 311 (Mont. 1979).

Prisons (a): Protection from violence, generally. In *Corpus Juris Secundum* (Volume 72, Section 77). (1987). St. Paul, MN: West Publishing.

Prisons (b): General considerations. In *Corpus Juris Secundum* (Volume 72, Section 80). (1987; Supplement 1998). St. Paul, MN: West Publishing.

Prisons (c): Liability for costs. In *Corpus Juris Secundum* (Volume 72, Section 89). (1987; Supplement 1998). St. Paul, MN: West Publishing.

Procunier v. Marinez, 416 U.S. 396, 404, 405 (1974).

Procunier v. Navarette, 434 U.S. 562, 98 S.Ct. 855 (1978).

Prushinowski v. Hambrick, 570 F. Supp. 863 (D.C. N.C. 1983).

Ramos v. Lamm, 693 F. Supp. 559 (10th Cir. 1980), cert. den., 101 S.Ct. 1759, two cases, 450 U.S. 1041, 68 L.Ed.2d 239, on remand, 520 F. Supp. 1059.

Roach v. Kligman, 412 F. Supp. 521, 525 (E.D. Pa. 1976).

Robbins v. South et al., 595 F. Supp. 785 (D. Mont. 1984).

Roe v. Wade, 410 U.S. 113 (1973), 35 L.Ed. 2d 147, 93 S.Ct. 75, rehearing denied, 410 U.S. 959, 35 L.Ed.2d 694, 93 S.Ct. 1409.

Sconier v. Jarvis, 458 F. Supp. 37 (U.S.D.C. Kansas, 1978).

Simpkins v. Bellevue Hospital, 832 F. Supp. 69 (S.D. N.Y.1993).

Sires v. Birman, 834 F.2d 9 (C.A.1 Mass. 1987).

Smith v. Sullivan, 553 F.2d 373 (C.A. Tex. 1977); 611 F.2d 1039, 1044 (5th Cir. 1980).

Sowell v. Israel, 500 F. Supp. 209 (D.C. Wis. 1980).

State v. Perry, 610 So.2d 746 (La. 1992).

Sudderth v. White, 621 S.W.2d. 33 (Ky. 1981), no writ.

Sundby v. Fiedler, 827 F. Supp. 580 (W.D. Wis. 1993).

Thomas v. Pate, 493 F.2d 151, 158 (7th Cir. 1974), certioari denied, 423 U.S. 877, 96 S.Ct. 149, 46 L.Ed.2d 110 (1975).

Thompson v. Burke, 556 F.2d 231 (3d. Cir. 1977).

Thor v. Superior Court (Andrews), 21 Ca.Rptr.2d 357, 855 P. 2d 375, 5 C.4th 725 (1993).

Todaro v. Ward, 431 F. Supp. 1129; 565 F.2d 48, 52 (S.D. N.Y. 1977).

Toussaint v McCarthy, 597 F. Supp. 1388 (D.C. Cal. 1984).

Turner v. Plageman, 418 F. Supp. 132 (D.C. Va. 1976).

United States v. Bundy, 587 F. Supp. 95 (1983).

United States v. County of Philadelphia, 413 F.2d 84,87 (3d Cir.), certioari denied, 396 U.S. 1046, 90 S.Ct. 696, 24 L.Ed. 691 (1969).

Vienneau v. Shanks, 425 F. Supp. 676 (D.C. Wis. 1977).

Vinnedge v. Gibbs, 550 F.2d 926 (C.A. Va. 1977).

Von Holden v. Chapman, 450 N.Y.S.2d 623, 87 A.D.2d 66 (1982).

Walker v. Fayette County, Pennsylvania, 599 F.2d 573 (C.A. Pa. 1979).

Walker v. Sumner, 917 F.2d 382, 8 F. 3d 33 (C.A.9 Nev. 1990).

Warren v. Missouri, 995 F.2d 130 (CA. 8 Mo. 1993).

Watson v. Carton, 984 F.2d 537 (C.A.1 Me. 1993).

Welch v. Sheriff, Lubbock County, 734 F. Supp. 765 (Tex. N.D. 1990).

Wellman v. Faulkner, 715 F. 2d 269, 272 (C.A. Ind. 1983).

White v. Napoleon, 897 F.2d 103 (C.A.3 N.J. 1990).

Wilkinson v. State, 667 P.2d 413 (1983).

Wood v. Strickland, 420 U.S. 308, 321, 95 S Ct, 992, 43. L.Ed.2d 214 (1975).

Wood v. Sun, 852 F.2d 1205 (C.A. Hawaii 1988).

Zant v. Prevatte, 248 Ga. 832, 286 S.E.2d. 715 (1982).

SUGGESTED READINGS

Bryson v. State, 793 S.W.2d 252 (Tenn. 1990).

The Rehabilitation Act, 29 U.S.C.A. § 504 (1973).

West v. Keve, 571 F.2d 158 (3d Cir. 1978).

AMERICAN JURISPRUDENCE

Penal and correctional: Medical care for inmates. Effect of over-crowding or funding limitations. In *American Jurisprudence* (Volume 60, Section 92). (1987; Supplement 1998). Rochester, NY: Lawyers Cooperative Publishing.

Penal and correctional: Medical care for inmates. Malpractice or accidental denial of medical care. In *American Jurisprudence* (Volume 60, Section 93) (1987; Supplement 1998). Rochester, NY: Lawyers Cooperative Publishing.

Penal and correctional: Medical care for inmates. Mental health care. In *American Jurisprudence* (Volume 60, Section 94). (1987; Supplement 1998). Rochester, NY: Lawyers Cooperative Publishing.

Penal and correctional: Medical care for inmates. Providing medical care in jails. In *American Jurisprudence* (Volume 60, Section 96). (1987; Supplement 1998). Rochester, NY: Lawyers Cooperative Publishing.

Penal and correctional: Searches on inmates. Generally; search of cell, locker, and related areas. In *American Jurisprudence* (Volume 60, Section 98). (1987; Supplement 1998). Rochester, NY: Lawyers Cooperative Publishing.

BODY CAVITY SEARCHES

McMath, T. (1987). Do prison inmates retain any Fourth Amendment protection from body cavity searches? *University of Cincinnati Law Review, 56*, 739.

CORPUS JURIS SECUNDUM

Prisons: Suicide and other self-inflicted harm. In *Corpus Juris Secundum* (Volume 72, Section 78). (1987). St. Paul, MN: West Publishing.

Prisons: Sanitation. In *Corpus Juris Secundum* (Volume 72, Section 79). (1987; Supplement 1998). St. Paul, MN: West Publishing.

Prisons: Standard of care, generally. In *Corpus Juris Secundum* (Volume 72, Section 81). (1987; Supplement 1998). St. Paul, MN: West Publishing.

Prisons: Nature and type of care. In *Corpus Juris Secundum* (Volume 72, Section 82). (1987; Supplement 1998). St. Paul, MN: West Publishing.

Prisons: Facilities, procedures, and staff in general. In *Corpus Juris Secundum* (Volume 72, Section 83). (1987; Supplement 1998). St. Paul, MN: West Publishing.

Prisons: Involuntary treatment. In *Corpus Juris Secundum* (Volume 72, Section 84). (1987; Supplement 1998). St. Paul, MN: West Publishing.

Prisons: Contagious diseases. In *Corpus Juris Secundum* (Volume 72, Section 85). (1987; Supplement 1998). St. Paul, MN: West Publishing.

Prisons: Drug and alcohol treatment. In *Corpus Juris Secundum* (Volume 72, Section 86). (1987; Supplement 1998). St. Paul, MN: West Publishing.

Prisons: Mental health care. In *Corpus Juris Secundum* (Volume 72, Section 87). (1987; Supplement 1998). St. Paul, MN: West Publishing.

Prisons: Right to particular physician or treatment. In *Corpus Juris Secundum* (Volume 72, Section 88). (1987; Supplement 1998). St. Paul, MN: West Publishing.

Prisons: Judicial intervention. In *Corpus Juris Secundum* (Volume 72, Section 90). (1987). St. Paul, MN: West Publishing.

CRUEL AND UNUSUAL PUNISHMENT

Friedman, M. (May, 1992). Cruel and unusual punishment in the provision of prison medical care: Challenging the deliberate indifference standard. *Vanderbilt Law Review, 45*(4), 921–949.

MEDICAL EXPERIMENTATION

Physician use of patient's tissue, cells, or bodily substances for medical research or economic purpose. *American Law Review* 5(16), 143.

MENTAL HEALTH CARE

The adaptation to prison by individuals with schizophrenia. *Bulletin of the American Academy of Psychiatry & Law, 21*, 427.

Preventing jailhouse suicides. *Bulletin of the American Academy of Psychiatry & Law, 22*(4), 477–488.

PRENATAL AND POSTNATAL CARE

Atwood, J. (October, 1997). Part I: Women and children behind bars. *Life Magazine*, pp. 76–84.

Atwood, J. (October, 1997). Part II: When Mom can't come home. *Life Magazine*, pp. 84–90.

Norz, F. (Spring, 1989). Prenatal and postnatal rights of incarcerated mothers. *Columbia Human Rights Law Review, 20*, S55–S73.

RIGHT TO MEDICAL CARE

Comment: The rights of prisoners to medical care and the implications for drug-dependent prisoners and pretrial detainees. *University of Chicago Law Review, 42*, 705, 708–709.

Court affirms prisoner's right to refuse life-sustaining treatment. *Journal of Legal Medicine & Ethics, 22*(1), 92.

George, B., Jr. (Winter, 1981). Standards governing the legal status of prisoners. *Denver Law Journal, 59*, 94–105.

Mental health screening and evaluation within prisons. *Bulletin of the American Academy of Psychiatry & Law, 22*(3), 451.

Moulding-Johnson, E. (Spring, 1989). The right to adequate medical care. *Columbia Human Rights Law Review, 20*, S3–S17.

Royston, W., & Weems, P. (February, 1981). Civil rights. *Texas Tech Law Review, 12* (1), 139–205.

Tuberculosis in correctional facilities: The tuberculosis control program of the Montefiore Medical Center Rikers Island Health Services. *Journal of Legal Medicine & Ethics, 21*, 342.

Tuberculosis in prison: Balancing justice and public health. *Journal of Legal Medicine & Ethics, 21*, 352.

SEARCH AND SEIZURE

Prisoner's search and seizure. (1993). In *American Law Review* (5th ed., Volume 14, p. 913). Rochester, NY: Lawyers Cooperative Publishing.

Urinalysis testing in correctional facilities. *Boston University Law Review, 68*, 475.

WEB SITES

Bureau of Justice Statistics. *Statistics on crime and punishment* [On-line]. Available: http://www.ojp.usdoj.gov/bjs/

Death row inmates [On-line]. Available: http://www.thelampofhope.com/

Inmate classified [On-line]. Available: http://www.inmate.com/

Prison law page: legal issues related to prisoners [On-line]. Available: http://www.wco.com~aerick/

Prison pen pals [On-line]. Available: http://www.prisonpenpals.com/

Texas Department of Criminal Justice. Statistics/information about the Texas corrections system [On-line]. Available: http://www.tdjc.state.tx.us/

Wisconsin super-max prison project: Maximum security prison project for violent offenders [On-line]. Available: http://www.supermax.jobsight

Abandonment: Leaving a nursing assignment without transferring responsibilities to appropriate personnel when continued nursing care is required by the condition of the client.

Abortion: The premature termination of a pregnancy.

Abrogated: The elimination of something, for example, a legal theory.

Abuse: Synonymous with neglect; nontherapeutic infliction of physical pain or injury or any persistent course of conduct intended to produce or resulting in mental or emotional distress; serious physical injury caused by another, which has not occurred by accidental means.

Access: A patient's ability to get to health care. Factors influencing access include availability, affordability, and acceptability.

Accountability: Responsible for maintaining the nursing standard of care.

Act Deontology: An ethical theory, which is duty based, and the duty depends on the situation; acts are based on personal moral values and rules.

Act Utilitarianism: Under this ethical theory, acts selected depend on their consequences, assessing the risks versus benefits; the action taken by the nurse depends on the situation. Synonymous with situational ethics.

Active Euthanasia: The facilitation of the patient's death by some direct intervention, such as with assisted suicide.

Activities of Daily Living (ADLs): Those everyday activities required to perform self-care, i.e., bathing, dressing, eating, toileting, getting around the house.

Actual Agents: One who has the authority to act on behalf of another e.g. nurses whose actions or details of work are controlled by the hospital.

Actual Damages: Also called compensatory damages; the amount of money that compensates the injured party for the injury sustained and nothing more.

Actual Knowledge: Real awareness, active agreement, and/or participation in actions or inactions that are at issue in a dispute or lawsuit.

Adhesion Contract: Standardized form agreements that do not allow the consumer to bargain on its terms and that must be agreed to on a "take it or leave it" basis or the consumer does not receive the services.

Administrative Law: Statutory laws and regulations designed to control government agencies, such as a professional licensing board, i.e. the board of nursing.

Advance Directives: Legal documents that set out the wishes of an individual in regard to health care in situations in which the individual is no longer capable of giving informed consent; the term can also include oral statement by the patient; a document that includes a living will and/or a durable power of attorney; synonymous with directive to physician. Synonymous with *individual instruction,* as identified under the Uniform Health Care Decisions Act of 1994; includes the following documents and/or instructions: (1) living will, (2) do not resuscitate (DNR) order, (3) euthanasia, (4) "right to die," and (5) "right to live."

Advanced Practice Nurse (APN): A registered professional nurse who is prepared for advanced nursing practice by virtue of knowledge and skills obtained through a post-basic or advanced educational program of study; acts independently and/or in collaboration with other health care professionals in the delivery of health care services. The American Association of Colleges of Nursing gives the following definition "Advanced Practice Nurse is an umbrella term appropriate for a licensed registered nurse prepared at the graduate degree level as either a Clinical Specialist, Nurse Anesthetist, Nurse-Midwife, or Nurse Practitioner" (AACN, Position Statement, Certification and Regulation of Advanced Practice Nurses, 1994). See Clinical Nurse Specialist (CNS) and Nurse Practitioner (NP).

Affirmative Defense: The burden is on the defendant to come forward to claim and prove the right to the defense.

Against Medical Advice (AMA): Description of situation in which the patient decides to leave the health care facility against the advice of the provider, or voluntarily admitted client initiates his or her own release via a request letter.

Age Discrimination and Employment Act (ADEA): Enforced by the EEOC, it prohibits discrimination by the employer against anyone 40 years old or older in decisions regarding hiring, promotions, and benefits.

Agency: A legal relationship wherein one person is authorized to act on behalf of another person; theory of law under which a hospital may be held liable for acts of independent contractors if they are held to be an agent or representative and/or acting on behalf of the hospital.

Agency for Health Care Policy Research (AHCPR): An agency whose purpose is to provide clinical practice guidelines.

Agent: An employee or independent contractor who has the authority to represent the organization.

Aggregate: The total amount of money that can be paid out by the insurance company in one year, under an individual insurance policy for nursing malpractice.

ALOS: Average length of stay; one of the standard measures of resource consumption in health care.

Alternate Dispute Resolution (ADR): Methods used to settle health care disagreements quickly and cost effectively outside the courtroom.

American Board of Nursing Specialization (ABNS): Established in 1991; serves as an umbrella organization that sets standards and requirements that certifying bodies for APN must meet.

American Law Institute (ALI) Standard: Most frequently used insanity determination requiring that the person is unable to appreciate the wrongfulness of an act or to conform his or her behavior to the requirements of the law; sociopathic individuals are excluded from using the ALI standard.

American National Standards Institute (ANSI): Organization that publishes accessibility standards that serve as a resource to life care planners regarding accessibility needs of patients.

American Nurse Credentialing Center: Founded in 1973, is an agency that provides advanced practice nurses with certification.

Americans with Disabilities Act (ADA): An act passed by Congress in 1990 to ensure that persons with disabilities are afforded equal opportunity in the workplace setting and full participation in the activities of daily living.

American Nurses Association Social Policy Statement: A statement by the ANA that addresses four features inherent in contemporary nursing practice, including: (a) assessing the person holistically, (b) integrating objective data provided by the patient, (c) scientific diagnosis and treatment, and (d) exhibiting a caring bond that promotes health and healing.

Amnesty International: A nongovernmental international human rights organization.

Anencephalic Infant: An infant born without cerebral hemispheres, but with a brain stem only.

Annotations: A short list of summaries that contain court cases in which the listed statutes were at issue.

Anti-Stalking Law: State criminal law that protects victims from stalkers; the victim need not prove that the stalker had the intent to carry out the threat.

Apparent Agency: Synonymous with *ostensible agency*; giving the impression the person is an agent of the organization.

Apparent Authority: Synonymous with *ostensible authority*; employees who appear to be agents of their employer but are not, e.g., independent contractor.

Appeal: One party to the lawsuit may challenge the trial court's decisions, and must show that the court committed an error during the trial ad that such error was harmful to or biased the outcome of the case.

Appeals Process for Utilization Review: Method by which the patient and/or physician disputes the utilization review (UR) decision of the managed care organization regarding the medical necessity of providing specific services.

Appraisement: A method of ADR through which the parties obtain a neutral person to conduct some duty that will assist in resolving their dispute, such as helping the parties determine certain facts about the case.

Arbitration: A method of ADR through which a dispute is submitted to one or more impartial or neutral persons who make a final, binding decision on the disputed issues.

Arrest Warrant: A legal document which gives the court the authority to detain someone.

Artificial Insemination: The insertion of a sperm into the womb of the female via artificial methods.

Assault: The attempt or threat to inflict injury on the person of another; "any willful attempt to threat to inflict injury upon the person of another, when coupled with the apparent ability to do so; and any intentional display of force, such as would give the victim reason to fear or expect immediate bodily harm" (*Black's Law Dictionary*, 1979).

Assault and Battery: A cause of action under tort law, which may involve the breach of a nursing duty, such as to provide undue nursing care.

Assisted-Living Facility: Synonymous with *personal care facility*; governed by state, not federal, law, requiring conditions such as (1) a safe, comfortable, and sanitary environment; (2) food service that provides wholesome and satisfying meals designed to meet nutritional needs; and (3) humane treatment.

Assisted Suicide: A form of active euthanasia, through which another person assists the patient with his or her death.

Assumption of the Risk: An affirmative defense pled by defendant; the patient is said to have known the risk of the procedure or treatment and willingly consented to have the procedure.

At Will Employment: The type of employment agreement under which the employee may be terminated with reasonable notice without cause.

Attorney-Client Relationship: A privileged relationship in which communications between attorney and client are confidential and cannot be disclosed without the client's consent, or unless there is a showing that the communications were made in furtherance of a crime or fraud.

Attorney Work Product: Any type of preparation by the attorney on behalf of their client, including thought processes and mental opinions.

Authorization for Release of Information: Written permission provided by the patient to disclose medical information, indicating what information, to whom, for what purpose, and for what period of time.

Autonomy: Ethical principle that provides for the freedom to be self-regulating.

Baclofen Pump: A device used to regulate the administration of medication prescribed to control and manage a patient with spastic extremities.

Bad Baby Case: Allows a cause of action to be filed after the child has reached a legal majority, or perhaps two years from the death after the alleged trauma.

Balanced Budget Act of 1997: Federal legislation that imposed dramatic reductions in reimbursement for home health services and resulted in major reductions in quantity of home health services.

Battery: The unlawful application of force to the person of another; an intentional touching without consent.

Beneficence: Ethical principle that provides for the nurse to "do good" for the patient.

Benefits: Under an individual insurance policy for nursing malpractice, additional advantages that may be obtained include: (a) legal fees and court costs, (b) reimbursement of defense costs, (c) reimbursement to the nurse for lost work time.

Bifurcation of the Trial: Separation of a trial is into two phases; the issue of liability tried first, and the issues of damages are tried after the verdict.

Bill of Resident's Rights: A requirement under the Medicare and Medicaid provisions of Chapter 42 of the United States Code; outlines the minimum standards of health, safety, patient autonomy, notice requirements, and fiduciary duties of facilities.

Bill of Rights: First 10 amendments to the Constitution, which identify basic rights.

Binding Arbitration: A method of ADR through which parties voluntarily agree to be bound by the decision of an impartial or neutral third person.

Bioethical Change Process: Process by which clinical concepts or realities become specific ethical and legal standards.

Bioethics: An ethical framework involving moral questions regarding the quality of life and death.

Biomedical Ethics: "The ethics of judgements made within the biomedical sciences" (Veatch, 1987, p. 1).

Blocked Account: Bank account that is blocked by the courts, with access only by person assigned by the court.

Board of Nurse Examiners (BNE): The administrative agency that regulates nursing practice on the state level.

Board of Nursing: The state regulatory agency given the authority to: (a) prescribe regulations setting forth educational requirements and admission standards for licensure of nurses, and in some states, for advanced practice nurses; (b) delineate the tasks that nurses and advanced practice nurses are permitted to carry out either independently or in collaboration with physicians; and, (c) establish criteria and administrative processes for disciplining nurses usually with authority to impose appropriate penalties.

Bona Fide: In good faith; true and genuine and without fraudulent intent.

Bona Fide Occupational Qualification (BFOQ): A qualification established by the employer that is deemed necessary to the daily operations of that business; usually have to do with safety concerns for patients or the public, such as health restrictions placed on pilots.

Bonded: Description of a person for whom insurance is provided who is managing the assets of another.

Borrowed Servant Doctrine: A legal theory of liability based on an employer's ability to control the actions of another employee.

Brain Death: Under the Natural Death Act, "the irreversible cessation of brain functioning accompanied by ongoing biologic functioning in all other parts of the body, maintained on life-support measures" (Andrews et al., 1996, p. 290).

Breach of Contract: In the employment setting, a failure on the employee's or employer's part to perform, without justification, all or a part of a contractual agreement.

Breach of Duty: The neglect or failure to fulfill, in an appropriate and proper manner, the duties of the job.

Burden of Proof: Evidence required to prove a specific issue.

Business Records: Records kept in the ordinary and usual course of business.

Cap of Damages: A statutory limit set on the amount of damages that may be recovered from a government entity, for example, $100,000 per incident.

Capacity: Possession of a set of values and goals; the ability to communicate and understand information; and the ability to reason and deliberate about one's choices.

Capitation: Specific dollar amount established to cover cost of health services delivered for a group of individuals for a specific time period.

Captain of the Ship Doctrine: A legal theory of vicarious liability whereby a physician who controls other persons (e.g., nurses) is responsible for their actions.

Care Map: A type of charting that is based on an integrated treatment plan, identifying services, patient outcomes, and length of stay.

Caring: The feeling that a person, place, thing, or event actually matters.

Cartesian Philosophy: An ethical theory under which the mind is separate from the body and must be treated differently.

Carveouts: Payers give the responsibility for managing the benefits for a specific portion of the care (psychiatric care, pharmaceuticals) in return for a portion of the pmpm fees; usually occurs in areas of health care benefits for which it is difficult to control costs.

Case Number: The number assigned to the lawsuit by the clerk of the designated court; also called a docket number.

Case Rate: A predetermined rate to be paid to a provider for a specified level of care; DRGs (diagnostic related groups) specify case rates that are paid according to the diagnosis.

Casuistry: An ethical decision-making model that uses paradigm cases to consider not only principles and rules of ethics but also consequences.

Categorical Imperative: A term composed of two definitions: *categorical* denotes a moral rule with no exceptions, such as a nursing standard; *imperative* denotes that this rule must be followed, such as the nursing standards established by the state board of nursing.

Causation: A direct relationship between the damages suffered and the negligence of the provider.

Cause in Fact: The next cause or actual cause of an event or injury; but for the negligence, the injury would not have occurred.

Cellular Pirates: Persons who use scanners and other technology to intercept and sell telephone communications.

Certification: Examinations developed by professional organizations which provide verification of a claim to competence at a certain level of practice.

Certified Agencies: Home health care agencies certified by Medicare.

Certified Nurse-Midwife (CNM): Advanced practice nurse who provides care to the pregnant woman before, during, and after the birth of the infant and administers care to the newborn infant, and who is involved in family planning and gynecology.

Certified Registered Nurse Anesthetist (CRNA): An advanced practice nurse whose practice involves evaluating the patient's overall physical health in anticipation of the administration of anesthesia and providing anesthesia to patients, which includes the selection and administration of drugs, intravenous fluids, and ventilator techniques.

Chain of Custody: A legal procedure by which the possession and storage of evidence is documented, from the moment it was obtained to its presentation in court.

Challenge for Cause: To dispute the ability of a person to act as a juror, stating the specific reason for exclusion, for example: (a) has a relationship with one of the parties, (b) is a friend of one of the attorneys, or, (c) a prejudice regarding one of the issues.

Charitable Immunity: Developed in response to the captain-of-the-ship doctrine; designed to protect specific persons and/or legal entities from liability; protects institutions that do charitable work from lawsuits that may bankrupt them.

Charting by Exception: To chart only abnormal findings.

Checks and Balances: The system built into the governmental framework via the Constitution that allows the Executive, Judicial, and Congressional branches of government to control the activities of one another.

Civil Law: The type of law that deals with wrong to individuals; regulations under which disputes between private parties are resolved, often resulting in monetary damages.

Civil Remedies: Judicial relief, which may be in the form of damages, awarded by the court, including money or orders to act or refrain from acting.

Civil Rights: Personal natural rights guaranteed and protected by the Constitution enjoyed by all citizens; right to vote, marry and divorce, enter into a contract, execute a will, obtain and maintain a professional license, and sue and be sued.

Claims Made Insurance: A type of insurance that provides coverage only for claims made during the time the policy is in force.

Clients: Terminology progression from *patients* when mentally ill persons returned to the communities for local outpatient treatments.

Clinical Ethics: A four-step ethical decision-making model that utilizes principled ethics, but organizes them in a different manner, considering the impact of socioeconomic factors on the decision.

Clinical Nurse Specialist (CNS): An advanced practice nurse whose focus of practice is not diagnosing the patient nor treating the patient with medications, but rather treating the patient through education, consultation, and therapy; advanced practice nurse with a master's degree in psychiatric-mental health nursing. Prepared for providing group or individual psychotherapy and may have prescriptive privileges. See Nurse Practitioner (NP).

Clinical Practice Guidelines: The clinical steps for patient management.

Code: Laws organized by legislatures into logical groups and systematically arranged into chapters, sections, and subsections.

Code of Ethics: A set of values and standards regulating a profession, such as nursing practice.

Code of Federal Regulations: Federal statutory law that establishes requirements for facilities receiving Medicare and Medicaid funding.

Collateral Source: Another source of payments for damages, such as insurance company payments for health care, paid prior to any recovery at trial.

Collective Bargaining: A method of ADR, established under the National Labor Relations Act of 1988, by which employees have the right to form and join unions, designate representatives, and participate in negotiation and bargaining with management on a collective basis.

Common Law: Law generated by judicial opinions, based on prior decisions and court cases.

Communication Right: Right of hospitalized mentally ill persons to visit with family and friends via unopened mail and telephone calls, unless the treatment team determines that to allow this right may be harmful to the patient.

Community Mental Health Legislation: Federal legislation in the 1960s that changed the care of the mentally ill. Large numbers of psychiatric patients were discharged from state-run hospital communities back to local communities, where they would live and attend local psychiatric treatment centers.

Compact: See Multistate Licensure Compact.

Comparative negligence: The legal theory of liability involving apportioning or dividing the amount of each party's fault or responsibility in causation of injury.

Compassion: "The ability to place oneself in the situation of another" (Burkhart, 1998, p. 35).

Compensation: Payment from an employer to an employee for services rendered. This includes salary and benefits.

Compensatory Damages: The amount of money the plaintiff asserts will be just compensation for the monetary loss that will be, or has been, incurred because of the defendant's wrongful action or inaction; also known as *actual damages*.

Competency: Presence of characteristics that make a patient legally fit and qualified to make independent decisions; of legal age, without mental disability or incapacity; legally fit and qualified to give testimony or execute legal documents..

Complaint: Also called Plaintiff's Petition; the initial legal document filed to initiate the lawsuit and state Plaintiff's claims and injuries.

Compromise: A win/win, amiable method of settling a dispute in which both parties give concessions; designed to prevent or terminate litigation.

Conciliation: Also known as *facilitation*, is an unstructured process of negotiation that involves promoting communication between the parties to the health care dispute.

Conclusions: Based on risk factors, statements of long-term needs, supported by records, assessment, and communication with the treatment team and other experts.

Concurrent Cause of Injury: Legal theory that maintains that plaintiff would not have been harmed but for acts of both defendants.

Concurrent Review: Utilization review done by either representatives of the payer or the provider to ensure that the care currently being provided is appropriate, consistent with the benefits available, and medically necessary.

Conditional Release: Outpatient court-ordered treatment or supervision after discharge requiring specific conditions outlined prior to discharge such as medication clinic visits, outpatient group or individual therapy sessions, or time spent in prescribed aftercare programs.

Conditions for Participation for Medicare and Medicaid Reimbursement: Federal regulations that require hospitals to report to the regional organ procurement agency every death and every severe neurological injury that may result in brain death.

Confidentiality: The right of a client to have any communications with a professional remain private or unshared with any other person; the client possesses the right to allow sharing of identified information.

Consent: Agreeing to the proposition of another.

Conservator: An individual, appointed by probate court, who manages a person and/or his or her estate when that person has been found incapable of managing his or her affairs.

Consideration: What the employer offers, bargains, and promises the contracted employee in exchange for the contracted employee's promise of service.

Consulting Exception: A method of telenursing licensure through which the nurse may practice telenursing for the sole purpose of consultation.

Consulting Experts: Nurses who do not directly participate in court proceedings, but serve as experts in the medicolegal area.

Consolidated Omnibus Budget Reconciliation Act (COBRA): Passed by Congress in 1992; implemented the Patient Self-Determination Act (PSDA).

Constructive Discharge: The employee leaves employment because the discrimination is so intolerable that no reasonable person could be expected to work in it.

Contingent: Possible but not absolute; conditional or provisional.

Continuing Education Requirement: Necessary academic credits, continuing nursing education credits, in-service training, or continuing education, which must be related to the area of specialization in which the applicant is seeking certification.

Continuing Tort: A tort that occurs over a period of time. For example, where the patient continues under a provider's care for a period of time, but the provider nevertheless negligently fails to detect the patient's illness.

Contract: An agreement involving legally enforceable promises between the employer and the contracted employee.

Contract Duties: Those duties and services set forth by the employer that are defined in the employment contract.

Contract Violations: An action or actions by the employer or employee that violate or break the contract stipulations as defined in the employment contract.

Contractual Arbitration: A method of ADR in which the parties have negotiated a contract to settle their dispute via arbitration, and the court will enforce the arbitrator's decision.

Contributory Negligence: A legal theory of liability whereby the amount of plaintiff's fault or responsibility in causing an injury is considered in calculation of reduction of damages.

Core Group: An identified group of providers known to offer efficient, effective care, who receive a large portion of the referrals from an HMO or PPO.

Core Requirements: Standards for the telenursing practice, which would be the basic requirements or standard adopted in all states.

Corporate Liability: The corporation's responsibility under various theories, including *respondeat superior*, agency, liability for negligent selection, hiring, firing, staffing, and so on.

Corporation: Legal structure that transfers legal responsibility from the individual shareholder to the entity.

Cost Containment: Actions of the managed care organization that involve cost sharing and price negotiation.

Course of Employment: The normal time, place, and/or circumstances of employment.

Court of Appeals: Panel of judges who review trial materials and determine whether an error has been made by the lower court i.e. trial court.

Court-Annexed ADR: ADR that is ordered by the court.

Court Reporter: A person who swears in witnesses and transcribes all the testimony during a legal proceeding.

Credentialing: Validation of the education, training, and experience of each provider; a voluntary form of self-regulation within a profession, which requires a higher standard of education, experience, and/or testing than licensure.

Crime: An injury that occurs as a result of intent to harm or a reckless disregard of whether harm will occur as a consequence of the action.

Criminal Justice: A professional field that encompasses the application of concepts from criminology, law enforcement, law adjudication, and corrections.

Criminal Law: The type of law that deals with acts that are considered to be against the people as a whole; regulations under which the state or federal government may deprive an individual of money, liberty, and/or life for acts considered offensive to society.

Critical Incident Stress Management (CISM): System in which persons are trained to offer additional assistance after incidents occur that are highly stressful, i.e., suicide of a patient.

Critical Pathways: A multidisciplinary care plan through which diagnosis and interventions are sequenced on a timeline.

Cross-examination: The attorney asks leading questions designed to elicit specific information, with a specific "yes" or "no" answer, without opportunity to explain or qualify.

Cruel and Unusual Punishment: Under the Eighth Amendment, the court asks the question: Is the action or inaction of such a nature that its effect (1) denies a constitutional right, (2) inflicts further penalty over and above that provided by law, and (2) results in the unnecessary or wanton infliction of pain.

Culpability: The degree of guilt.

Current Procedural Terminology (CPT) Codes: Codes used for reimbursement by third-party payers.

Cyber Liability: A form of liability for sexual harassment that occurs when sexually explicit computer images, messages, jokes, etc. can result in sexual harassment claims.

Cybercare: Nursing practice within cyberspace.

Damage Caps: Result of tort reform; amount plaintiff can recover from defendant is limited by statute, regardless of amount of jury award.

Damages: Injuries of a physical, emotional, psychological and/or economic nature.

Dangerousness: Criterion used to involuntarily commit mentally ill persons to a treatment center for psychiatric care, including (1) nature of harm, (2) magnitude of the behavior, (3) probability the behavior will occur, (4) imminence of the behavioral threat, and (5) frequency of the behavioral threat.

Debriefing: "A structured process integrating crisis intervention techniques with education. It is a peer driven, clinical guided discussion of a traumatic event designed to mitigate or resolve the psychological distress associated with a critical incident or traumatic event" (NMCISM, 1996).

Decryption: Decoding messages sent via the Internet/cyberspace.

"Deep Pocket": The defendant that has the most money from which plaintiff may recover damages.

Defamation: A quasi-intentional tort; a communication that holds someone up to ridicule, harms the reputation, and/or lessens the standing in the community; includes libel and slander.

Defendant: The person being sued in a civil trial.

Defense of Fact: Plaintiff and defendant disagree on how the event actually happened or who caused the injury, i.e., the facts of the case.

Defenses: Legal theories under which defendants may prove they are not liable for plaintiff's claim.

Delegation: The transfer of responsibility for the performance of a task from one person to another. The delegation of an activity passes on the responsibility for task performance but not the accountability for the process or the outcome of the task (ANA, 1996, p. 15).

Deliberate Deprivation: Intentional removal or denial of a constitutional right.

Deliberate Indifference: Intentional disregard of a constitutional right.

Demand Management: The type of nursing care that occurs when nurses are asked by the patients to help them manage their decisions in self-care, such as deciding when to physically enter the health care system.

Deontology: A theory of ethics based on the belief that the action of the nurse is right or wrong based on ethical principles or concepts of justice, autonomy, veracity, fidelity, and avoiding killing; duty based; also called *Kantian formalism or nonconsequentialism*.

Department of Health and Human Services: The federal agency in charge of Medicaid and Medicare programs.

Deposition: Questioning under oath of a witness by an attorney regarding issues relevant to a lawsuit.

Derivative Privilege: A privilege that comes from another privilege; for example, nurses may receive privileges from the privileges granted to physicians under their medical practice act.

Diagnosis: The conclusion reached on the condition of a patient, based on examination, history, and/or laboratory results.

Diagnostic Related Groups (DRGs): Case rates paid according to the diagnosis, rather than the units of service; established in 1983, provided a predetermined amount per diagnosis.

Direct Examination: The attorney asks the witness questions designed to elicit desired testimony, but may not ask leading questions.

Direct Liability: The managed care organization may become liable or responsible for the results of care unduly influenced by cost containment measures.

Direct Threat Standard: As defined by the EEOC, this standard involves a showing of the following elements by the employer, to demonstrate that accommodating the employee's disability in the workplace would pose a risk of undue hardship to the employer: (a) significant risk of substantial harm, (b) imminent threat, (c) dangerousness of the employee, (d) objective assessment that the potential for harm is significant and substantial, (e) duration of the risk, and (f) whether the risk can be reduced or eliminated by some reasonable accommodation.

Directive to Physician: Synonymous with *living will*; identifies life-sustaining procedures the person may or may not want withheld in the event the person is incapacitated, cannot make the decision, and in a terminal condition.

Disability: Any physical or mental impairment that limits a major life activity.

Disabled Nurse: Nurse in recovery, who is also protected by the Americans with Disabilities Act (ADA).

Discernment: "Sensitive insight involving acute judgment and understanding, and eventuates in decisive action" (Burkhart, 1998, p. 35).

Discharge Planner: Hospital employee who consults on, plans, and recommends home care services.

Discounts for Usual and Customary Fees: As a means of controlling costs, managed care organizations would negotiate discounts off the reasonable and customary fees in return for preferential treatment in referring patients.

Discovery Phase: First phase of the lawsuit, designed to uncover and gather information that will better define the issues of the case.

Discovery Rule: Legal doctrine that provides the statute of limitations does not begin to run until the plaintiff knew or should have known of the negligence or injury.

Discretionary Decisions: Decisions subject to the judgment of the decision-maker.

Discrimination: Unfair treatment or denial of privileges to persons because of their sex, age, race, nationality, or religion.

Distinguish: Identify the differences.

Distributive Justice: Ethical principle that provides for the fair and equitable distribution of health care goods and nursing services.

Do Not Resuscitate (DNR) Order: A directive written by the patient's physician, ordering the withholding of cardiopulmonary resuscitation if the patient goes into cardiac or respiratory arrest; a legal document that provides instructions to health care providers from the patient's doctor regarding the patient's right to receive or refuse life-sustaining and/or life-saving treatments.

Docket Number: The number assigned to the lawsuit by the clerk of the designated court; also called a case number.

Documentation: The written record of nursing care.

Drug Abuse: The use of a drug for a nontherapeutic purpose, especially one for which it was not prescribed or intended.

Duces Tecum: List of items the person must bring, when ordered by subpoena to appear before the court.

Durable Power of Attorney: A document that designates a substitute decision-maker; a legal document that allows a patient to designate an agent to make health care decisions for the patient in the event the patient is unable to.

Duty: Acts or interactions required after the presumption of a relationship between a provider and a patient.

Duty to Warn: The obligation of a health care provider who becomes aware of a client's intent to harm another person to notify the intended victim.

Elder Abuse Law: State mandatory reporting laws that protect men and women older than age 60 from abuse and neglect.

Electronic Media: All types of technology that transmit information, including but not limited to telephone, facsimile, computer, and satellite.

Elopement: Term used when a hospitalized client "escapes" or runs away from a treatment center.

Emancipated Minor: A minor who is financially independent, lives apart from his or her parents, is married, or is in the military service of the United States and is considered to have the same legal capacity as an adult.

Embryonic Stem Cells: Cells that have the power to develop into any kind of human cell or tissue.

Emergency: A threat to life and/or disability or serious aggravation of an existing disability.

Emergency Medical Treatment and Labor Act: Synonymous with *COBRA*; contains an "anti-dumping" provision under which hospitals must provide a medical screening examination and stabilize a patient before discharging and/or transferring him or her to another facility.

Emergency Nursing: The care of individuals of all ages with perceived or actual physical or emotional alterations of health that are undiagnosed or require further interventions.

Emergency Nursing Association (ENA) Code of Ethics: Published in 1989; provides a distinctive set of ideals and standards of conduct regarding research activities in emergency nursing.

Emergency Stay: Involuntary commitment of a person believed to be mentally ill for a period, generally 24 hours or so.

Empirical Absolutism: Acts are judged morally right based on what is known about the underlying scientific facts, following the natural law; for example, this position follows the foundations of Thomas Aquinas and traditional Catholic theology.

Employee Assistance Program (EAP): Program providing opportunities for employees to confide with counselors, e.g., about abuses they have experienced in the workplace.

Employee Retirement Income Security Act (ERISA): Federal law regulating employee benefits, including pensions and insurance plans; used to preempt malpractice suits against HMOs.

Employer: Person having control of payment of wages and job functions.

Employment Law: Specialty area of the law requiring knowledge of federal and state statutes, which regulate employment.

Empower: Encourage the patient to make the final decision regarding health care.

Empowerment: The ability of the patient to speak his or her own mind using personal power to make decisions for their own health care.

Encryption: A method of coding messages that are sent via the Internet/cyberspace.

Endorsement: A method of telenursing licensure through which the host state issues a license to practice to the nurse from another state with equivalent nursing standards.

Endpoint: The physician's and nurse's best guess of when skilled nursing services will be reduced to less than daily.

Enterprise Liability: A liability that has grown out of product liability claims, under which the payer or enterprise is liable for the actions of the provider.

Environment: "[Is composed of] three basic components: building(s), equipment and people. Effective management of the environment of care includes using processes and activities to a) reduce and control environmental hazards and risks; b) prevent accidents and injuries; and, c) maintain safe conditions for patients, visitors, and safety" (JCAHO, 1996).

Equal Employment Opportunity Commission (EEOC): The governmental agency that enforces Title VII guidelines, which provide protection from employment discrimination.

Equity: A system of law based on fairness; founded within common law.

Ethic of Care: Process of sharing relational stories of caregiving.

Ethical Dilemma: A choice between two or more alternatives with two or more equally unfavorable outcomes.

Ethics: Rules or principles that govern right conduct; a set of formal or informal rules that guide moral decisions; or choices between good and bad, right and wrong.

Euthanasia: An easy, painless, or good death.

Evidence: Pertinent information surrounding the client, the scene, or the suspect that might substantiate claims of innocence, guilt, or responsibility for outcomes.

Ex Parte Communications: Communicating with one party to a legal action while the other is not present.

Exclusionary Rule: Stems from the Fourth Amendment's prohibition on unreasonable search and seizure of evidence: (1) evidence obtained through an unlawful or unreasonable search cannot be used against the person whose rights the search violated; and (2) evidence in plain view could be confiscated, such as a weapon, drugs, or any item suspected of potential harm to others.

Exemplary or Punitive Damages: That amount of money assigned to the plaintiff that will stand as punishment of the defendant's actions.

Expert Forensic Nurse Witness: Nurses who by their competence and knowledge of current forensic nursing literature, active clinical forensic practice, attendance at forensic continuing education, research activity, publishing, teaching, consulting, membership in professional organizations, and/or peer review have demonstrated the expertise to testify in court on standards of forensic nursing practice.

Expert Testimony: A nurse who is familiar with the standard of care testifies about what a reasonable prudent nurse would have done, then render an opinion as to whether or not the nurse defendant acted accordingly.

Expert Witness: A witness who is considered by the court to be capable and qualified to summarize and explain complex and voluminous medical records ad medical terminology to the jury.

Exposure: The potential for a malpractice action to be filed against the insured party.

Exposure-prone Procedure: An invasive procedure that may directly expose or risk transmission of a disease to the patient.

Expressed Consent: Explicit acknowledgment of a health care provider's request to provide treatment; consent to medical treatment that takes the form of a specific verbal agreement and/or through a signed consent for treatment.

Extraordinary Medical Treatment: Synonymous with the term *heroic measures*; offers the patient little or no hope, with the prospect of a prolonged, expensive, and/or painful life (Andrews et al., 1996, p. 290).

Extrapyramidal Side Effects: Central nervous system side effects such as tardive dyskinesia that are related to major tranquilizer or neuroleptic drugs and are untreatable.

E-Zine: A magazine printed in cyberspace.

Fact-Finding: A method of ADR characterized by activities conducted by a neutral expert or fact-finder, including a hearing and a written report containing recommendations for settlement that are nonbinding suggestions.

Fact Witness: A witness who has actually been present to see or perceive a thing, and has been called an eyewitness.

Failure to Fire: Under this liability claim, the employer is held liable under the doctrine of *respondeat superior* only if the employee's act is considered to be one that is within the scope of employment or within the job description.

Fair Labor Standards Act of 1938 (FLSA): Legislation that allowed states to set minimum wage laws.

False Imprisonment: Restraining and/or detaining a person inappropriately or unlawfully.

Family and Medical Leave Act of 1993 (FMLA): Legislation enacted to protect the worker's balance between job and family; enables employees to take time from work for eligible reasons (as defined by law) without losing their jobs.

Feasibility: The legal concept that holds that but for the negligence, the injury would not have occurred.

Federal Common Law: Federal court holdings or decisions that become commonly held or repeated decisions in similar cases in other federal courts in other jurisdictions or locations.

Federal Emergency Medical Services System Act of 1973 (FEMA): Federal statutory law that provides guidelines for coordinating health care services during emergencies and disasters.

Feminist Ethics: An ethical decision-making model through which alternatives are considered that will best preserve existing relationships.

Fidelity: An ethical principle that embodies the nurse's duty to be loyal, faithful, and keep promises.

Fiduciary: An individual who can work with, or serve as, either a guardian or conservator and can handle coordination of needs and services for the person and the finances.

Focal Virtues: Character traits that are central to a virtuous person.

Forensic: Pertaining to or applied in legal proceedings.

Forensic Clients: Recipients of nursing assessments or interventions who have an actual or potential involvement with the legal system (enforcement or judicial); may include victims, perpetrators, the deceased, survivors, bystanders, and families or significant others.

Forensic Clinical Nurse Specialist: Advanced practice nurse, prepared at the master's level, who cares for forensic clients, e.g., the forensic psychiatric nurse.

Forensic Nursing: The application of the forensic aspects of health care combined with the biopsychological education of the registered nurse in the scientific investigation and treatment of trauma and/or death-related medicolegal issues (IAFN & ANA, 1997, p. 30).

Forensic Psychiatric Nurse: A nurse who practices in the psychiatric setting, who interfaces with clients and their legal issues, e.g., interacts with the judicial system to determine whether a forensic client is competent to stand trial.

Forensic Sciences: Fields of expertise in observation and interpretation of evidence involved in the investigation of legal cases; includes pathology, biology, toxicology, criminalistics, questioned documents, forensic odontology, forensic anthropology, physics, serology, jurisprudence, psychiatry, engineering, geology, microscopy, and nursing.

Foreseeability: A legal requirement that the general danger, not the exact sequence of events that produced the harm, be foreseeable.

Full Faith and Credit: Clause of the Constitution that provides that the courts of one state will recognize the laws of another state.

Fundamental Rights: Basic rights such as privacy, speech, religion, or liberty.

Gatekeeper: Individual in health care who must evaluate the patient's situation before authorizing the expenditure of funds on a treatment option.

General Duty Clause of the OSHA: Requires employers to provide a safe working environment.

Generalist Nurse Role: Direct care nurse role fulfilled by a nurse educated at the diploma, associate degree, or baccalaureate degree level.

Generations of Managed Care: Strategies for the step-by-step introduction of managed care in a geographic location.

Gerontological Nursing: Services provided for older persons, including the delivery of direct care, management and development of nonprofessional caregivers, and the evaluation of care and services.

Good Faith: Actions or inactions believed to be executed in the interest of and focused on the best outcome; total absence of intention (usually by the employer) to seek unfair advantage or defraud the employee.

Good Samaritan Act: Law that protects health care workers from being charged with negligence when they provide emergency treatment to those in immediate need.

Good Samaritan Statute: Laws that provide protection for a person who gives aid to an individual in imminent and serious peril and who acts with good faith and reasonable care to minimize or prevent injury, no matter the outcome.

Government Affairs Committee (GAC): A grassroots political action group initiated by the Texas Nurses Association that initiates legislation, drafts bills, identifies sponsors, and prepares backup materials.

Government Functions: Functions that can be performed only by a government unit, e.g. police, judicial.

Grassroots Organization: A political action group designed to quickly inundate legislators with information about a particular emerging health care issue.

Gross Negligence: Willful, intentional acts of negligence, for which punitive damages may be awarded.

Guardian: A person lawfully invested with the power and duty to take care of another person and manage his or her property rights.

Guardian Ad Litem: A guardian appointed by the court to prosecute or defend for an infant or child.

Guidelines: Recommended nursing practices designed to meet standards of care.

Guilty But Mentally Ill (GBMI): Criminal defense used in some states in place of the NGRI plea. When or if sanity is restored, the person serves his or her prison sentence.

Habeas Corpus: A claim regarding wrongful incarceration; written request for speedy release on the grounds that the individual is sane and able to be released.

Hacking: Intercepting electronic communications wired on the Internet, for example through "sniffing" or "spoofing."

Handicap: Physical or mental impairment that substantially limits one or more major life activities. May be long term or short term.

Hands-on Policy: The policy of assuming control; for example, placing laws regulating correctional facilities within the authority of the legislative and executive branches of the state and federal governments.

Harassment: The crime of willful and repeated interference with an employee; offensive behavior in the workplace that is directed toward an employee or group of employees based on discrimination because of race, color, religion, sex, or national origin.

Hazardous Agent: In relation to the perpetrator of workplace violence, synonymous with the term *human being*.

Health Care: Under the UHCIA, any care, service, or procedure administered by the provider, such as the diagnosis, treatment, and maintenance of the patient's physical or mental condition, and/or that affects the structure and/or any function of the body (UHCIA, 1997, § 1–101 & 102).

Health Care Communications: Health care information that is electronically wired.

Health Care Information: "Any information, whether oral or recorded in any form or medium, that identifies or can readily be associated with the identity of a patient and relates to the patient's health-care. The term includes any record of disclosure of health-care information" (ULCIA, 1997, § 1–101 & 102).

Health Care Provider: A member of the multidisciplinary treatment team who renders health care to the patient, for example, the nurse.

Health Care Quality Improvement Act of 1986: Legislation that created a national practitioner's data bank of information regarding health care practitioners who have been sanctioned.

Health Maintenance Organization (HMO): An entity that provides or arranges for the provision of coverage of specified health services needed by a plan member for a fixed, prepaid premium; a managed care organization.

Health Plan Employee Data and Information Setup (HEDIS): A data system that focuses on outcomes and documents effectiveness of managed care organizations.

Hill-Burton Act: Federal legislation requiring each state to provide adequate health care facilities for persons residing within its boundaries.

Holding: Final decision of the court.

Home Health Agency (HHA): Agency certified under Medicare to provide health care in the patient's home.

Home Health Nursing: The provision of nursing care to acute, chronically ill, and well clients of all ages in their homes while integrating community nursing principles that focus on health promotion and on environmental, psychosocial, economic, cultural, and personal health factors affecting an individual's and family's health status.

Home Health Providers: Those health care organizations that provide patient care in the home, i.e., visiting nurse associations, health departments, community-based nursing services, hospital-based agencies, nursing registries, hospices, independent professional practices, and proprietary agencies.

Home State: Under the Compact, the nurse's state of residence and the state that will grant the license, set the licensure standards, and take disciplinary action under that license.

Homebound: Requirement to receive home health.

Horizontal Violence: Violence that takes place by subtle yet very destructive methods; may include (1) acts of bullying, (2) physicians demeaning nurses or throwing objects, (3) being undermined by a coworker, or (4) threats.

Hospital (Clinical) Privileges: The American Hospital Association developed recommendations for nonphysician practitioners who provide care within a hospital setting; are usually extended by a committee review of applicant credentials on a regular basis.

Hospital-Based Agencies: Health care agencies that are owned by and located in close geographic proximity to the hospital.

Hospitals: Specialized entities that contain the equipment and employ the providers necessary to deliver health care.

Host State: Under the Compact, the state in which the patient resides and/or telenursing care is provided.

Hostile Working Environment: Working conditions in which an employee is subjected to harassment based on the employee's race, color, religion, sex, or national origin; is unlawful discrimination.

ICD-9 Codes: Codes listed in the International Classification of Diseases, 9th Revision, of the World Health Organization, used in billing insurance companies, by which diseases are classified according to medical diagnosis and then assigned a 6-digit number.

Immunity: Right to be free of any type of claim(s), including liability.

Impaired Nurse: The term used to describe a nurse abusing or addicted to alcohol or drugs.

Impairment: Under the ADA, a physiological disorder affecting one or more of a number of body systems, or a mental or psychological disorder.

Impasse: Occurs when the parties to ADR cannot reach a decision.

Impeach: To challenge the credibility of a witness by confronting the witness with prior inconsistent testimony.

Implied Consent: A nonverbal acknowledgment of a health care provider's request to provide treatment.

Implied Contract: A contract that has not been explicitly agreed to by the parties, but that the law nevertheless considers exists.

Imputed Negligence: The breach of a standard by one person is attributed to another; synonymous with the term *respondeat superior.*

In Loco Parentis: The principle by which another person who provides consent for the child in the absence of the parent.

***In Personam* Jurisdiction:** The court has jurisdiction over the parties to the dispute because they have had minimum contacts with the state.

In Vitro Fertilization: The insertion of a sperm into the egg within the laboratory setting.

Inadequate Staffing: Staffing that is inadequate to provide services contracted for and/or that does not meet an acceptable standard.

Incident Report: A report of special, unusual, or unexpected occurrences or outcomes that may become the subject of litigation.

Incompetency: Inability to understand information needed to reason and deliberate; an inability to make decisions in one's best interests.

Incompetency Determination: Legal decision that the mentally ill person is incapable of making personal or treatment decisions; designation used for a person charged with a crime who is unable to understand the charges and cannot assist the attorney with a defense.

Incompetent: Designation for a person who is unable to speak for himself or herself, comprehend and/or make decisions as a result of some incapacity, including but not limited to medical condition, age, deformity, or retardation.

Indemnified: One provider may cover the liability of another, for provision of health care stated within their contract for services.

Indemnity Insurance: A type of insurance under which the insured person is reimbursed for covered expenses.

Independent Contractor: A self-employed person who renders services to others, pays his or her own taxes, and has the final decision on how the work will be performed.

Independent Medical Examination: An examination used by the defense when physical and mental condition is an issue of the lawsuit; used in medical malpractice cases when the validity of the claims are at issue.

Indirect Liability: Legal liability based on the relationship to the provider; includes the doctrine of *respondeat superior.*

Informed Consent: The voluntary agreement by a person who is in possession and exercise of sufficient mental capacity to make an intelligent choice between proposed alternatives; may be expressed or implied; the acquisition of consent after providing the required elements detailing the proposed treatment or procedure; the right to adequate information on a level appropriate for the client's understanding in his or her primary language before treatment methods are initiated; the right to full disclosure of health care information that is a key patient right upon entering any health care agency. Information must be communicated by the physician, but may be discussed with clients by the nurse.

Inmates: Persons who have been convicted of a crime and who are incarcerated in a jail or prison.

Insane Asylums: Large warehouse-like buildings providing confinement for mentally ill persons.

Institutional Practice Guidelines: Clinical or critical pathways or patient care timelines that are designed to provide a health care program that addresses not only quality and clinical outcomes, but cost of care issues.

Instrumental Activities of Daily Living (IADLs): Daily activities of self-care, including preparing meals, shopping, managing money, using the telephone, doing housework, and taking medication.

Integrity: A central or focal virtue that is a combination of soundness, reliability, wholeness, fidelity, and consistency of convictions.

Intentional Assault Exception: Applies when an employer may be held liable for intentional torts that include an "actual intent to injure on the part of the employer" (*Gallegos v. Chastain,* 1981).

Intentional Infliction of Emotional Distress: Intending to cause emotional distress through outrageous conduct.

Intentional Injury: The consequences or harm caused by an action or inaction are intended.

Intentional Torts: Acts or inactions designed to bring about a particular result, including (1) assault, (2) battery, (3) false imprisonment, and (4) intentional infliction of emotional distress.

Interest of the Employer Test: A test under the National Labor Relations Act; used to determine whether the actions of the nurse were executed in the interest of the patient and, thus, the interest of the employer; including every nursing action of the employee acting within the terms of his or her job description.

Interim Payment System (IPS): Implemented by Congress under the Balanced Budget Act of 1997, provides for the payment of a per beneficiary limit.

Interlocutory Appeal: An appeal from the trial court entered during the course of litigation.

Intermediate Scrutiny: A test used by the courts to determine whether a law, that discriminates based on classifications such as gender, is substantially related to a legitimate state interest.

Interpretive Guidelines: A Medicare document that serves to interpret and clarify the conditions of participation of home health agencies.

Interrogatories: Written questions submitted by one party of a lawsuit to another; requires written responses under oath.

Interstate Compact for the Mutual Recognition Model on Nursing Regulation: Developed by the NCSBN, allows nurses to practice outside their state of licensure, as long as the nurse adheres to the nurse practice act in the state in which he or she practices.

Intuitionism: Synonymous with *non-naturalism;* acts are judged right based on intuition.

Invasion of Privacy: A quasi-intentional tort that takes one of the following three forms: (1) appropriation of name or likeness of another; (2) unreasonable and extremely offensive intrusion upon another or the personal affairs of another; and (3) placing another in a false light in the public eye.

Involuntary Commitment Admission: Legal procedure allowing friends, family, police officers, or physicians to initiate treatment via a petition for treatment.

Involuntary Community Treatment Commitment: Court-committed treatment for mentally ill individuals who have serious and persistent mental illness and a history of dangerousness to self or others.

Involuntary Euthanasia: Death results when treatment is withheld or withdrawn without informed consent.

Irresistible Impulse Test: Insanity determination broader in scope than the M'Naghten Rule; the person may avoid criminal responsibility even if he or she was able to distinguish between right and wrong and was fully aware of the nature and quality of the act by establishing that he or she was unable to refrain from acting.

Job Description: A written statement describing responsibilities of a specific job and the qualifications an applicant for that specific job should have.

Joint and Several Liability: A legal theory of liability whereby all of the persons deemed responsible for causing an injury may be held individually liable for all damages.

Joint Commission on Accreditation of Healthcare Organizations (JCAHO): Voluntary, independent accrediting agency for health care organizations; an independent nonprofit entity that establishes standards for the delivery of health care and conducts surveys to evaluate compliance.

Joint Tortfeasors: Persons who act in concert to cause an injury.

Judge: A person who acts as a neutral overseer of the proceedings and controls the parties' access to evidence under their opponents' controls, as well as their presentation of evidence to the jury; decides what issues will be presented to the jury; decides issues of law.

Judicial Arbitration: Arbitration that is ordered by the court; also referred to as *court-annexed arbitration*.

Judicial Review: The process by which a court reviews a decision of a lower court, a decision of an administrative body, or the constitutionality of a law passed by a legislature.

Jurisdiction: The authority of a court to hear a particular case.

Jurisprudence: The mechanism by which the American legal system makes and administers law.

Jury: Decides issues of fact and is the sole judge of the credibility of witnesses; decides issues of liability and damages.

Jury Instructions: Directions and explanations provided by the judge regarding laws that are relevant and apply to this particular case.

Justice: An ethical principle that encompasses the nurse's duty to be fair and equitable and provide access to and appropriate care to all patients.

Keep-Locking: Locking inmates in their cells.

Laches: A legal doctrine that can operate to bar a lawsuit even though the applicable statue of limitations has not run out because the plaintiff was a minor or was incompetent. Recognized at common law by many states, for it would be unfair to permit certain claims to go forward if it has been so long since the act that evidence has been lost, memories faded, and the defendant would be unduly prejudiced.

Law: A rule or regulation that is established and enforced by a government in the interest of its people; discipline addressing both individual behavior outcomes and rights as well as society safety; enables society to function as smoothly as possible; set of enforceable principles and/or rules established to protect society.

Least Restrictive Environment Standard: Providers have a duty to provide the patient as much freedom as possible.

Legal Entity: An organization created through a legal process, such as a corporation.

Legal Incapacity: Unable to bring suit, enter into contracts, or make any type of legal decision. For example, this includes minors under 18 and those who have been declared legally incompetent.

Liability: Legal responsibility for failing to properly perform required duties that subsequently cause harm to another person; the failure to meet professional and regulatory standards of care, resulting in harm to a patient.

Libel: Written defamatory statements.

Licensure: "A legal process by which a designated authority grants permission to a qualified individual to perform designated skills and service in a given jurisdiction" (Catalano, 1995, p. 82); mechanism by which a state establishes and verifies compliance with standards.

Life Care Plan: A dynamic document based on published standards of practice, comprehensive assessment, data analysis, and research, which provides an organized, concise plan for current and future needs, with associated costs, for individuals who have experienced catastrophic injury or have chronic health needs.

Life-Sustaining Medical Treatment (LSMT): Health care used to maintain the patient's life, which may be categorized as ordinary or extraordinary.

Life-Sustaining Procedure: A medical procedure or intervention that utilizes mechanical or other artificial means to sustain, restore, or supplant a vital function and that serves only to prolong the moment of death.

Limitations Period: The time frame in which a claim or lawsuit must be brought; see Statute of Limitations.

Limited Licensure: A method of telenursing licensure that limits the scope of nursing practice rather than the time period of practice; for example, may allow the nurse to perform only certain procedures.

Limiting Statutes: Statutes designed to limit the amount of damages (1) recoverable in a malpractice action; (2) to be paid by an individual health care provider, that is, the individual or hospital; and/or (3) by establishing a patient compensation board, similar to workers' compensation legislation, that screens damage awards.

Litigation: Adversarial contest in a court of justice for the purpose of enforcing a right; legal action or process.

Living Will: A document that states circumstances under which an individual prefers to have certain choices exercised on his or her behalf; synonymous with *directive to physician*; provided by state statute, allows any adult to sign a directive instructing the physician to withhold or withdraw life-sustaining procedures in the event of a terminal condition.

Lobbying: Actions that attempt to provide convincing information that results in a desired outcome from a public official.

Long Arm Statutes: Statutes that limit the reach or jurisdiction of the court in terms of other parties, states, and/or countries.

Long-Term Acute Care Hospital: Hospitals that are primarily engaged in providing medical services to patients whose average length of stay exceeds 25 consecutive days.

Long-Term Care: Health care services that provide physical, psychological, spiritual, social, and economic services to help people attain, maintain, or regain their optimum level of functioning.

Long-Term Care Facilities: Synonymous with *nursing facilities, skilled nursing facilities, long-term acute care hospitals*, and *assisted-living or personal care facilities*; overwhelming majority of patients are elderly.

Long-Term Stay: Involuntary commitment of a person believed to be mentally ill, generally, 90 days or so in length.

Loss of Consortium: A claim that the party is damaged because he/she is unable to carry on the normal marital relations.

Major Life Activity: Under the ADA, defined as the activities needed to care for oneself.

Major Tranquilizers: Neuroleptic drugs that came into use in the 1950s, which greatly reduced the bizarre behaviors of mentally ill

persons and allowed them to be amenable to talk and activity therapies; "miracle drugs."

Malice: Knowledge that the acts or inactions will likely cause harm; intent to cause serious harm.

Malpractice: Professional negligence; negligence committed by a person in a licensed, professional capacity, such as nurses, attorneys, accountants, and physicians.

Malpractice Insurance: The type of insurance that protects professional people against claims of negligence.

Managed Care: A system of managing and financing health care delivery to ensure that services provided to insurance plan members are necessary, efficiently provided, and appropriately priced.

Mandated: Ordered by state or federal statute.

Mandatory Licensure: Requires anyone practicing nursing to pass a licensure examination and become registered by the SBN; at the technical level, the individual must pass the licensed practical nurse (LPN) examination; at the professional level, the individual must pass the RN examination.

Mature Minor: An individual "judicially recognized as possessing sufficient understanding and appreciation of the nature and consequences of treatment despite their chronological age" and, thus, can give consent for treatment (Rozovsky, 1990).

Maximum Allowable Fees: A more stringent means of controlling costs that discounts; maximum allowable fees are the maximum amount of dollars the health plan will pay for a service, regardless of the charge by the provider.

Med-Arb: Mediation-arbitration; a method of ADR that is a two-step process, with mediation first, followed by formal arbitration to decide any issues not resolved in mediation.

Mediation: A method of ADR that is a process by which opposing parties submit their health care dispute to an impartial third party, the mediator, who attempts to help draw the parties together to agree on a mutual settlement.

Medical Durable Power of Attorney: A legal document that enables an individual to name another person to be a substitute decision-maker, under the circumstances of impaired functioning on the part of the person executing the document.

Medical Malpractice: Occurs when a doctor or nurse fails to do that which a reasonable, prudent doctor or nurse would do under the same or similar circumstances, or does that which a reasonable, prudent doctor or nurse would not do under the same or similar circumstances.

Medical Necessity: Determining that the care being received is appropriate for the symptoms exhibited by the patient receiving the care; a decision made by a physician according to established criteria.

Medical Records: Documentation designed to provide a summary of all observations made regarding nursing and medical diagnosis and to accurately reflect measures taken to alleviate identified problems as well as patient response to intervention.

Medical Savings Accounts (MSAs): Systems of payment for health care that refund to the employee the balance of the account not spent for health care at the end of the year.

Medically Futile Treatments: Treatments that will neither result in survival nor improve quality of life.

Medically Underserved Population: A population that has a shortage of health care providers or health care services.

Medicare Conditions of Participation (COP): Federal regulations that govern the provision of Medicare home health services.

Medicare Conditions of Payment: The requirements set forth under Medicare with which the home health agency must comply in order to be eligible to receive reimbursement for home health services rendered to eligible patients.

Medication Errors: The most common source of nursing negligence; occurs if the wrong patient receives the wrong medication, via the wrong route, at the wrong dosage, and/or at the wrong time.

Mental Impairment: Psychiatric diagnosis that are potentially covered under the Americans with Disabilities Act, for example: major depression, schizophrenia, anxiety disorders, bipolar disorders, and/or personality disorder.

Mentally Incompetent: One who is unable to provide consent for treatment and/or has a court-appointed guardian with the legal authority to provide consent for treatment.

Mere Possibility: Even the slightest chance of an occurrence.

Merits: Strengths and validity of the case.

Midlevel Providers: Term used to denote advanced practice nurses and physician's assistants.

Mini-Arbitration: A method of ADR that is a variation of the mini-trial, but the parties agree the arbitrator's decision will be binding.

Minimally Adequate: Standard or quality designed to meet only basic standards.

Minimum Contacts: Basic activity requirements of a party before they can be sued in a particular jurisdiction (Blacks, 1979, p. 897).

Minimum Data Set (MDS): The minimum information that must be included in the resident assessment instrument.

Mini-Trial: A method of ADR that is a court-annexed "mock" or simulated trial, adversarial in nature, intended to move opposing parties who are stuck in their position when negotiation and mediation have failed.

Minor: An individual whose age is below the age of majority, as determined in the specific state; all consent for medical treatment, testing and procedures must be obtained from the minor's parent or guardian, unless specified otherwise by state law.

Miracle Drugs: See neuroleptic drugs and major tranquilizers.

Miranda Rights: Basic rights that must be recited to someone who is taken into custody, including the following: (1) a right to remain silent, (2) a right to obtain an attorney, and (3) anything the person says may be used against them (*Miranda v. Arizona*).

Mitigate: The duty to lessen or reduce the amount of damages after an injury occurs.

M'Naghten Rule: Insanity determination regarding whether, at the time of the crime, the person had sufficient mental capacity to know and understand what he or she was doing and whether or not he or she knew and understood that the behavior was wrong and a violation of the rights of another.

Modified Responsibility: Plaintiff may recover in a negligence cause of action if plaintiff's negligence does not exceed that of defendant or if plaintiff's negligence is less than that of defendant.

Morals: One's sense of good and bad, right and wrong.

Motions In Limine: Requests filed by an attorney to limit inclusion of specified evidence.

Multidisciplinary Treatment Team (MDTT): A team of health care professionals that monitors and determines all aspects of the security, diagnosis, treatment, and rights of the health care consumer, through a shared decision-making process.

Multi-State Licensure Compact (Compact): A contract between states that is the mechanism by which the mutual recognition model of nursing licensure will be implemented by the NCSBN to provide telenursing across state lines.

Multi-State Licensure Privilege: Under the Compact, the authority to practice in any of the party states.

Mutual Recognition Model: A method of nursing licensure through which the host state agrees to legally recognize the standards under which the nurse practices telenursing; the nurse may be licensed in the home state but practice in other states, in compliance with their state laws.

Narrative Charting: Notes regarding the patient's status written in the nurse's own handwriting that provides an overview of the care of the patient for the shift.

National Council of State Boards of Nursing (NCSBN): A nonprofit organization, composed of the boards of nursing from the 50 states, the District of Columbia, and the five territories of the United States; organization through which boards of nursing act, including the development of licensing examinations.

National Licensure: A method of telenursing licensure that would create a national license, replacing the state license.

National Organ Transplant Act of 1984: Provides for the creation of a system for organ sharing on a national basis; prevents the sale of organs; and funds grants for agencies that obtain and provide organ transplantation services.

Natural Death Act: Legislation that allows competent persons to make life-saving decisions in advance of any situation in which they are unable to make independent decisions.

Negligence: Failure to exercise reasonable care; failure to use ordinary care; failure to use that degree of care that a reasonable and prudent person would use under the same or similar circumstances; breach of duty; wrongs that are not caused by intentional acts.

Negligence Per Se: Acts or inactions that are of such a nature that liability is automatic under law; negligence shown by virtue of violation of a statute or law intended to protect the class of persons of whom plaintiff is a member.

Negligent Hiring: Under this legal theory, the principal or health care organization is held liable for failing to ascertain the skills, references, licenses, and other attributes of the potential employee or medical staff person at the time of employment or admission to the staff.

Negligent Selection: Under this legal theory, the principal or health care organization is held liable for failing to ascertain the skills of the employee at the time of selection to perform a procedure.

Negotiation: A method of ADR that involves discussions on the terms of a proposed health care agreement and/or settlement of the terms and conditions of a health care transaction.

Networking: The art of connecting with a group that shares a common agenda and can collectively accomplish common goals.

Neuroleptics: Major tranquilizer drugs that came into use in the 1950s and greatly reduced the bizarre behaviors of mentally ill persons, allowing them to be amenable to talk and activity therapies; "miracle drugs."

Neutral Expert: A facilitator in the ADR process who is an expert.

Nonmaleficence: An ethical principle that contemplates that the nurse will do no intentional or unintentional harm to the patient.

Nonvoluntary Euthanasia: Death resulting when treatment is withheld or withdrawn, without knowledge of what the patient would have wanted.

Normative Decisions: Ethical decisions regarding rights and obligations to others that involve evaluations based on norms.

Not Guilty by Reason of Insanity (NGRI): Criminal defense for the purpose of avoiding responsibility by meeting one of three insanity standards: M'Naghten Rule, irresistible impulse test, or the American Law Institute (ALI) standard.

Notice of Intent to File Suit: A preliminary notice of the suit sent to defendant within a predetermined number of days before the lawsuit is filed with the court.

N-STAT: A grassroots lobbying group of nurses at the state or local level who belong to state and local nurses associations.

Nurse Death Investigator: A nurse who works collaboratively with the police department to investigate deaths, e.g., to notify the family of the death of the family member.

Nurse Manager: One who oversees the general effectiveness and efficiency of patient care and is concerned with organization, planning, operations, and supervision of nursing staff and the patient care provided.

Nurse-Midwife: Advanced practice nurse who manages the care of women and newborns.

Nurse-Patient-Relationship: The legal relationship that results when the patient seeks care from the nurse, and the nurse has performed some affirmative act for the patient; this relationship results in a duty by the nurse to the patient.

Nurse Practice Act: Under statutory law, the state's official document that defines and regulates the profession's scope of practice and allowable practicing parameters for an identified group.

Nurse Practitioner (NP): Advanced practice nurse with a master's degree in psychiatric-mental health nursing; has advanced physical diagnostic skills as well; provides primary health care and specialized health services to individuals, families, groups, and communities. See Clinical Nurse Specialist.

Nursing: The delivery of health care, for compensation, through use of the nursing process.

Nursing Care Plan: The plan of nursing interventions, including long- and short-term goals.

Nursing Code of Ethics: The professional values and standards of nursing practice.

Nursing Diagnosis: The conclusion of the nurse's assessments and findings by labeling the patient's responses.

Nursing Disciplinary Diversion Act: Provides to addicted nurses a diversion procedure as a voluntary alternative to disciplinary action.

Nursing Facilities: Commonly known as nursing homes; under federal law, must provide nursing care, services, and activities that maintain the highest practicable physical, mental, and psychosocial well-being of each resident.

Nursing Malpractice: A nurse's failure to use that degree of care that a reasonable and prudent nurse would use under the same or similar circumstances.

Nursing Negligence: A nurse's failure to use the degree of care that a reasonable and prudent nurse would use under the same or similar circumstances.

Nursing Social Policy: A document developed by a professional organization, e.g., the American Nurses Association for use in understanding nursing's relationship with society.

Nursing Supervisor: As defined under the NLRA, has the authority to recommend the performance of any of the following activities by a nursing employee, including hiring, transferring, suspending, laying off, recalling, promoting, discharging, assigning, rewarding, disciplining, adjusting grievances of, and/or directing the employee.

Obligation: Something owed to another.

Obstruction of Justice: Criminal liability that arises when the investigation is hampered in any manner, e.g., evidence is destroyed.

Occurrence Insurance Coverage: Type of policy that covers any occurrence of an injury or damage that occurs during the time the policy is in force.

Old Boy Network: Older more experienced nurses assist novice nurses in the political process.

Older Persons: Those individuals 65 and older.

Ombudsman: A neutral person who is an officer of the legislature, who: (a) supervises the administration of the health care agency board; (b) intervenes in specific complaints between the public and administrative agencies, such as

complaints between the nurse and the board of nursing; and/or (c) investigates, criticizes, and publicizes—but cannot reverse—the action of the agency or board.

Omnibus Budget Reconciliation Act of 1987 (OBRA): Federal legislation that governs providers of health care in long-term care facilities; forbids hospitals from turning away emergency room patients or dumping them on another institution for inability to pay for services.

On-line Service: An electronic Internet communication service.

Open Courts Provision: A provision that is found in some state constitutions, which precludes the state legislature from passing legislation that would cut off claims and causes of action that had been available to citizens at common law.

Opening Statement: Designed to give a comprehensive summary of the nature of the case by both defendant and plaintiff, including a: (a) succinct account of the evidence to be presented, and (b) explanation of the points that will be proven with the evidence.

Operation Restore Trust: A nationwide government antifraud initiative designed to scrutinize the compliance of home health agencies with Medicare guidelines for payment.

Order of Protective Custody: Involuntary commitment of a person believed to be mentally ill, generally for 1 month or so.

Ordinance: A rule or regulation passed by local government entities that affects the government and citizens within their borders.

Ordinary Care: That degree of care that a reasonable and prudent person would exercise under the same or similar circumstances.

Ordinary Medical Treatment: A treatment whose outcome offers the patient a good prognosis, without excessive pain or expense.

Ordinary Negligence: Failure to meet that standard of conduct required of reasonably prudent people.

Ostensible Agency: Synonymous with *apparent agency*; giving the impression that the person is an agent of the organization.

Otherwise Privileged: Health care communications categorized as privileged by other characteristics than just being a privately wired communication.

Outcome Assessment System Information Set (OASIS): Under the HCFA Conditions of Participation, the home health agency is required to collect data and report them to its state survey agency, i.e., sociodemographic, environmental, support system, health status, and functional status attributes of nonmaternity, adult patients.

Outcome Management: A management system to track and measure the outcomes of care using standard research methodologies.

Outcome Standards: Synonymous with *critical pathways and protocols*; used to establish standards of care for discharge.

Outpatient Commitment: Requires the client to follow a court-ordered course of treatment while continuing to live in the community.

Paradigm Cases: Classic cases used to illustrate an ethical issue about which everyone can agree; a standard example; used within the causuistry ethical decision-making model.

***Parens Patriae* Doctrine:** Legal doctrine enabling states to commit to treatment mentally ill persons who cannot care for themselves.

Party States: Under the Compact, those states that are members of the Compact and will allow Multistate Licensure of Nurses.

Passive Euthanasia: Facilitation of the patient's death by withdrawing life-preserving treatment that would prolong the life of one who is terminally ill and would not survive without it (E. K. Dvorak, personal communication, November 22, 1998).

Paternalism: An ethical principle under which health care decisions are made for the patient by the provider.

Patient: Under the UHCIA, the person who receives health care and who has received health care, including the deceased.

Patient Care Analysis Test: A test under the National Labor Relations Act used to determine whether the duties of the nurse were executed in the interest of the patient rather than the interest of the employer.

Patient Rights: A guarantee of certain rights and privileges to every hospitalized patient.

Patient Self–Determination Act (PSDA): A federal law that mandates hospitals and other health care agencies inform patients of their rights under state law to have living wills and durable powers of attorney for health care.

Payer: Person or entity that pays for the medical services, including insurance companies, managed care companies, employers, and/or the patient.

PDF Files: Computer files placed in a portable document format.

Pecuniary Damages: The amount of losses sustained by the patient; under the UHCIA, losses sustained because of the violation of the patient's right to confidentiality.

Peer Review: An established mechanism that allows professions to monitor the practice of its members.

Per Beneficiary Limit: Cap of $3500 in the amount home health agencies would be reimbursed annually per patient, regardless of medical need; established under the Balanced Budget Act of 1997, through IPS.

Per Member, Per Month (pmpm): The monthly payment capitated providers receive prospectively to cover the cost of health care needed for each beneficiary assigned to them.

Per Se Standard of Care: State statutes that require nurses to report negligence or abuse of dependent persons such as children, the aged, or the disabled.

Peremptory Challenge: Request by an attorney to excuse a potential juror without stating a cause.

Peripherals: Diagnostic equipment, such as the stethoscope or otoscope, that may be used to monitor the patient via a telehealth network.

Permissive Licensure: Allows individuals to practice nursing as long as they do not use the letters "RN" after their names; protects the registered nurse designation but not the practice of nursing itself.

Person: Under the UHCIA (1997), may be (1) an individual, or a patient; (2) a legal or commercial entity, such as a health care provider; or (3) a government entity or agency, such as a managed care organization or correctional facility (UHCIA, 1997, §1-101 & 102).

Personal Care Facility: See Assisted-Living Facility.

Personal Relativism: Determining that an act is morally right because it complies with the values of the person.

Petition: Legal request for involuntary commitment for persons in need of psychiatric treatment; outlines and describes behaviors evidencing need for treatment.

Physician's Assistant: Person who works with physicians, either under their supervision or via protocols or standing orders.

PIE: A method of charting that focuses on the *problem, intervention, and evaluation.*

Plaintiff: The party who brings a civil action or suit.

Plaintiff's Petition: Also called Plaintiff's Complaint; the initial legal document filed to initiate the lawsuit and state Plaintiff's claims and injuries.

Police Power Doctrine: Under the Tenth Amendment, the states are given the authority to regulate health care for the safety and security of their citizens (Gobis, 1997, p. 13); for example, states may protect citizens from dangerous acts of mentally ill persons by commitment for treatment.

Policy: Synonymous with *process standards.*

Political Action Committee (PAC): An organization of nurses that provides a mechanism for small contributors to have a collective strength and influence.

Political Networks: Organizations that allow the nurse to connect with the right influence; promote the deliberate use of politics to accomplish goals of the profession.

Politics: Process by which the decision-making of others is influenced regarding public issues, thereby changing situations and their course of events.

Practical Constraints: Limitations within which a service, such as health care, is offered.

Practice Guidelines: Protocols for nursing practice that direct the care to be provided; also called *clinical paths*, are written documents describing the optimal utilization, sequencing, and timing of interventions necessary to carry out a given procedure or treatment plan.

Precedent: Prior decisions that are followed when courts are presented with the same legal questions; in Latin, *stare decisis*, which means "let the decision stand"; basis for common law.

Precertification/Preadmission Certification: A review needed for hospitalization or other services prior to implementation, based on established review criteria.

Preferred Provider Organization (PPO): A program in which contracts exists between the health plan and providers; the plan provides incentives for members to use preferred providers as opposed to nonparticipating providers.

Prelitigation or Medical Review Panel: Before a lawsuit is filed, this panel of professionals decides whether or not negligence has occurred; the panel is designed to eliminate lawsuits with little or no merit.

Preponderance of the Evidence: Legal standard requiring that the outcome is more likely than not to have occurred as a result of a particular action or inaction; the patient more likely than not suffered the injury because the care provided fell below the standard.

Prescriptive Authority: Within the scope of professional practice, conditions under which the advanced practice nurse is given statutory permission to prescribe medications based on a medical diagnosis.

Preventive Commitment: Outpatient court-ordered treatment for persons who do not yet meet usual inpatient commitment criteria.

Prima Facie Case: A classic, textbook example that includes all the elements necessary to prove the claim; for example, contains the four elements of negligence.

Primary Care Providers (PCPs): Providers who give comprehensive care to an assigned group of patients or members; term usually reserved for family practice, pediatric, and internal medicine physicians; nurse practitioners; and physician's assistants.

Principled Ethics: Under this ethical decision-making model, the nurse assists in the determination of which of the following major ethical principles are in conflict, including patient autonomy, beneficence, nonmaleficence, or justice.

Prisoners: Persons who are confined or whose movements are restricted or monitored, because of crimes they have committed against the state.

Privacy Rights: The right of clients to keep personal information completely secret, although exceptions do exist under individual state and federal laws.

Privileged Communications: A communication between a client and a physician, lawyer, or clergyman that is protected from disclosure in a court of law.

Privileges and Immunities: The courts of one state recognize the privileges of another, e.g., licenses.

Proactive Law: Law applied in future cases.

Probate Court: The department of each county's court that deals with probate conservatorships, guardianships, and estates of people who have died.

Procedural Justice: A known, fair process within which distributive justice occurs, for example, the organ procurement system.

Procedural Law: Rules of civil procedure that seek to maintain an orderly and fair progression of the lawsuit, from filing to dismissal.

Procedure: Synonymous with *structure standards*.

Professional Liability: A legal requirement that a professional person pay a patient for harm suffered that was caused by failure to act properly and adhere to the standards of care.

Professional Nursing Legislative Agenda Coalition (PNLAC): A coalition of nursing organizations whose main goal is to build a consensus on legislative issues that affect all nurses.

Proprietary Agencies: Those agencies that are not owned or operated by a hospital, i.e., free-standing agencies.

Proprietary Functions: Services or functions provided by the government, but could also be provided by private industry, e.g., utility functions.

Protocols: Written guidelines, steps, or recommendations for care of a client with a specific disease, illness, and symptom.

Provider: Member(s) of the multidisciplinary treatment team (MDTT).

Provider Number: Number given to a health care provider in order to be paid for services under Medicare and Medicaid.

Provider Privileging: Ensures that individual providers are competent to perform the care that they are assigned to do.

Proximate Cause: The legal or direct cause of an event or injury; requires foreseeability.

Prudent Layperson: A person in the community who possesses an average level of understanding and medical knowledge.

Prudent Patient Standard: Also known as reasonable person; what a reasonable or prudent patient would have wanted to know in the same or similar situation.

Psychiatry: Discipline that addresses the meaning of individual behavior, life satisfaction, and quality-of-life issues.

Public Figure: Someone who has assumed a role of importance in the resolution of specific public affairs or affairs of general importance to the public.

Public Hospitals: Health care facilities funded by state and/or federal funds.

Public-Key Encryption: The most common form of computer encryption; the decryption key is kept secret by the receiver of the communication, but the encryption key is made public, and may be posted on the Internet or given to the sender by diskette or e-mail.

Public Law: Laws that govern relationships between citizens and the government.

Public Policy: Policy that is developed by governmental bodies, such as legislation passed by Congress.

Punitive Damages: An amount of money awarded to the plaintiff, designed to punish the defendant, if the wrongful action or inaction is found to have been performed with malice; also known as exemplary damages; may be used to force compliance with the arbitrator's decision.

Pure Responsibility: Plaintiff's damages are reduced or decreased in relation to portion of liability.

Qualified Immunity: Immunity from liability for an action or inaction based on certain qualifications or criteria.

Qualified Individual: Under the Americans with Disabilities Act, a person who can, with or without reasonable accommodation, perform the essential functions of the job.

Qualified Individual with Disability: An applicant or employee who can safely and properly perform all aspects of the job requirements with or without reasonable accommodations.

Quality Assurance: Process by which the total health care services provided to the patient are monitored for compliance with standards of care.

Quality of Care Program: Under managed care, the outcomes of care are documented, in addition to the results of monitoring of process indicators, for example, HEDIS.

Quasi-Intentional Torts: Torts involving speech.

Qui Tam: Synonymous with the term *whistle-blower.*

Quid Pro Quo Sexual Harassment: "Something for something"; occurs when a person in power over the employee (usually a supervisor) demands a sexual favor from the employee as a condition of employment.

Rape: A criminal act that is reportable and encompasses three general elements: (1) carnal knowledge of a woman, (2) lack of consent to this carnal knowledge, and (3) use of force to accomplish this act; includes the following acts of abuse: aggravated assault, attempted rape, indecent assault, involuntary sexual intercourse, sexual abuse, and statutory rape.

Rational Relationship Test: A legal test of the Supreme Court utilized where a challenged law regulates and affects only economic or property interests; the courts will strike down such a law only if it bears no rational relationship to a conceivable legitimate state purpose.

Realms: The levels on which ethical problems occur and ethical decisions are made; includes societal, institutional, and individual levels.

Reasonable Accommodation: The employer's legal responsibility to provide the disabled employee with the necessary restructuring, reassignment, equipment, training materials, interpreters, or other accommodations deemed reasonable.

Reasonable and Customary Fees: Schedule of fees paid by traditional fee-for-service health plans for services rendered; are based on the credentials of the providers and the usual charges for that geographic area.

Reasonable Doubt: The degree of doubt that would cause a reasonable person to hesitate to act if a decision involved the most important of his or her affairs.

Reasonable Person Standard: What a reasonable person or prudent patient would have done if placed in the same situation.

Reasonable Physician (Provider) Standard: What a reasonable health care provider in the local community would disclose during informed consent under the same or similar circumstances.

Reasonableness: The standard that governs the transmission of health care information under the UHCIA (1997), which requires reasonable safeguards to secure the confidentiality of all health care information maintained on behalf of the patient.

Rebuttal Evidence: Evidence is provided that is designed to contradict specific points raised by the defendant attorney.

Reciprocity: A method of telenursing licensure through which the nurse is granted equal privileges in the host state.

Reckless Disregard: Ignoring a substantial risk of danger that is either known or would be apparent to a reasonable person in the same position.

Recklessness: Actions or inactions characterized by highly unreasonable conduct or a gross departure from ordinary care, in a situation where a high degree of danger is apparent.

Referee: Within ADR, the person who conducts a reference or gathers the facts.

Reference: A method of ADR that is used in a pending lawsuit to obtain facts by order of the court.

Registration: The listing, or registering, of names of individuals on an official roster when they have met certain preestablished criteria (Catalano, 1996, p. 173); a mechanism by which the nurse submits, and the state accepts, documentation of training and competency.

Registration System: A method of telenursing licensure that would allow the nurse to register as a licensed professional nurse in one state, and notify the host state of the intent to practice telenursing in that state, and upon registering, agreeing to comply with the nursing standards of the host state.

Regulatory Bodies: Organizations and/or statutory laws that establish and monitor the standard of care delivered by the provider and/or received by the patient; for example, JCAHO.

Reimbursement: Payment for services rendered to a client by Medicare, Medicaid, managed care organizations, businesses, and indemnity insurers; depends on individual fee schedules, laws, and policies of each third-party payer (Buppert, 1998).

Release: The relinquishment or abandonment of a claim or lawsuit.

Religion: Organized faith.

Religious Tribunal: A method of ADR through which a religious authority or panel has the authority to modify the terms of an arbitration agreement and rule on issues that have not been specifically submitted to arbitration.

Remote State: Under the Compact, any state in which the nurse practices other than the home state.

Rent-a-Judge: A method of ADR also known as *consensual references* or *private judging*.

Reportable Situation: Occurrences that must be reported under law, including: (a) gunshot or stabbing wounds, (b) rapes or sexual assaults, (c) sexually transmitted diseases, and (d) abuse of children.

Request for Admission: A request to the opposing party, to either admit or deny the truth of certain statements of facts; typically used later in the discovery process to narrow issues over which there remains a dispute.

Request for Production: A request to the opposing party to disclose all documents and tangible items within their possession, custody or control that are relevant to the facts of the case.

Res Ipsa Loquitur: Latin term for "the thing speaks for itself;" a situation where the facts themselves provide the conclusion that the standard of care was not met. For example, where: (1) the event is of a kind that ordinarily does not occur in the absence of negligence; (2) other responsible causes, including the conduct of the plaintiff and third persons, are sufficiently eliminated by the evidence; (3) the indicated negligence is within the scope of the defendant's duty to plaintiff.

Resident Assessment Instrument (RAI): Consists of a minimum data set (MDS) of elements, common definitions, and coding categories needed to perform a comprehensive assessment of a long-term care facility resident.

Residents: Terminology used interchangably with *patients, clients,* and *consumers.*

Resignation at Will: The employee can terminate the relationship with the employer at any time.

Respondeat Superior: Under this legal doctrine, employers can be held liable for the acts or inactions of the employee, only if they knew, or should have known, of the negligent acts of the employee.

Restraint: The use of a chemical substance, mechanical device, and/or physical restriction by one or more persons that limits the activity of another.

Retrospective Review: Utilization review conducted, usually by representatives of the payer, after the patient has been discharged from service.

Right to Refuse Treatment: The right of the patient, verbally or through an advance directive, to refuse health care treatment.

Rights: Something claimed by/owed to another by virtue of legal, moral or ethical authority.

Risk Management: Process used to monitor and improve the quality of health care through prevention of injuries, by monitoring health care equipment, and early, prompt identification of negligent injuries by health care providers.

Risk Sharing: Various types of prepaid reimbursement mechanisms, such as case rates or capitation, in which the provider shares the risk of the medical care with the payer.

Rule Deontology: Ethical theories premised on the belief that duties are strictly based on nursing standards and/or rules of law.

Rule Utilitarianism: Ethical theories premised on the belief that actions are selected according to rules that will result in the greatest happiness and the least unhappiness.

Safe Harbor Law: Mechanism by which a nurse practice act may provide protection for the nurse who refuses to participate in acts or inactions that may potentially be detrimental to a patient and under which the registered nurse may not be suspended, terminated, disciplined, or discriminated against for refusing acts or inactions believed to be harmful to a patient.

Satisfaction: Payment of damages that have been awarded to a plaintiff.

Satisfaction of Outcome: Satisfaction with overall results of ADR.

Scope of Employment: The employee's job description.

Scope of Practice: "The nursing diagnosis and treatment of human responses to health and illness" (ANA, 1994, p. 2); "defined by the knowledge base of the nurse, the role of the nurse, and the nature of the client population within the practice environment" (ANA, 1994, p. 2).

Screening Examination: The minimum standard for examination of a patient, including at least vital signs and chief complaint.

Screening Panel: A method of ADR used for the purpose of reviewing and/or stating an opinion on the issues of liability and/or damages and encouraging settlement.

Serious Injury or Illness: An injury or illness occurring in the workplace, except for injury, illness or death caused by criminal actions.

Serious Medical Need: A condition diagnosed by a physician that requires a prescribed treatment; or a condition that is so obvious that a layperson would know that a doctor's attention is necessary.

Service of Process: The act of formally delivering lawsuit papers.

Settlement: Results when the remaining conditions at issue are finished and the claim may be discharged.

Severe Obesity: Under the ADA, body weight more that 100 percent over the norm.

Sexual Assault Nurse Examiner (SANE): A nurse with specialized education and practice in working with the sexual assault victim, including assessment; treatment, which may include immediate crisis intervention and provision of prophylactic drugs for pregnancy and sexually transmitted diseases; appropriate referral; and follow-up care.

Sexual Harassment: Unlawful employment discrimination consisting of harassment of the employee because of gender, whether or not the harassing conduct is of a sexual nature (hostile environment harassment); includes *quid pro quo* harassment.

Short-Term Stay: Involuntary commitment of a person believed to be mentally ill for a period of time, generally 1 month or so. See Order of Protective Custody.

Situational Right to Privacy: Privacy subject to the discretion or the decision-making authority of another.

Skilled Nursing Facilities (SNFs): Provide skilled nursing services to individuals who require extended inpatient care and are classified as hospital-based, free-standing, or swing-bed providers by Medicare for payment purposes; required under Medicare to have transfer agreements with hospitals.

Skilled Nursing Service: Those health care services provided by a registered nurse, or by a licensed practical or vocations nurse under the supervision of a registered nurse.

Slander: Oral defamatory statements.

Slow Code: An unwritten agreement between members of the MDTT to respond "slowly" to a cardiac or respiratory arrest.

Sniffing: A form of hacking, intercepting, or capturing electronic information as it travels through the intermediate or router's computer.

"So What" Defense: Defense to a lawsuit premised on the argument that although the nurse provided negligent care to plaintiff, plaintiff would have died anyway.

SOAP: A method of charting that documents the (S) subjective, (O) objective, (A) nursing assessment, and (P) planned nursing interventions.

Social Relativism: Decision-making that determines an act is morally right because it complies with the values of society.

Sovereign Immunity: "The king can do no wrong"; under this doctrine, state and federal governments, as well as various state and federal facilities such as hospitals and schools, are generally immune from tort liability.

Special Master: A fact-finder who assists in resolving a dispute in which the opinions of the parties' experts differ sharply.

Spoofing: A form of hacking, intercepting, or capturing electronic information by programming a router's computer to act as the recipient host.

Stalker: One who willfully, maliciously, and repeatedly follows or harasses another (the victim) and who makes a credible threat with the intent to place the victim or victim's immediate family in fear for their safety.

Standard of Care: That degree of care, expertise, and judgment exercised by a reasonable and prudent nurse under the same or similar circumstances; requires use of the nursing process.

Standard of Conduct: The stand of conduct in a negligence case; based on "what society demands generally of its members" (Keeton, Dobbs, Keeton & Owen, 1984, p. 169).

Standard of Employment: Would a reasonable prudent employer have fired such a nurse, before the nurse committed the tort that now is alleged, under the same or similar circumstances.

Standard of Practice: Serve as the framework for statements about competency levels and form the basis for outcomes for education and standards for the delivery of nursing care.

Standard of Reasonable Care: The right to receive health care under circumstances in which any reasonable person would seek medical care (*Bewer v. Perin*, 1984).

Standard of Review: Method by which the court analyzes all the facts of a lawsuit.

Standards of Professional Performance: Nursing process and activities directly surrounding patient care.

Stare decisis: Latin word for precedent; means "let the decision stand;" provides predictability to outcomes of legal disputes.

Stark Amendment Violation: Occurs when the provider invests in a telehealth project and also furnishes telecommunication equipment to smaller facilities.

State Board of Nursing: The official agency responsible for enforcing the state nurse practice act and regulating nursing practice.

Statute of Limitations: A specific time within which a lawsuit must be filed, set by state or federal law.

Statute of Repose: Statutes that do not allow the discovery rule to toll the statute of limitations.

Statutes: Laws passed by legislatures.

Stipulated: Describes facts that are agreed to without dispute.

Statutory Law: Rules and regulations known as statutes, created by state and federal legislators, which are designed to maintain social order and protect individual rights.

Strict Liability: May be held liable for acts of negligence without fault.

Strict Scrutiny: Under this test, a court decides whether a law alleged to impinge on fundamental rights is the least restrictive mechanism by which the state can accomplish a compelling state interest.

Subject Matter Jurisdiction: The court has authority to hear the particular issues or subjects at dispute; for example, the family court has authority to hear matters related to the subject of custody or divorce.

Subpoena: A legal device used to compel a person to appear before the court.

Subrogation: If an insurance company pays a patient's medical bills for injuries arising out of a nurse's malpractice, the insurance company will have a right to recover the amount from the patient when the patient recovers it from the nurse.

Substantial Factor in Causing Injury: Theory of liability under which all defendants are held liable, as acts of more than one defendant caused the injury, but it cannot be determined which was the actual cause.

Substantive Law: The actual law under which claims or lawsuits are brought and defended.

Summary Jury Trial: A method of ADR that is a variation of the mini-trial, during which the case is presented before a jury of people.

Supremacy Clause: Article VI of the Constitution; declares that the Constitution and laws of the United States are the supreme law of the land.

Surrogate Mother: One who carries for another an artificially implanted embryo or an embryo that has been created by artificial insemination by the sperm of a donor.

Tail: The extension of a medical malpractice insurance policy beyond the policy period, that would be in effect until there is no longer any possibility of a claim being made against his or her professional practice.

Tarasoff Duty: Duty to warn; a health care provider has a legal duty to warn another person if they are the intended victim of a client, which is being treated by the provider.

Team Nursing: A professional nurse leads a nursing team in delivering client-centered care; designed to eliminate the fragmentation of care resulting from a task-oriented approach to the delivery of nursing care.

Telecommunications: The electronic communication of information.

Telemedicine: "The provision of health-care consultation and education using telecommunication networks to communicate information ... [and] ... medical practices across distance via communications and interactive video technology" (Abke et al., 1997, p. 3).

Telenursing: Electronic transfer of nursing data, nursing information, and nursing expertise between two points.

Telepathology: The electronic transmission of pathology images.

Teleradiology: The electronic transmission of radiographic images.

Terminal Condition: Statutorily defined as an incurable or irreversible condition, such that it would produce death regardless of the application of life-sustaining procedures; certified in writing by the examining physician(s).

Termination for Cause: Termination of the employee for a valid reason.

Testifying Expert: The expert who testifies in court, to establish the applicable standard of care.

Testifying Witness: A forensic nurse who provides probative information about the facts of a particular case.

Testimonial Privilege: A right of communication applying to court-related proceedings, including communications between spouses, attorney and client, physician and patient, and clergy and parishioner.

Texas Peer Assistance Program for Nurses (TPAPN): An assistance program for impaired nurses in recovery for chemical addictions and/or mental illness.

Therapeutic Privilege: The right of the health care provider to decide, in his or her opinion and based on medical judgment, that it would be harmful to a patient to provide complete disclosure regarding the proposed treatment or procedure.

Tolled: The statute of limitations is suspended.

Tort: A civil wrong; a claim for malpractice, negligence, and/or damages.

Tort Reform: A revolution in common law designed to restrict and impose limits on monetary civil damages.

Totality of Conditions Test: Synonymous with the *totality of the circumstances test.*

Totality of the Circumstances Test: The standard or test under which the court considers all the facts surrounding the conditions or circumstances of a claim or lawsuit.

Transaction Costs: Costs of a dispute, including (1) out-of-pocket expenses; (2) the time and inconvenience of participating in the dispute; (3) resources consumed, such as neutral experts; and (4) lost opportunities.

Treatment: Health care procedures specifically designed to meet the patient's health care needs.

Trespass on the Case: Under early English law, this cause of action provided redress for injuries that were not necessarily done with force, as was the case in trespass.

Triage: Derived from the French word *trier,* which means "to sort."

Trial: The legal and factual issues are presented, heard and decided before a judge and jury.

Trial Court: The court in which a case is litigated.

Trial de Novo: A new trial.

Trust: Something managed by a fiduciary or guardian and/or attorney, given to him or her to be held and protected in the interest of another.

Trustworthiness: Moral actions that involve: (1) belief in and reliance on or by another, (2) acting within moral norms, (3) consistency and reliability, and (4) reputation.

Unavoidable Accident: An accident or event with injuries resulting without fault of anyone who could be held responsible.

Undue Hardship: Under the ADA, is "an action requiring significant difficulty or expense when considered in light of factors such as an employer's size, financial resources and the nature and structure of its operation" (U.S. Equal Employment Opportunity Commission, 1997).

Unfair Labor Practices: Actions taken by an employer to discourage or dissuade employees from taking part in union activities.

Uniform Anatomical Gift Act: A federal law that allows a patient to give informed consent to donate body organs; federal legislation that provides the following two ways to donate organs: (1) a person 18 years or older signs a card indicating a wish to donate, for example, on the back of a driver's license; and/or (2) a family member provides authorization by signing the appropriate document(s).

Uniform Controlled Substances Act of 1970: Federal law that defines addiction, classifies drug categories, and requires record keeping and reporting.

Uniform Determination of Death Act: A federal law that identifies the criteria for death, including brain death.

Uniform Health Care Information Act (UHCIA, 1997): A federal law that governs the flow of health-care information, and thus is one of the laws regulating telenursing. Legislation classifying drugs into five schedules, depending on their potential for abuse or usefulness (I, low usefulness/high abuse potential; V, less potential for abuse).

Universalism: Synonymous with *absolutism;* acts judged morally right on positions other than personal or societal values; for example, the application of universal theological values to the decision-making process.

Unlicensed Assistive Personnel (UAP): Individuals who are trained to function in an assistive role to the registered professional nurse in the provision of patient/client care activities as delegated by and under the supervision of the registered nurse (ANA, 1996, p. 5).

Unwelcome Conduct: Under the definition of sexual harassment, the conduct of the perpetrator was neither incited nor solicited, and the conduct was felt to be undesirable and/or offensive.

Use of Force: Any touching of an inmate.

Utilitarianism: An ethical theory based on the belief that a nursing action is judged on the outcomes or consequences, or risks versus benefits; also called *consequentialism.*

Utilization Management: The continual process of evaluating the necessity, appropriateness, and efficiency of health services.

Utilization Review: A utilization management (UM) technique whereby trained health care professionals evaluate the appropriateness, quality and medical necessity of service provided to plan members.

Valid Disclosure: Under the UHCIA, the release of health care information only with the written authorization of the patient.

Venue: The location of the court in which the lawsuit will be heard.

Veracity: An ethical and legal principle simply defined as truthfulness.

Vertical Integration: A single entity owns and controls both the provider components and the insurance business.

Vicarious Liability: A legal theory of liability under which one person is held responsible for the negligence or actions of another; those who benefit bear responsibility.

Vice Principal: An employee who is in an administrative position, such as a nursing supervisor.

Violence Against Women Act of 1994: Federal law that regulates and provides funding to states for domestic violence and sexual assault prevention, victim assistance, and prosecution of offenders.

Violent: "[A]cting with or characterized by extreme force, characterized by injurious or destructive force, an unjust or unwarranted exertion of force or power, rough or immoderate vehemence as of feeling or language" (*Random House Dictionary,* 1982).

Virtual Nursing : Providing nursing care via the Internet or cyberspace.

Virtual System: Managed care organizations or companies contract for services with physician groups, hospital systems, home nursing agencies, and other health care providers.

Voir Dire: Questioning of potential jurors by the attorneys for both sides of the case.

Voluntary Admission: Procedure allowing persons to admit that they are in need of treatment for mental illness.

Voluntary Euthanasia: Death occurs when the patient, after informed consent, refuses treatment.

Waive: To give up a legal right, such as the privilege of confidentiality in all health care information; for example, to refuse, relinquish, or forgo health care treatment.

Wanton and Willful Conduct: Conduct that shows a reckless disregard for the rights, welfare, or safety of others.

Wergild: Under Anglo-Saxon law, the precursor to the legal theory of vicarious liability, under which a murderer's family was held liable for compensation for the harm, e.g., paid to the crown for the subject, the lord for the vassal, and the family of the victim for their economic loss.

Whistleblower Laws: Laws that prohibit retaliation against persons who report unsafe health care practices.

Whistle-Blowing: Occurs when a provider reveals unsafe, unethical, illegal, and unprofessional or other behaviors within an organization that may be detrimental to the patient and/or delivery of health care.

Willful Conduct: Actions excluded under a malpractice insurance policy, including: (a) injury or damage sustained as a result of sexual abuse of a patient, (b) caused when the nurse is under the infuence of drugs or alcohol, or (c) occurring during the commission of criminal activity.

Willful Disclosure: Knowingly disclosing information without a valid authorization.

Wire Communication: "[A]ny communication made in whole or in part through the use of facilities for the transmission of communications by the aid of wire, cable, or the link connection between the point of origin and the point of reception furnished or operated by any person engaged as a common carrier in providing or operating such facilities for the transmission of interstate or foreign communications" [Federal Wiretap Statutes of 1968, § 2510(1)].

Workplace Violence: Occurs when a disgruntled coworker causes harm to the boss or another coworker; also includes, but is not limited to, harassment, sexual gestures, threatening remarks, objects being thrown, spitting or hitting, and/or pulling away in anger. "[V]iolent acts, including physical assaults and threats of assaults, directed toward persons at work or on duty" (CDC).

Writ of *Certiorari:* An order from the Supreme Court to a lower court to send the record of a case to them for review, i.e., for errors that implicate constitutional rights and duties.

Writ of *Habeas Corpus:* A written request to the court to release the petitioner from incarceration.

Wrongful Termination: Synonymous with wrongful discharge; the firing of an employee without lawful justification, e.g., firing an employee because of a personal grudge; the employee is fired based on causes that are discriminatory.

INDEX

An italic *"f"* following a page number indicates a figure; an italic *"t"* indicates a table.